Handbook of the Psychology of Aging

7th Edition

Editors

K. Warner Schaie and Sherry L. Willis

Associate Editors

Bob G. Knight, Becca Levy, and Denise C. Park

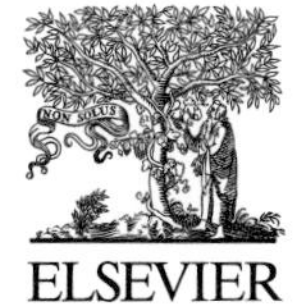

Amsterdam • Boston • Heidelberg • London • New York • Oxford • Paris
San Diego • San Francisco • Singapore • Sydney • Tokyo

Academic Press is an imprint of Elsevier

Academic Press is an imprint of Elsevier
32 Jamestown Road, London NW1 7BY, UK
30 Corporate Drive, Suite 400, Burlington, MA 01803, USA
525 B Street, Suite 1800, San Diego, CA 92101-4495, USA

Seventh edition, 2011

British Library Cataloguing-in-Publication Data
A catalogue record for this book is available from the British Library

Library of Congress Cataloging-in-Publication Data
A catalog record for this book is available from the Library of Congress

ISBN: 978-0-12-380882-0

For information on all Academic Press publications
visit our website at www.elsevierdirect.com

Typeset by MPS Limited, a Macmillan Company, Chennai, India
www.macmillansolutions.com

Printed and bound in the United States of America

11 12 13 14 15 10 9 8 7 6 5 4 3 2 1

Contents

Contributors ... vii
Foreword ... ix
Preface ... xi
About the Editors ... xiii

Part 1: Concepts, Theory, and Methods in the Psychology of Aging

1. Enduring Theoretical Themes in Psychological Aging: Derivation, Functions, Perspectives, and Opportunities ... 3
   Roger A. Dixon
2. Methodological and Analytical Issues in the Psychology of Aging ... 25
   Emilio Ferrer, Paolo Ghisletta
3. Historical Influences on Aging and Behavior ... 41
   K. Warner Schaie

Part 2: Neuroscience, Cognition and Aging

4. Executive Function and Cognitive Aging ... 59
   Mary Luszcz
5. The Cognitive Consequences of Structural Changes to the Aging Brain ... 73
   Karen M. Rodrigue, Kristen M. Kennedy
6. Behavior Genetics of Aging ... 93
   William S. Kremen, Michael J. Lyons
7. Neuroplasticity, Aging, and Cognitive Function ... 109
   Denise C. Park, Gérard N. Bischof
8. Memory Changes and the Aging Brain: A Multimodal Imaging Approach ... 121
   Lars Nyberg, Lars Bäckman
9. Age Differences in Complex Decision Making ... 133
   Ellen Peters, Nathan F. Dieckmann, Joshua Weller
10. Cognitive Interventions ... 153
    Elizabeth A. L. Stine-Morrow, Chandramallika Basak

Part 3: Social and Health Factors that Impact Aging

11. The Relevance of Control Beliefs for Health and Aging ... 175
    Margie E. Lachman, Shevaun D. Neupert, Stefan Agrigoroaei
12. The Speedometer of Life: Stress, Health and Aging ... 191
    David M. Almeida, Jennifer R. Piazza, Robert S. Stawski, Laura C. Klein
13. Health Disparities, Social Class, and Aging ... 207
    Keith E. Whitfield, Roland Thorpe, Sarah Szanton

14. Relationships between Adults and their Aging Parents 219
Karen L. Fingerman, Kira S. Birditt

15. Intergenerational Communication Practices 233
Howard Giles, Jessica Gasiorek

16. Age Stereotypes and Aging 249
Mary Lee Hummert

17. Aging in the Work Context 263
Catherine E. Bowen, Martin G. Noack, Ursula M. Staudinger

18. Wisdom, Age, and Well-Being 279
Monika Ardelt

Part 4: Complex Behavioral Processes and Psychopathology of Aging

19. Emotional Experience and Regulation in Later Life 295
Susan Turk Charles

20. Psychopathology, Bereavement, and Aging.. 311
Susan Krauss Whitbourne, Suzanne Meeks

21. Assessment of Emotional and Personality Disorders in Older Adults.. 325
Barry A. Edelstein, Daniel L. Segal

22. Neuropsychological Assessment of the Dementias of Late Life 339
Stephanie Cosentino, Adam M. Brickman, Jennifer J. Manly

23. Family Caregiving for Cognitively or Physically Frail Older Adults: Theory, Research, and Practice........................ 353
Bob G. Knight, Andres Losada

24. Decision Making Capacity 367
Jennifer Moye, Daniel Marson, Barry Edelstein, Stacey Wood, Aida Saldivar

Author Index..381
Subject Index 413

Contributors

Numbers in parentheses indicate the page number on which the author's contribution begins

Stefan Agrigoroaei (175), Department of Psychology, Brandeis University, Waltham, Massachusetts

David M. Almeida (191), Department of Human Development and Family Studies, The Pennsylvania State University, University Park, Pennsylvania

Monika Ardelt (279), Department of Sociology and Criminology & Law, University of Florida, Gainesville, Florida

Lars Bäckman (121), Aging Research Center, Karolinska Institute, Stockholm, Sweden

Chandramallika Basak (153), Beckman Institute, University of Illinois, Champaign, Illinois

Kira S. Birditt (219), Institute for Social Research, University of Michigan, Ann Arbor, Michigan

Gérard N. Bischof (109), The Center for Vital Longevity, University of Texas, Dallas, Texas

Catherine E. Bowen (263), Jacobs Center on Lifelong Learning and Institutional Development, Jacobs University Bremen, Bremen, Germany

Adam M. Brickman (339), Gertrude H. Sergievsky Center, Taub Institute for Research on Alzheimer's Disease and the Aging Brain, Department of Neurology at Columbia University Medical Center, New York

Susan Turk Charles (295), School of Social Ecology, University of California, Irvine, California

Stephanie A. Cosentino (339), Gertrude H. Sergievsky Center, Taub Institute for Research on Alzheimer's Disease and the Aging Brain, Department of Neurology at Columbia University Medical Center, New York

Nathan F. Dieckmann (133), Decision Research, Eugene, Oregon

Roger A. Dixon (3), Department of Psychology, University of Alberta, Edmonton, Alberta, Canada

Barry Edelstein (325, 367) Department of Psychology, West Virginia University, Morgantown, West Virginia

Emilio Ferrer (25), Department of Psychology, University of California, Davis, California

Karen L. Fingerman (219), Child Development and Family Studies, Purdue University, West Lafayette, Indiana

Jessica Gasiorek (233), Department of Communication, University of California Santa Barbara, Santa Barbara, California

Paolo Ghisletta (25), Faculty of Psychology and Educational Sciences, University of Geneva, Genève, Switzerland; Distance Learning University, Sierre, Switzerland

Howard Giles (233), Department of Communication, University of California Santa Barbara, Santa Barbara, California

Mary Lee Hummert (249), Vice Provost for Faculty Development, University of Kansas, Lawrence, Kansas

Kristen M. Kennedy (73), School of Behavioral and Brain Sciences, University of Texas, Dallas, Texas

Laura C. Klein (191), Department of Human Development and Family Studies, The Pennsylvania State University, University Park, Pennsylvania

Bob G. Knight (353), School of Gerontology, University of Southern California, Los Angeles, California

William S. Kremen (93), Department of Psychiatry, Center for Behavioral Genomics, University of California, San Diego, La Jolla, California; VA San Diego Healthcare System, La Jolla, California

Margie E. Lachman (175), Department of Psychology, Brandeis University, Waltham, Massachusetts

Andres Losada (353), Department of Psychology, Universidad Reg Juan Carlos, Madrid, Spain

Contributors

Mary Luszcz (59), Department of Psychology, Flinders Centre for Ageing Studies, Flinders University, Adelaide, South Australia, Australia

Michael J. Lyons (93), Department of Psychology, Boston University, Boston, Harvard Institute of Epidemiology and Genetics, Boston

Jennifer J. Manly (339), Gertrude H. Sergievsky Center, Taub Institute for Research on Alzheimer's Disease and the Aging Brain, Department of Neurology at Columbia University Medical Center, New York

Daniel Marson (365), Department of Neurology, University of Alabama-Birmingham, Birmingham, Alabama

Suzanne Meeks (311), Department of Psychological and Brain Sciences, University of Louisville, Louisville, Kentucky

Jennifer Moye (367), Geriatric Mental Health, VA Boston Healthcare System, Massachusetts

Shevaun D. Neupert (175), Department of Psychology, North Carolina State University, Raleigh, North Carolina

Martin G. Noack (263), Jacobs Center on Lifelong Learning and Institutional Development, Jacobs University Bremen, Bremen, Germany

Lars Nyberg (121), Department of Integrative Medical Biology and Radiation Sciences, Umeå University, Umeå, Sweden

Denise C. Park (109), The Center for Vital Longevity, University of Texas, Dallas, Texas

Ellen Peters (133), Department of Psychology, The Ohio State University, Columbus, Ohio

Jennifer R. Piazza (191), Department of Human Development and Family Studies, The Pennsylvania State University, University Park, Pennsylvania

Karen M. Rodrigue (73), School of Behavioral and Brain Sciences, University of Texas, Dallas, Texas

Aida Saldivar (365), Boston VA Medical Center, Boston, Massachusetts

K.Warner Schaie (41), Department of Psychiatry and Behavioral Sciences, University of Washington, Seattle, Washington

Daniel L. Segal (325), Department of Psychology, University of Colorado, Colorado Springs

Ursula M. Staudinger (263), Jacobs Center on Lifelong Learning and Institutional Development, Jacobs University Bremen, Bremen, Germany

Robert S. Stawski (191), Department of Human Development and Family Studies, The Pennsylvania State University, University Park, Pennsylvania

Elizabeth A.L. Stine-Morrow (153), Beckman Institute, University of Illinois, Champaign, Illinois

Sarah L. Szanton (207), School of Public Health, Johns Hopkins University, Baltimore, Maryland

Roland Thorpe (207), School of Public Health, Johns Hopkins University, Baltimore, Maryland

Joshua Weller (133), Decision Research, Eugene, Oregon

Susan Krauss Whitbourne (311), Department of Psychology, University of Massachusetts-Amherst, Amherst, Massachusetts

Keith E. Whitfield (207), Department of Psychology and Neuroscience, Duke University, Durham, North Carolina

Stacey Wood(365), Department of Psychology, Scripps College, Claremont, California

Foreword

Advances in science and technology in the 20th century reshaped 21st century life in industrialized nations around the world. Living conditions so improved that infant and childhood mortality were profoundly reduced and medical advances in the prevention and treatment of leading causes of death among adults, such as heart disease and cancer, further extended the lives of older individuals. As a result, in the course of a single century, the average life expectancy in developed countries nearly doubled. For the first time in human history, old age became a normative stage in life. Not only are individuals living longer on average, but populations have begun to age as a result of this increase in life expectancy along with a precipitous drop in fertility rates. Countries in the developed world are rapidly reaching the point where there will be more people over 60 than under 15. Thus, the status of older people holds ramifications for the functioning of entire societies.

Even though the near-doubling of life expectancy was a spectacular achievement, there were not concurrent advances in our ability to alleviate the disabling conditions of later life. Nor were there sociological advances to create a world as responsive to the needs of very old people as to the very young. In order to realize the enormous potential of longer life, scientists must come to a more comprehensive understanding of human aging and the social, psychological and biological factors that contribute to optimal outcomes. Along with the phenomenal advances in the genetic determinants of longevity and susceptibility to age-related diseases has come the awareness of the critical importance of environmental factors that modulate and even supersede genetic predispositions. This series provides a balanced perspective of the interacting factors that contribute to human aging.

The Handbooks of Aging series, comprised of three separate volumes, *The Handbook of the Biology of Aging, The Handbook of the Psychology of Aging,* and *The Handbook of Aging and the Social Sciences,* is now in its seventh edition and has provided a foundation for an understanding of the issues of aging that are relevant both to the individual and to societies at large. Because discoveries in these fields have been both rapid and broad, the series has played a uniquely important role for students and scientists. By synthesizing and updating progress, they offer state-of-the-art reviews of the most recent advances. By continually featuring new topics and involving new authors, they have pushed innovation and fostered new ideas. With the explosion of information and research on aging in recent decades, there has been a concomitant increase in the number of college and university courses and programs focused on aging and longevity. *The Handbook of Aging* series has provided knowledge bases for instruction in these continually changing fields.

Indeed, *The Handbooks* are resources for teachers and students alike, providing information for didactics and inspiration for further research. Given the breadth and depth of the material covered, they serve as both a source of the most current information and as an overview of the various fields. One of the greatest strengths of the chapters in *The Handbooks* is the synthesis afforded by authors who are at the forefront of research and thus provide expert perspectives on the issues that current define and challenge each field. The interdisciplinary nature of aging research is exemplified by the overlap in concepts in chapters ranging from basic biology to sociology.

We express our deepest thanks to the editors of the individual volumes for their incredible dedication and contributions. It is their efforts to which the excellence of the products is largely credited. We thank Drs. Edward J. Masoro and Steven N. Austad, editors of *The Handbook of the Biology of Aging*; Drs. K. Warner Schaie and Sherry L. Willis, editors of *The Handbook of the Psychology of Aging*; and Drs. Robert H. Binstock and Linda K. George, editors of *The Handbook of Aging and the Social Sciences*. We would also like to express our appreciation to Nikki Levy, our publisher at Elsevier, whose profound interest and dedication has facilitated the publication of *The Handbooks* through their many editions. And, finally, we extend our deepest gratitude to James Birren for establishing and shepherding the series through the first six editions.

Thomas A. Rando, Laura L. Carstensen
Center on Longevity, Stanford University

Preface

The *Handbook of the Psychology of Aging* provides a basic reference source on the behavioral processes of aging for researchers, graduate students, and professionals. It also provides perspectives on the behavioral science of aging for researchers and professionals from other disciplines.

The present edition involves at least a partial generational turnover in the editorial leadership for this major handbook. James E. Birren, who was the founding editor of this handbook, decided that this project could no longer continue as a major focus of his remaining energy. Hence, he turned over the senior editorship to K. Warner Schaie, who had been the co-editor for all previous editions of the *Handbook*. He in turn invited Sherry L. Willis who had been a frequent contributor to earlier editions, to become the co-editor. Given the many new directions in our field, we next invited a new group of associate editors to help us in our efforts. We recruited the help of Denise C. Park to assist in the planning and editing of the expanded section on topics related to neuroscience, Becca Levy for the section on health and social influences on behavior, and Bob G. Knight for the section on psychopathology and complex processes.

The seventh edition of the *Handbook* continues to reflect both the continuing interest of the scientific community as well as the needs and worldwide growth of the older portion of the population as well as their expanding total and active life expectancy. The growth of the research literature provides new opportunities to replace the index of chronological age as the primary independent variable with other variables that represent causal mechanisms, and hence present the potential for control or experimental modification. Both academic and public interests have been contributing to the emergence of the psychology of aging as a major subject in universities and research institutions. Issues of interest to the psychology of aging touch upon many features of daily life, from the workplace and family life to public policy matters covering health care, retirement, social security, and pensions.

The psychology of aging is complex and many new questions keep being raised about how behavior is organized and how it changes over the course of life. Results of the markedly increasing number of longitudinal studies are providing new insights into the casual factors in behavior changes associated with adult development and aging. They are contributing to our understanding of the role of behavior changes in relation to biological, health, and social interactions. Parallel advances in research methodology particularly directed toward the problems of studying change allow us to explicate in greater detail, patterns and subpatterns of behavior over the life span.

Facing the rapidly accelerating growth of the relevant research literature, the editors once again have had to make choices about what new topics should be included in the handbook. But the growth in research activity does not occur uniformly across all fields. Hence, some topics covered in earlier editions of the *Handbook* are not included in the present edition. In this edition we have markedly expanded coverage of the section on Neuroscience, Cognition, and Aging. Other new topics first introduced in this edition include relationships between adults and their aging parents, intergenerational communication practices, assessment of emotional and personality disorders in older adults, neuropsychological assessment of the dementias of late life, and family caregiving for cognitively or physically frail older adults.

We continue the editorial principle of not inviting previous contributors to revise their earlier contribution. Instead, if we felt that a topic needed updating we asked a new approach to the topic from a different perspective. When a previous contributor reappears in a subsequent edition, it is typically on a different topic in which the contributor has developed expertise. For these reasons, readers are advised to consult earlier volumes of the *Handbook*, both for data and for interpretations. The previous editions should be consulted for a perspective on the development of the subject matter of the psychology of aging.

The chapters are organized into four divisions: Part 1: Concepts, Theory, and Methods in the Psychology of Aging; Part 2: Neuroscience, Cognition, and Aging; Part 3: Social and Health Factors that Impact Aging; and Part 4: Complex Behavioral Processes and Psychopathology of Aging.

The review process recommended many changes in the draft manuscripts. The draft of each chapter was reviewed by one associate editor and by the two senior editors. The senior editors thank the associate editors, Bob G. Knight, Becca Levy, and Denise C. Park for their advice on the selection of topics, authors, and their reviews of the chapter drafts. Their careful reading of the manuscripts and their detailed editorial suggestions are gratefully acknowledged.

K. Warner Schaie
Sherry L. Willis

About the Editors

K. Warner Schaie

K. Warner Schaie is the Evan Pugh Professor Emeritus of Human Development and Psychology at the Pennsylvania State University. He also holds an appointment as Affiliate Professor of Psychiatry and Behavioral Sciences at the University of Washington. He received his Ph.D. in psychology from the University of Washington, an honorary Dr. phil. from the Friedrich-Schiller University of Jena, Germany, and an honorary Sc.D. degree from West Virginia University. He received the Kleemeier Award for Distinguished Research Contributions and the Distinguished Career Contribution to Gerontology Award from the Gerontological Society of America, the MENSA lifetime career award, and the Distinguished Scientific Contributions award from the American Psychological Association. He is a past president and council representative of the APA Division of Adult Development and Aging. He is author or editor of 58 books including the textbook *Adult Development and Aging* (5th edition, with S. L. Willis) and all previous editions of the *Handbook of the Psychology of Aging* (with J. E. Birren). He has directed the Seattle Longitudinal Study of cognitive aging since 1956 and is the author of more than 300 journal articles and chapters on the psychology of aging. His current research interest is in the life course of adult intelligence, its antecedents and modifiability, the impact of cognitive behavior in midlife upon the integrity of brain structures in old age, and the early detection of risk for dementia, as well as methodological issues in the developmental sciences.

Sherry L. Willis

Sherry L. Willis is a Research Professor in the Department of Psychiatry and Behavioral Sciences at the University of Washington. She previously held an appointment as Professor of Human Development at the Pennsylvania State University. Dr. Willis' research has focused on age-related cognitive changes in later adulthood. In particular she is known for her work on behavioral interventions to remediate and enhance cognitive performance in community-dwelling normal elderly. Currently, she is a Principal Investigator on the ACTIVE study, a randomized controlled trial to examine the effects of cognitive interventions in the maintenance of everyday functioning in at-risk community-dwelling elderly, funded by NIA. She has been the co-director of the Seattle Longitudinal Study. In addition to her cognitive intervention research, Dr. Willis has conducted programmatic research on changes in everyday problem-solving competence in the elderly and cognitive predictors of competence. She and colleagues have developed several measures of Everyday Problem Solving. She is the co-author of the textbook *Adult Development and Aging*, (with K. W. Schaie, now in its 5th edition). She has edited 10+ volumes on various aspects of adult development and cognition and has authored over a hundred publications in adult development. She has served as President of Division 20, Adult Development and Aging, American Psychological Association. She was a Fulbright Fellow in Sweden. She received a Faculty Scholar Medal for Outstanding Achievement and the Pauline Schmitt Russell Distinguished Research Career Award from the Pennsylvania State University, and the Paul and Margret Baltes award from Divison 20 of the American Psychological Association She currently has funding from NIA (MERIT Award) to examine midlife predictors of cognitive risk in old age.

Bob G. Knight

Bob G. Knight is Associate Dean of the USC Davis School of Gerontology, the Merle H. Bensinger Professor of Gerontology and Professor of Psychology at the Andrus Gerontology Center, University of Southern California. He also serves as Director of the Tingstad Older Adult Counseling Center. He helped to organize and served as founding Chair of the Council of Professional Geropsychology Training Programs (2008). He has served as the president of both the Society for Clinical Geropsychology and the APA Division of Adult Development and Aging. His research interests include cross-cultural issues in family caregiving, age difference in the effects of emotion on cognition, and the development of wisdom. Dr. Knight received his Ph.D. in clinical psychology from Indiana University, Bloomington, IN.

Becca Levy

Becca Levy is an Associate Professor in the Department of Epidemiology and Public Health and the Department of Psychology at Yale University. She received her doctoral training in Social Psychology, with a focus on the Psychology of Aging, from Harvard University. She was awarded a Brookdale National Fellowship, a Margret M. Baltes Early Career Award in Behavioral and Social Gerontology from the Gerontological Society of America, the Springer Award for Early Career Achievement on Adult Development and Aging from the American Psychological Association, and an Investigator Award from the Donaghue Medical Research Foundation. Dr. Levy's research explores psychosocial influences on aging. Ongoing projects explore psychosocial determinants of longevity, psychosocial factors that contribute to elders' successful cognitive and physical functioning, and interventions to improve aging health. She has provided testimony to the United States Senate on ageism in the media.

Denise C. Park

Denise Park is Distinguished University Professor of Behavioral and Brain Sciences as well as Regents Research Scholar at the University of Texas at Dallas where she directs the Center for Vital Longevity. Dr. Park is interested in not only how the function of the brain and mind changes with age, but also is focused on interventions that can be used to delay cognitive aging and support cognitive function in every day life. Using both brain scans and behavioral studies, Dr. Park tries to understand the role of age-related changes in memory function.. Before joining UT Dallas, she was a professor at the University of Illinois, Urbana-Champaign, where she was director of the Center for Healthy Minds. She received her Ph.D. from the State University of New York at Albany. She is a fellow of the American Association for the Advancement of Science; received the American Psychological Association's award for Distinguished Contributions to the Psychology of Aging, and has served on the Board of Directors of the American Psychological Society as well as chaired the Board of Scientific Affairs of the American Psychological Association.

Part 1

Concepts, Theory, and Methods in the Psychology of Aging

1 Enduring Theoretical Themes in Psychological Aging: Derivation, Functions, Perspectives, and Opportunities *3*

2 Methodological and Analytical Issues in the Psychology of Aging *25*

3 Historical Influences on Aging and Behavior *41*

Chapter | 1 |

Enduring Theoretical Themes in Psychological Aging: Derivation, Functions, Perspectives, and Opportunities

Roger A. Dixon
Department of Psychology, University of Alberta, Edmonton, Canada

CHAPTER CONTENTS

Introduction 4
Characterizing the Theoretical Landscape in Psychological Aging 4
Featured Theorists: Identifying and Integrating Enduring Theoretical Themes 5
Selections from James E. Birren 6
Overview 6
Approach to Theoretical Considerations in Psychological Aging 7
Theoretical Themes: Global-Local, Complexity, Aging Change, Differential Role 7
Special Attention to the Role of Chronological Age 7
Conclusions about Birren 8
Selections from Paul B. Baltes 8
Overview 8
Prominent Themes 1: Aging Change, Balancing Trajectories, Complexity, Differential Role, Global-Local 8
Prominent Themes 2: Linking Global-Local with Chronological Age 9
Conclusion: Special Emphases of Baltes 9
Selections from Timothy A. Salthouse 9
Overview 9
Nature of the Field and Definitions 9
Key Themes: Complexity, Global-Local, and Aging Change 10
Promoting Theoretical Development in Psychological Aging 10
Selections from Other Theoretical Reviews 10
The Themes Appear in Other General Commentaries 10
The Six Themes Appear in Process-Specific or "Local" Theories 11
Summary 12
"Populations" of Theoretical Themes and Perspectives in Psychological Aging 12
A Population of Theories of Psychological Aging 12
Contributions of Developmental Epidemiological Perspectives 14
Illustrations: Selected Future Directions for Psychological Theories of Aging 16
Whither Cognitive/Social/Affect Neurosciences of Aging? 16
Whither Chronological-Biological-Age Indexes: Has BioAge Come of Age? 16
Whither Theoretical Implications of Genetic-Epigenetic-Environment-Process Studies? 17
Toward Explanation in Psychological Aging: Do "Causes" Hunt in Packs? Do "Effects" Assemble in Patterns or Disperse and Flee? 17
Conclusions 18
Acknowledgments 18
References 19

DOI: 10.1016/B978-0-12-380882-0.00001-2

INTRODUCTION

From its earliest editions, the editors of the *Handbook of the Psychology of Aging* (hereafter, *Handbook*) series have wisely included informative theoretical, methodological, and historical chapters. On one recent autumn afternoon, I oriented to my upper-level bookshelf containing most editions of this archival series, closed my eyes, and randomly pulled one volume from the shelf. By chance, it was the 20-year-old third edition (Birren & Schaie, 1990), which I opened to the table of contents. As expected, this volume features three chapters in this influential tradition, including contributions to (a) theories and history of the developmental approach to aging (Birren & Birren, 1990), (b) novel (then, but still relevant) methods for analyzing differential and common developmental change (McArdle & Anderson, 1990), and (c) the still important (and unresolved) concepts of chronological age and developmental time in human aging theory and research (Schroots & Birren, 1990). Notably, these three chapters welcomed a reprised inspection, for they had tapped into persistently important themes, issues, and characteristics of psychological aging scholarship. Understandably, the content chapters reflect the texture of the era (e.g., Hultsch & Dixon, 1990). Still curious, I repeated this exercise on several *Handbook* editions, with the same outcome. To the credit of the field of psychological aging and of the *Handbook* editors, successive volumes have regularly and systematically presented chapters examining (a) wide-ranging theoretical derivations, underpinnings, and implications; (b) methodological principles and practices relevant to the theoretical study of aging-related change and variability; and (c) illuminative historical roots, conceptual tendencies, and evolutionary trajectories (e.g., Birren & Schroots, 2001; Schaie, 2011).

The overall purpose of this chapter is to fill a niche in the well-established ecology of psychological theories of aging. Four main goals are pursued. First, I note a perspective on the theoretical context of theories of psychological aging. The tenor of this section is more pragmatic-theoretical than global-metatheoretical. Second, I selectively and briefly review theoretical writings from the past 50 years, focusing on the chapter authors previously featured in this *Handbook* series. Six historically valid, recurring themes or lessons are identified, each of which provides points of contact across developmental processes, theoretical perspectives, and historical periods. Subsequently, I briefly adumbrate several other recent contributions to the literature on theories of psychological aging with attention to the six enduring themes previously identified. Third, these coordinated perspectives and enduring themes provide a foundation upon which to evaluate current theoretical efforts and evolve new and more adaptive ones. Fourth, compelling opportunities for new theoretical advances in psychological aging are provided by new developments in neighboring disciplines, a selection of which are noted in this section. The general goal of this chapter is not one of producing a global or unified theory of psychological aging. Instead, it aims to (a) explain why such a goal may not be among the principal standards or objectives for researchers in this field, and (b) support the contention that theoretical opportunities and advances based on a population of adapted themes and theories are nevertheless plentiful, functional, and promising.

CHARACTERIZING THE THEORETICAL LANDSCAPE IN PSYCHOLOGICAL AGING

Just as no history of a science is without the influence of the historian and his or her historiography, no review of scientific theory exists independently of the filtering lens through which the theorists read, interpret, and write (Hanson, 1958) or the historically evolving conceptual, social, professional, and scientific circumstances of the era (e.g., Kuhn, 1962; Pepper, 1970; Toulmin, 1972). In the past in life-span psychological research, such observations have often led to discussion of scientific paradigms, metatheories, and world views, as they applied to the study of individual development and aging (e.g., Baltes & Willis, 1977; Dixon & Lerner, 1999; Reese & Overton, 1970). This is not the present purpose for three related reasons. First, the general lesson has been learned in that it is probably apparent to most contemporary readers that theories and research methods are informed by underlying (and often untestable) assumptions, models, metaphors, and perspectives (Overton & Reese, 1973). Second, for this reason this particular line of theoretical-historical inquiry has not been particularly active or overtly influential in recent years, at least in the field of psychological aging. Third, one reason it has become both an acknowledged background condition and yet rarely cited or targeted for research is that the field may have moved to a post-paradigmatic period of interdisciplinary, integrative, and even pragmatic perspectives and research. Perhaps in the earlier paradigmatic-centered period metatheoretical differences were accentuated (if not magnified). If so, in a post-paradigmatic period metatheoretical differences (if relevant) may be less likely to restrict or interrupt the pragmatic reconnaissance of (even small) plots of common ground and the probing expansion of these commonalities along shared conceptual and empirical boundaries.

Nevertheless, to recap briefly, the paradigmatic view has held that, because the underlying tendencies of different meta-approaches may be in fundamental conceptual competition, the derived theories may be incommensurable and the associated data collected to test the theories may be mutually unacceptable. This systemic and often static incommensurability may exist even when the research is addressed to common levels of analysis or evidently similar developmental phenomena (Dixon et al., 1991). As a brief illustration, scholars studying the intriguing phenomena of late-life potential or adaptive success can address different (even nonoverlapping) aspects from a variety of largely unshared conceptual and methodological perspectives. These include (a) post-formal or dialectical operations; (b) naturally occurring differential trajectories and protection factors; (c) social-emotional regulation, adaptivity, and influences; (d) cognitive or self reserve, plasticity, or expertise; (e) pragmatic cognitive-personal resilience or compensation; and (f) multiple forms of healthy or successful aging (e.g., Baltes & Baltes, 1990; Ericsson & Smith, 1991; Labouvie-Vief, 1980; Pushkar et al., 1998; Schaie & Carstensen, 2006; Vaillant, 2002). However, paradigm-level perspectives are viewed also as changing, fallible, modifiable, responsive to data, and adaptive (or not). In addition, such metatheoretical perspectives may be inextricably interdisciplinary, theories may be more flexible and pluralistic, methods are definitely more comprehensive and powerful, and the research goals may become more pragmatic and integrative. Specifically, research may become less characterized by how it contributes to a covering metatheory or global theory. Instead, theoretically and clinically significant research may be evaluated in terms of how functional they are, regardless of the academic sources of ideas, levels of analyses (biological, individual–psychological, social–cultural), or the simplicity–complexity of results.

FEATURED THEORISTS: IDENTIFYING AND INTEGRATING ENDURING THEORETICAL THEMES

The *Handbook* chapters (and related work) of three previous contributors are reviewed and tapped as source material for identifying and integrating key enduring themes of psychological theories of aging. The three contributors are James E. Birren, Paul B. Baltes, and Timothy A. Salthouse. Six common and enduring theoretical themes were identified inductively from these authors' *Handbook* (and other) chapters. These themes are used as points of contact and complementarity in the discussion of each contributor's theoretical work (see also Table 1.1). To preview, the themes are (a) *global-local*, or the relative theoretical goal of broader or more narrow theories; (b) *complexity*, or the tendency

Table 1.1 Six enduring themes in the last half-century of research on theories of psychological aging

THEME AND SUB-THEMES	TREND?	ILLUSTRATIVE REFERENCES
Global-Local: Continua from Global to Relatively Local Theories • Population of changing and adapting relatively local theories • Less emphasis on formally structured global theories of "aging"? • More emphasis on moderate but integrative (local) theories of domains of aging? • Balance of focus (with evidence) and scope (with latitude) • Balance of breadth (with qualification) and depth (with precision)	Local	Baltes (1987), Baltes et al. (2006a), Bengtson et al. (1999), Birren (1999), Birren & Cunningham (1985), Cavanaugh (1999), Dixon & Hertzog (1996), Salthouse (2006)
Complexity: Continua from Complexity (Diversity) to Simplicity (Uniformity) • Global theories powerful in their breadth and simplicity • Local theories effective in recognition of complexity • Complexity and multiplicity of influences, contexts, predictors, precursors, causes • Multidirectionality of trajectories • Diversity and multidimensionality of outcomes and patterns • Trend to interdisciplinary or epidemiological approaches	Complexity	Baltes et al. (2006a), Bengtson et al. (1999), Birren (1999), Cavanaugh (1999), Dixon (2010), Hendricks & Achenbaum (1999), Li (2002), Park et al. (1999)

(*Continued*)

Table 1.1 (Continued)

THEME AND SUB-THEMES	TREND?	ILLUSTRATIVE REFERENCES
Aging Change: **Focus on Aging (Change) versus Aged (Status)** • Aging as continuous with life span development and change • Description/explanation of actual aging change processes • Complementary and comparative descriptions of aged groups • Methodological interest in intraindividual designs • Theoretical and clinical importance of longitudinal research	Aging	Baltes & Carstensen (1999), Baltes & Willis (1977), Nesselroade & Baltes (1979), Schaie & Hofer (2001), Schroots & Birren (1990)
Chronological Age: **Status of Chronological Age versus Alternatives** • Chronological age as limited index, not cause/explanation • Search for alternative aging indices (functional or social age) • Emergence of attention to biological vitality or "BioAge" • Challenges in identifying alternative indices that are as simple, valid, available, generalizable, as chronological age	Challenge	Anstey (2008), Baltes & Willis (1977), Birren (1999), Birren & Cunningham (1985), Klemera & Doubal (2006), MacDonald et al. (2004), Nakamura & Miyao (2007), Spiro & Brady (2008), Wahlin et al. (2006)
Differential: **Differential versus Universal Theories and Methods** • Marked individual differences in onset, trajectory/slope, rate, final level • Individual difference "variables" from neurobiological, genetic, health/disease, lifestyle, and other domains • Mean-level trajectories versus intra-individual variability in change • Cultural or social differences in aging changes and variability • Status group differences in aging changes and variability	Differential	Baltes & Willis (1977), Ghisletta et al. (2006), Hertzog (2008), Kramer et al. (2005), Li (2003), Schaie (1996, 2005)
Balance of Trajectory: **Attention to Decline (Losses), Maintenance, and Improvement (Gains)** • Robust evidence for aging declines across domains and processes • Complementary interests in sustained, maintained, resilient performance • Contingent interests in improvement, gains, advances, plasticity • Mechanisms of reserve, compensation, selection, and optimization • Interest in psychological health, cognitive health, successful aging	Balance	Ball et al. (2002), Baltes (1987), Baltes & Baltes (1990), Cabeza et al. (2002), Carstensen et al. (2006), Dixon (2000, 2010), Einstein & McDaniel (2004), Park & Reuter-Lorenz (2009), Stern & Carstensen (2000)

Note. *Trend* = Estimated historical trend according to review (see text). *Illustrative References*: Not a comprehensive list; for further citations see text.

to represent or emphasize complex processes, dynamic phenomena, or multiple influences, levels, and determinants; (c) *aging change,* or the relative emphasis on aging as life span development or the aged as a status or phase in life; (d) *chronological age,* referring to the much discussed status of age as an index of aging; (e) *differential role,* or the theoretical and methodological impact of notions of differential change with aging; and (f) *balance of trajectory,* or the extent to which theories treat or permit multiple directions of aging, including decline, stability, and growth.

Selections from James E. Birren

Overview

In one of the longest running serial commentaries integrating theoretical, methodological, and historical aspects of psychological aging, Birren and colleagues (e.g., Birren, 1959; Birren, 1999; Birren & Birren, 1990; Birren & Cunningham, 1985; Birren & Schroots, 2001) identified several key issues that are still relevant. Fifty years after his first gerontological paper, Birren (1999) observed that the study of aging (in general) and psychological aging (in particular) have been revealed as among the most inherently complex phenomena of the human sciences. In Birren's (1999) review, researchers were successful in investigating segments of the factors and dynamics involved in psychological aging, but the essential balance between data and theory had yet to be struck. In fact, he ventured a colorful expression to describe the field as "data-rich and theory-poor" (Birren, 1999, p. 459). In the discussion of this expression he conveyed several points, all of which are relevant to the psychological theories of aging.

Approach to Theoretical Considerations in Psychological Aging

In their history of the field of psychological aging, Birren and Schroots (2001, p. 3) characterized the field as focusing on "manifest changes or transformations that occur in human and animal behavior related to length of life." Unpacking the key terms and relating the overall characteristics to the current field results in several important points. First, derivable from their extensive historical work is the notion that a prominent emphasis in the field of aging is the study of changes, transformations, and transitions. Aging is not just about the aged per se (as a group or category), it is also about the processes that lead to and through the 70% of the life span typically covered by adulthood (the theme of aging change). Parenthetically, this may be one reason some modern observers prefer the term "psychology of aging" rather than terms such as "geropsychology." The former term includes the notion of change and development explicitly (e.g., Baltes & Willis, 1977). Second, reflecting the complexity theme, the term "behavior" is used to demarcate the system of targeted aging-related processes as those that are mediated by the central nervous system (CNS). This likely covers most behavioral processes of theoretical interest in psychological aging (see Bengtson & Schaie, 1999), but other mediators are listed briefly including skeletal and muscular fitness, non-CNS health conditions (e.g., Type 2 diabetes), and even institutions. A spectrum of modulators (including the CNS but also more distal mechanisms such as health, institutions, and genetic and epigenetic functions) are of current theoretical interest, as are many of the underlying disciplines such as neurosciences and molecular biology (noted in Birren & Cunningham, 1985). Third, promising theoretical opportunities may be presented when (a) the "black box" of the mediating CNS is opened to direct investigation of its functions in modulating behavioral aging; (b) the mediating CNS is investigated for associations with cognitive, emotional, social, personality, and other behavioral processes of aging; and (c) the ancillary mediating systems (e.g., health, peripheral biology) are included in psychological aging studies (e.g., Cabeza et al., 2004; Craik & Bialystok, 2006; Dixon et al., 2004; Stern & Carstensen, 2000). These considerations are consistent with several key theoretical themes of psychological aging.

Theoretical Themes: Global-Local, Complexity, Aging Change, Differential Role

Birren expressed (a) admiration and satisfaction at the accelerating increase in published literature in the field since the 1950s, and (b) appreciation of the growing challenges associated with both local and larger (global) theories in the field (e.g., Birren & Cunningham, 1985; Birren et al., 1983). This field continues to be provoked by the dynamic interplay among these two associated profiles. Nevertheless, however palpable, manageable, and uncluttered the phenomena of psychological aging may have seemed historically (Birren & Schroots, 2001), it had become increasingly apparent through methodological advances (e.g., Baltes, 1968; Schaie, 1965; Schaie, 2010) and accumulating observed phenomena that psychological aging was dynamic, complex, differential, and interactional across multiple levels of analysis (Birren, 1999). Although many successful theories of specific aging phenomena were accumulating, most theories were constrained by their specificity and most theorists were suitably qualified in their expressions of theoretical ambition and breadth.

Special Attention to the Role of Chronological Age

In the field of psychological aging, chronological age has been a traditional variable for organizing research and theory. Nevertheless, it has become increasingly understood to be an index of aging-related change but not necessarily (or even feasibly) a cause or source of theoretical explanations. Birren (1999) and Birren & Cunningham (1985) argued explicitly that the novel, if not game-changing, theoretical advances would come only when chronological age was integrated with (or replaced by) variables that reflected theoretically significant causes of psychological aging. Many of these potential causal variables would likely come from the underlying biological and health domains (i.e., biomarkers). They would replace or supplement chronological age due to their causal proximity, ambient qualification, and functional relationships with many psychological processes. However, Birren also argued that the search for theoretical explanations of specific processes of psychological aging could be viewed as a search for "long causal chains" (1999, p. 463) of contributing variables and sequences leading to psychologically relevant trajectories, statuses, interactions, or outcomes (see also Baltes & Willis, 1977; Birren, 1959). Accordingly, he noted that these factors would derive from biological and health domains as well as from the behavioral, social, environmental, and institutional realms (see also Schaie & Carstensen, 2006). To be sure, there are advantages to the chronological age approach. These include the fact that theories relevant to specific variables can be easily produced, tested, revised, and further developed (Birren, 1999). In addition, chronological age is reliably measureable and a powerful index of passage of lifetime. Corresponding disadvantages of the chronological age approach are that the pertinent data, theories, and segments are infrequently additive, collateral, or mutually concomitant. This deficiency in complementarity can lead to disciplinary and theoretical fractionation, rather than to integration or advancement. Some observers view age as a potentially crude marker of the changes that occur in the mediators and targets of psychological aging — but it may indeed remain the "meat and potatoes" index variable for much psychological aging research.

Conclusions about Birren

Birren's work addresses all of the six key theoretical themes of psychological aging. Even the early *Handbook* chapter (Birren & Cunningham, 1985) attended to themes such as complexity and aging change. In fact, the authors discuss the importance of time (aging), both methodologically (employing time-structured designs, collecting temporal-based data, and using change-sensitive analyses) and theoretically (using time as an organizing concept in explanations). However, one of the strongest sustained arguments about the theoretical role of chronological age in psychological aging research is also presented in this chapter (and is echoed in contemporary literature; Anstey, 2008; Spiro & Brady, 2008). First, chronological age may serve productively as a surrogate variable, especially if researchers understand that (a) it simply (and vaguely) represents an undifferentiated host of influences, and (b) new nonchronological, change-sensitive indices should be developed. In contemporary context, one suggestion is that these new nonchronological age approaches will likely supplement and qualify chronologically based findings. How well they will replace chronological age, overturn chronological-age-based findings, or qualify chronological-age-based theories is not yet known. Second, as Birren had noted in previous contributions, the 1985 chapter reviewed his perspective on alternative indicators of age and time, including functional age, biological age, social age, and psychological age. The goal of these renditions of change indices is to develop markers that more closely represent the "conglomeration of influences" that predict or mediate target processes of psychological aging. There is still theoretical interest in these alternative markers.

Selections from Paul B. Baltes

Overview

Reaching for an uncommonly broad and interdisciplinary perspective on psychological theories of aging, the work of Baltes and colleagues (e.g., Baltes et al., 2005; Baltes et al., 2006a; Baltes & Smith, 1997) merits featured attention. Baltes and Willis (1977) contributed the first theoretical chapter appearing in the initial edition of the *Handbook* series. Over 30 years ago, the authors covered basic issues in scientific theories, including procedures for evaluation (e.g., precision, scope, and deployability) and characteristics of psychologically scientific theories (e.g., metatheory), but also contributed early and cogent statements pertaining to all six key theoretical themes. In subsequent contributions, Baltes and colleagues expanded (a) the range of psychological processes considered from their theoretical–developmental perspective (e.g., intelligence, wisdom, personality, memory, success), (b) the mechanisms of influence and determination (cultural, biological, interactional), and (c) the trajectories, forms, and outcomes of psychological change with aging (selection, optimization, compensation, impairment, successful aging). Their treatment of these issues evolved programmatically in both convergent and divergent ways. Based on both historical and mature perspectives (e.g., Baltes et al., 2006a), the architecture (Baltes' term) of his theoretical approach reveals numerous points of contact with the key enduring themes of psychological aging.

Prominent Themes 1: Aging Change, Balancing Trajectories, Complexity, Differential Role, Global-Local

Baltes' (e.g., 1987) concept of development emphasizes several themes relevant to theories of psychological aging: (a) aging change, in that he argues that development occurs throughout the life span, (b) balance of trajectories, in that life span change includes processes interpretable as both growth and decline, and (c) complexity, in that these developmental changes are influenced by multiple contexts and interact continuously and dynamically to produce patterns of gains, losses, stability, variability, reversibility, plasticity, and adaptivity (Baltes, 1987; Baltes et al., 2006b; Dixon & Baltes, 1986). Regarding complexity, Baltes and colleagues frequently noted that psychological aging is influenced from multiple levels of analysis ranging from the biological to the cultural (Baltes et al., 2005;

Li, 2003), including psychological, social, environment, and their interactions (Baltes et al., 2006b). The Differential Role theme is readily detectable in the *Handbook* chapter (Baltes & Willis, 1977), as revealed in the notion that the study of psychological aging focuses on changes that are often multidirectional, variable, and differential. In addition, they highlighted the methodological corollary that designs and strategies for directly observing intra-individual change (e.g., longitudinal) are crucial for assessing the dynamics of psychological aging (Hofer & Sliwinski, 2006; Schaie & Hofer, 2001). When such designs are implemented in the service of examining the complexities of aging dynamics, antecedent or explanatory variables will be found from a "multitude" (Baltes & Willis, 1977, p. 143) of factors, systems, precursors, influences, chains of precipitating events, and causes (recall Birren, 1999). Thus, even in 1977, Baltes and Willis invoked the global-local theme, indicating that the literature to date did "not support the notion of a monolithic, single-agent explanatory position" (p. 143).

Prominent Themes 2: Linking Global-Local with Chronological Age

A global and all encompassing theory of psychological aging seemed elusive in 1977, and Baltes studiously avoided such claims. In fact, a common thread in Baltes' (e.g., 1987) theoretical work was a series of efforts to develop systems, taxonomies, metaframes, theoretical families, metatheoretical propositions, and other types of flexible organizing structures — seeking common conceptual ground but eschewing claims of universal theories. Of specific interest were the dynamic interactions among both static elements and changing processes of biology and culture in producing dynamic and interactive psychological aging changes. Although the authors acknowledged that contemporary methods (including large-scale longitudinal studies and computational modeling) could contribute to explanations (and therefore theory development), they noted it was not possible to completely isolate or disentangle all contributing causes (Baltes & Smith, 1997; Li, 2002).

Even in 1977, Baltes and Willis articulated the point that chronological age is only one of several potential ways to organize time trajectories in psychological aging. Moreover, they argued that chronological age is especially (and perhaps only) useful when intra-individual change patterns are sufficiently homogeneous to yield high relationships between age and processes of psychological development. To the extent that there are individual differences in various aspects of long-term change patterns (e.g., trajectory or shape, timing and severity of inflection or change points, directionality and slope), the theoretical power of chronological age is reduced. Still plaguing researchers today is the identification of viable alternative indices of aging, although Baltes and Willis point to both the terminal decline phenomenon (e.g., MacDonald et al., 2008; Rabbitt et al., 2002; Sliwinski et al., 2006) and social age (involving class, life course, and cultural indicators) as two potential alternatives.

The search for determinants of development has been an important objective for theoretical work in psychological aging. Baltes and colleagues (2006a) identified some candidate determinants, including such fundamental aspects of cognition as speed or slowing (Salthouse, 1996), inhibition or distractibility (Darowski et al., 2008; Lustig et al., 2007), sensory-related common cause (Baltes & Lindenberger, 1997), and various neurological indices (Cabeza et al., 2004; Hedden & Gabrieli, 2005). Their life span functional perspective attributed the potential for aging-related adaptivity to personality or other self-systems, with the possibility of multiple determinants, dynamic interactions among levels of analyses, and consequent individual differences in trajectories and variability over long periods of aging.

Conclusion: Special Emphases of Baltes

Although Baltes and Willis (1977) aver in defining age and aging, they do so in the service of making their main points that (a) aging will continuously be redefined, (b) aging is linked with development in that both occur throughout the life span, (c) aging is not tantamount to decline, and (d) despite the fact it can be easily measured and is conventional in the literature, chronological age is suboptimal as a standby explanatory category. They encourage the development of alternative procedures for indexing, charting, and accounting for the multitude of determinants — from the biological to the cultural — of psychological aging processes.

Selections from Timothy A. Salthouse

Overview

A complementary but different approach to the tradition of theoretical chapters was provided by Salthouse (2006) in the sixth and immediately previous edition of the *Handbook* series. Not since Baltes and Willis (1977) had a chapter in this series reviewed basic characteristics of scientific theories as they apply to the psychology of aging. Salthouse's presentation, which is fine-grained and grounded in a fertile version of philosophy of science, is recommended for further study.

Nature of the Field and Definitions

Salthouse noted that successful scientific theories organize and guide research for both descriptive and explanatory questions. Whereas descriptive questions can be tested with a variety of research designs and evaluated in terms of fit with theory-based predictions, explanatory questions are intrinsically theoretical in that they address questions of causality or mechanisms. With respect to psychological aging, the latter may include precursors of psychological change, covariates of differential change, mediators of relationships, and determinants of group differences. All require systematic procedures of evaluation.

Key Themes: Complexity, Global-Local, and Aging Change

Consistent with positions established by Birren and Baltes, Salthouse noted that multiple "causal" factors may be operating in the prediction of many interesting and complex aging-related psychological functions. Salthouse's (2006) suggestions for future theoretical development in psychological aging are consistent with those of previous *Handbook* reviewers. In a note concordant with the global-local theme, he indicated that there is no unified theory of psychological aging, but offered clear recommendations for future theory development.

Promoting Theoretical Development in Psychological Aging

Salthouse offered several memorable recommendations. First, researchers in psychological aging should sample across a broader population of variables that may control or contribute to theoretically relevant psychological processes (complexity). Second, researchers should continually explore novel linkages among new data and associated testable theories. In this way, theories, which are in transition (also emphasized by Baltes & Willis, 1977) can be updated, clarified, improved, and lead to even newer studies and data and tests of theories. Third, researchers may ensure that these dynamic data-theory linkages are not conducted in multiple isolations, but are articulated in the context of other related research programs, both concurrent and historical. To the credit of the field, all previous theoretical chapters have demonstrated these integrations with other researchers, neighboring fields, and historical contributions. Notably, Salthouse's own theoretical contributions to psychological aging research have been among the most scholarly, systematic, influential, and productive programmatic efforts to implement these three recommendations (e.g., Salthouse, 1991, 1996).

Selections from Other Theoretical Reviews

The foregoing section focused on contributions from previous *Handbook* authors. Six theoretical themes were identified as (a) appearing in remarkably similar terminology and connotations across the authors and (b) enduring over time. Although the pool of published theoretical analyses is limited, other reviewers in disparate venues have commented on psychological aging theory. In this section, writings from selected authors are explored both for (a) validation of the key theoretical themes and (b) affirmation of unique perspectives and applications.

The Themes Appear in Other General Commentaries

Cavanaugh (1999, p. 1) began his review of theories of aging with a simple but deceptively elegant query: "Why do people grow old?" The search for answers to this perplexing query is essentially a search for explanations (or theories) of aging. Moreover, this search has occupied the interest of a multitude of observers for centuries, including philosophers, novelists, poets, theologians, and scientists at many levels of analysis. Cavanaugh hastened to clarify, however, that this abiding but seemingly uncomplicated root question did not imply that one should expect to arrive at a single or comprehensive theory of aging — thus invoking the global-local theme at the outset of his review. In fact, he noted that a broad assortment of qualitatively distinct explanations is due to the inscrutable and interacting diversity of complex and dynamic process of aging (e.g., the complexity theme). For Cavanaugh, the complexity derived from the fact of multiple "developmental forces," (e.g., biological, psychological, sociocultural, life cycle) affecting human aging. Cavanaugh also alluded to the chronological age theme, noting that researchers and theorists should attend to several meanings of age (e.g., problems with chronological age, as well as alternatives such as biological age, psychological age, social age) and aging (e.g., primary aging, secondary aging, tertiary aging). The differential and balance of trajectories themes were embodied in his proposal that theories of aging should target not only typical patterns of aging-related change (often decline), but also individual differences in those patterns (Hertzog, 2008), as well as the possibility that some combinations of influences may lead to extended periods of stability, maintenance, or even "gains" or "successful" aging (Baltes & Baltes, 1990; Dixon, 2000, 2010).

Two chapters from an important theoretical collection (Bengtson & Schaie, 1999) addressed relevant issues of general aging theories. Hendricks and Achenbaum (1999) cast the study of aging — and the development and testing of theories about aging — as a "hybrid" (p. 30) and "multifaceted" (p. 28) endeavor, requiring "broadly based theories" (p. 26) to guide and interpret multidisciplinary epidemiological data. Accordingly, both the global-local and complexity themes were endorsed. These authors emphasized the special relevance of theories and data pertaining to changes in (and linked across) domains such as biology, psychology, and culture (e.g., Baltes et al., 2006a; Park, 1992). Given the growing base of available multidisciplinary information, the authors contemplated whether the depth and breadth of the multiple disciplines involved in aging research required teams of complementary experts not only to conduct the research but to develop broader theoretical models to represent it.

The global-local theme was addressed directly in a corresponding chapter by Bengtson et al. (1999). The authors posed a provocative question regarding whether general theories of aging are possible and even important: Are global theories of aging "archaic" in an increasingly differentiated field. Specifically, they argued that such general theories seemed to be of diminishing relevance across the constituent disciplines of gerontology. Instead, more local and process-specific theories (with firm empirical foundations) were thriving. For example, in social psychological aging, ambitious and general approaches to explaining a wide range of aging phenomena, such as disengagement theory, were less in evidence at their writing (1999) than in previous decades. In contrast, specific theories aimed at less global phenomena, such as socioemotional selectivity theory (e.g., Carstensen et al., 2006), were being developed with intensified explications of the mechanics and implications of basic empirical relationships. The improved empirical base of more specific theories could lead to enhanced explorations of theoretical range, multidisciplinary interactions, and even breadth of everyday application. In the context of emerging local and empirically informed theories, little room was left for grander theories of modest evidentiary base. One qualifying note regarding the global-local theme is that there may be fewer publication outlets for explicating global theories of psychological aging, whereas progress in local theories can be charted in the typical research literature.

Consistent with the aging change and complexity themes, Bengtson and Schaie (1999) also noted that there is some disagreement, if not confusion, about the question of just what gerontological researchers are trying to explain. To them, aging theories must be (a) explicitly developmental in nature and (b) incorporate multiple levels of influence and interaction (from biological, psychological, and the social domains). They lamented that although intra-individual data are required to advance and test all levels of theories of aging, the proportion of longitudinal studies was still relatively small. Improvements have occurred in the intervening period (e.g., Hofer & Sliwinski, 2006; Hultsch, 2004). In sum, the authors cautioned that the goal of achieving a grand or global theory of aging may not be reasonable, but theoretical advances at more local levels can certainly be reached in the short term.

The Six Themes Appear in Process-Specific or "Local" Theories

Historically, many successful and influential examples of theories regarding specific phenomena have appeared. These include (a) processing speed theories of cognitive aging (Salthouse, 1991, 1996); (b) neurocognitive resources, reserve, or interrelation theories (Cabeza et al., 2002; Craik & Byrd, 1982; Stern, 2007); (c) inhibition theory of memory aging (Lustig et al., 2007; Zacks et al., 2000); (d) organization or systems of memory in aging (Light, 1992; Nyberg et al., 2003); (e) personality structure and stability in aging (McCrae & Costa, 1994; Roberts et al., 2006); (f) learned dependency theory of social adjustment and aging (M. Baltes, 1996); and (g) socioemotional selectivity theory (Carstensen et al., 2006). Two of these theories were reviewed in a memorably instructive chapter by M. Baltes and Carstensen (1999). Consistent with the enduring theoretical themes, the theory of learned dependency in old age is recast as a developmental-aging phenomenon (aging change) influenced by biological change and social conditions (complexity). As such, it serves as both an aging-related deficit and a functional-adaptive control mechanism. Similarly, socioemotional selectivity theory begins with the oft noted deficit of social interactions in the everyday lives of many North American older adults (leading to former theories such as mutual disengagement of older adult and society), but confers functional or motivated life-span-related decisions to some of these older adults who proactively manage their social worlds to optimize personal social and emotional goals. In fact, the difference (or paradox) between the robust deficits observed in cognitive and physiological aging is contrasted with the late-life competence displayed in emotion regulation. Subsequently, the authors associated both theories to the organizing notion of "selective optimization with compensation" at both the individual-developmental and the group- or couple-developmental levels of analysis (Carstensen et al., 2006; Charles & Carstensen, 2007). In general, these are examples of local theories expanding in purview and enhancing their potential theoretical and empirical impact.

In recent publications, the enduring theoretical themes may appear in slightly different terms and nuances. For example, in their conceptual framework, Stern and Carstensen (2000) identified key components of psychological aging. These included both (a) a focus on a wide range of pragmatic and adaptive everyday functions (balancing trajectories), and (b) a broad "conjunction" of interacting and influential factors from multiple levels of analyses, including the biological, neurological, and psychological (complexity).

The differential role theme has also appeared in multiple recent publications (e.g., Dixon & Hertzog, 1996; Hertzog, 2008). Specific issues associated with the notion of examining multiple patterns and trajectories of psychological aging have also appeared (e.g., Baltes et al., 2006a; Carstensen et al., 2006; Dixon, 2010).

Summary

Over the last several decades the intellectual ecology of psychological theories of aging displayed a notable degree of consistency in identifying, exploring, and evaluating a set of six key theoretical themes. Considerable overlap was observed across both historical and current reviews, multiple authors in various collections, and substantive developmental domains such as social, personality, self, memory, and cognition. The number of points of contact and shared borders of complementarity and commensurability are remarkable. Notably, this review was open to the possibility that such commonality would not be detected. For example, this review could have resulted in a population of essentially contradictory or incompatible issues, but it did not. Similarly, this review could have resulted in commonality only among relatively weak concepts with little or no relevance to empirical research in modern psychological aging, but it did not. Moreover, this review could have resulted in little or no common ground, furthering debate about metatheories, global theories, and contradictory local theories, but it did not. Taken together, these reviews provide a foundation or structure for continuing theoretical developments in psychological aging. In the next section, some aspects to consider when pursuing theoretical work in psychological aging are presented based on this foundation.

"POPULATIONS" OF THEORETICAL THEMES AND PERSPECTIVES IN PSYCHOLOGICAL AGING

The six enduring theoretical themes (Table 1.1) are consequential to the field because they (a) are consensually and historically established as conceptually prominent matters of essential contention; (b) convey promise for future theoretical advances as they evolve from less to more resolved status; and (c) function to organize current knowledge and to promote further developments in methodological or theoretical guidelines, research protocols, evaluation criteria, and benchmarks for adaptation and success. However, taken together, these themes may be better characterized as a cluster of themes representing a population of local theories than as a global, well-structured, or unified metatheory of general psychological aging. Implications of this population view of scientific theories include the notion that informal collections of formal local theories may be an appropriate scientific goal for complex, evolving, adapting, and dynamically interactive research enterprises such as psychological aging. In the case of psychological aging, one concrete example is represented by developmental epidemiological approaches.

A Population of Theories of Psychological Aging

Scientific theories often cluster in populations of related or complementary doctrines, some of which may provide fertile pools of shareable ideas, perspectives, questions, and methods. For example, in aging some theories of cognitive plasticity (e.g., Lövden et al., 2010) are complementary to perspectives on cognitive compensation (e.g., Dixon et al., 2008), which are in turn related to concepts of selection and optimization (e.g., Baltes et al., 2006a), and conceptual neighbors with socioemotional selectivity theory (e.g., Carstensen et al., 2006a). In the theoretical reviews previously noted, there was little overt interest expressed in expectations or requirements that such "local" scientific theories display (or be evaluated in terms of) the extent of their (a) global reach or ambition, (b) immutable or universal principles, or (c) logical structure or formal systematicity. Instead, the focus was typically on the extent to which theories functioned to reflect or account for the crucial challenges of a given evolving content or process domain of aging (e.g., self, emotion, memory) and its potential integration with selected domain neighbors in the field (Baltes & Willis, 1977; Salthouse, 2006). This focus on theoretical functionality, integrativeness, and adaptability is common in scientific disciplines, especially those involving complexities of time and change (Toulmin, 1972). Accordingly, the field of psychological aging can be assured that the theoretical situation is at least (a) not less formal or inferior to that of many other disciplines and (b) not less successful for the lack of global reach and formal systematicity. Moreover, this perspective is not in contrast to some views of the theoretical situation in related disciplines such as biological aging or sporadic Alzheimer's disease (AD). In each of these disciplines there are important qualifications, areas of incompleteness, points of contention, controversial aspects, and a rapidly evolving evidentiary base affecting theoretical stability.

Table 1.2 illustrates three dimensions shared by a population of the theoretical themes. The first shared dimension (see segment 1) indicates that it is typical and functional that a population of local theories in psychological aging has features of independence, overlap, complementarity, and (often marginal) coexisting awareness. It is often the changing

Table 1.2 Three characteristics of the population of psychological aging theories that are typical of populations of scientific theories in other disciplines

1. Typical Characteristics of a Population of Coexisting Relatively "Local" Theories
    - Some theories function as independent local theories (e.g., theories of a single aging process, theories with narrow or specific explanans)
    - Some theories function as local theories but with shared boundaries (conceptual territory, research goals, and methods) with neighboring local theories
    - Local theories are pragmatic, expand geographically, grow geometrically, but rarely seek or become global, formal logical, static structural theories
    - Local theories are historical and may have their own genealogies, traditions, scientific protocols, professional cultures
    - A population of local theories may share and generate variations, mutations, innovations; these may lead to theoretical change, survival, and adaptation
    - Within populations (and within most local theories), theoretical change is gradual, continuous, multidirectional, multidetermined, with open end points
2. Characteristics of Successful Local Theories in a Disciplinary Population
    - Local theories establish and test the limits of received or apparent boundaries of the theory's share of the population or discipline
    - Successful local theories find and push the margins of complementarity with intra- and extra-disciplinary neighbors (leading to theoretical growth)
    - Driving theoretical advances are methodological novelties, conceptual variations, and pertinent empirical evidence (plus some serendipity)
    - Successful theories generate, transmit, test, adapt, and incorporate advances from events driving theoretical advances
    - Successful theories foster a research environment that facilitates local independent theory development, integrative local theory development, connections to the disciplinary population of theories
3. The Rationality of a Population of Disciplinary Theories Includes Logical Coherence, Research Fertility, Empirical Validation and Nonrational but Knowable Influences
    - Includes consensually established key concepts, historically enduring theoretical issues, methodological technology and criteria
    - Includes influences of people (researchers) actively involved in the discipline (personality, preferences, ambitions, persuasion, idiosyncrasies, vision)
    - Includes professional networks and societies that organize, guide, or shape research preferences, project funding, public presentations, publication
    - Influences on the concurrent success or failure of concepts and theoretical issues may include intrinsic intellectual merit, professional-level vision, personal-level persuasion
    - The rationality or logical coherence of the discipline is dynamic, interactive, and influenced by all the factors noted herein
    - Concurrent or enduring prominence of concepts or theoretical issues may be related to ultimate theoretical significance in the discipline (or not)
    - Rationality of local theories may be evaluated "cross-sectionally" (comparing alternate theories of similar phenomena or adequacy of a single theory in accounting for relevant phenomena)
    - Rationality of local theories may be evaluated "longitudinally" by tracing logic, influences, and adaptiveness of particular concepts or issues over historical time, examining the conditions and factors that lead to their trajectories and outcomes

local theories, especially those at the integrative or disciplinary boundaries, that generate variations and innovations that lead to theoretical advances. Second (see segment 2 of Table 1.2), successful local theories identify and push the margins or boundaries of complementarity within the population. This process is often facilitated by methodological novelties, conceptual variations, empirical evidence (for and against), and serendipity (the standby of scientific progress). Successful disciplines or populations of theories foster research ecologies that facilitate independence and integration (interdisciplinarity) of local theories, thereby facilitating theoretical growth. Third (see segment 3 in Table 1.2), like other scientific disciplines, the "rationality" of the field of psychological aging is characterized and influenced by much more than the objective or logical structure of its explanations, theories, accumulating evidence, and detached criteria.

Although these are important characteristics, the field is also guided and evaluated by influences deriving from a variety of less analytical, less abstract, and less tangible characteristics of its researchers, leaders, professional networks, societies, and research cultures. Accordingly, the rationality of the field of psychological aging includes some minor but inevitable components of irrationality, and it is up to the population of researchers (and their cultural tools) to separate the wheat from the chaff — a continuous project for any evolving theoretical enterprise. In sum, these three dimensions are common characteristics of the theoretical ecology of fields addressing complex and dynamic phenomena. Although a population of theories does not constitute a global or unified theory, it may contribute to the development of ever-advancing and generalized theories.

Contributions of Developmental Epidemiological Perspectives

In their *Handbook* chapter, Birren and Cunningham (1985; Birren & Birren, 1990) commented on the accelerating pace of research in psychological aging (during the previous 40 years). That pace of productivity is, if anything, even more dazzling in the intervening 25 years. A veritable explosion of information in psychological aging has occurred, and much of it has pushed the boundaries of inquiry to include contexts and influences on psychological aging that could only be imagined during the formative years of the field. Impressive is the precision and sheer breadth of current contributions, including such new intellectual neighbors as the clinical/cognitive neurosciences, health sciences, genetics/epigenetics, pharmacology, life course social science, psychiatry, as well as quantitative and computational methods (e.g., Baltes et al., 2006a; Cabeza et al., 2004; Dixon et al., 2004; Hofer et al., 2003; National Institute on Aging, 2008; Ram & Nesselroade, 2007; Stern & Carstensen, 2000). Among other observers, we have urged consideration of a "pluralistic and epidemiological agenda" (Dixon & Nilsson, 2004, p. 5) as applied to the program of integrating diverse influences in understanding psychological aging. From this perspective, an intellectually healthy discipline is one that promotes scientifically competitive interdisciplinary efforts to understand complex, dynamic, and interrelated phenomena (Dixon & Nesselroade, 1983; Toulmin, 1972).

As we have seen in this chapter, psychological changes of aging are occasioned (preceded, caused, promoted, coupled, led or lagged) by a host of influences and contexts, unique combinations of which may be responsible for different collections of trajectories and outcomes (Baltes & Smith, 1997; Dixon, 2010; Park et al., 1999; Stern & Carstensen, 2000). Among the useful procedures for investigating multidimensional and multidetermined changes that occur over long periods are large-scale studies, often with epidemiological characteristics (National Institute on Aging, 2008). Indeed, in recent years, more integrative research efforts have been launched with various processes of psychological aging linked with biological, health, neurological, genetic/epigenetic, sociocultural domains (Anstey, 2008; Dixon et al., 2004; Li, 2003; Schaie & Carstensen, 2006; Spiro & Brady, 2008; Wahlin, 2004; Waldstein, 2000), often (but not necessarily) in the context of large-scale longitudinal studies. Among the key interests in this effort have been identifying precursors of the principal sets of possible trajectories for a wide range of aging-related changes: (a) normal decline or losses (e.g., Craik & Bialystok, 2006; Craik & Salthouse, 2007), (b) cognitively healthy maintenance or stability or preservation of performance over notably long periods of adulthood and aging (e.g., Dixon, 2010; Schaie, 1996, 2005), as associated in all cases with (c) interactive contributions from pools of risk factors (neurobiological or other disease-related influences; e.g., Cabeza et al., 2004; Wahlin, 2004) and protective factors (e.g., cognitive reserve and lifestyle activities; Stern, 2007). As shown in Figure 1.1, among the guiding theoretical questions are those that point toward discovering the identity and function of precursor factors that individually and interactively, across multiple levels of analysis, may lead differentially to a variety of psychological process trajectories and psychological health-related outcome conditions.

In the figure, the first panel presents the epidemiological contexts of psychological aging in four provisional clusters. These provisional clusters correspond roughly to "bio-psycho-social-temporal" contexts often referred to as sources of influences on psychological aging (e.g., Baltes et al., 2006a; Schaie & Carstensen, 2006; Whitbourne, 2001). Figure 1.1 refers to the clusters with the informal labels biological vitality, neurocognitive vitality, dimensions of life experience, and levels and facts of temporal changes. For research practice, any number or variety of variables derived from these contexts may operate to influence psychological trajectories of aging through the prism of the middle panel of Figure 1.1 (i.e., epidemiological function). Some psychological trajectories of aging may be influenced heavily by a given risk factor, but many other individual profiles may be influenced by the combined or interactive effects of multiple risk factors, perhaps even as qualified by specific protection factors. The third panel summarizes the four categories of potential change and outcome patterns associated with psychological aging. Although the most common trajectory is some manner of decline and the most frequent outcome is some level of lesser success, developmental epidemiological studies could also address the sources of

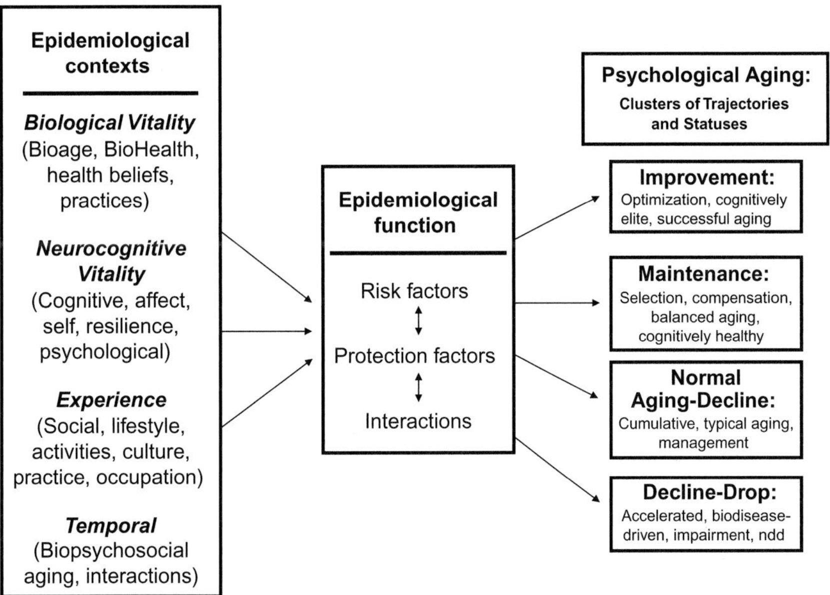

Figure 1.1 Template for identifying developmental-epidemiological contexts, functions, trajectories, and outcomes in psychological aging (NDD: neurodegenerative disease).

influences, the protection factors operating, and the outcomes that may be characterized in more favorable terms. As one example, consider the case of sporadic (as contrasted with familial) AD. Even for this relatively well-defined outcome, there is no known single factor (e.g., genetic, epigenetic, environmental) that conveys preclinical certainty upon a process of neurodegeneration leading to a formal diagnosis of sporadic AD. Instead, there are several (and a growing known number of) factors that confer a qualified risk for AD. Notably, most trajectories and outcomes of psychological aging processes are less defined or diagnosable than sporadic AD, thus inviting even greater qualification. Therefore, two complementary avenues of research and theory are evident. One direction is to identify both single and combinatorial risk factors (e.g., from multiple clusters) and investigate how they may act and interact in leading to defined or probable outcomes such as sporadic AD (National Institute on Aging, 2008). The second and complementary direction is to identify temporally interacting influences (e.g., protection factors) or systems of influence (whether crossed, coupled, decoupled, leading, or lagging) that operate in producing cognitive maintenance or psychological health with aging. Arguably, theoretical advances will occur when these two directions are merged.

The central goal of epidemiological approaches to the development and distribution of health and illness has aspects of both theoretical (e.g., explanation of normal decline and disease-based phenomena) and practical (e.g., implications for remedial intervention, avoiding unhealthy trajectories, promoting healthier outcomes) considerations. For all eventualities, some attention to potential risk factors (which hinder maintenance, accelerate decline, and are associated with less propitious outcomes) or protection factors (which promote maintenance, buffer decline, and are associated with promoting health) would benefit from guidance from local domain-related theories. At the level of a population of theories of psychological aging, a valuable characteristic would be the implementation of time-structured research designs that have intervals and overall durations reflecting the expected change rates in the target processes.

Unfortunately, with aging, while the risk factors are accumulating and growing in intensity, the protective resources are typically diminishing in number and vitality (Baltes et al., 2006b). Nevertheless, to fully understand the interactive dynamics that could typify some long-term changes in psychological health, it may be important not only to have intra-individual theories and data, but also measures that represent multiple relevant risk and protection factors. Moreover, according to the population of theoretical themes described in this chapter — because of the dynamic, interactive, complex, open-ended, and multiply determined nature of many processes of psychological aging — the resulting theories will be continuing, incomplete, unfinished, adaptive, and improved but not final, and likely not global or unified.

ILLUSTRATIONS: SELECTED FUTURE DIRECTIONS FOR PSYCHOLOGICAL THEORIES OF AGING

This section provides an overview of the current status and expected future directions of four particularly promising, active, and integrative movements in research and theory in psychological aging. The four illustrations of fertile and promising research directions are (a) the integration of cognitive, social, and affective neuroscience in aging; (b) the coordinating agendas of chronological and biological age; (c) the emerging studies on genetic, epigenetic, and environmental influences; and (d) new epidemiological perspectives on the concept and pursuit of explanation in aging theories.

Whither Cognitive/Social/ Affect Neurosciences of Aging?

There can be no doubt that neurological integrity — and a variety of morphological, functional, and neuromodulation indicators — is directly related to concurrent cognitive performances, social behaviors and relationships, and affective or emotional attributes. Developmentally, neurological factors are also implicated in virtually all directions and rates of changes among these processes with aging (e.g., Cabeza et al., 2004; Knight & Mather, 2006; Raz et al., 2005; Tadorov et al., in press). The recent technological, empirical, and theoretical progress in the applied neurosciences of aging has been impressive. Consistent with the complexity and balance of trajectories themes, many theories of psychological aging — even local theories of memory, attention, executive functions, emotion regulation, well-being, personality — are incorporating multiple aspects of the neurological substrate in their research programs. Notably, researchers are increasingly shifting from description-intensive work (e.g., documenting relatively simple associations) to tackling key explanatory (and therefore theoretical) issues relevant to a variety of domains of aging. Examples include aging-related (a) theories of neurocognitive reserve and brain health (e.g., Hedden & Gabrieli, 2005; Park & Reuter-Lorenz, 2009; Persson et al., 2006; Reuter-Lorenz & Lustig, 2005; Stern, 2007); (b) brain, cognitive, and social mechanisms of resilience and adaptation, such as plasticity and compensation (e.g., Cabeza et al., 2002; Dixon, Garrett et al., 2008; Lövden et al., 2010; Raz, 2009; Reuter-Lorenz & Cappell, 2008); (c) neural mechanisms associated with well-being and emotional regulation (e.g., Blanchard-Fields 2005; Cacioppo et al., in press; St. Jacques et al., 2010); (d) neuroanatomical correlates of personality (e.g., Wright et al., 2007); (e) linkages to a variety of neurobiological and biological health makers (e.g., white matter degradation, volumetric indices, dopaminergic status, homocysteine levels, hypertension and vascular effects; e.g., Anstey, 2008; Bäckman et al., 2006; Raz, 2009; Spiro & Brady, 2008); and (f) linkages to genetic or epigenetic markers (e.g., National Institute on Aging, 2008). Longitudinal studies and sophisticated techniques for analyzing increasingly multivariate data are also coming on line, as this field becomes ever more interdisciplinary and addresses ever more complex, dynamic, and interactive relationships with aging.

Whither Chronological-Biological-Age Indexes: Has BioAge Come of Age?

As we have seen, the chronological age theme emerged historically in the context of dissatisfaction with the conceptual status of chronological age (e.g., Birren, 1999). Biological or functional age (e.g., BioAge) has received considerable research attention in the past decade and, although very promising in concept, it too has revealed some limitations in implementation (e.g., Anstey, 2008; Anstey et al., 2005; Hofer et al., 2003; Jackson et al., 2003; Lindenberger & Ghisletta, 2009; MacDonald et al., 2004; Salthouse, Hambrick, & McGuthry, 1998). What is the current theoretical status of the chronological age versus biological age discussion? Where is the debate and research likely heading? First, it would be a challenge to find many observers who do not concur with the basic premise that chronological age is merely an index of developmental time; one that carries few causal implications and little explanatory weight. Second, many of these observers would probably also concur with the notion that finding mechanism-related functional markers of aging could in principle advance our theoretical understanding of specific psychological changes. Third, observers would also agree with the corollary idea that multiple candidate markers exist in the biological realm. Fourth, a corresponding goal is to produce an estimate of BioAge that could lead to more (a) precise descriptive understanding of many aspects of psychological aging and (b) integrated and sharpened theories of relevant aging-related psychological processes.

Five key recent advances that auger well for future theoretical developments are adumbrated. First, some progress in honing the concept and defining principal candidate markers has been made. For example, attention to examining BioAge has usefully emphasized functional biomarkers (e.g., Anstey, 2008), although this is not to diminish probable interactive contributions of neurobiological indicators (e.g., Raz, 2004), general health burden indicators (e.g., Spiro & Brady,

2008; Wahlin, 2004), specific non-neurological aging-related disease indicators (e.g., Type 2 diabetes, hypertension), or genetic and epigenetic indicators (e.g., National Institute on Aging, 2008). Second, functional biomarkers (e.g., pulmonary, muscle, motor health) are designed to reflect a construct of biological vigor or vitality that, when rendered in progressive decrements with biological aging, could represent a distribution along which individuals can be measured in terms of (a) relative biological age or aging and (b) probability of biological mortality (e.g., Nakamura & Miyao, 2003). Third, increasing numbers of epidemiological and longitudinal studies of psychological aging are including functional biomarkers in their protocols, and thus the number of datasets, operational definitions, and publications of perspectives on BioAge has multiplied. Fourth, given that BioAge is considerably more complicated to estimate than chronological age, considerable attention has been devoted to developing viable and replicable multivariate representations (e.g., Klemera & Doubal, 2006; MacDonald et al., 2004; Nakamura & Miyao, 2003, 2007). Fifth, it is becoming clearer that useful markers of BioAge may include certain neurocognitive, sensory, and fluid intelligence indicators (e.g., Anstey, 2008; Lindenberger & Ghisletta, 2009; MacDonald et al., 2008). Sixth, BioAge may be usefully explored for its contributions along continua of risk factors consistent with a developmental epidemiological perspective (e.g., Goffaux et al., 2005), one of which (it should not be overlooked) is indeed chronological age (Klemera & Doubal, 2006). In sum, BioAge is coming of age in psychological aging research and theory that early featured theorists (e.g., Baltes and Birren) would probably endorse. It is one composite indicator of biological vitality that will play an expanded role in future explanations of a wide range of psychological aging phenomena.

Whither Theoretical Implications of Genetic-Epigenetic-Environment-Process Studies?

The notion of candidate genes and gene–gene interactions (epistasis) holding theoretical potential was rarely mentioned in the early historical-theoretical context of psychological aging. Moreover, the notion of polygenic and gene–environment interactions (e.g., Deary et al., 2004) and epigenetic factors (e.g., Liu et al., 2009) potentially offering theoretically important contributions in psychological aging have only recently emerged. In fact, the theoretical legacy of the "neurogenetics" of psychological aging is unknown. However, the field has (a) grown rapidly in empirical technologies, bases, and accumulated observations; (b) begun to cross the threshold of collecting disconnected (and small-effect) single associations to generating theoretical rationales and testing theoretical predictions concerning aging-related associations; and (c) been increasingly incorporated into epidemiological and longitudinal studies.

Conceivably, a conspicuous historical moment in the transition from the descriptive to more theoretical genetic–epigenetic research in psychological aging may have occurred in 2008. The National Institute on Aging workshop summary, Genetic Methods and Life Course Development, addressed numerous ways in which genetic and epigenetic variations (and their interactions) can be related to (and contribute to explanations of) a variety of phenotypic variations relevant to psychological aging. Included in the discussion were (a) prominent cognitive aging phenomena (e.g. executive functions, episodic memory, AD), (b) processes of psychosocial aging (e.g., mental health, depression, personality, emotion regulation), and (c) concepts of psychological adaptation (e.g., successful aging, positive aging). Important opportunities and challenges are noted, including methodological (e.g., small candidate gene effect sizes, complex traits are underpinned by multiple genes and epigenetic factors), theoretical (e.g., developing standard "arsenals" of candidate genes and epigenetic markers for given processes, recognizing that many aging-related phenotypes are conceptually complex, if not syndrome-like), and logistical (identifying and coordinating multidisciplinary teams, assembling large-scale longitudinal and epidemiological data) issues. At this juncture, a growing number of theoretically and methodologically sophisticated forays into these areas of psychological research have been offered (e.g., Deary et al., 2004; Green et al., 2008; Shanahan & Hofer, 2005; Zubenko et al., 2007). For example, McClearn (2006) argued that a "contextual genetics" approach is advisable because most theoretically interesting psychological phenotypes are complex, nonreducible, subject to time-related changes, and a function of a "pluralism" of causes, and are therefore "moving targets." A theoretically guided integrative approach is recommended in which longitudinal epidemiological research designs play a role similar to gene–gene interactions, gene–environment interactions, epigenetic factors, and even interactions with other biological and age-related factors. Obviously, these perspectives are consistent with the enduring theoretical themes identified in this chapter.

Toward Explanation in Psychological Aging: Do "Causes" Hunt in Packs? Do "Effects" Assemble in Patterns or Disperse and Flee?

Description and explanation are crucial aspects of theoretical research in any scientific endeavor (Salthouse, 2005, 2006). Although explanations can select and integrate information from multiple sources and multiple occasions, a cause per se can only be identified with experimental procedures. Experimental (and quasi-experimental) procedures have contributed abundantly to theoretical advances in the study of a wide array of psychological aging phenomena (e.g., Craik & Salthouse, 2007; Schaie, 1977). What is the status of theoretical explanation in a field that is increasingly understood to address some research questions in a manner related to the six theoretical themes? This is a viable concern as the research questions often involve multivariable complexity, dynamically interactional levels and processes, interdisciplinarity, multidirectionality, and long-term change and variability (e.g., Baltes et al., 2006a; Dixon et al., 2004; Hertzog, 2004; Nesselroade & Baltes, 1979; Schaie & Hofer, 2001). One concession is that the term "cause" (used in the section head) refers loosely to a collection of theoretical functions including precursors, risk or protection factors, predictors, leading indicators, or antecedents. Similarly, the term "effects" in the section head is used loosely to refer to theoretically important information concerning associated outcomes, subsequent trajectories, lagging indicators, or consequent conditions.

With the terminology clarified, what is the potential theoretical meaning of the expression in the section head: How is it that "causes hunt in packs" and "effects flee in patterns"? The first expression is adapted from the declaration of McClearn (2006, p. 315) and Roberts (1967) that "genes hunt in packs", by which it is meant that in the determination of complex phenotypes genes typically operate (hunt, predict, associate) in the interactive and temporal context of other genes. As we have seen, of theoretical importance in psychological aging is the distinct possibility that "causes" or precursors from multiple domains (e.g., genetic, environment, health burden, biological vitality, neurological integrity, social integration, institutional or historical characteristics) may be selectively but interactively contributing members of the "packs" that affect the aging of particular complex phenotypes. A challenging theoretical task is to determine (a) which domains may be involved in the aging of specific psychological processes; (b) which indicators of these domains should be assembled and tested for their potential contributing role; (c) how the indicators and domains may interact in their contributions at any static point in time; and (d) how the indictors and domains may operate as dynamic "packs" in "hunting" or contributing to the risk-protection profile that leads to a complex trait. The second expression is intended to underscore the theoretically important corollary notion that the complex phenotypes (the "effects") are also not always or necessarily static, trait-like, unidimensional, or non-interacting entities. Instead, they could be sets of subphenotypes, trajectories of change, status transitions, transitory states, syndromes or composites, or other patterned changes and outcomes.

Two cautionary summary observations are in order. First, the overall application to description and explanation in psychological aging would include the possibilities that (a) dynamic but multidomain packs of precursors may (b) hunt or contribute to risk-protection profiles, in (c) detectable schemes of interactions to (d) produce or lead to complex phenotypes that (e) may be outcomes, patterns, or trajectories that are (f) of theoretical interest in psychological aging. Second, such an approach implies the importance of time-structured epidemiologically related theories and methods that have been noted by featured and other reviewed theorists in psychological aging, as well as numerous other recent observers (e.g., Dixon, 2010; Goffaux et al., 2005; Hofer et al., 2003; McClearn, 2006). However, this does not imply that only these large-scale and complex research methods can lead to viable descriptions and explanations in psychology and aging. To the contrary, complementary experimental work identifying specific candidates and mechanisms of biological, environmental, sociocultural, institutional, genetic, or neurological systems of aging-related performance or change will continue to make theoretical and methodological contributions to this vibrant and booming field.

CONCLUSIONS

A review of featured and notable contributions to the study of theoretical issues in psychological aging has identified a set of core characteristics and enduring themes. These characteristics and their research implications may apply differentially across aging populations and psychological processes, but generally share multiple points of contact and complementarity. This *Handbook* series has served as a vital historical depository for progress in articulating theoretical perspectives in psychological aging. Accordingly, future reviews in forthcoming editions will clarify the continuing evolution of this singularly challenging aspect of the field.

ACKNOWLEDGMENTS

I appreciate research support from the National Institute on Aging (R37 AG008235-20) and from the Canada Research Chairs program. For their technical assistance I thank Jill Friesen and Bonnie Geall. I thank the editors for helpful reviews of an earlier version of this chapter.

REFERENCES

Anstey, K. (2008). Cognitive aging and functional biomarkers: What do we know, and where to from here? In S. M. Hofer & D. F. Alwin (Eds.), *The handbook of cognitive aging: Interdisciplinary perspectives* (pp. 327–339). Thousand Oaks, CA: Sage.

Anstey, K., Dear, K., Christensen, H., & Jorm, A. F. (2005). Biomarkers, health, lifestyle and demographic variables as correlates of reaction time performance in early, middle and late adulthood. *Quarterly Journal of Experimental Psychology, 58A*, 5–21.

Bäckman, L., Nyberg, L., Lindenberger, U., Li, S-C., & Farde, L. (2006). The correlative triad among aging, dopamine, and cognition: Current status and future prospects. *Neuroscience and Biobehavioral Reviews, 30*, 791–807.

Ball, K., Berch, D. B., Helmers, K. F., Jobe, J. B., Leveck, M. D., Marsiske, M., et al. (2002). Effects of cognitive training interventions with older adults: A randomized control trial. *Journal of the American Medical Association, 288*, 2271–2281.

Baltes, M. M. (1996). *The many faces of dependency in old age*. New York: Cambridge University Press.

Baltes, M. M., & Carstensen, L. L. (1999). Social-psychological theories and their applications to aging: From individual to collective. In V. L. Bengtson & K. W. Schaie (Eds.), *Handbook of theories of aging* (pp. 209–226). New York: Springer.

Baltes, P. B. (1968). Longitudinal and cross-sectional sequences in the study of age and generation effects. *Human Development, 11*, 145–171.

Baltes, P. B. (1987). Theoretical propositions of life-span developmental psychology: On the dynamics between growth and decline. *Developmental Psychology, 23*, 611–626.

Baltes, P. B., & Baltes, M. M. (Eds.), (1990). *Successful aging: Perspectives from the behavioral sciences*. New York: Cambridge University Press.

Baltes, P. B., Freund, A. M., & Li, S-C. (2005). The psychological science of human ageing. In M. L. Johnson (Ed.), *The Cambridge handbook of age and ageing* (pp. 47–71). Cambridge, UK: Cambridge University Press.

Baltes, P. B., & Lindenberger, U. (1997). Emergence of a powerful connection between sensory and cognitive functions across the adult life span: A new window at the study of cognitive aging? *Psychology and Aging, 12*, 12–21.

Baltes, P. B., Lindenberger, U., & Staudinger, U. M. (2006a). Life span theory in developmental psychology. In W. Damon & R. M. Lerner (Eds.), *Handbook of child psychology: Vol. 1. Theoretical models of human development* (6th ed.) (pp. 569–664). New York: Wiley.

Baltes, P. B., Reuter-Lorenz, P. A., & Rosler, F. (Eds.), (2006b). *Lifespan development and the brain: The perspective of biocultural co-constructivism*. Cambridge: Cambridge University Press.

Baltes, P. B., & Smith, J. (1997). A systemic-wholistic view of psychological functioning in very old age: Introduction to a collection of articles from the Berlin Aging Study. *Psychology and Aging, 12*, 395–409.

Baltes, P. B., & Willis, S. W. (1977). Toward psychological theories of aging and development. In J. E. Birren & K. W. Schaie (Eds.), *Handbook of the psychology of aging* (pp. 128–154). New York: Van Nostrand Reinhold.

Bengtson, V. L., Rice, C. J., & Johnson, M. L. (1999). Are theories of aging important? Models and explanations in gerontology at the turn of the century. In V. L. Bengtson & K. W. Schaie (Eds.), *Handbook of theories of aging* (pp. 3–20). New York: Springer.

Bengtson, V. L., & Schaie, K. W. (Eds.), (1999). *Handbook of theories of aging*. New York: Springer.

Birren, J. E. (1959). Principles of research on aging. In J. E. Birren (Ed.), *Handbook of aging and the individual: Psychological and biological aspects*. Chicago: University of Chicago Press.

Birren, J. E. (1999). Theories of aging: A personal perspective. In V. L. Bengtson & K. W. Schaie (Eds.), *Handbook of theories of aging*. New York: Springer.

Birren, J. E., & Birren, B. A. (1990). The concepts, models, and history of the psychology of aging. In J. E. Birren & K. W. Schaie (Eds.), *Handbook of the psychology of aging* (3rd ed.) (pp. 3–20). San Diego: Academic Press.

Birren, J. E., & Cunningham, W. R. (1985). Research on the psychology of aging: Principles, concepts, and theory. In J. E. Birren & K. W. Schaie (Eds.), *Handbook of the psychology of aging* (2nd ed.) (pp. 3–34). New York: Van Nostrand Reinhold.

Birren, J. E., Cunningham, W. R., & Yamamato, K. (1983). Psychology of adult development and aging. *Annual Review of Psychology, 34*, 543–575.

Birren, J. E., & Schaie, K. W. (Eds.), (1990). *Handbook of the psychology of aging* (3rd ed.). San Diego, CA: Academic Press.

Birren, J. E., & Schroots, J. J. F. (2001). The history of geropsychology. In J. E. Birren & K. W. Schaie (Eds.), *Handbook of the psychology of aging* (5th ed.) (pp. 3–28). San Diego, CA: Academic Press.

Blanchard-Fields, F. (2005). Introduction to the special section on emotion-cognition interactions and the aging mind. *Psychology and Aging, 20*, 539–541.

Cabeza, R., Anderson, N. D., Locantore, J. K., & McIntosh, A. R. (2002). Aging gracefully: Compensatory brain activity in high-performing older adults. *Neuroimage, 17*, 1394–1402.

Cabeza, R., Nyberg, L., & Park, D. C. (Eds.), (2004). *Cognitive neuroscience of aging: Linking cognitive and cerebral aging*. New York: Oxford University Press.

Cacioppo, J. T., Berntson, G. G., Bechara, A., Tranel, D., & Hawkley, L. C. Could an aging brain contribute to subjective well being? The value added by a social neuroscience perspective. In A. Tadorov, S. T. Fiske, & D. Prentice (Eds.), *Social neuroscience: Toward understanding the underpinnings of the social mind.* New York: Oxford University Press, in press.

Carstensen, L. L., Mikels, J. A., & Mather, M. (2006). Aging and the intersection of cognition, motivation, and emotion. In J. E. Birren & K. W. Schaie (Eds.), *Handbook of the psychology of aging* (6th ed.) (pp. 343–362). Burlington, MA: Elsevier Academic Press.

Cavanaugh, J. C. (1999). Theories of aging in the biological, behavioral, and social sciences. In J. C. Cavanaugh & S. K. Whitbourne (Eds.), *Gerontology* (pp. 1–32). New York: Oxford University Press.

Charles, S. T., & Carstensen, L. L. (2007). Emotion regulation and aging. In J. J. Gross (Ed.), *Handbook of emotion regulation*. New York: Guilford Press.

Craik, F. I. M., & Bialystok, E. (Eds.), (2006). *Life-span cognition: Mechanisms of change*. Oxford, UK: Oxford University Press.

Craik, F. I. M., & Byrd, M. (1982). Aging and cognitive deficits: The role of attentional resources. In F. I. M. Craik & S. Trehub (Eds.), *Aging and cognitive processes* (pp. 191–211). New York: Plenum Press.

Craik, F. I. M., & Salthouse, T. A. (Eds.), (2007). *Handbook of aging and cognition* (3rd ed). New York: Psychology Press.

Darowski, E. S., Helder, E., Zacks, R. T., Hasher, L., & Hambrick, D. Z. (2008). Age-related differences in cognition: The role of distraction control. *Neuropsychology, 22*, 638–644.

Deary, I. J., Wright, A. F., Harris, S. E., Whalley, L. J., & Starr, J. M. (2004). Searching for genetic influences on normal cognitive aging. *Trends in Cognitive Science, 8*, 178–184.

Dixon, R. A. (2000). Concepts and mechanisms of gains in cognitive aging. In D. Park & N. Schwarz (Eds.), *Cognitive aging: A primer* (pp. 23–41). Philadelphia, PA: Psychology Press.

Dixon, R. A. (2010). An epidemiological approach to cognitive health in aging. In L. Bäckman & L. Nyberg (Eds.), *Memory, aging, and the brain* (pp. 144–166). London, UK: Psychology Press.

Dixon, R. A., Bäckman, L., & Nilsson, L-G. (Eds.), (2004). *New frontiers in cognitive aging*. Oxford, UK: Oxford University Press.

Dixon, R. A., & Baltes, P. B. (1986). Toward life-span research on the functions and pragmatics of intelligence. In R. J. Sternberg & R. K. Wagner (Eds.), *Practical intelligence: Nature and origins of competence in the everyday world* (pp. 203–234). Cambridge, UK: Cambridge University Press.

Dixon, R. A., Garrett, D. D., & Bäckman, L. (2008). Principles of compensation in cognitive neuroscience and neurorehabilitation. In D. T. Stuss, G. Winocur, & I. H. Robertson (Eds.), *Cognitive neurorehabilitation* (2nd ed.) (pp. 22–38). Cambridge, UK: Cambridge University Press.

Dixon, R. A., & Hertzog, C. (1996). Theoretical issues in cognitive aging. In F. Blanchard-Fields & T. M. Hess (Eds.), *Perspectives on cognitive change in adulthood* (pp. 25–65). New York: McGraw-Hill.

Dixon, R. A., & Lerner, R. M. (1999). A history of systems in developmental psychology. In M. H. Bornstein & M. E. Lamb (Eds.), *Developmental Psychology: An advanced textbook* (4th ed.) (pp. 3–45). Mahwah, NJ: Erlbaum.

Dixon, R. A., Lerner, R. M., & Hultsch, D. F. (1991). The concept of development in the study of individual and social change. In P. van Geert, & L. Mos (Eds.), *Annals of theoretical psychology: Developmental psychology: Vol. 7* (pp. 279–323). New York: Plenum.

Dixon, R. A., & Nesselroade, J. R. (1983). Pluralism and correlational analysis in developmental psychology: Historical commonalities. In R . M. Lerner (Ed.), *Developmental psychology: Historical and philosophical perspectives* (pp. 113–145). Hillsdale, NJ: Erlbaum.

Dixon, R. A., & Nilsson, L-G. (2004). Don't fence us in: Probing the frontiers of cognitive aging. In R. A. Dixon, L. Bäckman, & L-G. Nilsson (Eds.), *New frontiers in cognitive aging* (pp. 3–15). Oxford, UK: Oxford University Press.

Einstein, G. O., & McDaniel, M. A. (2004). *Memory fitness: A guide for successful aging*. New Haven, CT: Yale University Press.

Ericsson, K. A., & Smith, J. (Eds.), (1991). *Toward a general theory of expertise: Prospects and limits*. Cambridge, UK: Cambridge University Press.

Ghisletta, P., Bickel, J-F., & Lövdén, M. (2006). Does activity engagement protect against cognitive decline in old age? Methodological and analytical considerations. *Journals of Gerontology: Psychological Sciences, 61B*, P253–P261.

Goffaux, J., Friesinger, G. C., Lambert, W., Shroyer, L. W., Moritz, T. E.,McCarthy, M., et al. (2005). Biological age — A concept whose time has come: A preliminary study. *Southern Medical Journal, 98*, 985–993.

Green, A. E., Munafo, M. R., DeYoung, C. G., Fossella, J. A., Fan, J., & Gray, J. R. (2008). Using genetic data in cognitive neuroscience: From growing pains to genuine insights. *Nature Reviews Neuroscience, 9*, 710–720.

Hanson, N. R. (1958). *Patterns of discovery: An inquiry into the conceptual foundations of science*. Cambridge, UK: Cambridge University Press.

Hedden, T., & Gabrieli, J. D. E. (2005). Healthy and pathological processes in adult development: New evidence from neuroimaging of the aging brain. *Current Opinion in Neurology, 18*, 740–747.

Hendricks, J., & Achenbaum, A. (1999). Historical development of theories of aging. In V. L. Bengtson & K. W. Schaie (Eds.), *Handbook of theories of aging* (pp. 21–39). New York: Springer Publishing Co.

Hertzog, C. (2004). Does longitudinal evidence confirm theories of cognitive aging derived from cross-sectional data? In R. A. Dixon, L. Bäckman, & L-G. Nilsson (Eds.), *New frontiers in cognitive aging* (pp. 41–64). Oxford, UK: Oxford University Press.

Hertzog, C. (2008). Theoretical approaches to the study of

cognitive aging: An individual-differences perspective. In S. M. Hofer & D. F. Alwin (Eds.), *The handbook of cognitive aging: interdisciplinary perspectives* (pp. 34–49). Thousand Oaks, CA: Sage.

Hofer, S. M., Berg, S., & Era, P. (2003). Evaluating the interdependence of aging-related changes in visual and auditory acuity, balance, and cognitive functioning. *Psychology and Aging, 18*, 285–305.

Hofer, S. M., & Sliwinski, M. J. (2006). Design and analysis of longitudinal studies on aging. In J. E. Birren & K. W. Schaie (Eds.), *Handbook of the psychology of aging* (6th ed.) (pp. 15–37). San Diego, CA: Elsevier.

Hultsch, D. F. (Ed.), (2004). *Special issue: Longitudinal Studies of Cognitive aging. Aging, Neuropsychology, and Cognition: 11* (2–3) 101–376.

Hultsch, D. F., & Dixon, R. A. (1990). Learning and memory in aging. In J. E. Birren & K. W. Schaie (Eds.), *Handbook of the psychology of aging* (3rd ed.) (pp. 258–274). San Diego, CA: Academic Press.

Jackson, S. H. D., Weale, M. R., & Weale, R. A. (2003). Biological age: What is it and can it be measured? *Archives of Gerontology and Geriatrics, 36*, 103–115.

Klemera, P., & Doubal, S. (2006). A new approach to the concept and computation of biological age. *Mechanisms of Ageing and Development, 127*, 240–248.

Knight, M., & Mather, M. (2006). The affective neuroscience of aging and its implications for cognition. In T. Canli (Ed.), *The biological bases of personality and individual differences* (pp. 159–183). New York: Guilford.

Kramer, A. F., Colcombe, S. J., McAuley, E., Scalf, P., & Erickson, K. I. (2005). Fitness, aging and neurocognitive functioning. *Neurobiology of Aging, 26*, 124–127.

Kuhn, T. S. (1962). *The structure of scientific revolutions*. Chicago, IL: University of Chicago Press.

Labouvie-Vief, G. (1980). Beyond formal operations: Uses and limits of pure logic in life span development. *Human Development, 23*, 141–161.

Li, S-C. (2002). Connecting the many levels and facets of cognitive aging. *Current Directions in Psychological Science, 11*, 38–43.

Li, S-C. (2003). Biocultural orchestration of developmental plasticity across levels: The interplay of biology and culture in shaping the mind and behavior across the lifespan. *Psychological Bulletin, 129*, 171–194.

Light, L. L. (1992). The organization of memory in old age. In F. I. M. Craik & T. A. Salthouse (Eds.), *The handbook of aging and cognition* (pp. 111–165). Hillsdale, NJ: Erlbaum.

Lindenberger, U., & Ghisletta, P. (2009). Cognitive and sensory declines in old age: Gauging the evidence for a common cause. *Psychology and Aging, 24*, 1–16.

Liu, L., van Groen, T., Kadish, I., & Tollefsbol, T. O. (2009). DNA methylation impacts on learning and memory in aging. *Neurobiology of Aging, 30*, 549–560.

Lövdén, M., Bäckman, L., Lindenberger, U., Schaefer, S., & Schmiedek, F. (2010). A theoretical framework for the study of adult cognitive plasticity. *Psychological Bulletin*, 136, 659–676.

Lustig, C., Hasher, L., & Zacks, R. T. (2007). Inhibitory deficit theory: recent developments in a "new view." In D. S. Gorfein & C. M. MacLeod (Eds.), *The place of inhibition in cognition* (pp. 145–162). Washington, DC: American Psychological Association.

McArdle, J. J., & Anderson, E. (1990). Latent variable growth curve models for research on aging. In J. E. Birren & K. W. Schaie (Eds.), *Handbook of the psychology of aging* (3rd ed.) (pp. 21–44). San Diego, CA: Academic Press.

McClearn, G. E. (2006). Contextual genetics. *Trends in Genetics, 22*, 314–319.

McCrae, R. R., & Costa, P. T. (1994). The stability of personality: Observation and evaluations. *Current Directions in Psychological Science, 3*, 173–175.

MacDonald, S. W. S., Dixon, R. A., Cohen, A-L., & Hazlitt, J. E. (2004). Biological age and 12-year cognitive change in older adults: Findings from the Victoria Longitudinal Study. *Gerontology, 50*, 64–81.

MacDonald, S. W. S., Hultsch, D. F., & Dixon, R. A. (2008). Predicting impending death: Neurocognitive inconsistency is a selective and early marker. *Psychology and Aging, 23*, 595–607.

McGue, M., & Johnson, W. (2008). Genetics of cognitive aging. In F. I. M. Craik & T. A. Salthouse (Eds.), *The handbook of aging and cognition* (3rd ed.) (pp. 55–96). New York: Psychology Press.

Nakamura, E., & Miyao, K. (2003). Further evaluation of the basic nature of the human biological aging process based on a factor analysis of age-related physiological variables. *Journals of Gerontology: Biological Sciences, 58A*, 196–204.

Nakamura, E., & Miyao, K. (2007). A method for identifying biomarkers of aging and constructing an index of biological age in humans. *Journals of Gerontology: Biological Sciences, 62A*, 1096–1105.

National Institute on Aging. (2008). Workshop Summary: Genetic methods and life course development. Washington, DC: National Institutes of Health.

Nesselroade, J. R., & Baltes, P. B. (Eds.), (1979). *Longitudinal research in the study of behavior and development*. New York: Academic Press.

Nyberg, L., Maitland, S. B., Rönnlund, M., Bäckman, L., Dixon, R. A., Wahlin, Å, et al. (2003). Selective adult age differences in an age-invariant multi-factor model of declarative memory. *Psychology and Aging, 18*, 149–160.

Overton, W. F., & Reese, H. W. (1973). Models of development: Methodological implications. In J. R. Nesselroade & H. W. Reese (Eds.), *Life-span developmental psychology: Methodological issues* (pp. 65–86). New York: Academic Press.

Park, D. C. (1992). Applied cognitive aging research. In F. I. M. Craik & T. A. Salthouse (Eds.), *The handbook of aging and cognition* (pp. 449–493). Hillsdale, NJ: Erlbaum.

Park, D. C., Nisbett, R. E., & Hedden, T. (1999). Aging, culture, and cognition. *Journals of Gerontology: Psychological Sciences, 54B*, 75–84.

Park, D. C., & Reuter-Lorenz, P. (2009). The adaptive brain: Aging and neurocognitive scaffolding. *Annual Review of Psychology, 60*, 173–196.

Pepper, S. C. (1970). *World hypotheses.* Berkeley, CA: University of California Press.

Persson, J., Nyberg, L., Lind, J., Larsson, A., Nilsson, L.-G., Ingvar, M., et al. (2006). Structure-function correlates of cognitive decline in aging. *Cerebral Cortex, 16*, 907–915.

Pushkar, D., Bukowski, W. M., Schwartzman, A. E., Stack, D. M., & White, D. R. (Eds.), (1998). *Improving competence across the lifespan*. New York: Plenum.

Rabbitt, P., Watson, P., Donlan, C., McInnes, L., Horan, M., Pendleton, N., et al. (2002). Effects of death within 11 years on cognitive performance in old age. *Psychology and Aging, 17*, 1–14.

Ram, N., & Nesselroade, J. R. (2007). Modeling intraindividual and intracontextual change: Rendering developmental context operational. In T. D. Little, J. A. Bouvaird, & N. A. Card (Eds.), *Modeling contextual effects in longitudinal studies* (pp. 325–342). Mahwah, NJ: Erlbaum.

Raz, N. (2004). The aging brain: Structural changes and their implications for cognitive aging. In R. A. Dixon, L. Bäckman, & L-G. Nilsson (Eds.), *New frontiers in cognitive aging* (pp. 115–133). Oxford, UK: Oxford University Press.

Raz, N. (2009). Decline and compensation in aging brain and cognition: Promises and constraints. *Neuropsychology Review, 19*, 411–415.

Raz, N., Lindenberger, U., Rodrigue, K. M., Kennedy, K. M., Head, D., et al. (2005). Regional brain changes in aging healthy adults: General trends, individual differences and modifiers. *Cerebral Cortex, 15*, 1676–1689.

Reese, H. W., & Overton, W. F. (1970). Models of development and theories of development. In L. R. Goulet & P. B. Baltes (Eds.), *Life span developmental psychology: Research and theory* (pp. 115–145). New York: Academic Press.

Reuter-Lorenz, P., & Cappell, K. (2008). Neurocognitive aging and the compensation hypothesis. *Current Directions in Psychological Science, 17*, 177–182.

Reuter-Lorenz, P. A., & Lustig, C. (2005). Brain aging: Reorganizing discoveries about the aging mind. *Current Opinion in Neurobiology, 15*, 245–251.

Roberts, B. W., Walton, K. E., & Viechtbauer, W. (2006). Personality traits change in adulthood: Reply to Costa and McCrae (2006). *Psychological Bulletin, 132*, 29–32.

Roberts, R. C. (1967). Some concepts and methods in quantitative genetics. In J. Hirsch (Ed.), *Behavior-genetic analysis.* New York: McGraw-Hill.

Salthouse, T. A. (1991). *Theoretical perspectives on cognitive aging.* Hillsdale, NJ: Erlbaum.

Salthouse, T. A. (1996). The processing-speed theory of adult age differences in cognition. *Psychological Review, 103*, 403–428.

Salthouse, T. A. (2005). From description to explanation in cognitive aging. In R. J. Sternberg, J. Davidson, & J. Pretz (Eds.), *Cognition and intelligence*. New York: Cambridge University Press.

Salthouse, T. A. (2006). Theoretical issues in the psychology of aging. In J. E. Birren & K. W. Schaie (Eds.), *Handbook of the psychology of aging* (6th ed.) (pp. 3–13). San Diego, CA: Elsevier.

Salthouse, T. A., Hambrick, D. Z., & McGuthry, K. E. (1998). Shared age-related influences on cognitive and noncognitive variables. *Psychology and Aging, 13*, 486–500.

Schaie, K. W. (1965). A general model for the study of developmental problems. *Psychological Bulletin, 64*, 92–107.

Schaie, K. W. (1977). Quasi-experimental designs in the psychology of aging. In J. E. Birren & K. W. Schaie (Eds.), *Handbook of the psychology of aging* (pp. 39–58). New York: Van Nostrand Reinhold.

Schaie, K. W. (1996). *Intellectual development in adulthood: The Seattle Longitudinal Study*. New York: Cambridge University Press.

Schaie, K. W. (2005). *Developmental influences on adult intelligence: The Seattle Longitudinal Study*. New York: Oxford University Press.

Schaie, K. W. (2011). Historical influences on aging and behavior. In K. W. Schaie & S. L. Willis (Eds.), *Handbook of the psychology of aging* (7th ed.). Oxford, UK: Elsevier.

Schaie, K. W., & Carstensen, L. L. (Eds.), (2006). *Social structures, aging, and self-regulation in the elderly*. New York: Springer Publishing Co.

Schaie, K. W., & Hofer, S. M. (2001). Longitudinal studies in aging research. In J. E. Birren & K. W. Schaie (Eds.), *Handbook of the psychology of aging* (5th ed.) (pp. 53–77). San Diego, CA: Academic Press.

Schroots, J. J. F., & Birren, J. E. (1990). Concepts of time and aging in science. In J. E. Birren & K. W. Schaie (Eds.), *Handbook of the psychology of aging* (3rd ed.) (pp. 45–64). San Diego, CA: Academic Press.

Shanahan, M. J., & Hofer, S. M. (2005). Social context in gene-environment interactions: Retrospect and prospect. *Journals of Gerontology: Series B, 60B*, 65–76.

Sliwinski, M. J, Stawski, R. S., Hall, C. B., Katz, M., Verghese, J., & Lipton, R. (2006). On the importance of distinguishing pre-terminal and terminal cognitive decline. *European Psychologist, 11*, 172–181.

Spiro, A., III, & Brady, C. B. (2008). Integrating health into cognitive aging research and theory: Quo vadis? In S. M. Hofer & D. F. Alwin (Eds.), *The handbook of cognitive aging: Interdisciplinary perspectives* (pp. 260–282). Thousand Oaks, CA: Sage.

Stern, P. C., & Carstensen, L. L. (Eds.), (2000). *The aging mind: Opportunities in cognitive research.* Washington, DC: National Academy Press.

Stern, Y. (Ed.), (2007). *Cognitive reserve: Theory and applications.* New York: Taylor & Francis.

St. Jacques, P., Dolcos, F., & Cabeza, R. (2010). Effects of aging on functional connectivity of the amygdale during negative evaluation: A network analysis of MRI data. *Neurobiology of Aging, 31*, 315–327.

Tadorov, A., Fiske, S. T., & Prentice, D. (Eds.). *Social neuroscience: Toward understanding the underpinnings of the social mind*. New York: Oxford University Press, in press.

Toulmin, S. (1972). *Human understanding: The collective use and evolution of concepts*. Princeton: Princeton University Press.

Vaillant, G. E. (2002). *Aging well*. Boston: Little Brown.

Wahlin, Å. (2004). Health, disease, and cognitive aging. In R. A. Dixon, L. Bäckman, & L-G. Nilsson (Eds.), *New frontiers in cognitive aging* (pp. 279–302). Oxford, UK: Oxford University Press.

Wahlin, Å., MacDonald, S. W. S., de Frias, C. M., Nilsson, G-G., & Dixon, R. A. (2006). How do health and biological age influence chronological age and sex differences in cognitive aging: Moderating, mediating, or both? *Psychology and Aging, 21*, 318–332.

Waldstein, S. R. (2000). Health effects on cognitive aging. In P. C. Stern & L. L. Carstensen (Eds.), *The aging mind: Opportunities in cognitive research*. Washington, DC: National Academy Press.

Whitbourne, S. K. (2001). *Psychology of adult development and aging: Biopsychosocial perspectives*. New York: Wiley.

Wright, C. I., Feczko, E., Dickerson, B., & Williams, D. (2007). Neuroanatomical correlates of personality in the elderly. *Neuroimage, 35*, 263–272.

Zacks, R. T., Hasher, L., & Li, K. Z. H. (2000). Human memory. In F. I. M. Craik & T. A. Salthouse (Eds.), *The handbook of aging and cognition* (2nd ed.) (pp. 293–358). Mahwah, NJ: Erlbaum.

Zubenko, G. S., Hughes, H. B., Zubenko, W. N., & Maher, B. S. (2007). Genome survey for loci that influence successful aging: Results at 10-cM resolution *American Journal of Geriatric. Psychiatry, 15*, 184–193.

Chapter | 2 |

Methodological and Analytical Issues in the Psychology of Aging

Emilio Ferrer[1], *Paolo Ghisletta*[2]

[1]Department of Psychology, University of California, Davis, USA; [2]Faculty of Psychology and Educational Sciences, University of Geneva, Switzerland and Distance Learning University, Sierre, Switzerland

CHAPTER CONTENTS

Introduction 25
Research Designs in Studies of Adulthood 25
Incomplete Data and Attrition in Aging Research 27
Methodological Approaches for Dealing with Incomplete Data 27
Planned Incomplete Data as a Design Feature 28
Summary on Incomplete Data 29
Methodological Issues Associated with Research in Aging 29
Measurement Invariance Over Time 29
Retest Effects 30
Alternative Definitions of Time 31
Statistical Models for Assessing Change in Aging Research 32
Statistical Models for Change Processes 32
Latent Growth Models 32
Multilevel Models 32
Multivariate Models for Change and Dynamics 32
Statistical Models for Intra-Individual Variability 33
Statistical Models for Survival and Long-Term Predictions in Aging Research 34
Summary of Data Analysis in Aging Research 34
Future Directions and Methodological Recommendations in Aging Research 34
Matching Model Parameters to Theoretical Aging Mechanisms 34
Identifying Time-Related Sequences and Discontinuities in Aging Processes 35
Concluding Remarks 35
Acknowledgments 35
References 36

INTRODUCTION

The goal of this chapter is to provide a review of some central methodological and analytical issues in current aging research. Instead of an exhaustive review covering every single topic, we offer a selection of issues that, in our opinion, play a fundamental role in the study of the psychology of aging. Some of these issues concern longitudinal designs and methodology, while others concern the description of various forms of incomplete data as well as techniques for dealing with such incompleteness. In addition, we review a number of analytical procedures that have the potential to capture the complex changes associated with aging. Besides reviewing the current status of methodology in aging research, it is our desire to describe recent challenges in this area, highlight some potential solutions, and raise new questions to stimulate further research.

RESEARCH DESIGNS IN STUDIES OF ADULTHOOD

There is a long history in the study of human development, especially in adulthood, advocating longitudinal designs (e.g., Nesselroade & Baltes, 1979). It is

DOI: 10.1016/B978-0-12-380882-0.00002-4

commonly agreed upon that investigating any changing phenomenon requires longitudinal data. This is also the case in aging research. Studying the various changes (i.e., growth and decline) associated with the multiple dimensions of aging necessitates longitudinal designs in which individuals are assessed repeatedly in time.

Longitudinal designs are preferred to cross-sectional designs, in which there is one measurement occasion only. The advantages of these designs include the possibility of directly estimating within-person change, differences in those changes across individuals, and associations between rates of change and other variables of interest (e.g., Schaie, 1983; Schaie & Hofer, 2001). In spite of these desirable benefits, however, longitudinal designs also give rise to a number of issues of a logistic, methodological, and practical nature. Important among those issues are attrition, cohort effects, and retest effects (Nesselroade & Baltes, 1979). We review each of these issues in this chapter.

An obvious obstacle to the implementation of longitudinal designs is cost. Assessing participants repeatedly will inevitably increase the time length of a study as well as its financial costs. This is arguably the major reason behind the still greater popularity of cross-sectional designs in the psychology of aging. Bleszner and Sanford (2010), in their editorial for the 65th anniversary of the *Journals of Gerontology: Psychological Sciences*, reviewed all 437 articles published in the journal between 2000 and 2008. Of these, 400 articles were empirical, 256 (64%) of which made use of cross-sectional methodology, whereas 138 (34.5%) articles used longitudinal designs. Almost 20 years earlier, Nelson and Dannefer (1992) reviewed 185 articles published in prominent journals about aging and development during the 1980s. The gerontological studies were 127, and of those only 10 used a longitudinal design. While the proportion of longitudinal studies in the aging literature increased strongly from a meager one tenth to a low one third, we are still far from the desirable methodological situation where most studies about change are longitudinal rather than cross-sectional.

Although the need to use longitudinal designs in aging research is unambiguous, longitudinal designs vary and the choice should be aligned with the research question. Probably the most common design consists of the collection of a battery of measures on a number of individuals at multiple occasions, typically over several years. In some cases, such longitudinal studies span for a large period of time. In other instances, because following a cohort of individuals over a long time is expensive and time-consuming, multiple cohorts of different ages are followed over time in what is called a cohort-sequential design (Bell, 1953, 1954; Schaie, 1996). From its inception, the goal of longitudinal designs has been to identify age-related changes at the person level and compare these changes across individuals (for examples of such designs see the extensive review by Schaie & Hofer, 2001). Efforts now exist to integrate multiple studies into a comprehensive assembly of data used to address pertinent questions with greater accuracy and precision. An example of these efforts includes the Integrative Analysis of Longitudinal Studies of Aging (Hofer & Piccinin, 2009). Our knowledge of human development, especially during adulthood, has greatly benefited from these designs. Many of the most relevant findings from this research have been replicated across multiple studies and now constitute part of the empirical evidence of theories of cognitive aging.

In addition to the standard longitudinal design, other types of plans for collection of repeated data are possible. For example, Nesselroade (1991) proposed the measurement-burst design, in which individuals are repeatedly assessed over time, and at each occasion data are collected with a more rapid frequency than the intervals of the overall study. For instance, consider a study spanning over three years with one assessment per year. At each assessment, participants complete a battery of measures intended to capture systematic long-term changes over time such as intra-individual change over the years. In addition, at each data collection period, individuals participate in repeated assessments over multiple occasions, typically multiple consecutive days, to assess short-term, reversible variations such as intra-individual variability (IV). An empirical example is provided by Sliwinski et al. (2009).

Short-term fluctuations are indeed valuable indicators of aging, as they represent measures of variability (Nesselroade, 1991). In many instances, such measures can be highly informative, perhaps even more so than measures of central tendency. For example, individuals show differences in variability in many attributes, and the degree of that variability can be a reliable trait of the individual (Fiske & Rice, 1955; Nesselroade, 1991). Consider changeable attributes such as mood or anxiety. Aspects of such changeable factors may differ across individuals in a reliable way that allows predicting other inter-individual differences. One prominent example here includes variability in perceived control as predictive of mortality (Eizenman et al., 1997).

Designs aimed at capturing short-term variability and fluctuations often involve daily diaries. In some instances, participants are asked to complete measures, tasks, and so forth, several times a day. Some modern applications of this design involve technology such as beepers and cell phones, which prompts participants at random times throughout the day. Other applications involve ambulatory devices (e.g., blood pressure) that allow researchers to collect data continuously while the participants go on with their lives.

The study of IV has recently gained popularity in cognitive aging (for a recent review see Hultsch et al.,

2008). Indeed, empirical evidence points to differences in IV between young and old individuals, groups with normative versus altered neurological status, healthy individuals and head injury patients, demented and healthy older adults and others. Many studies on IV in cognition are relatively simple and administer simple cognitive tasks (e.g., simple or choice reaction time tasks) repeatedly, up to over 100 times. Given the simplicity and brevity of such tasks, the repeated administration lasts only a few minutes and usually does not imply fatigue or reduction in participants' motivation. Intra-individual variability in cognition also seems related to brain-based measurements.

Studying intra-individual change and variability usually requires a heavier methodology for data collection. An example is the COGITO study, where over 100 individuals are measured over 100 days on a relatively large cognitive battery (Brose et al., in press). Such a study, although allowing for stronger substantive conclusions, must be very carefully planned to avoid typical drawbacks of longitudinal studies — such as strategy acquisition by participants to ameliorate their performance, their decrease in motivation, and attrition — a topic to which we turn next.

INCOMPLETE DATA AND ATTRITION IN AGING RESEARCH

One of the most ubiquitous problems in longitudinal studies of aging is incomplete data. Arguably, the first step in a typical study at which incomplete data are encountered is during the initial sampling and the process of contacting participants. Nonresponse and refusal by individuals are important forms of missing data often overlooked. Indeed, the ability of the initial sample to represent the underlying population can be strongly hindered by this first form of selectivity. Once participants become involved in the study, there are multiple factors that lead to missing data. Many times, participants in longitudinal studies chose not to complete questions in a questionnaire or perform specific tasks in an experiment. In addition, they often decide to discontinue participation altogether. Such dropout from the study can be due to a variety of factors including fatigue, relocation, dislike of the measurement protocols, forgetting to attend the assessment, or, particularly important in studies of older adults, deteriorating health and subsequent death. Dropout is likely to be selective because individuals who decide to continue in a study are typically healthier, more motivated, and more highly functioning than those who discontinue their participation.

Whatever the reason, dropout implies a loss of data with a potential loss of statistical power. Even more important, dropout can lead to a resulting sample that is no longer representative of the intended population and to subsequent bias of the parameter estimates. This is particularly the case when data are lost in a nonrandom fashion. In some instances, the missing data are not related to the study and can be ignored. In other cases, the incomplete data are related to outcomes of the study but the reasons for missing data are related to the measured variables and, thus, can be accounted for in the analyses. In other, yet more problematic cases, the missing data are related to outcomes of the study and at the same time there is a lack of information which could help account for the incompleteness. Following the work of Rubin and colleagues (Little & Rubin, 1987; Rubin, 1987), these conditions were typically labeled *missing completely at random* (MCAR), *missing at random* (MAR), and *not missing at random* or *nonignorable* (NMAR), respectively (e.g., Graham, 2009; Schafer & Graham, 2002).

Methodological Approaches for Dealing with Incomplete Data

There are multiple approaches available to deal with incomplete data ranging from simple techniques to more sophisticated methods. For a long time, the most common solution to any type of missing data was to ignore the problem; that is, the researcher would delete the cases with any incomplete data (i.e., case wise or pair wise) and would analyze the complete cases only. This approach is simple and easy to implement but it could lead to (a) the loss of potentially large amounts of data, especially when using multivariate analysis; (b) decrease in precision, via increased standard errors; and (c) parameter bias, if they are not missing completely at random (Allison, 2002).

Recognizing the potential limitations of analyses based on incomplete data motivated statisticians and methodologists to develop methods for dealing with such data in a more satisfactory way. Some of these techniques include the use of sample weights to adjust for any known sample biases. Other approaches rely on sample information to adjust for missing data with the goal of increasing the number of cases to be included in the analysis.

In the last two decades, a number of statistical techniques have been developed for dealing with incomplete data directly (e.g., Little & Rubin, 1987). The goal of these methods is to obtain unbiased parameter estimates even if some of the data are missing. Two major approaches include likelihood-based estimations of a structural model about the data and imputation of missing data. The major difference between these approaches is that the former assumes a structural model is known and correctly specified. This approach neither reduces the analyses to participants with complete data only nor replaces missing data. The latter approach, alternatively, is not preoccupied with a model to explain the structure of the data. Rather, it replaces any missing datum with educated guesses as to what the missing piece of information should have been had it been measured.

An essential aspect for applying likelihood-based estimation methods to make valid inferences concerns the relationship between the reasons for dropout (or missing data) and the outcomes of the study. When the dropout mechanisms are known, measured, and included in the analyses, estimates from likelihood-based methods are unbiased (Little & Rubin, 1987). The idea under this approach is to obtain estimates as if everybody had been measured on all variables at all time points. This technique can also be implemented using structural equation modeling with multiple groups in which the groups of participants follow different yet complementary patterns of incompleteness, such that all the data are fully covered across all groups (Ghisletta & McArdle, 2001; McArdle, 1994; McArdle & Hamagami, 2001).

One important starting point in this type of analysis is to describe the different patterns of missing data as accurately as possible. Such a task can be accomplished, for example, by defining groups of cases as a function of the available data in each group. The idea behind these analyses is to identify differences between those individuals with all the available data and those individuals with data missing. Detecting and understanding such differences between the groups can help determine whether the missing data are related to important variables in the study.

Likelihood-based methods specify an initial model for all cases in the data, irrespective of the incomplete information. Then, the same structural model is fitted to each group representative of the various patterns of missingness. Such specification assumes metric invariance across the groups, but this assumption is rarely tested. Under such assumptions, the model parameters are computed using all the available data. This approach is appropriate when the data are MAR (Rubin, 1987; Schafer, 1997). Under reasonable MAR assumptions, SEM with multiple groups are sometimes used as ways to deal with missing data, including the design of studies with planned incomplete data. To increase the probability that the MAR assumption is acceptable, the structural model can be augmented to include so-called auxiliary variables, which are correlated with the reasons for missingness but are not important elements of the phenomenon under investigation (Graham, 2003). The impetus of this procedure is not to obtain estimates of new parameters, but to ameliorate the estimation quality of all previously existing parameters.

The likelihood-based approach is now the default estimation method in several structural equation modeling programs. The researcher, however, still has duties of utmost importance: discussing and trying to assess the feasibility of the MCAR or MAR assumptions, specifying an adequate structural model, and planning ahead to be able to include appropriate auxiliary variables. Other analytic approaches that consider incomplete data are based on raw data. These approaches calculate the parameters from the model likelihood for each individual in the sample, and then compute the individual misfit from the data likelihood for each individual separately. Most modern computer programs implement this estimation method by default, either as a maximum likelihood or full-information maximum likelihood. Under conditions of MCAR or MAR, the Expectation-Maximization (EM) algorithm, part of these estimation methods, produces consistent and efficient parameter estimates (Little & Rubin, 1987).

The second approach to missing data is imputation, which has undergone several refinements in the last two decades. At first, any missing datum was simply replaced by a single pretender, and most often this was the mean on that same variable across the participants who had been assessed. Then more sophisticated single-imputation methods were developed (e.g., regression-based). In recent years, statisticians and methodologists concentrated on multiple imputation (MI; Schafer, 1999a), by which each missing datum is replaced not by a unique value, but by few (typically at least 5) possible values. This technique consists of replacing each missing or deficient value with a number of reasonable estimates (usually at least 5 or 10), representing a distribution of possibilities (Rubin, 1987). The sets of new values create a number of datasets, from which multiple estimates can be generated for each parameter by repeating the same statistical procedure. Appropriate summaries of these estimates are then created for each parameter, considering the uncertainty about the missing mechanism within and across datasets, leading to unbiased parameter estimates and reasonable standard errors.

MI typically consists of two steps. In the first step, the EM algorithm is used to impute missing information in the dataset and estimate model parameters using the log-likelihood of the new dataset. This iterative procedure converges when the elements of the covariance matrix do not change across iterations. In the second step, Data Augmentation, data are generated through an iterative Markov chain. Convergence is achieved when parameters become independent across iterations. MI can easily be implemented using specialized software (NORM; Schafer, 1999b) or via functions in more general programs (PROC MI in SAS, MICE in R, AMELIA).

Planned Incomplete Data as a Design Feature

Incomplete data are not necessarily a problem. In many studies, assessments include a very extensive battery of measurements, and having participants complete all the measures is unreasonable due to fatigue, time availability, and so on. In these cases, researchers could randomly assign variables to participants such that no single participant needs to be assessed on all variables, but overall assessments exist on each variable. For instance, rather than administering an 8-hour battery of cognitive tasks to all participants, only half the tasks are administered to each participant. As discussed in detail by McArdle (1994), care must be taken to exhaust all appropriate permutations and to implement them on any randomly chosen subsample. Because of the random assignment in this design, the resulting incomplete data are missing at random (by design; Graham et al., 2006; McArdle, 1994; McArdle & Hamagami, 1991). Any statistical technique for dealing with MAR data is applicable here. The incomplete data design not only applies to measures at a given assessment but to the number of occasions throughout the study, time interval between assessments, or any other feature of the design. Although more researchers are now considering this type of design, it is still underused in studies of aging. An interesting application of this design feature is for typical two-occasion designs in which the most appropriate time interval is unknown. Rather than arbitrarily choosing a time interval for all participants, a set of possible alternative intervals are selected, and each is applied to a distinct subsample of randomly chosen participants (McArdle & Woodcock, 1997).

Summary on Incomplete Data

Although all these recent methods for dealing with incomplete data produce parameter estimates that are consistent and efficient under MCAR and MAR conditions, when the data are NMAR (nonignorable), they can fail to generate unbiased and efficient parameter estimates. It is important to recognize that any given technique for incomplete data is based on a set of assumptions — models of behaviors — that may or may not be met in any specific dataset. One implication from this notion is that specific studies based on specific datasets may be needed to determine the utility of any given technique. It is sometimes a good idea to combine various techniques on the same dataset to examine the robustness and reliability of the results across the different methods.

METHODOLOGICAL ISSUES ASSOCIATED WITH RESEARCH IN AGING

Measurement Invariance Over Time

In addition to attrition, studies in aging research are associated with a number of methodological issues (for an extensive overview, see Hertzog & Nesselroade, 2003). Some of these issues are related to the measurement and psychometric properties of variables and their underlying constructs. This is sometimes overlooked, as oftentimes researchers focus their efforts on the analyses without questioning whether the variables are measured in a psychometrically sound manner. Here, researchers should pay attention to the various forms of validity, reliability, and dimensionality of variables and constructs (e.g., Little et al., 1999). In some instances, to guarantee a number of these properties techniques such as factor analyses, structural equation modeling with latent variables, or item response theory models may need to be used.

An important aspect related to ensuring the measurement of the proper construct is factorial invariance (Meredith, 1964, 1993). Measurement equivalence and construct invariance are essential in longitudinal studies examining changes across time as well as in comparisons across groups. In either situation, ensuring the same construct is measured across occasions (or across groups) is necessary to identify quantitative changes over time or differences across groups. The concept of factorial invariance is often used to investigate measurement invariance in reference to the common factor model (Bontempo & Hofer, 2007). Here, we focus on longitudinal invariance or measurement invariance across time. This type of invariance refers to the situation in which the numerical values across measurement occasions are obtained on the same measurement scale (Meredith, 1993). In this condition, each indicator with the same characteristics (i.e., identical scaling and wording) must relate to the underlying construct in the same fashion over time, thus ensuring an equal definition of a latent construct over time (Ferrer et al., 2008; Hancock et al., 2001; Sayer & Cumsille, 2001).

Based on the work by Meredith and colleagues (Meredith, 1993; Meredith & Horn, 2001), Widaman and Reise (1997) distinguished between configural and metric factorial invariance. Configural invariance indicates that the same observed variables of the latent construct are specified at each occasion, independent of the numerical values. Metric factorial invariance presupposes configural invariance and refers to the measurement structure. There are three levels of increasingly restrictive assumptions: weak, strong, and strict factorial invariance. In weak factorial invariance the factor loading of each indicator takes the same numerical value across measurement occasions. In strong factorial invariance, the previous restriction is increased by requiring the intercept for each indicator to be invariant across time. Finally, in strict factorial invariance, the unique variance for each manifest variable is fixed to be equal over time. Some researchers also use the term "partial invariance" to denote that some of the relevant parameters in the model are not invariant across occasions (e.g., some of the factor loadings do not present metric invariance). This type of invariance, however, is sometimes considered an insufficient compromise of proper measurement.

In addition to what is known about factorial invariance and group selection (Meredith, 1964, 1993), factorial invariance has important implications with regard to longitudinal studies. For example, longitudinal factorial invariance allows the possibility of assessing change over time at the level of the construct — or latent variable — rather than at the level of the observed variables. Quantifying change in this way, however, requires that the constructs are measured using various indicators (i.e., observed variables) at each occasion. When factorial invariance over time can be demonstrated in this fashion, the estimates from such a second-order model lead to the same expected trajectories than those from a first-order model (i.e., using composites). When such an assumption is not reasonable, however, the estimates can lead to very different estimated trajectories (Ferrer et al., 2008). Moreover, when factor loadings and intercepts fail to exhibit longitudinal invariance (i.e., they vary freely across occasions), one cannot ensure that the same construct is measured over time. In this situation, any observed changes across occasions are of a qualitative, rather than quantitative, nature. In other words, the changes represent shifts in the nature of the construct rather than quantitative growth in the construct.

Longitudinal factorial invariance is particularly important in those studies in which the scales for assessing constructs change across assessments. This is sometimes the case when researchers decide to add new variables or change scales during a study due to refinements in testing or changes in the meaning of a construct for the population under study. In all these cases, the researcher's goal remains to assess change over time, although the constructs are not measured with the same variables across occasions. In these situations, ensuring longitudinal factorial invariance becomes more complex. Linkage among the variables through some anchor indicator (i.e., a variable measured throughout the study or connects the different variables) is needed to ensure construct equivalence across time (see McArdle et al., 2009).

In empirical applications, however, it is often hard to obtain even weak factorial invariance. In such cases researchers may be discouraged in seeking invariance and choose to abandon the factor analysis model to define a given construct. They may instead calculate a simple composite score of less desirable psychometric properties and contaminate any subsequent analyses. This has partially motivated Nesselroade and colleagues to propose that invariance be sought for at the level of the inter-factor relationships via idiographic filters and not at the level of indicators (Nesselroade et al., 2007). Invariance at this level is tantamount to traditional invariance for the loadings of second-order factors derived from the initial inter-factor relationships. This approach to construct definition is particularly promising when several variables have been assessed on a large number of occasions across multiple individuals. It is then possible to apply an individually oriented approach to construct definition where the focus is not that the relationships between indicators and the constructs are invariant across individuals. Rather, invariance is sought on the relationships among the latent constructs across individuals.

Retest Effects

Longitudinal studies can be characterized as quasi-experimental designs (as in Campbell & Stanley, 1963) in which random assignment of subjects to age conditions is unfeasible (see Schaie, 1977). Instead, comparisons are made of individuals at different ages, as if randomly selected from the population of interest. A major threat to validity in such studies is represented by possible retest effects. In many situations, the repeated measurements are independent of the attribute to be measured. Consider, for example, physical growth. Individuals will grow irrespective of the number (or method) of assessments used to measure growth. In other situations, however, the repeated measurements may get in the way of the attribute itself. Now consider memory. At each assessment, participants in a longitudinal study complete a battery of measures related to memory. It is possible that completing the memory tasks at a given occasion may help the participants improve their performance at the next assessment. If so, the repeated testing interferes with the normal time course of the attribute under investigation. The extent of this contamination will be a function of a number of factors, including the nature of the attribute measured, the number of repeated assessments, and the retest interval between assessments (e.g., Cattell, 1957; McArdle & Woodcock, 1997). Note that when large batteries of similar tasks are administered, retest effects may also emerge in cross-sectional designs (e.g., working on a spatial orientation task may influence the performance on a subsequent similar, yet different, spatial orientation task). In this case, counterbalancing task administration order may neutralize retest effects.

The issue of retest effects has been well documented in psychological studies of aging, particularly in the area of cognitive abilities (e.g., Horn, 1972; McArdle & Woodcock, 1997; Schaie, 1996; Thorndike, 1933). A common finding in this area is that performance in a cognitive test improves over occasions with differences in magnitude of improvement across variables (e.g., Lowe & Rabbitt, 1998; Rabbitt et al., 2001; Wilson et al., 2002; cf. Schaie, 1988) and, across persons (Ferrer et al., 2004). In particular, both the means and the variances have been found to increase from the first to the second assessment (Jones, 1962; McArdle & Woodcock, 1997) and practice effects have been detected over multiple occasions, although decreasing in magnitude across occasions (Lövdén et al., 2004; Rabbitt et al., 2001).

When the research goal is examining the time course of attributes, the age-related changes, supposedly reflecting development or maturation, need to be separated from the changes due to retest, presumably reflecting practice and experience. Such separation can be carried out either methodologically or statistically. Using the former approach, so-called refreshment samples can be included in longitudinal studies. Such samples have the same characteristics and structure with respect to important variables (e.g., age, sex, socioeconomic status) than the initial sample did at study inception and are added to any subsequent occasion. By doing this, it is possible to compare samples with equal structure that differ only with respect to the number of previous test exposures. For instance, the original's sample second assessment can be compared with the initial performance of the first refreshment sample. If the two samples are indeed parallel with respect to important sampling characteristics, any potential difference in performance between them is to be attributed to retest effects in the original sample (cf. Schaie, 1989).

Typical longitudinal studies, however, do not include refreshment samples but simply assess the original sample repeatedly. Then, the only alternative to counteract retest effects is to estimate how their effects separately change (e.g., Ferrer et al., 2004; McArdle & Woodcock, 1997; Rabbitt et al., 2001). For example, Ferrer et al. (2004) examined the separate effects associated with age and retest on changes in memory, spatial reasoning, and processing speed through adulthood (40 to 70 years). All three cognitive abilities revealed declines associated with increased age and improvements related to each of the four measurement occasions. Although the age-related effects were similar across variables, the retest effects were largest for memory and smallest for speed. When the retest effects were not included in the statistical model, the age-related parameters were underestimated with more severe bias when retest effects were larger. Furthermore, for memory and space reasoning, both age and retest effects were similar across groups of different ages. For processing speed, however, pronounced age effects were found for older individuals (i.e., aged 60 years or more) and retest effects were evident for younger individuals with variability in such retest effects manifested at all ages.

It is important to recognize that retest effects can be confounded with other factors such as attrition and cohort effects (Schaie, 1988). For example, with both the methodological and the statistical approach, the existence of substantial cohort effects may jeopardize any estimation of retest effects. This occurs because both approaches assume that the samples compared differ only with respect to the number of previous test exposures and age (and eventually other demographic variables considered, such as sex). If cohort effects further differentiate the samples they will confound the estimation of retest effects.

Alternative Definitions of Time

Classical statistical models for dealing with repeated measures, such as repeated-measures analysis of variance, force a single definition of time. The phenomenon under investigation can only be described and analyzed as a function of occasions of measurement, and this may or may not fit the theoretical background. Hence change can only be described and analyzed as a function of occasions of measurement. Recent analytical methods, however, allow researchers to define with greater flexibility the time basis on which the phenomenon investigated unfolds. Change can thus be studied over different time bases, such as age, time elapsed since a particular event (e.g., marriage, loss of a spouse, preclinical dementia diagnosis), and as a function of different definitions of event time (Schaie, 2006). With recent analytical techniques the dimension across which the repeated measurements were collected need not be the same as that used to analyze the data (cf. Schaie, 2006).

Wohlwill (1970) urged researchers to consider explicit definitions of the variable age when describing any developmental phenomenon. The automatic equation behavior-as-a-function-of-age, unfortunately, remains prominent today in the psychology of aging. However, recent applications of advanced statistical models to repeated measures data have provided empirical evidence that other time bases may describe a change phenomenon more accurately. For example, Sliwinski et al. (2003) studied memory decline in initially nondemented older adults, one fourth of whom eventually developed preclinical dementia during the duration of their longitudinal study. For the preclinical subgroup, memory decline was not adequately described by their chronological age. Instead, numbers of years to the prediction of preclinical dementia accounted for virtually all individual differences in memory decline in that subgroup. The statistical comparison of the two time bases (chronological age vs. years to preclinical dementia diagnosis) was possible by applying a latent growth curve model (LGC; described under statistical model for assessing change in aging research). Wohlwill's (1970) suggestion that age ought to be treated as the dependent variable can be directly implemented via statistical techniques such as survival analysis (Schaie, 1989). The typical survival or event history paradigm, however, uses time rather than age as the dependent variable. Other techniques such as latent change models (described under statistical models for assessing change in aging research) may include changes in age as the dependent variable.

STATISTICAL MODELS FOR ASSESSING CHANGE IN AGING RESEARCH

Research in the psychology of aging encompasses a wide range of questions with varied designs, complex datasets, and unique goals. Discussing statistical models that could be applied to each of these questions and datasets would require scope and space beyond this chapter. Instead, we focus on statistical models that, in our view, can be helpful to elucidate change and dynamics related to aging. This choice is necessarily limited but was motivated by our desire to concentrate on models with potential for identifying the complex changes associated with aging.

Statistical Models for Change Processes

Latent Growth Models

Latent growth curve models are a standard method to analyze longitudinal data related to within-person changes (Bollen & Curran, 2006; Browne & DuToit, 1991; McArdle & Anderson, 2000; McArdle & Epstein, 1987; Meredith & Tisak, 1990), and have been used extensively in aging research (see Hertzog & Nesselroade, 2003).

A basic growth curve model for a variable Y measured over time ($t = 1$ to T) on the same individual ($i = 1$ to N) can be written as

$$Y_{i,t} = \gamma_{i,0} + A_t \cdot \gamma_{i,s} + e_{i,t}$$

where $Y_{i,t}$ is the observed score on person i at measurement t; $\gamma_{i,0}$ is the latent initial level score of person i; A_t is the group basis coefficients that represent the timing or shape of the growth (e.g., age); $\gamma_{i,s}$ is a latent score of person i, representing the slope, or the individual change over time; and $e_{i,t}$ is the latent error score of person i at measurement t. This model includes sources of individual differences in the level and slope, as

$$\gamma_{0i} = \mu_0 + e_{0i} \quad \text{and}$$

$$\gamma_{si} = \mu_s + e_{si},$$

where the level and slope scores have fixed group means (μ_0 and μ_s) and residuals (e_{i0} and e_{is}), and these residuals have variance components (σ_{02}, σ_{s2} and σ_{0s}; $u_i \sim N(0, G)$). Similarly, the error term associated with the within-person residual eit has also a zero mean and a variance term σe2 [ei ~ N(0, R)]. The basic model described here can take different specifications depending on the researcher's hypotheses. By setting the basis coefficients (At) to specific values one can test alternative hypotheses of growth. These can include specifications of no change, linear growth (or decline), and nonlinear change in the form of polynomials or latent basis.

Latent Growth Curve models can also be extended to include covariates, both time-invariant and time-varying covariates (e.g., McArdle & Epstein, 1987), as well as other slopes representing retest effects (Ferrer et al., 2004; McArdle & Woodcock, 1997; McArdle et al., 2002; Rabbitt et al., 2001). They can also be used to compare among multiple groups, both when such groups are observed or latent (as in mixture models), and include latent variables with multiple indicators as second-order factors (e.g., Ferrer et al., 2008; McArdle, 1988). There is vast literature on LGC models, their specification, multiple applications for examining change, and their limits (e.g., Bollen & Curran, 2006; Hertzog et al., 2006; McArdle, 2009; Singer & Willett, 2003).

Multilevel Models

Multilevel models (MLM) — also labeled hierarchical linear models or random-effect models — are a very popular technique for analyzing data that have a hierarchical structure (e.g., students nested within classrooms, repeated measures nested within individuals; Bryk & Raudenbush, 1987). Under certain assumptions, LGC and MLM are equivalent, but practical software implementation differences may exist (Ghisletta & Lindenberger, 2004). One advantage of MLM over LGC is that the specification of time basis is easier to implement. With current developments in software (e.g., M*plus*, Muthén & Muthén, 2007), however, such differences are alleviated.

MLM are particularly suited to the analyses of nonlinear change (McArdle et al., 2002). Their flexibility also makes them useful for detecting discontinuities in the data. Oftentimes, patterns of change are characterized by a function that takes on different values before and after a transition point (e.g., Cudeck & Klebe, 2002). For example, the age-related decline in a given cognitive ability may be linear before and after a given point (e.g., onset of a disease), but with a much steeper slope after the transition. Moreover, such transition points could be unknown and, thus a target of the model.

Multivariate Models for Change and Dynamics

Many questions in aging research concern potential interrelations between two or more processes through adulthood, as the processes unfold over time. Consider, for example, the relations among processing speed, working memory, and fluid reasoning throughout adulthood. Consider also the emotional exchanges between husbands and wives during old age as they help each other to cope with daily stressors. The goal in this research is to identify the interrelations among the processes over time. For this, methods are needed that can capture the dynamic interplay among the various within- or between-individual processes. One such approach includes the latent change score (LCS) models (McArdle & Nesselroade, 1994; McArdle, 2001; McArdle & Hamagami, 2001). There are several reviews of the many modeling possibilities using LCS models (Ferrer & McArdle, 2010; McArdle, 2009).

Consider two observed variables Y and X measured over time ($t = 1$ to T) on individuals ($i = 1$ to N). The trajectory equations for observed variables Y and X for person i at time t can be defined as a function of an initial latent score (y_0 and x_0) and a linear accumulation of latent changes (i.e., changes in the unobserved variables Δ_y and Δ_x) up to time t, plus residuals (e_y and e_x), as

$$Y_{i,t} = y_{i,0} + \left(\sum_{k=1}^{t} \Delta y k i\right) + e_{yi,t}, \quad \text{and}$$

$$X_{i,t} = x_{i,0} + \left(\sum_{k=1}^{t} \Delta x k i\right) + e_{xi,t}.$$

This trajectory equation defines the time course of the two variables from their initial conditions up to a given time point t. Included is a general expression of changes in the variables (Δ_y and Δ_x) that can be specified in different ways, depending on the hypothesis of change and dynamics. One possible specification is as following

$$\Delta y_{i,t} = \alpha_y \cdot y_{i,s} + \beta_y \cdot y_{i,t-1} + \gamma_y \cdot x_{i,t-1}, \quad \text{and}$$

$$\Delta x_{i,t} = \alpha_x \cdot x_{i,s} + \beta_x \cdot x_{i,t-1} + \gamma_x \cdot y_{i,t-1},$$

where α is the coefficient associated with additive scores at each occasion $y_{i,s}$ and $x_{i,s}$; β is a self-feedback parameter representing the influence of the same variable at the previous time $t-1$; and γ is a coupling coefficient, representing the influence of the other variable at the previous state $t-1$ on the change of the variable of focus. This last component represents forces from one variable at time $t-1$ that lead to changes in the other variable between the occasions $t-1$ and t, as the system unfolds over time. In aging research, LCS models have mainly been used to study the dynamics of cognitive functioning (e.g., Ghisletta & Lindenberger, 2003, 2005; McArdle et al., 2000).

Statistical Models for Intra-Individual Variability

As noted before, one area of study in aging research that is still underused, but is quickly gaining popularity, is IV. This is an important methodology for understanding individual processes and inter-individual differences in such processes. Individuals show differences in variability in many important characteristics, and the degree of that variability can be a reliable trait of the individual that can be stable and help predict other inter-individual differences (Fiske & Rice, 1955; Nesselroade, 1991). Many approaches have been developed to capture an individual's fluctuations over time (Cattell et al., 1947; Hultsch et al., 2008; Zevon & Tellegen, 1982). Such pursuits began with Cattell's P-technique (Cattell et al., 1947), a factor analysis of multivariate time series data consisting of multiple observed variables measured on a single individual across multiple time points. P-technique was originally developed to measure individual traits and has been used in aging research (see Jones & Nesselroade, 1990 for a review). This technique, however, is limited in that it does not specify lagged relations among the variables, thus not capturing any time-related dependencies among manifest or latent variables.

Dynamic factor analysis (DFA; see Browne & Nesselroade, 2005) is a generalization of the P-technique that incorporates lagged effects, thus, overcoming the limitations of P-technique. DFA is used to identify a lagged structure in covariance matrices, which presumably accounts for time-related dependencies among manifest and latent variables. DFA models were developed precisely to account for such dependencies, as they can be revealing of mechanisms associated with dynamic processes. In DFA models, the relations of factors and variables are defined across time intervals to describe time-related processes. This method can be useful when the researcher is interested in examining the fluctuations of a given attribute considering both the factorial structure of the observed variables (i.e., how are the observed variables related to the presumed factors) as well as the time organization of the latent factors (i.e., are the factors related over time).

DFA models have been specified and applied in different ways, depending primarily on the way lagged relations among manifest and latent variables are expressed (Molenaar, 1985; see Browne & Nesselroade, 2005; Ferrer & Zhang, 2009; Nesselroade et al., 2002; and Wood & Brown, 1994, for reviews). One specification suited to research in aging (e.g., burst measurement designs) is the so-called process factor analysis model formulated by Browne and colleagues (Browne & Nesselroade, 2005; Browne & Zhang, 2007). This particular formulation can be expressed as a function of two equations, one relating the manifest variables to the factors and another expressing the time-relations of the factors. The first equation is written as

$$\mathbf{y}_t = \Lambda \mathbf{f}_t + \mathbf{u}_t,$$

where, y_t is a matrix of manifest variables measured at time t, Λ is a matrix of factor loadings invariant over time, f_t is a vector of common factors at time t, and u_t is a vector of unique factors at time t assuming $u_t \sim (0, D_\varepsilon)$. The second equation of the model can be written as

$$f_t = \sum_{i=1}^{p} A_i f_{t-i} + \sum_{j=1}^{q} B_j z_{t-j} + z_t,$$

where A_i represents autoregressive weight matrices, B_j includes the moving average weight matrices, and $z_t \sim (0, \Psi)$ is a random shock vector. This DFA specification is a variable autoregressive moving average, or VARMA (p, q) model, where p stands for the number of autoregressive lags, and q represents the number of moving average terms in the model. When $q = 0$, this VARMA (p, q) model becomes a variable autoregressive, or VAR (p, 0) DFA model.

DFA models have not been used in aging research very often. Most psychological studies using DFA models have focused on mood and affect. Some examples include investigations of daily mood changes in dyads (Ferrer & Nesselroade, 2003) and pregnant women (Nesselroade et al., 2002), the mood structure among individuals with Parkinson's disease (Shifren et al., 1997), and the relations of cognitive performance to biomedical variables (Nesselroade & Molenaar, 1999).

Statistical Models for Survival and Long-Term Predictions in Aging Research

Survival analysis, also called event history or duration modeling, involves the modeling of time up to a certain event, given that the event has not yet occurred. In a sense, this technique augments the logistic regression model, typically used to predict dichotomous outcomes such as dead versus alive, ill versus healthy, and so on, by conditioning the event upon time. Typical applications in the psychology of aging are the prediction of the time of death or of age at disease onset (e.g., dementia, functional dependence). Although this set of techniques originated in disciplines such as demography, epidemiology, sociology, and economics, its use in psychological research has increased in recent decades. The empirical relevance of several psychological hypotheses, such as the terminal decline hypothesis (Kleemeier, 1962) predicting a sudden drop in cognitive functioning a few years prior to death, has been repeatedly assessed with this methodology (see Schaie, 1989 for an early application of survival analysis in aging research).

When the timing of an event is to be predicted not only by a single measurement but by change occurring throughout repeated measurements, typical applications did not use LGC or MLM to describe the change process. Instead, simple difference scores (e.g., $Y_{i,t} - Y_{i,t-1}$) were employed. Recent developments in statistics, paralleled by software applications, have allowed merging advanced statistical models about change with survival models. The so-called joint longitudinal + survival analysis predicts the timing of a given event based on individuals' latent level and slope scores, which theoretically are not contaminated by measurement error (Henderson et al., 2000). Although not yet very popular, this promising analytical model can be fairly easily implemented with existing software (Guo & Carlin, 2004; Muthén & Muthén, 2007; see Singer & Willett, 2003). A few applications in psychology of aging research exist (Ghisletta et al., 2006; McArdle et al., 2005). Recent developments of the joint + survival analysis also estimate the effects of multiple predictors simultaneously in a truly multivariate setup (Ghisletta, 2008).

Summary of Data Analysis in Aging Research

As we mentioned previously, many other statistical approaches exist to examine group differences and to model change. Because of space constraints and emphasis on change and dynamics, we selected a number of modeling techniques that we believe can more adequately investigate processes associated with aging. Readers whose research and data characteristics do not match those described in this chapter may want to focus their attention to other relevant techniques.

FUTURE DIRECTIONS AND METHODOLOGICAL RECOMMENDATIONS IN AGING RESEARCH

Matching Model Parameters to Theoretical Aging Mechanisms

A primary goal in aging research is to identify mechanisms underlying aging processes. This goal requires sophisticated methodology to collect data that can then be accurately described with statistical models whose parameters match theoretical mechanisms. A first step in this arduous task involves describing the processes under study. Once such processes are described in detail, one can proceed to testing theoretical hypotheses to understand the underlying mechanisms. One possible way to accomplish this undertaking is mapping the parameters of a given statistical model to a given theoretical process (e.g., cognition, emotion). In this chapter we have focused on methodologies and statistical models usually applied by researchers who collected behavioral data. A promising complimentary perspective entails investigating the neural changes involved during particular processes examined with behavioral data. Combining these two approaches will produce a more accurate and complete understanding of any aging process.

A fundamental choice in this plan is the selection of statistical models that most closely match the theoretical hypotheses of interest. For this, the researcher must first rely on a given theory of change and then express a model in which the parameters represent the desired hypothesis of change. Oftentimes, a number of models are fitted to data and one candidate is selected based on statistical fit. Frequently, however, such models lack a theoretical basis, which impedes the mapping of the model parameters onto theoretical mechanisms of change and, thus, generate new hypotheses. An example of an attempt to match model parameters to conceptual mechanisms is given by Kail and Ferrer (2007). Ram and Grimm (2007) also addressed this issue by describing how simple and complex LGC models can be used to articulate theories of change. In sum, we believe that a systematic examination of statistical models and their parameters in the light of the underlying theoretical paradigm should lead to a better understanding of aging processes.

Identifying Time-Related Sequences and Discontinuities in Aging Processes

Another chief goal in aging research is to identify time-related sequences among processes of interests. It is of crucial importance to determine which components of a complex process lead and which ones lag as they unfold over time. Although LCS models were described as potentially informative of such sequences, such information is not equivalent to causal inferences given that such models are typically applied to correlational data. To obtain stronger evidence in favor of causal mechanisms, researchers need to use experimental designs with randomized groups (Pearl, 2000; Shadish et al., 2008). Only with that methodology, will researchers be able to increase their confidence about the lack of previous systematic group differences and third variables.

Another important goal for future research is the identification of discontinuities in the aging processes (e.g., onset of disease, stability and sudden change in a process). For this, researchers will need to combine complex techniques, including nonlinear models, with designs that include intense measurements. With proper combinations of data and statistical techniques, researchers will be able to characterize discontinuities in a given process and identify the number and location of nonlinear features in the data as well as the transitions across discontinuities. Although some research exists along these lines (e.g., Cudeck & Klebe, 2002), more studies are needed to further our knowledge of how best to model such discontinuities, in particular regarding models that can account for effects that vary (i.e., dampening or amplifying) over time (Boker, 2001).

Finally, we advocate a more rigorous focus on the individual, with a stronger reliance on intra-individual change and variability studies. Molenaar and colleagues (e.g., Hamaker et al., 2005; Molenaar, 2004) demonstrated that the analysis of aggregate data cannot correctly characterize information about intra-individual change over time in disaggregated data. A pending question then is how to aggregate information across individuals that allows discussing inter-individual differences while preserving information about intra-individual change over time. This is an old question concerning the idiographic-nomothetic debate. However, it still remains an unsolved issue that deserves further research and can generate important information in aging research.

CONCLUDING REMARKS

Our goal in this chapter was to review some important methodological and analytical issues in current aging research. We selected those questions that, in our opinion, are essential to the quest of furthering our knowledge about aging processes and that can generate new research questions. We hope we were able to accomplish such goals and that the information in this chapter can help to raise new questions and stimulate further studies in aging research.

ACKNOWLEDGMENTS

This work was supported in part by grants from the National Science Foundation (BCS-05-27766 and BCS-08-27021) and NIH-NINDS (R01 NS057146-01) to Emilio Ferrer, and from the Swiss National Science Foundation (100014-107764 and 100014-120510) to Paolo Ghisletta.

REFERENCES

Allison, P. D. (2002). *Missing data*. Thousand Oaks, CA: Sage.

Bell, R. Q. (1953). Convergence: An accelerated longitudinal approach. *Child Development, 24*, 145–152.

Bell, R. Q. (1954). An experimental test of the accelerated longitudinal approach. *Child Development, 25*, 281–286.

Bleszner, R., & Sanford, N. (2010). Looking back and looking ahead as Journal of Gerontology: Psychological Sciences turns 65. *Journals of Gerontology: Psychological Sciences, 65B*, 3–4.

Boker, S. M. (2001). Differential structural equation modeling of intra-individual variability. In L. Collins & A. Sayer (Eds.), *New methods for the analysis of change* (pp. 3–28). Washington, DC: APA Press.

Bollen, K., & Curran, P. J. (2006). *Latent curve models: A structural equation perspective*. Hoboken, NJ: Wiley.

Bontempo, D., & Hofer, S. M. (2007). Assessing factorial invariance in cross-sectional and longitudinal studies. In A. D. Ong & M. v. Dulmen (Eds.), *Handbook of methods in positive psychology* (pp. 153–175). Oxford, UK: Oxford University Press.

Brose, A., Schmiedek, F., Lövdén, M., Molenaar, P. C. M., & Lindenberger, U. Adult age differences in covariation of motivation and working memory performance: Contrasting between-person and within-person findings. *Research in Human Development, 7*, 61–78.

Browne, M., & Du Toit, S. H. C. (1991). Models for learning data. In L. Collins & J. L. Horn (Eds.), *Best methods for the analysis of change* (pp. 47–68). Washington, DC: APA Press.

Browne, M. W., & Nesselroade, J. R. (2005). Representing psychological processes with dynamic factor models: Some promising uses and extensions of ARMA time series models. In A. Maydeu-Olivares & J. J. McArdle (Eds.), *Advances in psychometrics: A festschrift to Roderick P. McDonald* (pp. 415–451). Mahwah, NJ: Erlbaum.

Browne, M. W., & Zhang, G. (2007). Developments in the factor analysis of individual time series. In R. C. MacCallum & R. Cudeck (Eds.), *Factor analysis at 100: Historical developments and future directions*. Mahwah, NJ: Erlbaum.

Bryk, A. S., & Raudenbush, S. W. (1987). Application of hierarchical linear models to assessing change. *Psychological Bulletin, 101*, 147–158.

Campbell, D. T., & Stanley, J. C. (1963). Experimental and quasi-experimental designs for research on teaching. In N. L. Gage (Ed.), *Handbook of research on teaching* (pp. 171–246). Chicago, IL: Rand McNally.

Cattell, R. B. (1957). *Personality and motivation structure and measurement*. New York: World.

Cattell, R. B., Cattell, A. K. S., & Rhymer, R. M. (1947). P-technique demonstrated in determining psychophysical source traits in a normal individual. *Psychometrika, 12*, 267–288.

Cudeck, R., & Klebe, K. J. (2002). Multiphase mixed-effects models for repeated measures data. *Psychological Methods, 7*, 41–63.

Eizenman, D., Nesselroade, J., Featherman, D., & Rowe, J. (1997). Intraindividual variability in perceived control in an older sample: The MacArthur successful aging studies. *Psychology and Aging, 12*, 489–502.

Ferrer, E., Balluerka, N., & Widaman, K. F. (2008). Factorial invariance and the specification of second-order latent growth models. *Methodology, 4*, 22–36.

Ferrer, E., Hamagami, F., & McArdle, J. J. (2004). Modeling latent growth curves with incomplete data using different types of structural equation modeling and multilevel software. *Structural Equation Modeling, 11*, 452–483.

Ferrer, E., & McArdle, J. J. Longitudinal modeling of developmental changes in psychological research. *Current Directions in Psychological Science. 19*, 149–154.

Ferrer, E., & Nesselroade, J. R. (2003). Modeling affective processes in dyadic relations via dynamic factor analysis. *Emotion, 3*, 344–360.

Ferrer, E., Salthouse, T. A., Stewart, W. F., & Schwartz, B. S. (2004). Modeling age and retest processes in longitudinal studies of cognitive abilities. *Psychology and Aging, 19*, 243–259.

Ferrer, E., & Zhang, G. (2009). Time series models for examining psychological processes: Applications and new developments. In R. E. Millsap & A. Maydeu-Olivares (Eds.), *Handbook of quantitative methods in psychology* (pp. 637–657). London: Sage Publications.

Fiske, D. W., & Rice, L. (1955). Intra-individual response variability. *Psychological Bulletin, 57*(3), 217–250.

Ghisletta, P. (2008). Application of a joint multivariate longitudinal-survival analysis to examine the terminal decline hypothesis in the Swiss Interdisciplinary Longitudinal Study on the Oldest Old. *Journals of Gerontology: Psychological Sciences, 63B*, P185–P192.

Ghisletta, P., & Lindenberger, U. (2003). Age-based structural dynamics between perceptual speed and knowledge in the Berlin Aging Study: Direct evidence for ability dedifferentiation in old age. *Psychology and Aging, 18*, 696–713.

Ghisletta, P., & Lindenberger, U. (2004). Static and dynamic longitudinal structural analyses of cognitive changes in old age. *Gerontology, 50*, 12–16.

Ghisletta, P., & Lindenberger, U. (2005). Exploring structural dynamics within and between sensory and intellectual functioning in old and very old age: Longitudinal evidence from the Berlin Aging Study. *Intelligence, 33*, 555–587.

Ghisletta, P., & McArdle, J. J. (2001). Structural modeling of children's height. *Structural Equation Modeling, 10*, 19–39.

Ghisletta, P., McArdle, J. J., & Lindenberger, U. (2006). Longitudinal cognition-survival relations in old and very old age: 13-year data from the Berlin Aging Study. *European Psychologist, 11*, 204–223.

Graham, J. W. (2003). Adding missing-data-relevant variables to FIML-based structural equation models. *Structural Equation Modeling, 10*, 80–100.

Graham, J. W. (2009). Missing data analysis: Making it work in the real world. *Psychological Review, 60*, 549–576.

Graham, J. W., Taylor, B. J., Olchowski, A. E., & Cumsille, P. E. (2006). Planned missing data designs in psychological research. *Psychological Methods, 11*, 323–343.

Guo, X., & Carlin, B. P. (2004). Separate and joint modeling of longitudinal and event time data using standard computer packages. *The American Statistician, 58*, 16–24.

Hamaker, E. L., Dolan, C. V., & Molenaar, P. C. M. (2005). Statistical modeling of the individual: Rationale and application of multivariate stationary time series analysis. *Multivariate Behavioral Research, 40*, 207–233.

Hancock, G. R., Kuo, W., & Lawrence, F. R. (2001). An illustration of second-order latent growth models. *Structural Equation Modeling, 8*(3), 470–489.

Henderson, R., Diggle, P. J., & Dobson, A. (2000). Joint modeling of longitudinal measurements and event time data. *Biostatistics, 1*, 465–480.

Hertzog, C., Lindenberger, U., Ghisletta, P., & von Oertzen, T. (2006). On the power of multivariate latent growth curve models to detect correlated change. *Psychological Methods, 11*, 244–252.

Hertzog, C., & Nesselroade, J. R. (2003). Assessing psychological change in adulthood: An overview of methodological issues. *Psychology and Aging, 18*, 639–657.

Hofer, S. M., & Piccinin, A. M. (2009). Integrative data analysis through coordination of measurement and analysis protocol across independent longitudinal studies. *Psychological Methods, 14*, 150–164.

Horn, J. L. (1972). State, trait, and change dimensions of intelligence. *British Journal of Educational Psychology, 42*, 159–185.

Hultsch, D. F., Strauss, E., Hunter, M. A., & MacDonald, S. W. S. (2008). Intraindividual variability, cognition, and aging. In T. A. Salthouse & F. I. M. Craik (Eds.), *The handbook of aging and cognition* (3rd ed.), (pp. 491–556). New York, NY: Psychology Press.

Jones, M. (1962). Practice as a process of simplification. *Psychological Review, 69*, 274–294.

Jones, C. J., & Nesselroade, J. R. (1990). Multivariate replicated, single-subject, repeated measures designs and P-technique factor analysis: A review of intraindividual change studies. *Experimental Aging Research, 16*, 171–183.

Kail, R. V., & Ferrer, E. (2007). Processing speed in childhood and adolescence: Longitudinal models for examining developmental change. *Child Development, 78*, 1760–1770.

Kleemeier, R. W. (1962). Intellectual changes in the senium. *Proceedings of the American Statistical Association, 1*, 290–295.

Little, T. D., Lindenberger, U., & Nesselroade, J. R. (1999). On selecting indicators for multivariate measurement and modeling with latent variables: When "good" indicators are bad and "bad" indicators are good. *Psychological Methods, 4*, 192–211.

Little, R. T. A., & Rubin, D. B. (1987). *Statistical analysis with missing data.* New York: Wiley.

Lövdén, M., Ghisletta, P., & Lindenberger, U. (2004). Cognition in the Berlin Aging Study (BASE): The first ten years. *Aging, Neuropsychology, and Cognition, 11*, 104–133.

Lowe, C., & Rabbitt, P. M. A. (1998). Test/re-test reliability of the CANTAB and ISPOCD neuropsychological batteries: Theoretical and practical issues. *Neuropsychologia, 36*, 1–8.

McArdle, J. J. (1988). Dynamic but structural equation modeling of repeated measures data. In J. R. Nesselroade & R. B. Cattell (Eds.), *The handbook of multivariate experimental psychology: Vol. 2* (pp. 561–614). New York: Plenum Press.

McArdle, J. J. (1994). Structural factor analysis experiments with incomplete data. *Multivariate Behavioral Research, 29*, 409–454.

McArdle, J. J. (2001). A latent difference score approach to longitudinal dynamic structural analysis. In R. Cudeck, S. du Toit, & D. Sörbom (Eds.), *Structural equation modeling: present and future. A Festschrift in honor of Karl Jöreskog* (pp. 341–380). Lincolnwood, IL: Scientific Software International.

McArdle, J. J. (2009). Latent variable modeling of differences in changes with longitudinal data. *Annual Review of Psychology, 60*, 577–605.

McArdle, J. J., & Epstein, D. B. (1987). Latent growth curves within developmental structural equation models. *Child Development, 58*, 110–133.

McArdle, J. J., Ferrer-Caja, E., Hamagami, F., & Woodcock, R. W. (2002). Comparative longitudinal structural analyses of the growth and decline of multiple intellectual abilities over the life-span. *Developmental Psychology, 38*, 115–142.

McArdle, J. J., Grimm, K. J., Hamagami, F., Bowles, R. P., & Meredith, W. (2009). Modeling lifespan growth curves of cognition using longitudinal data with multiple samples and changing scales of measurement. *Psychological Methods, 14*, 126–149.

McArdle, J. J., & Hamagami, E. (1991). Modeling incomplete longitudinal and cross-sectional data using latent growth structural models. In L. M. Collins & J. L. Horn (Eds.), *Best methods for the analysis of change: Recent advances, unanswered questions, future directions* (pp. 276–304). Washington, DC: American Psychological Association.

McArdle, J. J., & Hamagami, F. (2001). Linear dynamic analyses of incomplete longitudinal data. In L. Collins & A. Sayer (Eds.), *New methods for the analysis of change* (pp. 137–176). Washington, DC: APA Press.

McArdle, J. J., Hamagami, F., Meredith, W., & Bradway, K. P. (2000). Modeling the dynamic hypotheses of *Gf-Gc* theory using longitudinal life-span data. *Learning and Individual Differences, 12*, 53–79.

McArdle, J. J., & Nesselroade, J. R. (1994). Structuring data to study development and change. In S. H. Cohen & H. W. Reese (Eds.), *Life-span developmental psychology: Methodological innovations* (pp. 223–267). Hillsdale, NJ: Erlbaum.

McArdle, J. J., Small, B. J., Bäckman, L., & Fratiglioni, L. (2005). Longitudinal models of growth and survival applied to the early detection of Alzheimer's Disease. *Journal of Geriatric Psychiatry and Neurology, 18*, 234–241.

McArdle, J. J., & Woodcock, R. W. (1997). Expanding test-retest design to include developmental time-lag components. *Psychological Methods, 2*, 403–435.

Meredith, W. M. (1964). Notes on factorial invariance. *Psychometrika, 29*, 177–185.

Meredith, W. M. (1993). Measurement invariance, factor analysis, and factorial invariance. *Psychometrika, 58*, 525–543.

Meredith, W., & Horn, J. (2001). The role of factorial invariance in modeling growth and change. In L. M. Collins & A. G. Sayer (Eds.), *New methods for the analysis of change* (pp. 203–240). Washington, DC: American Psychological Association.

Meredith, W., & Tisak, J. (1990). Latent curve analysis. *Psychometrika, 55*, 107–122.

Molenaar, P. C. M. (1985). A dynamic factor model for the analysis of multivariate time series. *Psychometrika, 50*, 181–202.

Molenaar, P. C. M. (2004). A manifesto on psychology as idiographic science: Bringing the person back into scientific psychology — this time forever. *Measurement, 2*, 201–218.

Muthén, L. K., & Muthén, B. O. (2007). *Mplus user's guide* (5th ed.). Los Angeles, CA: Muthén & Muthén.

Nelson, E. A., & Dannefer, D. (1992). Age heterogeneity: Fact or fiction? The fate of diversity in gerontological research. *The Gerontologist, 32*, 17–23.

Nesselroade, J. R. (1991). The warp and woof of the developmental fabric. In R. M. Downs, L. S. Liben, & D. S. Palermo (Eds.), *Visions of aesthetics, the environment, & development: The legacy of Joachim F. Wohlwill* (pp. 213–240). Hillsdale, NJ: Lawrence Erlbaum Associates, Inc..

Nesselroade, J. R., & Baltes, P. B. (1979). *Longitudinal research in the study of behavior and development*. New York: Academic Press.

Nesselroade, J. R., Gerstorf, D., Hardy, S., & Ram, N. (2007). Idiographic filters for psychological constructs. *Measurement, 5*, 217–235.

Nesselroade, J. R., McArdle, J. J., Aggen, S. H., & Meyers, J. M. (2002). Alternative dynamic factor models for multivariate time-series analyses. In D. M. Moscowitz & S. L. Hershberger (Eds.), *Modeling intraindividual variability with repeated measures data: Advances and techniques* (pp. 235–265). Mahwah, NJ: Erlbaum.

Nesselroade, J. R., & Molenaar, P. C. M. (1999). Pooling lagged covariance structures based on short, multivariate time-series for dynamic factor analysis. In R. H. Hoyle (Ed.), *Statistical strategies for small sample research* (pp. 224–251). Newbury Park, CA: Sage.

Pearl, J. (2000). *Causality: Models, reasoning, and inference*. Cambridge: Cambridge University Press.

Rabbitt, P., Diggle, P., Smith, D., Holland, F., & McInnes, L. (2001). Identifying and separating the effects of practice and of cognitive ageing during a large longitudinal study of elderly community residents. *Neuropsychologia, 39*, 532–543.

Ram, N., & Grimm, K. J. (2007). Using simple and complex growth models to articulate developmental change: Matching method to theory. *International Journal of Behavioral Development, 31*, 303–316.

Rubin, D. B. (1987). *Multiple imputation for nonresponse in surveys*. New York: Wiley.

Sayer, A. G., & Cumsille, P. E. (2001). Second-order latent growth models. In L. M. Collins & A. G. Sayer (Eds.), *New methods for the analysis of change* (pp. 179–200). Washington, DC: American Psychological Association.

Schafer, J. L. (1997). *Analysis of incomplete multivariate data*. London: Chapman & Hall.

Schafer, J. L. (1999a). Multiple imputation: A primer. *Statistical Methods in Medical Research, 8*, 3–15.

Schafer, J. L. (1999b). *NORM: Multiple imputation of incomplete multivariate data under a normal model* [Computer Software]. University Park: Pennsylvania State University. Department of Statistics.

Schafer, J. L., & Graham, J. W. (2002). Missing data: Our view of the state of the art. *Psychological Methods, 7*, 147–177.

Schaie, K. W. (1977). Quasi-experimental designs in the psychology of aging. In J. E. Birren & K. W. Schaie (Eds.), *Handbook of the psychology of aging* (pp. 39–58). New York: Van Nostrand Reinhold.

Schaie, K. W. (1983). The Seattle Longitudinal Study: A 21-year exploration of psychometric intelligence in adulthood. In K. W. Schaie (Ed.), *Longitudinal studies of adult psychological development* (pp. 64–135). New York: Guilford Press.

Schaie, K. W. (1988). Internal validity threats in studies of adult cognitive development. In M. L. Howe & C. J. Brainard (Eds.), *Cognitive development in adulthood: Progress in cognitive development research* (pp. 241–272). New York: Springer-Verlag.

Schaie, K. W. (1989). The hazards of cognitive aging. *The Gerontologist, 29*, 484–493.

Schaie, K. W. (1996). *Intellectual development in adulthood: The Seattle Longitudinal Study*. Cambridge: Cambridge University Press.

Schaie, K. W. (2006). The concept of event time in the study of aging. In J. Baars & H. Visser (Eds.), *Concepts of time and aging* (pp. 121–135). Amityville, NY: Baywood Publishing Co.

Schaie, K. W., & Hofer, S. M. (2001). Longitudinal studies in aging research. In J. E. Birren & K. W. Schaie (Eds.), *Handbook of the psychology of aging* (5th ed.) (pp. 53–77). San Diego, CA: Academic Press.

Shadish, W. R., Clark, M. H., & Steiner, P. M. (2008). Can nonrandomized experiments yield accurate answers? A randomized experiment comparing random to nonrandom assignment. *Journal of the American Statistical Association, 103*, 1334–1343.

Shifren, K., Hooker, K., Wood, P., & Nesselroade, J. R. (1997). Structure and variation of mood in individuals with Parkinson's disease: A dynamic factor analysis. *Psychology and Aging, 12*, 328–339.

Singer, J. D., & Willett, J. B. (2003). *Applied longitudinal data analysis.* New York, NY: Oxford University Press.

Sliwinski, M. J., Almeida, D. M., Smyth, J., & Stawski, R. S. (2009). Intraindividual change and variability in daily stress processes: Findings from two measurement-burst diary studies. *Psychology and Aging, 24*, 828–840.

Sliwinski, M. J., Hofer, S. M., Hall, C., Buschke, H., & Lipton, R. B. (2003). Modeling memory decline in older adults: The importance of preclinical dementia, attrition, and chronological age. *Psychology and Aging, 18*, 658–671.

Thorndike, R. L. (1933). The effect of the interval between test and retest on the constancy of the IQ. *Journal of Educational Psychology, 24*, 543–549.

Widaman, K . F., & Reise, S. P. (1997). Exploring the measurement invariance of psychological instruments: Applications in the substance use domain. In K. J. Bryant, M. Windle, & S. G. West (Eds.), *The science of prevention: Methodological advances from alcohol and substance abuse research* (pp. 281–324). Washington, DC: American Psychological Assocation.

Wilson, R. S., Beckett, L. A., Barnes, L. L., Schneider, J. A., Bach, J., Evans, D. A., et al. (2002). Individual differences in rates of change in cognitive abilities of older persons. *Psychology and Aging, 17*, 179–193.

Wohlwill, J. F. (1970). The age variable in psychological research. *Psychological Review, 77*, 49–64.

Wood, P., & Brown, D. (1994). The study of intraindividual differences by means of dynamic factor models: Rationale, implementation, and interpretation. *Psychological Bulletin, 116*, 166–186.

Zevon, M. A., & Tellegen, A. (1982). The structure of mood change: An idiographic/nomothetic analysis. *Journal of Personality and Social Psychology, 43*, 111–122.

Chapter | 3 |

Historical Influences on Aging and Behavior

K. Warner Schaie

Department of Psychiatry and Behavioral Sciences, University of Washington, Seattle, Washington, USA

CHAPTER CONTENTS

Introduction	**41**
Theories and Concepts	**42**
Conceptual Frameworks	**43**
Three Environmental Systems	43
A Co-Constructive Framework	45
Selected Neurobiological and Sociocultural Influences	45
Secular Cohort Trends in Cognition	45
Generational Differences in Cognition	46
Educational Influences	**46**
The Impact of the GI Bill	46
National Defense Education Act	47
Historical Change in Educational Curriculum and Pedagogy	47
Changes of Occupational Status and Work Complexity	**48**
Changes in Healthcare, Chronic Disease and Lifestyles	**48**
Hypertension	48
Cardiovascular Disease	48
Diabetes	48
Health Behaviors	49
The Role of Immigration	**49**
Societal Interventions to Reduce Poverty in Targeted Populations	**49**
Summary and Future Directions	**50**
References	**50**

INTRODUCTION

Like most American psychologists trained in the middle of the twentieth century in the tradition of Midwestern dust-bowl empiricism, I began my work on aging and behavior by treating behavior as a "black box" that could be studied without much attention to the environment or the biological infrastructure of the individual. But my concerns were soon broadened by exposure to the interdisciplinary community of gerontologists (cf. Schaie, 2000). My initial interest in considering historical influences on aging and behavior were stimulated primarily by methodological concerns related to disentangling of the different components of developmental change occurring over the life span and clarifying the distinction of inferences that can be drawn from the study of cross-sectional age differences and longitudinal age changes (cf. Schaie, 1965, 1977, 1988, 1994, 2005b, 2007). While the historical influences implicit in the cohort and period effects were first seen primarily as confounds in both cross-sectional or longitudinal research of aging parameters that needed to be controlled (also see Kuhlen, 1940), these influences sooner or later began to intrigue me as substantive issues worth study in their own right. My exposure to the substantive issues of cohort effects was sharpened by my long and fruitful interaction with the eminent sociologist Matilda Riley (Riley et al., 1972; Riley & Riley, 1994). My interaction with her also led to my launching a series of interdisciplinary conferences on social structures and aging that led to a 20-volume series of topical monographs charting the influence of macro-social structure on individual

DOI: 10.1016/B978-0-12-380882-0.00003-6

aging, beginning with a volume on social structures and psychological processes (Schaie & Schooler, 1989) and ending with a volume on social structure and aging individuals (Schaie & Abeles, 2008).

In trying to explicate my general developmental model I also began to specify broader substantive meaning for cohort beyond simply defining it as a common range of years of birth or defining period as the time of the measurement event (cf. Schaie, 1984, 1986, 2006a). Spurred by the work of the New Zealand political scientist Joseph Flynn (1984, 1987, 1999; Dickens & Flynn, 2001) who rediscovered the cohort effects in human abilities first introduced into sociology by Norman Ryder (1965) and into psychology by this author (1965), I began to think more seriously about the importance of historical influences upon behavior and aging. This interest increased even further during my collaboration with Glen Elder in organizing a conference on the historical influences on lives and aging (Schaie & Elder, 2005).

Since my aging research has largely focused on the adult life-span trajectory of cognitive abilities, I decided to become more focused also in my thinking about historical influences on cognitive abilities as my dependent variables. I therefore began to identify the various historical changes occurring over the past century that might reasonably be sources of major impact (Schaie, 2005a, 2006b, 2008b; Schaie & Achenbaum, 1993; Schaie et al., 2005; Willis & Schaie, 2006a).

In this chapter, I will first marshal some theoretical arguments on why one should pay attention to historical influences in studying the aging process of various psychological constructs as individuals develop from young adulthood to old age to the end of their lives, and I will lay out some of the principal concepts that require attention when studying such historical influences.

I will then examine historical changes in some of the major societal structures that I judge to be particularly prominent in influencing and constraining adult psychological development. The most prominent of these structures is the influence of educational attainment and changes in access to educational opportunities (such as caused by the GI bill, cf. Laub & Sampson, 2005). Second, I will examine the influence of changes in occupational structure caused by the shift from an agricultural and manufacturing economy to one that is highly technologically and service-oriented. Third, I will consider changes in healthcare and lifestyles that favorably impact level and change in optimal psychological functioning or compensate for declines that were common in earlier historical periods (cf. Leventhal et al., 2008). Fourth, I will discuss the influence of historical changes in immigration patterns as they affect the composition of the adult population and hence modify patterns of psychological aging in a given society (cf. Rumbaut, 2005). Fifth, I will briefly mention some other social interventions that have influenced the aging of psychological processes by major social interventions in the United States designed to reduce poverty in various specially targeted population segments (cf. Huston et al., 2005).

Finally, I will summarize the effects of changes in the above historical influences and how they affect the psychological characteristics and rate of change in old age of the elderly and then engage in some modest speculation about how these trends might develop over the next decade or two.

THEORIES AND CONCEPTS

It should be noted that this chapter might have taken a very different form if the editors had elected to commission it to an historian or a sociologist. In the first case the emphasis might have been upon the history of aging as a topic worthy of interest to psychologists and begun with an analysis of G. Stanley Hall's seminal opus (1922) as well as focusing upon the meaning of historical events that may have impacted psychological inquiry (cf. Cole, 1993; Cole et al., 2008). In the second case, the theoretical focus might well have begun with the work of Mannheim (1952; Pilcher, 1994) on the problem of generations and then shifted to the more recent work of the Rileys (1994) on generations moving as convoys through time.

Instead I decided that as a chapter for a handbook that emphasized psychological change over adulthood as its prime dependent variables, it would be more appropriate to have a psychologist address the impact of historical changes in our society that have had important impact on many of the substantive variables typically studied by psychologists interested in the human aging process (cf. James, 2005; Schaie et al., 2005).

Much of the interest by psychologists in historical influences on behavior has been stimulated by the literature on generational or cohort differences in both level and developmental trajectories of many psychological constructs. Particularly in the field of cognitive psychology it was found early on that the disassociation between the findings from studies of cross-sectional age differences and longitudinal age changes could best be understood by considering what was called the age-cohort-period model in sociology (Ryder, 1965), and the age-cohort-time model in psychology (Schaie, 1965).

The age-cohort-period model suggests that given observation R in a developmental or age-related study of inter-individual differences or intra-individual change is characterized by the form: $R = f(A, C, P)$; where A is the chronological age, C is the birth cohort, and P is the calendar time at which the observation is conducted. These components are confounded, much as temperature, pressure, and volume in the physical sciences, such that when two of the components are known the third is determined, even though all three may be of interest to the investigator. For the researcher of aging the major issue is that in age difference research (cross-sectional studies) age is confounded with cohort, and in age change research (longitudinal studies) age is confounded with period or time of measurement. Except in animal research, convergence of findings from cross-sectional and longitudinal study only occurs under very special circumstances (also see Ferrer & Ghisletta, Chapter 2; Zelinski et al., 2009).

A number of research designs have been proposed that allow at least partial unconfounding of these components by means of replicated cross-sectional or longitudinal sequences (cf. Schaie, 1977, 2005a, 2007; Willis, 1989). Less attention, however, has been given to provide alternate solutions by freeing the confounded components from their rigid identification by calendar time (Schaie, 1986). This could be accomplished by treating age as a dependent rather than an independent variable to determine the age at which a behavior or event of interest is first observed or the span of ages over which a given behavior endures (cf. Wohlwill, 1970). On the other hand cohort would need to be defined as referring to the common entry into a similar environment at a common point in time, whereas time could be redefined as the event density characterizing a particular period (cf. Schaie, 1984, 1986, 2006a).

When these issues were first identified for students of the psychology of aging, the immediate concerns were to determine how they might confound our understanding of age changes and differences over large periods of the life standing. More recently researchers in the psychology of aging have become more interested in how historical changes in societal influences

CONCEPTUAL FRAMEWORKS

I have previously suggested a conceptual framework for the understanding of cohort differences in intelligence to identify those influences in the historical cultural context that might impact cohort differences in both the mean level and trajectory of mental abilities across adulthood (cf. Schaie et al., 2005). This conceptual framework, adapted from Bronfenbrenner (1986; Bronfenbrenner & Crouter, 1983), is designed for the study of the major domains of influence that would provide possible mechanisms for cohort or generational differences in intellectual performance. While Bronfenbrenner's model is ordinarily presented as a series of concentric circles, our framework is presented as a matrix (see Table 3.1). This conceptual structure is necessary to make explicit multiple systems of influence at different developmental phases (childhood, adolescence, young adulthood, middle age, and old age) across the life span. At the core of our framework are the physical and psychological characteristics of the individual.

Three Environmental Systems

The proposed framework includes three systems of influence at each developmental phase: chronosystem, exosystem, and mesosystem. In the Bronfenbrenner model, after the family, the nearest and most direct environmental system, the *mesosystem*, is given first and primary consideration among the extra-familial systems. However, the ordering of environmental systems is reversed in our framework, given our primary concern with the impact of broad sociocultural events on cohort differences. Thus, we first consider the *chronosystem* that is concerned with the changes and continuities over time in environments that impact the individual's development. Two dimensions of the chronosystem are considered. First, the simplest form of chronosystem focuses on domain-specific life transitions. Two types of transitions have been distinguished in the psychological and sociological literatures (Baltes, 1979; Riley et al., 1972): normative (school entry, puberty, work entry, marriage, child bearing, retirement) and non-normative (death or severe illness, divorce, winning the lottery). These transitions are usually specific to a particular life domain (marriage, work), although there may be spillover to other domains. These transitions are usually defined by a circumscribed relatively brief time period during which they occur. In contrast, a second dimension of the chronosystem deals with cumulative effects of an entire sequence of transitions or events occurring over a more extended time period in the individual's life (e.g., war, depression, technological advances). The impact of such historical or sociocultural life course events on individual development has been an important focus of the work of social psychologists such as Elder (1974), Stewart (2003), and Helson and Moane (1987). However, the developmental outcomes of interest in the prior work have primarily been factors such as well-being, stability, and success in work and marriage, rather than cognitive performance. Of critical importance is the expectation that the relative impact of these long-term historical or sociocultural events will vary depending on the developmental phase of the individual. Thus, the same historical event may result in very different outcomes for different cohorts experiencing the event at different developmental phases.

The *exosystem* deals with environments that are not directly experienced by the individual, but are important environments for significant others, such as the target individual's parents, spouse, or friends. Such environments "external" to the developing individual are referred to as exosystems. As the Kahn and Antonucci

Table 3.1 Framework for the study of environmental influences

DEVELOPMENTAL PHASE	MESOSYSTEM CONTEXTS OF THE INDIVIDUAL	EXOSYSTEM CONTEXTS OF SIGNIFICANT OTHERS	CHRONOSYSTEM SINGLE-DOMAIN TRANSITIONS & LIFE COURSE OR CUMULATIVE EVENTS
Childhood	1) Family 2) Academic 3) Leisure/Social 4) Media	1) Parents 2) Extended family and Friends	1) Single domain transitions normative and non-normative 2) Life course/cumulative events (economic, political, social, etc.)
Adolescence	1) Family 2) Academic 3) Work 4) Leisure/Social 5) Media	1) Parents 2) Extended family, friends and colleagues	1) Single domain transitions normative and non-normative 2) Life course/cumulative events (economic, political, social, etc.)
Young adulthood	1) Family 2) Academic 3) Work 4) Leisure/Social 5) Media	1) Parents 2) Spouse or significant other 3) Extended family, friends and colleagues	1) Single domain transitions normative and non-normative 2) Life course/cumulative events (economic, political, social, etc.)
Middle age	1) Family 2) Academic 3) Work 4) Leisure/Social 5) Media	1) Parents 2) Spouse or significant other 3) Extended family, friends and colleagues	1) Single domain transitions normative and non-normative 2) Life course/cumulative events (economic, political, social, etc.)
Young-old age	1) Family 2) Academic 3) Work 4) Leisure/Social 5) Media	1) Parents 2) Spouse or significant other 3) Extended family, friends and colleagues	1) Single domain transitions normative and non-normative 2) Life course/cumulative events (economic, political, social, etc.)
Old-old age	1) Family 2) Academic 3) Work 4) Leisure/Social 5) Media	1) Spouse or significant other 2) Extended family, friends and colleagues	1) Single domain transitions normative and non-normative 2) Life course/cumulative events (economic, political, social, etc.)

From Schaie et al., 2005. Reproduced by permission.

(1980) model of convoys of social support suggests, the significant others in the individual's life would be expected to change across the life course, progressing from parents, to spouses and extended family, friends, and colleagues. The external environments in the exosystem that impact individual development would thus vary across the life course as the significant others change. In the child literature, the parents' work environment has been shown to impact childrearing practices (Kohn & Schooler, 1983), occupational aspirations of adolescents (Mortimer & Kumka, 1982), and curricular activities (Morgan et al., 1979).

In the Bronfenbrenner model, the exosystem focuses primarily on the concurrent environments of significant others (e.g., parent's work environment) that may impact the developing individual. However, our framework also includes transitions occurring across the adult lives of significant others that may influence the individual. For example, the father's educational or occupational experiences as a young adult and occurring in a particular historical may influence subsequent intellectual functioning of the offspring (Hauser & Featherman, 1976).

The mesosystem involves the principal contexts or environments in which individual development takes place. Given the focus on childhood, the family is considered the primary context of development in the Bronfenbrenner model. However, in our framework, we include the family as one of the facets of the environments within the mesosystem. Other environments experienced directly by the individual include work, leisure/social context, and media or technology-based contexts. The relative impact of these various environments is expected to vary across the life course and to interact with the personal characteristics of the individual.

It is assumed that long-term cumulative events primarily impact individual development indirectly as mediated by environmental factors in the meso- and exosystem and interact with the personal characteristics (e.g., personality, attitudes, lifestyles) of the individual who is a member of the cohort under investigation.

A Co-Constructive Framework

An alternative theoretical approach to the study of historical influences on psychological aging with particular application to cognition has been presented by Willis and Schaie (2006; see also Schaie, 2008a). Both neurobiological and sociocultural influences on development have long been recognized. Co-evolutionary theorists (Boyd & Richerson, 1985; Cavalli-Sforza & Feldman, 1981; Dunham, 1991; Tomasello, 1999) maintain that both biological and cultural evolution has occurred and that recent, cohort-related advances in human development in domains such as intelligence can be attributed largely to cumulative cultural evolution. Cultural activities impact the environment influencing mechanisms such as selection processes; thus allowing humans to co-direct their own evolution (Cavalli-Sforza & Feldman, 1981; Dunham, 1991). Baltes' co-constructionist approach imposes a life span developmental perspective on co-evolutionary theory and provides principles regarding the timing of the varying contributions of neurobiology and culture at different developmental periods and across different domains of functioning perspective proposed by Baltes and colleagues (Baltes, 1997; Li, 2003; Li & Freund, 2005).

Three principles are proposed regarding the relative contributions of biology and culture influences across the life span: (1) The beneficial effects of the evolutionary selection process occur primarily in early life and are less likely to optimize development in the latter half of life. (2) Further advances in human development depend on ever increasing cultural resources. From a historical perspective, increases in cultural resources have occurred via cumulative cultural evolution and have resulted in humans reaching higher levels of functioning. At the individual level, increasing cultural resources are required at older ages for further development to occur or to prevent age-related losses. (3) In old age, the efficacy of increasing cultural resources is diminished due to decline in neurobiological functions.

In a related co-evolutionary approach, Tomasello and others (Dawkins, 1989; Dunham, 1991; Tomasello, 1999) have proposed mechanisms for social transmission of cultural knowledge. Humans have evolved forms of social cognition unique to humans, which have enabled them not only to create new knowledge and skills but more important to preserve and socially transmit these cultural resources to the next cohort/generation. Cultural learning thus involves both social transmission of cultural knowledge and resources developed by one person, and also sociogenesis or collaborative learning and knowledge creation.

Selected Neurobiological and Sociocultural Influences

I shall next briefly review relevant literature documenting cohort and generational trends in cognition and consider sociocultural and neurobiological influences that have been found to account for inter-individual differences in intra-individual cognitive change. I draw upon the conception (Gauvain, 1998; Li, 2003; Tomasello, 1999) of culture to focus on two sociocultural domains: accumulated cultural resources and concurrent culture-based activities. Expanding upon Li's triarchic view of cultural domains, we view accumulated cultural resources as represented by structural variables such as educational level, occupational status, and ability level. These variables reflect the individual's prior acquisition and accumulation of cultural knowledge and skills. In contrast, the second component of the triarchic view of culture focuses on current activities, habits, and beliefs of the individual that are shaped by concurrent social dynamics and processes. The individual's current activities in domains such as health behaviors, cognitive engagement, and the complexity of one's work tasks are viewed as aspects of social dynamics that impact cognitive functioning and cohort differences in cognition. With regard to neurobiological influences, we focus on the two domains of chronic diseases and biomarkers, shown in the next section to impact cognitive change in adulthood.

Secular Cohort Trends in Cognition

For several decades there has been an intensive debate on the nature and directionality of cohort differences in cognition (Alwin, 2009). Cross-sectional data from several Western societies indicate the occurrence of "massive IQ gains on the order of 5 to 25 points in a single generation" (Flynn, 1987, p. 171; 1999). The "Flynn effect" has been documented primarily for post-World War II cohorts born in the 1950s. This massive cohort gain has been documented most clearly for fluid abilities, rather than crystallized abilities. Relatively little rationale has been offered for why fluid rather than crystallized abilities would show these positive trends for post-World War II cohorts.

In contrast, cross-sectional reports on college admission tests indicate negative cohort trends for certain birth cohorts of young adults (Astin & Henson, 1977; Wilson & Gove, 1999). Likewise, Alwin (1991; Alwin & McCammon, 2001), and Glenn (1994) reported negative cohort trends in verbal ability.

To examine cohort-related shifts in the domains of intelligence impacted by culture, an extensive database of multiple cohorts studied over the same developmental ages is needed, such as is present in the Seattle Longitudinal Study (SLS; Schaie, 2005a). Studies, such as Flynn's, highlight some of the serious limitations in prior cohort studies of cognition — focusing only on *level*, rather than developmental *change* in cognitive functioning, on a limited number of cohorts, over a single age period, and with no consideration of cohort-related differences in trajectory patterns (cf. Schaie, 2008b; Schaie et al., 2005; Schaie & Zanjani, 2006).

Generational Differences in Cognition

Studies of secular trends in cognition have focused almost exclusively on unrelated cohorts. The study of biologically related generations is important for several reasons. First, comparison of cohort versus generational data permit examination of whether a similar increase in prevalence of positive developmental trajectories hypothesized to occur across cohorts is also found across generations. More important, the comparison of the relative impact of neurobiological versus sociocultural influences, in biologically related individuals versus cohorts, would inform the relative potency of cultural and genetic influences on intelligence at various developmental periods. For example, the co-constructionist perspective posits that the influence of neurobiological factors increases in old age and exceeds the impact of cumulative cultural influences. A more stringent test of the increased impact of neurobiological factors in old age should be a study of successive family generations in contrast to successive unrelated cohorts given the shared genetics and environment across generations. The increased influence of neurobiological factors in old age is based in part on the assumption among evolutionary theorists that positive selection effects are most clearly manifested early in the life span and that the expression of deleterious genes in old age has been less constrained by the evolutionary process (Finch & Kirkwood, 2000).

EDUCATIONAL INFLUENCES

Educational level is the most consistent nonbiological predictor of both cognitive level and rate of change in prior longitudinal studies and meta-analyses (Albert et al., 1995; Anstey & Christensen, 2000; Schaie, 2005a). Moreover, education predicts cognitive change not only in old age but also throughout adulthood (Farmer et al., 1995; Lyketsos et al.,1999; Schaie, 2008b). Consistent with co-constructionist approaches, education is reported to most consistently predict change in crystallized abilities, memory, and mental status, and is less consistently predictive of change in fluid abilities and speed. The effects of education on cognitive change remain when controlling for factors such as age, gender, race, and health. In the MacArthur study of successful aging, education best predicted change in cognition (Albert et al., 1995).

Secular trends in education are well documented. Educational attainment, particularly in post-secondary education, has increased significantly across birth cohorts in the first half of the twentieth century. In 2000 15% of 65+ elders had attended college, compared to almost 50% of Baby Boomers. Hauser and Featherman (1976) reported a total increase of about 4 years of education from birth cohorts 1897 to 1951. Intergenerational differences in schooling peaked among men born shortly after World War I, and a deceleration has occurred across more recent cohorts. Intergenerational differences between successive generations, approximately 20 to 30 years apart, range from 2 to 4 years (cf. also Willis & Schaie, 2006b).

The Impact of the GI Bill

One of the major historical influences that led to marked increases in educational attainment for a broad segment of the population was the GI Bill, which benefited veterans of World War II and the Korean War (Laub & Sampson, 2005; Sampson & Laub, 1996; Segal, 2005).

Further educational training was provided through GI Bills for veterans of World War II, the Korean War, and the Vietnam War. Study of the effects of the GI Bill on World War II veterans is of particular interest, because a greater proportion of the U.S. male population was involved in World War II than in the Korean or Vietnam wars. The effects of the GI Bill on post-secondary education were most pronounced. Almost half of all veterans of World War II and the Korean conflict used the benefits for education and training, and 82 percent of those veterans who had attended college before the war made use of GI benefits to continue their education (Nam, 1964). Approximately one-third of veterans whose college work was interrupted by military service finished college or went on to graduate or professional school. For veterans who had just completed high school or had barely started college, one-fifth went on to get a college degree and a larger proportion took at least some college work. In comparison, only 10 percent of those who were working at the time of military service acquired at least an academic year of schooling after the war. Sampson and Laub (1996) reported that GI Bill training as well as in-service schooling enhanced subsequent occupational status, job stability, and economic well-being, independent of childhood differences and socioeconomic background. The benefits of the GI Bill were larger for younger veterans and for those who had evidence of delinquency in military service records.

Moreover, the dramatic numbers of veterans on college campuses after World War II and the Korean War significantly altered academic protocol and curriculum. In 1947, seven out of ten men enrolled in college or universities were veterans of World War II. Similarly, in 1956 one-fourth of all male college students were veterans of the Korean conflict (Nam, 1964). These veterans not only challenged prewar assumptions of who could benefit from a college education, but also challenged the very definition of what higher education should offer. Feeling as though the war had delayed their entry into adult life, veterans demanded streamlined education and that the curriculum be geared to real life in contrast to the more traditional emphasis in higher education on liberal arts and humanities. These veterans pressed academia with the view that the main duty of the university was to train individuals for adult participation in the modern world and to be the vehicle toward a secure job in a large corporation (Vinocour, 1947). Of course, military service may also have other developmental consequences such as effecting subsequent rates of maturation (cf. Aldwin & Levenson, 2005).

National Defense Education Act

In 1957 the Soviet Union launched Sputnik. The national panic generated by this event resulted in Congress passing a federal-aid-to-education bill, known as The National Defense Education Act of 1958. A major provision of the law involving a $15 million grant was the provision of funds to identify talented students and encourage them to pursue higher education. In the 1957–1958 term alone, Congress proposed over 80 laws to establish programs that would seek out bright students and provide them with financial support for schooling.

Historical Change in Educational Curriculum and Pedagogy

There have also been historical shifts in educational pedagogy and curriculum throughout the past century. A marked shift in educational philosophy was the Progressive movement in education that peaked in the 1920s and whose most noted proponent was John Dewey (Emirbayer, 1992). The goal of the movement was development of a "demographic character" equipped for responsible citizenship. This new citizen was to be developed from the "melting pot" represented in the United States during the early 1900s as a result of a large number of immigrants and the movement of the population from rural to urban areas and the growth of industrial centers such as Boston. These educational processes have undergone several trends from the basics to "progressive" to "tracking" and back to basics time and again. In the late 1800s, education was a structured curriculum that included rigid recitations of the 3 Rs: reading, writing, and arithmetic. High schools were not typical and most children ended their education after eight years. Kindergarten did not become the norm until the 1920s.

Tracking continued through the 1940s and the curriculum became even more split between college preparatory classes and industrial training. By the end of World War II, the Scholastic Aptitude Test (SAT) was beginning to replace IQ tests for college admissions and are still used. The SATs were similarly biased against minorities and immigrant children who did not have the same level of language skills or experience the same culture as the white, middle- and upper-middle class students. The Cold War caused another major shift in American public schools. Progressive curriculums had evolved into "life adjustment" courses by the early 1950s.

The Progressive movement advocated what might seem as contradictory initiatives (Emirbayer, 1992). On the one hand, due to the increased number of pupils because of child labor laws and compulsory school attendance, the educational practices of standardized testing and tracking of students was introduced. Standardized testing was viewed as a more "scientific" way of determining children's likely occupational attainment and allocating them into different educational channels (Ackerman, 1995). On the other hand, the Progressive movement also advocated movement away from teacher-directed lecture and rote recitation to increased student–teacher interaction, group exercises, and critical reflection. The Progressive movement also involved the introduction of the kindergarten, manual and vocational education, and evening classes.

Further support for extensive historical changes in curricula taught at different ages is shown in the recent work of Blair and colleagues (Blair et al., 2005). Findings of this research are particularly relevant to discussions of Flynn IQ effects, where the claim is made that IQ gain for the post-World War II cohorts has been primarily in the fluid abilities. Blair and colleagues have documented cohort differences in the age at which students were introduced to visuospatial skills such as traditionally taught in geometry. An 1894 college textbooks included a problem that required the student to draw and cut out a two-dimensional triangle and to fold the triangle to develop a three-dimensional polyhedron. By 1955 this type of problem was included in the seventh-grade textbook. By 1971 the same concept was taught to third graders, and by 1991 a first-grade textbook included a simplified version of the concept.

CHANGES OF OCCUPATIONAL STATUS AND WORK COMPLEXITY

Major historical changes in the U.S. workforce have occurred across cohorts (cf. Schaie & Schooler, 1998). Currently 20% of workers are in professional occupations, compared to 7% in 1950, while farmers have decreased from 10% in 1950 to 0.6%. The median age of retirement is now 62 years with only 18% of men 65+ working, compared to 46% in 1950. Women's work participation has increased with 52% of women aged 55 to 64 working compared to 27% in 1950 (Blau & Duncan, 1967; Farr & Schwall, 2008).

Occupational experience is related to maintenance of cognitive abilities at older ages (Owens, 1966). Avolio and Waldman (1990) reported that occupational status moderated the relationship between age and cognitive ability with a negative relationship for unskilled workers and no relationship for skilled workers. Salthouse (1990) reported that architects preserved higher levels of spatial ability later in the life span when compared with non-architects of similar ages. Historical shifts in work organization have resulted in fewer hierarchical levels and increased worker self-direction and responsibility for a broader range of tasks. As a result, job complexity has increased. Job conditions involving self-directed, substantively complex work are associated with increased intellectual flexibility and self-direction (Kohn & Schooler, 1983; Schooler, 1990, 1998). Findings indicate that the reciprocal relation between substantively complex work and cognition are even stronger in older men than was found in younger men (Schooler & Caplan, 2008; Schooler et al., 2004). Schooler's work also suggested age/cohort differences in work complexity; older workers, on average, were found to do less substantively complex work. For a theoretical discussion of cognitive plasticity see Willis et al. (2009).

CHANGES IN HEALTHCARE, CHRONIC DISEASE AND LIFESTYLES

I focus here on the chronic diseases of hypertension, cardiovascular disease, and diabetes not only due to their high prevalence in old age, but because of the related changes in lifestyles expressed through improved health behaviors (cf. also Leventhal et al., 2008; Schaie et al., 2002).

Hypertension

Hypertension is associated with poorer cognitive performance at all adult ages, primarily on fluid-type tests (e.g., attention, learning, memory, executive functions; Elias & Robbins, 1991; Elias et al., 1987; P. Elias et al., 1995; Waldstein & Elias, 2001); crystallized abilities are less affected. Chronic hypertension is associated not only with level of cognition but also with accelerated longitudinal decline (Elias et al., 1996; Elias et al., 1998; Knopman et al., 2000). Hypertension impacts cognitive decline in young adults as well as the aged (P. K. Elias et al., 2004). In a 20-year longitudinal study, cognitive decline was 12.1 percent greater for hypertensives compared to normotensives. Prospective cohort studies reported that the higher blood (Swan et al., 1992). Moreover, antihypertensive therapy has increased two- to threefold in recent cohorts and consideration of the impact of long-term antihypertensive therapy on the relation between hypertension and cognition is critical in longitudinal studies (Elias et al., 1998).

Cardiovascular Disease

Atherosclerosis contributes to mild but consistent deficits in cognitive performance in midlife and old age (Waldstein & Elias, 2001). Community-based studies of dementia (Lim et al., 1999) have found that cerebrovascular pathology often co-occurs with Alzheimer's disease (AD) pathology (Snowdon et al., 1997). Up to 45 percent of community-based incident dementia cases with autopsy-proven AD have co-occurring cerebral infarctions (Lim et al., 1999). In cases with vascular disease, less AD neuropathology is necessary for similar severity of clinical dementia (Snowdon et al., 1997), especially at earlier stages of the disease (Esiri et al., 1999). However, most of this evidence comes from cross-sectional studies with few longitudinal studies relating cognitive performance and atherosclerosis.

Diabetes

Case control studies of Type 2 diabetes in older adults have found cognitive impairment, most commonly for fluid-type abilities of learning and memory (Hassing et al., 2004a,b; Strachan et al., 1997). Large-scale epidemiological studies support the findings of case control studies, but most have been cross-sectional. An exception is the Framingham Health Study, which reported evidence of a causal relationship between diabetes and cognitive dysfunction (Elias et al., 1997). Duration of diabetes was related to poorer performance on verbal memory and abstract reasoning tests.

Health Behaviors

Health behaviors are considered sociocultural influences since these behaviors are acquired through socialization and are highly related to education (Markus et al., 2004). Substantial similarity in health behaviors across generations within families has also been reported (cf. Maitland, 1997). Self-regulatory health behaviors also differ markedly across ethnic and racial groups (cf. Jackson & Knight, 2006). The impact of health behaviors such as exercise, smoking, and alcohol consumption on maintenance of cognitive ability has been mixed (Anstey & Christensen, 2000). Colcombe and Kramer (2003) reported fitness effects to be selective with aerobic fitness training having a greater positive impact on tasks associated with executive control. In the MacArthur successful aging study (Albert et al., 1995) strenuous daily physical activity was a significant predictor of positive cognitive change. There is a paucity of studies on cigarette smoking and cognition. A systematic review found decreased AD risk in case-control studies but increased risk in prospective cohort studies (Kukull et al., 2002). Obesity has been associated with atherogenesis, hypertension, and diabetes and was found to increase risk for cognitive decline or AD (Sarkisian, 2000). More recent studies indicated that a U- or J-shaped curve may describe the relationship between level of alcohol use and cognitive functioning (Hendrie et al., 1996). Some studies find the association between cognition and moderate drinking stronger for women than for men. The MIDUS midlife study found educational differences in health behavior practices with college educated reporting a higher rate of exercise and lower rates of smoking (Markus et al., 2004), suggesting positive cohort trends in health behaviors. Support for healthier lifestyles appears also to be offered by participation in religious communities (Krause, 2008; Schaie et al., 2004). More recent cohorts of elderly have also experienced increased access to activities and resources that provide healthier lifestyles and better healthcare (cf. Schaie & Pietrucha, 2000; Schaie et al., 2003). The evidence seems clear that historical trends in extending preventive health practices and positive lifestyle changes have led to substantial health benefits for successive generations of elderly individuals (cf. Leventhal et al., 2008; Schaie et al., 2002). A large number of laboratory studies that showed the effectiveness of cognitive training interventions to slow cognitive decline in the elderly have now reached the level of clinical trials (e.g., Willis et al., 2006).

THE ROLE OF IMMIGRATION

Particularly in view of the dramatic decline of the American fertility rates in recent cohorts, the role of immigration has once again increased in importance in determining our society's age structure, as well as determining many characteristics of the aging population (DeJong, 2005; Fuligni, 2005; Gibson & Lennon, 1999; Rumbaut, 2005; Treas & Batalova, 2007). The recent interest in projecting the proportion of elderly immigrants as well as the aging of the immigrant of the American populations has led to some interesting conclusions.

First, it appears that current projections of the foreign-born population represent underestimates of the proportion of foreign-born within the elderly populations. Second, immigrants in general and older immigrants in particular contribute to the increasing racial and ethnic diversity in American society. Third, social and cultural incorporation of older immigrants appears to be a function of the length of time they have spent in the United States. Hence relatively recent older immigrants tend to be disadvantaged as compared to immigrants who have spent a major portion of their lives in the United States (Hirschman, 2007). They are less likely to be fluent in English, are less likely to live in homes they own, and they have much lower incomes. On the other hand, long-term immigrants are more similar to their native-born counterparts (cf. Treas & Batalova, 2007).

SOCIETAL INTERVENTIONS TO REDUCE POVERTY IN TARGETED POPULATIONS

Until fairly recently reaching advanced ages was limited to the socioeconomically favored and powerful in society (e.g., Achenbaum, 1993). But as life expectancy has increased for larger segments of the population, poverty has often characterized advanced old age (Haber, 1993). Therefore, beginning in the late nineteenth century, most industrial nations began to implement public retirement and pension systems to provide some income security for that period of life when increasing frailty, chronic disease, and disabilities ended participation in the world of work for most individuals (Gratton, 1993; Hayward, 2005; Plakans, 1989; Ransom et al., 1993; Vinovskis, 1989, 2005b). Most of the public plans providing reliable financial support for older persons are based on some understanding of an intergenerational contract that assumes that succeeding generations will provide for the old age of those who preceded them (Street & Quadagno, 1993).

Other interventions that have targeted earlier life stages and specific geographic areas have also had indirect effects on leading to the targeted cohorts reaching old age in better health, with fewer disabilities, and greater educational and financial resources. Such programs have included President Lyndon Johnson's attempts to reducing Appalachian poverty, the Head Start program (Vinovskis, 2005a), and the changes in welfare and employment policies enacted under the Clinton administration (cf. also Duncan, 2005; Hayward, 2008; Huston et al., 2005).

SUMMARY AND FUTURE DIRECTIONS

In this chapter I have tried to identify and discuss some of the major historical influences that might provide explanatory mechanisms for a better understanding of cohort and period differences in psychological aging processes. To do so within the confines of a single chapter I had to be selective rather than exhaustive in my inclusion of possible influences. Hence, I first proposed some theoretical arguments for why one should pay attention to historical influences in studying the aging process of various psychological constructs as individuals develop from young adulthood to old age and the end of their lives, and I then laid out some of the principal concepts that require attention when studying such historical influences. I next focused on historical changes in educational attainment, occupational structures, healthcare and lifestyles, the role of immigration, and the impact of social interventions to reduce poverty.

Out of necessity, I primarily covered historical influences that occurred in the United States. This, of course, led to a major omission by not attending to some of the major political changes that have transformed life and made a major impact upon psychological aging in other countries. Here I refer the reader to other more recent contributions that have discussed the impact on individual development by political events such as the German reunification (Silbereisen et al., 2005) or the collapse of the Soviet Union (Smyth, 2005; Titma & Tuma, 2005). Other historical influences that I slighted in this chapter and that deserve future exploration in relation to their influence on aging processes include changes in family structure (Hagestad & Uhlenberg, 2007; Hughes & Waite, 2007), and the cultural transformation of the meaning of the aging experience (cf. Fry, 2008), as well as the dramatic changes in retirement expectations and practices (cf. Eckerdt, 1998, 2008). I have also not attended to historical transformations of the meaning of adult development in non-Western cultures (e.g., Ikels, 1989; Sangree, 1989; Usui, 1989).

REFERENCES

Achenbaum, W. A. (1993). (When) did the papacy become a gerontocracy? In K. W. Schaie & W. A. Achenbaum (Eds.), *Societal impact on aging: Historical perspectives* (pp. 204–231). New York: Springer Publishing Co.

Ackerman, M. (1995). Mental testing and the expansion of educational opportunity. *History of Education Quarterly, 35*, 279–300.

Albert, M. S., Jones, K., Savage, C. R., Berkman, L., Seeman, T., Blazer, D., et al. (1995). Predictors of cognitive change in older persons: MacArthur studies of successful aging. *Psychology and Aging, 10*, 578–589.

Aldwin, C. M., & Levenson, M. R. (2005). Military service and emotional maturation: The Chelsea pensioners. In K. W. Schaie & G. Elder (Eds.), *Historical influences on lives and aging* (pp. 235–251). New York: Springer Publishing Co.

Alwin, D. F. (1991). Family of origin and cohort differences in verbal ability. *American Sociological Review, 56*, 625–638.

Alwin, D. F. (2009). History, cohorts, and patterns of cognitive aging. In H. B. Bosworth & C. Hertzog (Eds.), *Aging and cognition* (pp. 9–38). Washington, DC: American Psychological Association.

Alwin, D. F., & McCammon, R. J. (2001). Aging, cohorts, and verbal ability. *Journals of : Social Sciences, 56B*, S151–161.

Anstey, K., & Christensen, H. (2000). Education, activity, health, blood pressure and Apolipoprotein E as predictors of cognitive change in old age: A review. *Gerontology, 46*, 163–177.

Astin, A. W., & Henson, J. W. (1977). New measure of college selectivity. *Research in Higher Education, 6*, 1–9.

Avolio, B. J., & Waldman, D. A. (1990). An examination of age and cognitive test performance across job complexity and occupational types. *Journal of Applied Psychology, 75*, 43–50.

Baltes, P. B. (1979). Life-span developmental psychology: Some converging observations on history and theory. In P. B. Baltes, & O. G. Brim (Eds.). *Life-span development and behavior: Vol. 2* (pp. 256–281). New York: Academic Press.

Blair, C., Gamson, D. A., Thorne, S., & Baker, D. P. (2005). Rising mean IQ: Cognitive demand of mathematics education for young children, population exposure to formal schooling, and the neurobiology of the prefrontal cortex. *Intelligence, 33*, 93–106.

Blau, P. M., & Duncan, O. D. (1967). *The American occupational structure*. New York: Wiley.

Boyd, R., & Richerson, P. J. (1985). *Culture and the evolutionary process*. Chicago, IL: University of Chicago Press.

Bronfenbrenner, U. (1986). Ecology of the family as a context for human development research perspectives. *Developmental Psychology, 22*, 723–742.

Bronfenbrenner, U., & Crouter, A. (1983). The evolution of environmental models in developmental research. In P. H. Mussen (Ed.), *Handbook of child psychology*. (4th ed., Vol. 1, W. Kessen [Ed.], History, theory, and methods, pp. 357–414). New: York Wiley.

Cavalli-Sforza, L. L., & Feldman, M. W. (1981). *Cultural transmission and evolution: a quantitative approach*. Princeton, NJ: Princeton University Press.

Colcombe, S., & Kramer, A. F. (2003). Fitness effects on the cognitive function of older adults: A meta-analytic study. *Psychological Science, 14*, 25–130.

Cole, T., Achenbaum, W. A., & Carlin, N. C. (2008). Aging, history, and the course of life: Social structures and cultural meaning. In K. W. Schaie & R. P. Abeles (Eds.), *Social structures and aging individuals* (pp. 233–254). New York: Springer Publishing Co.

Cole, T. R. (1993). The prophecy of *senescence:* Stanley Hall and the reconstruction of old age in twentieth-century America. In K. W. Schaie & W. A. Achenbaum (Eds.), *Societal impact on aging: Historical perspectives* (pp. 165–181). New York: Springer Publishing Co.

Dawkins, R. (1989). *The selfish gene* (2nd ed.). Oxford, UK: Oxford University Press.

DeJong, G. F. (2005). Immigration of older adults: Extending the incorporation typology. In K. W. Schaie & G. Elder (Eds.), *Historical influences on lives and aging* (pp. 99–107). New York: Springer Publishing Co.

Dickens, W. T., & Flynn, J. R. (2001). Heritability estimates versus large environmental effects: The IQ paradox resolved. *Psychological Review, 108*, 346–369.

Duncan, D. J. (2005). Welfare reform and well-being. In K. W. Schaie & G. Elder (Eds.), *Historical influences on lives and aging* (pp. 286–298). New York: Springer Publishing Co.

Dunham, W. H. (1991). *Coevolution: Genes, culture, and human diversity.* Palo Alto, CA: Stanford University Press.

Eckerdt, D. J. (1998). Work place norms for the timing of retirement. In K. W. Schaie & C. Schooler (Eds.), *Impact of work on older adults* (pp. 101–123). New York: Springer Publishing Co.

Eckerdt, D. J. (2008). No career for you: Is that a good or bad thing? In K. W. Schaie & R. P Abeles (Eds.), *Social structures and aging individuals* (pp. 193–212). New York: Springer Publishing Co.

Elder, G. H., Jr. (1974). *Children of the great depression*. Chicago, IL: University of Chicago Press.

Elder, G. H., Jr., & *Conger, D.* (2000). *Children of the land*. Chicago, IL: University of Chicago Press.

Elias, M. F., Elias, P. K., D'Agostino, R. B., Silbershatz, H., & Wolf, P. A. (1997). Role of age, education, and gender on cognitive performance in the Framingham Heart Study: Community-based norms. *Experimental Aging Research, 23*, 201–235.

Elias, M. F., & Robbins, M. A. (1991). Cardiovascular disease, hypertension, and cognitive function. In A. Shapiro & A. Baum (Eds.), *Behavioral aspects of cardiovascular disease* (pp. 249–285). Hillsdale, NJ: Erlbaum.

Elias, M. F., Robbins, M. A., & Elias, P. K. (1996). A 15-year longitudinal study of Halstead-Reitan neuropsychological test performance. *Journals of Gerontology: Psychological Sciences, 451B*, P331–334.

Elias, M. F., Robbins, M. A., Elias, P. K., & Streeten, D. H. (1998). A longitudinal study of blood pressure in relation to performance on the Wechsler Adult Intelligence Scale. *Health Psychology, 17*, 486–493.

Elias, M. F., Robbins, M. A., Schultz, N. R., Streeten, D. H., & Elias, P. K. (1987). Clinical significance of cognitive performance by hypertensive patients. *Hypertension, 9*, 192–197.

Elias, P. K., D'Agostino, R. B., Elias, M. F., & Wolf, P. A. (1995). Blood pressure, hypertension, and age as risk factors for poor cognitive performance. *Experimental Aging Research, 21*, 393–417.

Elias, P. K., Elias, M. F., Robbins, M. A., & Budge, M. M. (2004). Blood pressure-related cognitive decline: Does age make a difference? *Hypertension, 44*, 1–6.

Emirbayer, M. (1992). Beyond structuralism and voluntarism: the politics and discourse of progressive school reform, 1890–1930. *Theory and Society, 21*, 621–664.

Esiri, M. M., Nagy, Z., Smith, M. Z., Barnetson, L., & Smith, A. D. (1999). Cerebrovascular disease and threshold for dementia in the early stages of Alzheimer's disease. *The Lancet, 354*, 919–920.

Farmer, M. E., Kittner, S. J., Rae, D. S., Barko, J. J., & Regier, D. A. (1995). Education and change in cognitive function: The Epidemiologic Catchment area Study. *Annals of Epidemiology, 5*, 1–7.

Farr, A. L., & Schwall, A. R. (2008). New employment structures — varieties of impact on ageing workers. In K. W. Schaie & R. P. Abeles (Eds.), *Social structures and aging individuals* (pp. 213–230). New York: Springer Publishing Co.

Finch, C. E., & Kirkwood, T. B. (2000). *Chance, development, and aging.* New York: Oxford University Press.

Flynn, J. R. (1984). The mean IQ of Americans: Massive gains 1932 to 1978. *Psychological Bulletin, 95*, 29–51.

Flynn, J. R. (1987). Massive IQ gains in 14 nations: What IQ tests really measure. *Psychological Bulletin, 101*, 171–191.

Flynn, J. R. (1999). Searching for Justice: The discovery of IQ gains over time. *American Psychologist, 54*, 5–20.

Fry, C. L. (2008). Cultural transformations, history and the experiences of aging. In K. W. Schaie & R. P Abeles (Eds.), *Social structures and aging individuals* (pp. 255–284). New York: Springer Publishing Co.

Fuligni, A. J. (2005). Convergence and divergence in the developmental contexts of immigrants in the United States. In K. W. Schaie & G. Elder (Eds.), *Historical influences on lives and aging* (pp. 89–98). New York: Springer Publishing Co.

Gauvain, M. (1998). Cognitive development in social and cultural context. *Psychological Science, 7*, 188–192.

Gibson, C. J., & Lennon, E. (1999). Historical census statistics on the foreign-born population of the United States: 1850–1950. *Population Division Working Paper No. 29*. Washington, DC: U.S

Bureau of the Census. Online at http://www.census.gov/population/www/documentation/twps0029/twps0029.html#data.

Glenn, N. D. (1994). Television watching, newspaper reading, and cohort differences in verbal ability. *Sociology of Education, 67,* 216–230.

Gratton, B. (1993). The creation of retirement: Families, individuals and the social security movement. In K. W. Schaie & W. A. Achenbaum (Eds.), *Societal impact on aging: Historical perspectives* (pp. 45–73). New York: Springer Publishing Co.

Haber, C. (1993). Over the hill to the poorhouse: Rhetoric and reality in the institutional history of the aged. In K. W. Schaie & W. A. Achenbaum (Eds.), *Societal impact on aging: Historical perspectives* (pp. 90–114). New York: Springer Publishing Co.

Hagestad, G. O., & Uhlenberg, P. (2007). The impact of demographic changes on relations between age groups and generations: A comparative perspective. In K. W. Schaie & P. Uhlenberg (Eds.), *Social structures demographic changes and the well-being of older persons* (pp. 239–261). New York: Springer Publishing Co.

Hall, G. S. (1922). *Senescence, the last half of life.* New York: Appleton & Co.

Hassing, L. B., Hofer, S. M., Nilsson, S. E., Berg, S., Pedersen, N. L., McClearn, G. E., et al. (2004b). Comorbid Type 2 diabetes mellitus and hypertension acerbates cognitive decline: Evidence from a longitudinal study. *Age and Ageing, 33,* 355–361.

Hauser, R. M., & Featherman, D. L. (1976). Equality of schooling: Trends and prospects. *Sociology of Education, 49,* 99–120.

Hayward, M. D. (2005). What happened to America's elderly population? In K. W. Schaie & G. Elder (Eds.), *Historical influences on lives and aging* (pp. 35–42). New York: Springer Publishing Co.

Hayward, M. D. (2008). How have social institutional forces shaped family structures and well-being over the past 50 years? In K. W. Schaie & R. P. Abeles (Eds.), *Social structures and aging individuals* (pp. 335–344). New York: Springer Publishing Co.

Helson, R., & Moane, G. (1987). Personality change in women from college to midlife. *Journal of Personality and Social Psychology, 53,* 176–186.

Hendrie, H. C., Gao, S. J., Hall, K. S., & Hui, S. L. (1996). The relationship between alcohol consumption, cognitive performance, and daily functioning in an urban sample of older Black Americans. *Journal of the American Geriatrics Society, 44,* 1158–1165.

Hirschman, C. (2007). Immigration and an aging America: Downward spiral or vicious circle. In K. W. Schaie & P. Uhlenberg (Eds.), *Social structures demographic changes and the well-being of older persons* (pp. 37–51). New York: Springer Publishing Co.

Hughes, M. H., & Waite, L. J. (2007). The aging of the second demographic transition. In K. W. Schaie & P. Uhlenberg (Eds.), *Social structures demographic changes and the well-being of older persons* (pp. 179–211). New York: Springer Publishing Co.

Huston, A. C., Mistry, R. S., Bos, J. M., & Shim, M. S. (2005). Well-being of low-income adults in a period of historical changes in welfare and employment policies. In K. W. Schaie & G. Elder (Eds.), *Historical influences on lives and aging* (pp. 252–285). New York: Springer Publishing Co.

Ikels, C. (1989). Becoming a human being in theory and practice: Chinese views of human development. In D. I. Kertzer & K. W. Schaie (Eds.), *Age structuring in comparative perspective* (pp. 109–134). New York: Springer Publishing Co.

Jackson, J. S., & Knight, K. M. (2006). Race and self-regulatory health behaviors: The role of the stress response and the HPA axis in physical and mental health disparities. In K. W. Schaie & L. L. Carstensen (Eds.), *Social structures, aging, and self-regulation in the elderly* (pp. 189–208). New York: Springer Publishing Co.

James, J. B. (2005). This American life: A discussion of the role of history in developmental outcomes. In K. W. Schaie & G. Elder (Eds.), *Historical influences on lives and aging* (pp. 21–34). New York: Springer Publishing Co.

Kahn, R. L., & Antonucci, T. C. (1980). Convoys over the life course: Attachment, roles and social support. *Life Span Development, 3,* 253–286.

Kertzer, D. I., & Schaie, K. W. (Eds.), (1989). *Age structuring in comparative perspective.* New York: Springer Publishing Co.

Knopman, D. S., Boland, L. L., Folsom, A. R., Mosley, T. H., McGovern, P. G., Howard, G., et al. (2000). Cardiovascular risk factors and longitudinal cognitive changes in middle age adults. *Neurology, 54*(Suppl. 3).

Kohn, M. L., & Schooler., C. (1983). *Work and personality: An inquiry into the impact of social stratification.* Norwood, NJ: Ablex.

Krause, N. (2008). Religion, health, and health behaviors. In K. W. Schaie & R. P. Abeles (Eds.), *Social structures and aging individuals* (pp. 73–96). New York: Springer Publishing Co.

Kuhlen, R. G. (1940). Social change: A neglected factor in psychological studies of the life span. *School and Society, 52,* 14–16.

Kukull, W. A., Higdon, R., Bowen, J. D., McCormick, W. C., Teri, L., & Schellenberg, G. C. (2002). Dementia and Alzheimer disease incidence: a prospective cohort study. *Archives of Neurology, 59,* 1737–1746.

Laub, J. H., & Sampson, R. J. (2005). Coming of age in wartime: How World War II and the Korean War changed lives. In K. W. Schaie & G. Elder (Eds.), *Historical influences on lives and aging* (pp. 151–208). New York: Springer Publishing Co.

Leventhal, H., Musumeci, T. J., & Leventhal, E. A. (2008). To act or not to act: Using statistics or feelings to reduce disease risk, morbidity and mortality. In K. W. Schaie & R. P. Abeles (Eds.), *Social structures and aging individuals* (pp. 25–72). New York: Springer Publishing Co.

Li, S.-C. (2003). Biocultural orchestration of developmental plasticity across levels: The interplay of biology and culture in shaping the mind and behavior across the life span. *Psychological Bulletin, 129*, 171–194.

Li, S.-C., & Freund, A. M. (2005). Advances in lifespan psychology: A focus on biocultural and personal influences. *Research in Human Development, 2*, 1–23.

Lim, A., Tsuang, D., Kukull, W., Nochlin, D., Leverenz, J., McCormick, W., et al. (1999). Clinico-neuropathological correlation of Alzheimer's disease in a community-based case series. *Journal of the American Geriatric Society, 47*, 564–569.

Lyketsos, C. G., Chen, L. S., & Anthony, J. C. (1999). Cognitive decline in adulthood: An 11.5-year follow-up of the Baltimore Epidemiologic Catchment Area Study. *American Journal of Psychiatry, 156*, 58–65.

Maitland, S. B. (1997). *Factorial invariance and concordance of health behaviors and health status: A study of individual differences in familial context.* Unpubl. doctoral dissertation. University Park, PA: The Pennsylvania State University.

Mannheim, K. (1952). The problem of generations. In K. Mannheim (Ed.), *The sociology of knowledge*. London, UK: Rutledge, Kegan, and Paul.

Markus, H. R., Ryff, C. D., Curham, K. B., & Palmersheim, K. A. (2004). In their own words: Well-Being in midlife among high school-educated and college educated adults. In O. G. Brim, C. D. Ryff, & R. C. Kessler (Eds.), *How healthy are we? A national study of well being in midlife.* Chicago, IL: University of Chicago Press.

Morgan, W. R., Alwin, D. F., & Griffin, L. J. (1979). Social origins, parental values and the transmission of inequality. *American Journal of Sociology, 85*, 156–166.

Mortimer, J. T., & Kumka, D. (1982). A further examination of the "occupational link hypothesis." *Sociological Quarterly, 23*, 3–16.

Nam, C. B. (1964). Impact of the "GI Bills" on the educational level of the male population. *Social Forces, 43*, 26–32.

Owens, W. A. (1966). Age and mental abilities: A second adult follow-up. *Journal of Educational Psychology, 57*, 311–325.

Pilcher, J. (1994). Mannheim's sociology of generations: An undervalued legacy. *British Journal of Sociology, 45*, 481–495.

Plakans, A. (1989). Stepping down in former times: A comparative assessment of "retirement" in traditional Europe. In D. I. Kertzer & K. W. Schaie (Eds.), *Age structuring in comparative perspective* (pp. 175–195). New York: Springer Publishing Co.

Ransom, R. L., Sutch, R., & Williamson, S. H. (1993). Inventing pensions: The origin of the company-provided pension in the United State, 1900–1940. In K. W. Schaie & W. A. Achenbaum (Eds.), *Societal impact on aging: Historical perspectives* (pp. 1–38). New York: Springer Publishing Co.

Riley, M. W., Johnson, M. J., & Foner, A. (1972). *Aging and society: Vol. 3: A sociology of age stratification*. New York: Russell Sage.

Riley, M. W., & Riley, J. W. (1994). Age integration and the lives of older people. *The Gerontologist, 34*, 110–115.

Rumbaut, R. G. (2005). Immigration, incorporation and generational cohorts in historical contexts. In K. W. Schaie & G. Elder (Eds.), *Historical influences on lives and aging* (pp. 43–88). New York: Springer Publishing Co.

Ryder, N. B. (1965). The cohort as a concept in the study of social changes. *American Sociological Review, 30*, 843–861.

Sampson, R. J., & Laub, J. H. (1996). Socioeconomic achievement in the life course of disadvantaged men: Military service as a turning point, circa 1940–1965. *American Sociological Review, 61*, 347–367.

Sangree, W. H. (1989). Age and power: Life-course trajectories and age structuring on power relations in East and West Africa. In D. I. Kertzer & K. W. Schaie (Eds.), *Age structuring in comparative perspective* (pp. 23–46). New York: Springer Publishing Co.

Sarkisian, C. A., Liu, H., Gutierrez, P. R., Seeley, D. G., Cummings, S. R., & Mangione, C. M. (2000). Modifiable risk factors predict functional decline among older women: A prospectively validated clinical prediction tool. The study of osteoporotic fractures research group. *Journal of the American Geriatric Society, 4*, 170–178.

Schaie, K. W. (1965). A general model for the study of developmental problems. *Psychological Bulletin, 64*, 92–107.

Schaie, K. W. (1977). Quasi-experimental designs in the psychology of aging. In J. E. Birren & K. W. Schaie (Eds.), *Handbook of the psychology of aging* (pp. 39–58). New York: Van Nostrand Reinhold.

Schaie, K. W. (1984). Historical time and cohort effects. In K. A. McCluskey & H. W. Reese (Eds.), *Life-span developmental psychology: Historical and generational effects* (pp. 1–15). New York: Academic Press.

Schaie, K. W. (1986). Beyond calendar definitions of age, time, and cohort: The general developmental model revisited. *Developmental Review, 6*, 252–277.

Schaie, K. W. (1988). The impact of research methodology on theory building in the developmental sciences. In J. E. Birren & V. L. Bengtson (Eds.), *Emergent theories of aging: Psychological and social perspectives on time, self and society* (pp. 41–58). New York: Springer Publishing Co.

Schaie, K. W. (1994). Developmental designs revisited. In S. H. Cohen & H. W. Reese (Eds.), *Life-span developmental psychology: Methodological issues revisited* (pp. 45–64). Hillsdale, NJ: Erlbaum.

Schaie, K. W. (2000). Living with gerontology. In J. E. Birren & J. J. F. Schroots (Eds.), *A history of geropsychology in autobiography* (pp. 233–248). Washington, DC: American Psychological Association.

Schaie, K. W. (2005a). *Developmental influences on adult intelligence; The Seattle Longitudinal Study*. New York: Oxford University Press.

Schaie, K. W. (2005b). What can we learn from longitudinal studies of adult intellectual development? *Research in Human Development, 2*, 133–158.

Schaie, K. W. (2006a). The concept of event time in the study of aging. In J. Baars & H. Visser (Eds.), *Concepts of time and aging* (pp. 121–135). Amityville, NY: Baywood Publishing Co.

Schaie, K. W. (2006b). Societal influences on cognition in historical context. In K. W. Schaie & L. L. Carstensen (Eds.), *Social structures, aging, and self-regulation in the elderly* (pp. 13–24). New York: Springer Publishing Co.

Schaie, K. W. (2007). Generational differences; the age-cohort-period model. In J. E. Birren (Ed.), *Encyclopedia of gerontology: Age, aging, and the aged* (2nd ed.) (pp. 601–609). Oxford, UK: Elsevier.

Schaie, K. W. (2008a). A lifespan developmental perspective of psychological aging. In K. Laidlaw & B. G. Knight (Eds.), *The Handbook of emotional disorders in late life: Assessment and treatment* (pp. 3–32). Oxford, UK: Oxford University Press.

Schaie, K. W. (2008b). Historical processes and patterns of cognitive aging. In S. M Hofer & D. F. Alwin (Eds.), *Handbook on cognitive aging: Interdisciplinary perspective* (pp. 368–383). Thousand Oaks, CA: Sage.

Schaie, K. W., & Abeles, R. A. (Eds.), (2008). *Social structures and aging individuals: Continuing challenges.* New York: Springer Publishing Co.

Schaie, K. W., & Achenbaum, W. A. (Eds.), (1993). *Societal impact on aging: Historical perspectives.* New York: Springer Publishing Co.

Schaie, K. W., & Elder, G. H., Jr. (Eds.), (2005). *Historical influences on lives and aging.* New York: Springer Publishing Co.

Schaie, K. W., Krause, N., & Booth, A. (Eds.), (2004). *Religious influences on health and well-being in the elderly.* New York: Springer Publishing Co.

Schaie, K. W., Leventhal, H., & Willis, S. L. (2002). *Social structures and effective health behaviors in the elderly.* New York: Springer Publishing Co.

Schaie, K. W., & Pietrucha, M. (Eds.), (2000). *Mobility and Aging.* New York: Springer Publishing Co.

Schaie, K. W., & Schooler, C. (Eds.), (1989). *Social structure and aging: Psychological processes.* Hillsdale, NJ: Erlbaum.

Schaie, K. W., & Schooler, C. (Eds.), (1998). *Impact of work on older adults.* New York: Springer Publishing Co..

Schaie, K. W., & Uhlenberg, P. (Eds.), (2007). *Social structures demographic changes and the well-being of older persons.* New York: Springer Publishing Co.

Schaie, K. W., Wahl, H.-W., Mollenkopf, H., & Oswald, F. (Eds.), (2003). *Aging independently: Living arrangements and mobility in the elderly.* New York: Springer Publishing Co.

Schaie, K. W., Willis, S. L., & Pennak, S. (2005). A historical framework for cohort differences in intelligence. *Research in Human Development, 2,* 43–67.

Schaie, K. W., & Zanjani, F. A. K. (2006). Intellectual development across adulthood. In C. Hoare (Ed.), *Handbook of adult development and learning* (pp. 99–122). New York: Oxford University Press.

Schooler, C. (1990). Psychosocial factors and effective cognitive functioning in adulthood. In J. E. Birren & K. W. Schaie (Eds.), *Handbook of the psychology of aging* (3rd ed.) (pp. 347–358). San Diego, CA: Academic Press.

Schooler, C. (1998). Environmental complexity and the Flynn effect. In U. Neisser (Ed.), *The rising curve: Long term gains in IQ and related measures* (pp. 67–79). Washington, DC: American Psychological Association.

Schooler, C., & Caplan, L. J. (2008). Them who have, get: Social structure, environmental complexity, intellectual functioning and self-directed orientation in the elderly. In K. W. Schaie & R. P. Abeles (Eds.), *Social structures and aging individuals* (pp. 131–154). New York: Springer Publishing Co.

Schooler, C., Mulatu, M. S., & Oates, G. (2004). Occupational self-direction, intellectual functioning, and self directed orientation in older workers: Findings and implications for individuals and societies. *American Journal of Sociology, 110,* 161–197.

Segal, D. R. (2005). Time, race, and gender differences in the effects of military service on veteran outcomes. In K. W. Schaie & G. Elder (Eds.), *Historical influences on lives and aging* (pp. 229–234). New York: Springer Publishing Co.

Silbereisen, R. K., Reitzle, M., & Pinquart, M. (2005). Social change and individual development: A challenge-response approach. In K. W. Schaie & G. Elder (Eds.), *Historical influences on lives and aging* (pp. 148–165). New York: Springer Publishing Co.

Smyth, R. (2005). The more things change: Coping with transition in the new Russia. In K. W. Schaie & G. Elder (Eds.), *Historical influences on lives and aging* (pp. 199–207). New York: Springer Publishing Co.

Snowdon, D. A., Greiner, L. H., Mortimer, J. A., Riley, K . P., Greiner, P. A., & Markesbery, W. R. (1997). Brain infarction and the clinical expression of Alzheimer disease: The Nun Study. *Journal of the American Medical Association, 277,* 813–817.

Stewart, A. J. (2003). Gender, race and generation in a Midwest high school: Using ethnographically informed methods in psychology. *Psychology of Women Quarterly, 27,* 1–11.

Strachan, M. W. J., Deary, I. J., Ewing, F. M. E., & Frier, B. M. (1997). Is Type II diabetes associated with an increased risk of cognitive dysfunction? *Diabetes Care, 20,* 438–445.

Street, D., & Quadagno, J. (1993). The state, the elderly, and the intergenerational contract: Toward a new political economy of aging. In K. W. Schaie & W. A. Achenbaum (Eds.), *Societal impact on aging: Historical perspectives* (pp. 130–150). New York: Springer Publishing Co.

Swan, G. E., LaRue, A., Carmelli, D., Reed, T. E., & Fabsitz, R. R. (1992). Decline in cognitive performance in aging twins, heritability and biobehavioral predictors from the National Heart, Lung, and Blood Twin Study. *Archives of Neurology, 49,* 476–483.

Titma., M., & Tuma, N. B. (2005). Human agency in the transition from Communism: Perspectives on the life course and aging. In K. W. Schaie & G. Elder (Eds.), *Historical influences on lives and aging* (pp. 108–143). New York: Springer Publishing Co.

Tomasello, M. (1999). *The cultural origins of human cognition.* Cambridge, MA: Harvard University Press.

Treas, J., & Batalova, J. (2007). Older immigrants. In K. W. Schaie & P. Uhlenberg (Eds.), *Social structures demographic changes and the well-being of older persons* (pp. 1–24). New York: Springer Publishing Co.

Usui, I. (1989). Can Japanese society promote individualism. In D. I. Kertzer & K. W. Schaie (Eds.), *Age structuring in comparative perspective* (pp. 143–166). New York: Springer Publishing Co.

Vinocour, S. M. (1947, November). The veteran and college. *Newsweek, 80*, 140.

Vinovskis, M. A. (1989), Stepping down in former times: The view from colonial and 19th-century America. In D. I. Kertzer & K. W. Schaie (Eds.), *Age structuring in comparative perspective* (pp. 215–225). New York: Springer Publishing Co.

Vinovskis, M. A. (2005a). *The birth of Head Start: Pre-school education policies in the Kennedy and Johnson administrations*. Chicago, IL: University of Chicago Press.

Vinovskis, M. A. (2005b). Historical change and the American life course. In K. W. Schaie & G. Elder (Eds.), *Historical influences on lives and aging* (pp. 1–20). New York: Springer Publishing Co.

Waldstein, S. R., & Elias, M. F. (2001). *Neuropsychology of cardiovascular disease*. Mahwah, NJ: Erlbaum.

Willis, S. L. (1989). Cohort differences in cognitive aging: A sample case. In K. W. Schaie & C. Schooler (Eds.), *Social structure and aging: Psychological processes* (pp. 94–112). Hillsdale, NJ: Erlbaum.

Willis, S. L., & Schaie, K. W. (2005). Cognitive trajectories in midlife and cognitive functioning in old age. In S. L. Willis & M. Martin (Eds.), *Middle adulthood: A lifespan perspective* (pp. 243–276). Thousand Oaks, CA: Sage.

Willis, S. L., & Schaie, K. W. (2006a). A co-constructionist view of the third age: The case of cognition. *Annual Review of Gerontology and Geriatrics, 26*, 131–152.

Willis, S. L., & Schaie, K. W (2006b). Cognitive functioning in the Baby Boomers: Longitudinal and cohort effects. In S. K. Whitbourne & S. L. Willis (Eds.), *The baby boomers grow up* (pp. 205–234). Mahwah, NJ: Lawrence Erlbaum Associates.

Willis, S. L., Schaie, K. W., & Martin, M. (2009). Cognitive plasticity. In V. Bengtson, M. Silverstein, N. Putney, & D. Gans (Eds.), *Handbook of theories of aging* (2nd ed.) (pp. 295–322). New York: Springer Publishing Co.

Willis, S. L., Tennstedt, S. L., Marsiske, M., Ball, K., Elias, J., Koepke, K. M., et al. (2006). Long-term effects of cognitive training on everyday functional outcomes in older adults. *Journal of the American Medical Association, 296*, 2805–2814.

Wilson, J. A., & Gove, W. R. (1999). The intercohort decline in verbal ability: Does it exist? *American Sociological Review, 64*, 253–266.

Wohlwiil, J. F. (1970). The age variable in psychological research. *Psychological Review, 77*, 49–64.

Zelinski, E. M., Kennison, R. F., Watts, A., & Lewis, K. L. (2009). Convergence between cross-sectional and longitudinal studies: Cohort matters. In H. B. Bosworth & C. Hertzog (Eds.), *Aging and cognition* (pp. 101–118). Washington, DC: American Psychological Association.

Part | 2 |

Neuroscience, Cognition and Aging

4 Executive Function and Cognitive Aging *59*

5 The Cognitive Consequences of Structural Changes to the Aging Brain *73*

6 Behavior Genetics of Aging *93*

7 Neuroplasticity Aging, and Cognitive Function *109*

8 Memory Changes and the Aging Brain: A Multimodal Imaging Approach *121*

9 Age Differences in Complex Decision Making *133*

10 Cognitive Interventions *153*

Chapter | 4 |

Executive Function and Cognitive Aging

Mary Luszcz
Department of Psychology, Flinders Centre for Ageing Studies, Flinders University, Adelaide SA, Australia

CHAPTER CONTENTS

Introduction	**59**
Purpose, Scope, and Aims	**60**
Conceptualizing EF	**60**
Evolution of the Construct	60
The Confluence of Neuropsychology and Cognitive Psychology	61
The Dominance of Task-Based Approaches	61
Structural Approaches to Executive Function "Unity and Diversity"	**62**
Diversity of EF in Older Adults	63
Unity of EF	63
Interim Conclusion	63
Cognitive Approaches to EF	**63**
Switching Tasks	64
The Process-Dissociation Approach	64
Mediation and Moderation in EF	65
Cognitive Neuroscience and Prefrontal Involvement in EF	**66**
Volumetric Work and a Specific Frontal Task	66
Diffuse Brain Integrity and Frontal/ Executive Function	66
Frontal Activation Patterns	67
Event-Related Potentials and Executive Functioning	67
Interim Conclusion	68
Looking Forward	**68**
Conclusions	**69**
References	**69**

INTRODUCTION

Parsimony is the ultimate goal of attempts to explain human behavior. This has led to a search for unifying generic constructs or brain areas that are widely applicable across domains, that is, cognitive aging. During the closing decade of the last century, executive function (EF),[1] and its associated "frontal-executive" theorizing captured the imagination of scholars of cognitive aging. EF refers to "domain-general control processes that monitor and regulate other cognitive processes to guide the attainment of future goals" (Head et al., 2008, p. 492). According to the frontal-executive hypothesis, early age-related changes located in the frontal lobe are associated with deficient executive control processes (ECPs; see West, 1996 for details and Phillips & Henry, 2009 for a critique). In short, neurodegeneration localized to the prefrontal cortex (PFC) is functionally linked to EF: early and marked structural or volumetric deterioration within the PFC (e.g., Raz, 2000) has been posited to be responsible for EF failures.

From a cognitive perspective, EF features prominently in efforts to understand *mechanisms* that underlie complex thought and behavior in late life. It coexists with conceptualizations invoking depletion of resources (e.g., processing efficiency or speed) or capacity limitations but as the evidence from neuroimaging becomes more compelling, it is increasingly difficult to invoke a single cognitive primitive (Luszcz & Bryan, 1999) to explain behavioral performance. This notion is reflected in the emergence of several more general cognitive theories such as the *scaffolding theory of aging and cognition* (STAC) from Park and Reuter-Lorenz (2009), Stern's (2009) notion of *cognitive reserve*, or Greenwood's (2007) *functional plasticity*

DOI: 10.1016/B978-0-12-380882-0.00004-8

account. The theorizing of these authors converges on broadly analogous conceptualizations that attempt to resolve the paradox of decreasing cognitive performance with age in a range of domains, "many of which are also executive in nature" (Park & Reuter-Lorenz, p. 177), concurrent with increases in the amount and extent of prefrontal activation (Buckner, 2004; Spreng et al., 2010). Other chapters in this volume deal explicitly with theories of aging (Chapter 1), brain imaging (Chapter 5), and neurocognitive plasticity in aging (Chapter 7). In contrast, this chapter introduces these rapid shifts in theorizing in order to illustrate their intersection with EF.

PURPOSE, SCOPE, AND AIMS

The purpose of this chapter is to set out the basics and encapsulate the nuances of EF by reviewing some of the behavioral and cognitive neuroscience research it has given rise to, and its relevance to the field of cognitive aging. Comprehensive treatment of all the intricacies of what has come to be known as EF is beyond the scope of this chapter. Several extant reviews provide insightful perspectives on EF (e.g., Daniels et al., 2006; Luszcz & Lane, 2008; Phillips & Henry, 2005, 2008; Rabbitt, 1997) and these inform this chapter. Of necessity, important areas are omitted or mentioned in passing. For instance, little heed is paid to developmental change (see Juardo & Roselli, 2007) across the life span. Indeed, because the majority of extant research is cross-sectional, the reader is cautioned that some effects are likely to reflect cohort differences or secular trends in EF, rather than its development or change. This chapter focuses on EF in primary aging, hence pathology-related decline in EF is not discussed (but see Buckner, 2004; Head et al., 2004). Finally, limited attention is given to the concept of *regulation* that is characteristic of contemporary theories of aging (e.g., socioemotional selectivity; Carstensen et al., 2006). This is not to deny the significance of these topics, but rather reflects constraints on the scope of the chapter, and coverage of these topics by other contributors to this volume.

The broad aims guiding the chapter are (1) to provide a road map for the reader pointing out some of the trends emerging in recent literature on the construct and its proposed neurological underpinnings, to set them on the path to exploring aspects most relevant to their own work; (2) to raise some of the more vexing quandaries that beset the field; and (3) to highlight emerging directions in EF research and theorizing.

These aims course through the chapter, and will unfold, firstly, by canvassing the varied ways in which EF is conceptualized and, the related issue of level or grain of analysis, in the context of EF representing a unitary or multifactorial construct. Approaches to EF at the micro-level of fractionated processes, the macro-level of a homunculus-like regulator of cognition, and also at a meso-level of meta-analysis are also documented. Both correlational and experimental laboratory approaches are canvassed. Then evidence of frontal involvement in EF characteristic of the cognitive neuroscience of aging will be considered. This chapter closes by looking forward to possible future directions and conclusions.

CONCEPTUALIZING EF

This section comprises two parts. First, the construct of EF is introduced in an historical context. Its origins within neuropsychology and cognitive psychology are articulated. Then the initial dominance within these traditions of task-based approaches is described and critiqued. Finally, structural approaches to defining EF and identifying their "unity and diversity" (Miyake et al., 2000) are presented.

Evolution of the Construct

Most fundamentally, EFs encompass controlled processing (Cohen, 2004). More than a century ago, it was proposed that "higher centers" of the brain *controlled* "lower centers" (Jackson, 1884 as cited in Daniels et al., 2006). Historically, the term also can be linked to the basic distinctions made decades ago between *structural components* and *control processes* (Atkinson & Shiffrin, 1968). These constitute a fundamental division of human memory into "learned or inherent structural components" in contrast to "labile" strategies used to execute a task such as encoding, rehearsal, or search. Control processes were further elaborated in dual-process theories of memory and attention that distinguish between cognitively *controlled*, in contrast to more *automatic* processing of information (Shiffrin & Schneider, 1977). Controlled processing refers to the deliberate activation of cognitive processes that require attention or effort to perform well on a given task. Automatic processing, on the other hand, is involuntary and initiated by the nature of the input, without deliberate intervention or control. According to Shiffrin and Schneider (1977) controlled processing is capacity-limited, but automatic processing is not. Hasher and Zacks (1979) drew out the implications of this model for cognitive aging. More recently, Daniels et al. (2006) concurred that cognitive control processes are "coextensive" with executive processes (p. 100). Control processes include *inter alia* rehearsal, coding, retrieval, decision making, and other deliberate strategies. Almost by definition, executive functions are many and varied.

The Confluence of Neuropsychology and Cognitive Psychology

Contemporarily, interest in EF and aging stems from the confluence of neuropsychology and cognitive psychology. Both approaches have subscribed to some extent to the frontal hypothesis or frontal-executive hypothesis of cognitive aging (Luszcz & Lane, 2008; Phillips & Henry, 2008).

From a neuropsychological perspective, the focus is on *executive dysfunction*: impairment in behavior or cognitive performance that is a direct consequence of neurological insult to the frontal lobes. The neuropsychologist's fundamental task is formally capturing the behavioral features of executive dysfunction to make, or confirm, a diagnosis. Hence, many of the psychometric tasks used to identify age-related differences in EF have been sourced from neurology and this tradition takes a more "global" view of what constitutes EF. EF is the metaphoric umbrella under which numerous variants or subcomponents shelter.

From a cognitive perspective, EF refers to a range of mental control processes associated with neuroanatomical integrity of the brain. Age-related differences in these processes are of interest in their own right (e.g., Salthouse et al., 2003) and also in terms of the extent to which they could serve as predictors of other aspects of cognition, mediators between aging and cognition (e.g., Bryan & Luszcz, 2000a; Head et al., 2008), or moderators of cognitive outcomes of interventions designed to enhance activity (e.g., Carlson et al., 2008). Viewed in this way, it is not surprising that EF constitutes a collection of interdependent higher order, strategic processes; that is a system of control processes (Luszcz & Lane, 2008).

In part, it is the dual lineage of the EF construct that is at the heart of the confusion concerning the variety of terms, concepts, and elements that appear in the literature. Salthouse (2005), who uses the term *executive functioning,* illustrates well the confusion that has arisen in the nomenclature attributed to both the tasks purported to measure executive functioning, and the way EF has been delineated by different writers. In general, neuropsychologists tend to refer to executive (or frontal) "function" (or functions). In contrast, within cognitive psychology or cognitive neuroscience executive *functioning* is used, putatively capturing the "processing" postulated to be *executive* (also referred to as "cognitive- control processes" or "executive control processes" or ECPs. Broadly, the two groups are referencing essentially the same *construct.*

The ambiguity is exacerbated when considering the terminology used to differentiate among EFs or processes. They have been described in a multitude of ways in the literature. For instance, Salthouse et al. (2003, p. 566) stated they may be "responsible for planning, assembling, coordinating, sequencing, and monitoring other cognitive operations." Friedman et al. (2008, p. 201) expanded considerably in their account:

> ***executive control may be more accurately characterized as a collection of related but separable abilities… arguably the three most frequently studied executive functions are response inhibition (the ability to inhibit dominant, automatic, or prepotent responses), updating working memory representations (the ability to monitor incoming information for relevance to the task at hand and then appropriately update by replacing old, no longer relevant information with newer, more relevant information, and set shifting (the ability to flexibly switch back and forth between tasks or mental sets).***

The common feature here, and elsewhere, is the notion of *control* or "the ability to direct mental function and behavior in accord with an internally represented set of intentions" (Cohen, 2001, p. 2089). The imperfect solution adopted in this chapter is to employ terminology in line with the source of the work. However, the neuropsychological versus cognitive approaches are not mutually exclusive, which, again, adds confusion.

Adding to the complexity, EF also has a part to play in regulating emotions and impulses, dealing with life's novelty and risks, and maintaining autonomy (Daniels et al., 2006); that is, it is crucial to adaptation (Hess, 2006 for a review). Thus EF plays a central role in psychosocial functioning (Henry et al., 2009) and motivation (Carstensen et al., 2006; Germain & Hess, 2007). The intersection of EF and these latter areas is only beginning to be explored in cognitive aging and warrants extensive further research.

The Dominance of Task-Based Approaches

Much of the initial research on EF has been task-driven with lean theoretical motivation apart from linking deleterious executive functioning to changes in neural substrates in the PFC (Hogan, 2004; Phillips & Henry, 2005 for critique).

The cross-fertilization between neuropsychological and cognitive approaches to understanding EF is evident in the relatively frequent use of psychometrically sound neuropsychological tests. Psychometric soundness, however, is not a sufficient basis for assuring that the underlying construct assessed is indicative of ECPs (Salthouse, 2005). It is fundamental also to demonstrate construct, convergent and discriminant validity of chosen measures (see Luszcz & Lane, 2008; Rabbitt, 1997; Salthouse et al., 2003 for more extended discussions) and, in longitudinal research, factorial invariance (de Frias et al., 2009).

Neuropsychologists, and much of the correlational research done by cognitive aging researchers, use psychometric tests that are likely to be multifaceted and hence reliant on multiple ECPs, as well as non-executive processes. Thus, they are assessing EF at a *macroanalytic* level and several studies have shown that when this is done, tasks are often found to be only moderately related to each other, and, quite often, also likely to be more related to non-executive than executive control processes (Salthouse, 2005). There also are pronounced differences in the level at which EF is operationalized within the cognitive aging literature, as will be discussed in the section on cognitive approaches to executive function.

As already discussed, there is no clear consensus about the number and nature of EFs. They, and the class of purportedly EF tasks used to assess them, tend to be described as "impure," multiply determined, and overlapping (Luszcz & Lane, 2008; Rabbitt, 1997). Previous writers have provided abundant coverage of various executive tasks. Articles that provide balanced and well-informed distillations of the utility of various instruments and their associated psychometric properties deal with detecting adult age differences in EF (Bryan & Luszcz, 2000b), detecting frontal deficits (Crawford & Henry, 2005), and provide details about and critiques several widely used tests of EF (Salthouse et al., 2003).

STRUCTURAL APPROACHES TO EXECUTIVE FUNCTION "UNITY AND DIVERSITY"

The ensemble of higher order processes already mentioned is far from an exhaustive inventory, but it illustrates the complexity inherent in attempts to delineate the fundamental nature of EF and the structure of the construct (Rabbitt, 1997 and/or Daniels et al., 2006 provide particularly lucid accounts of a range of complexities). Evidence reviewed next is illustrative of studies showing multiple (Hedden & Yoon, 2006; Hull et al., 2008) and unitary dimensions of EF (de Frias et al., 2006).

The work of Miyake et al. (2000) has been influential in shaping the focus of much of the contemporary research on EF, including cognitive aging. In their individual differences study, they used latent variables and confirmatory factor analysis to assess the organization and roles of a variety of executive functions in young adults. They concluded that EF could be characterized both by *unity*, suggesting complementarity among subcomponents of EF, and also *diversity*, suggesting that subcomponents could nonetheless be separable. Three proposed executive functions were confirmed as separable subcomponents of EF: *shifting* between tasks or mental sets, *updating* and monitoring of working memory, and *inhibition* of prepotent responses. Separability was considered indicative of the diversity of EF. Each subcomponent differentially predicted performance on more complex executive tasks: shifting contributed to Wisconsin Card Sorting Test (WCST) performance, inhibition to solving the Tower of Hanoi puzzle, and updating the Operation Span Task (a measure of verbal working memory capacity); this adds strength to the notion of diverse ECFs.

While separable, the subcomponents also were moderately correlated with each other. The authors explain the latter, in the face of the former, in terms of possible shared task requirements, the impure nature of even putatively basic EF tasks, or the necessity, regardless of the specific task, to keep goal-relevant information available in working memory. Miyake et al. (2000) concluded that it is simplistic to think of unity–diversity as a dichotomy, rather both seem to coexist. This conclusion is in accord with approaches to EF operating at different grains of analysis. That is, taking a *molar level* approach to EF is consistent with unity, while computational models involving fractionation of EF are characteristic of *microanalytic* approaches to EF, reflecting diversity. Strikingly, the coexistence of unity and diversity in EF is consistent with a genetic twin study done with Miyake's colleagues (Friedman et al., 2008). They demonstrated that inhibition, updating, and shifting were "correlated because they [each] are influenced by highly heritable (99%) common factor..." yet separable due to "additional genetic influences unique to particular executive functions" (56%: updating; 42%: shifting; variance in inhibition was entirely explained by the common EF factor). This level of heritability is greater than that for intelligence and strongly implicates an innate source for the coextensiveness of separable ECPs and a common EF factor. It also implies that the origin of individual differences in EF is hardwired.

Particularly pertinent to this chapter, Hull et al. (2008) adopted the Miyake et al. (2000) study as a model in their confirmatory factor analytic work with older adults. Results provided robust evidence for a shifting and an updating factor, but only one marker of an inhibition factor was extracted. The latter result adds to the debate about the distinctiveness of an inhibition construct, which is echoed by Daniels et al. (2006) and Salthouse (2005; Salthouse et al., 2003).

Inhibition gained prominence from the early work of Hasher and Zacks (1988) on inhibitory control in aging and continues as an important research heuristic (Darowski et al., 2008; Witthöft et al., 2009). While some (Hedden & Yoon, 2006) considered that inhibition is a "unifying principle of executive function" (p. 511), this conclusion seems premature. Inhibition is probably the least understood, although intuitively appealing, of Miyake et al.'s (2000) EF subcomponents.

Diversity of EF in Older Adults

Hedden and Yoon (2006) included multiple markers of shifting, updating, and inhibition in their study of older adults, along with measures of verbal and visual memory and perceptual speed. They adopted a correlated factors approach to determine if a unitary or multicomponent EF dimension emerged, and if it could be differentiated from memory and perceptual speed dimensions. The original model fit the data well, but in testing further models, the shifting and updating variables were defined as one EF dimension, with resistance to proactive interference (inhibition) as a second one. These EF constructs were distinct from the measures of verbal and visual memory and perceptual speed. However, the Stroop and antisaccade task loaded on the speed construct, rather than the intended inhibition construct, making this statement somewhat of an oversimplification of the findings. Salthouse's work (2003, 2005) showed that a variety of Stroop measures are strongly influenced by speed. Overall the results are consistent with the "diversity" of EF and its differentiation, although the fractionation of EF components was not entirely consistent with Miyake et al. (2000) or Hull et al. (2008).

Unity of EF

Other work has supported a single factor solution (unity), despite including tasks deemed to be tapping into discrete dimensions of EF. Taking data from the Victoria Longitudinal Study, de Frias et al. (2006) used newer (Brixton and Hayling tests developed by Burgess & Shallice, 1997) and traditional (WCST and Stroop) tests intended to predominantly measure shifting and inhibition, respectively. All four loaded on a single EF "factor". The same authors (de Frias et al., 2009) replicated a single factor solution, even though additional updating tasks were included.

What is innovative about the more recent report is that it addressed individual differences by classifying participants into three groups, along a continuum of cognitive functioning (impaired, normal, and elite). For the elite group only, the underlying three-factor structure emerged, which was consistent with Miyake et al. (2000). More important for all groups, their respective single-factor structures remained invariant over a three-year period. These results highlight the need to know more about the initial level of cognitive ability of participants under examination. They also may have theoretical implications for broader cognitive aging debates such as that surrounding dedifferentiation (see Anstey et al., 2003 for a combined, cross-sectional and longitudinal look at dedifferentiation, taking into account individual differences in age, ability, and attrition).

Interim Conclusion

These studies give a flavor of attempts to establish the structure of EF. They should be read in conjunction with Salthouse et al.'s (2003) thorough analyses of EF tasks putatively marking inhibition, updating, and shifting. They argue that these are elements required for many complex cognitive tasks, which ECPs are meant to orchestrate. For instance, they may obviate the "default option" in information processing; keep track of what is going on at a given time, and update adaptive responses accordingly; or coordinate multiple cognitive activities. Their findings provide only weak evidence for *unique* EF constructs or ones that are more related to EF than they are to other cognitive processes. Their findings also suggest caution on a number of levels, particularly in relation to construct and discriminant validity. Luszcz and Lane (2008) elaborated caveats about the utility of the EF construct in cognitive aging.

At this stage of theoretical development concerning EF, a task-driven approach may not be without merit. However, when using neuropsychological tests to operationalize EF much more attention needs to be paid to some of the basics of psychometrics (Luszcz & Lane, 2008). An alternative to reliance on blunt and multiply determined neuropsychological tests is to use more circumscribed and well-delineated experimental tasks to assist in advancing the field. It is to this approach that we next turn.

COGNITIVE APPROACHES TO EF

This section comprises both experiments and multivariate, correlational models that examine EF. Cognitive psychologists adopting experimental approaches implement a more fine-grained componential or *microanalytic approach* to executive functioning, compared to the *macroanalytic* approach associated with correlational studies of frontal tasks (Luszcz & Lane, 2008). A microanalytic approach aims to identify particular facets of EF that are operative or sensitive to aging, or likely to mediate relationships between aging and other aspect(s) of cognitive function under scrutiny (Head et al., 2008). In some cases, neuropsychological tasks are used as individual differences indicators of EF, along with an experiment designed to manipulate aspects of EF (e.g., Bryan & Luszcz, 2000a; Bryan et al., 1999). Task-switching paradigms and the process-dissociation procedure (PDP) are covered in this section to illustrate this alternative approach to isolating specific ECPs. It closes by addressing individual differences in EF based on mediation and moderation in EF.

Switching Tasks

Switching tasks lend themselves to fine-grained analysis. They necessitate maintaining and coordinating information across a series of trials. They generate both latency and accuracy data, although typically the data on speed of responding (latencies) are central to establishing age-related differences in ECP. This is because most often the "cost" of making (or failing to make) a switch is taken to indicate good (or poor) shifting of response or mental set, and coordinating the appropriate response depends on it. Costs can be calculated by subtracting a baseline response time from that observed on switch trials or by looking at the times taken to generate the two different types of responses.

This literature differentiates between *global* and *local* switches. Global switch costs are additive and arise from the effort to maintain a mental set, while local switch costs are those that occur as a response is made. In its simplest form, a switching task may require switching between two mental sets (A, B) equally often, and there are many parametric variants. In general, age differences are observed for global, but not local, task switches (e.g., Kray & Lindenberger, 2000). The difficulty is more one of holding competing sets in mind so that correct global switches can be made, rather than executing the actual (local) switch. This pattern varies as the number of sets to be maintained increases, with the cost for local switches rising (Kray et al., 2002) or when the need to switch is unpredictable (van Asselen & Ridderinkhof, 2000).

Verhaeghen and Cerella (2008) reviewed a vast body of work on switching tasks, much of which is covered in their previous meta-analyses (Verhaeghen & Cerella, 2002). They derived Brindley plots and state traces across studies. By aggregating smaller studies, general patterns emerge that may assist in resolving some of the inconsistencies when comparing individual studies. Aggregation should increase the sensitivity of data to demonstrating underlying cognitive, possibly executive, control processes. They refer to their meta-analytic approach to cognitive aging as operating at a *mesoanalytic level;* that is, in more detail than that of the macro-level characteristic of a task-based approach, but more coarsely than obtained in a micro-level analysis of individual experiments.

Their approach requires accepting the assumption that the tasks examined in the aggregate dataset represent similar processes. The plausibility of this assumption seems to have gone largely unchallenged. The feature of Verhaeghen and Cerella's review (2008) most pertinent to this chapter relates to tasks involving *multiple processing streams,* which they refer to as *compound* tasks (p. 140). These include the Stroop and switching tasks, among others, which require ECP of suppressing (i.e., inhibition of) prepotent responses (for local switching), and maintaining and coordinating (i.e., updating) two processing streams (for global switching), respectively. The control processes are quantified indirectly by contrasting the latencies for the simple and compound (multiple) processing streams.

With respect to aging, the aim is to compare any deficit on a simple task with that on a compound task to identify the deficit on the ECP. The compounding effect could be either *additive* (analogous to a fixed set-up charge associated with the extra processing element) or *multiplicative* (more time is required at each step along the way). Through their analyses Verhaeghen and Cerella (2008) sought to address two questions concerning aging-related effects attributable to ECP manipulations; one pertains to whether the control costs are additive or multiplicative and the other is whether any associated aging-related deficits are reliable.

They observed a multiplicative compounding effect in resistance to interference and in local switching, but an additive effect for global switching. The more striking results were that the magnitude of the multiplicative compounding effect was equivalent in younger and older adults, which contrasts with much of the literature, although additive compounding effects (local task switching) did show the usual age-related deficits. In processing terms, this means that when tasks required active selection of relevant information and ignoring irrelevant information, or shifting attention away from one aspect of a task to direct it to another, control-specific deficits did not emerge. It was only under conditions that required maintenance of two distinct mental sets, which added a step to the information-processing stream, that age differences emerged. Verhaeghen and Cerella (2008) suggested that the disparity between their findings and those seen across single studies in the literature may derive from failure to take into account baseline cognitive slowing, and they encouraged researchers to design studies that do so. They go on to suggest that their conclusions provided both a simpler and a more positive outlook for cognitive aging. Taken a step further, they, like Salthouse, called into question the need for a separate EF construct, and, it follows, the unity–diversity debate.

The Process-Dissociation Approach

Daniels et al. (2006) eloquently discussed the dilemma of attempting to disentangle specific executive processes from each other or other cognitive processes. Put simply, performance on most cognitive tasks (executive or otherwise) is likely to be dependent on multiple ECPs and efforts to isolate or partition variance associated with purported EFs have produced mixed results, both within and across studies (e.g., de Frias et al., 2006; Friedman & Miyake, 2004; Miyake et al., 2000; Salthouse et al., 2003; Salthouse, 2005). Instead Daniels et al. (2006) advocated a more computational (microanalytical) approach, using Jacoby's (1991)

PDP, which is redolent of dual process models (e.g., Hasher & Zacks, 1979; Shiffrin & Schneider, 1977) of memory and attention.

The goal of the PDP is to isolate and measure ECP within a range of cognitive tasks, rather than relying on "executive" tasks that may be driven by a combination of automatic and controlled processes. It generates parameter estimates that can then be used as valid indices of individual differences in EF (Salthouse et al., 1997). To do so, for example in the context of an episodic memory task, they differentiate between parameters of *recollection* (a controlled form of memory, showing age-related differences) and *familiarity* (a more automatic form of memory, such as a guess based on how accessible information is). Older adults typically show lower estimates of recollection than younger adults, but estimates of familiarity do not differ (e.g., Jacoby, 1991). Proactive interference, which has been characterized as an executive process reflecting inhibition (Hedden & Yoon, 2006), is another construct amenable to the PDP approach. In the case of proactive inhibition, the PDP distinguishes between recollection and the more automatic process associated with *accessibility bias* (based on familiarity and akin to guessing, in common parlance). If recollection fails, accessibility bias may provide a sufficient basis for remembering.

Jacoby et al. (2001) had older and younger adults study cue-target pairings of typical and atypical words for a pair-associates memory task. These were varied across study trials on a 50:50 or 75:25 basis, and at test the cue occurred with a word fragment that could be completed with either of the initially studied targets. When accessibility bias was varied (i.e., it was higher in the 75:25 than the 50:50 condition) during initial training, dissociations were observed that strongly supported their dual-process model. Moreover, in a second experiment, recollection, but not accessibility bias, was negatively influenced by age. So although older adults' recollection failed more often, older adults were no more influenced by accessibility bias than younger adults. These results, in combination with finding greater accessibility bias in a 75:25 condition, suggest that deficits in recollection, not inhibition of proactive interference, are producing the effect.

In relation to studies seeking to identify an EF factor associated with interference, these results suggest two things. It seems that a non-executive process (accessibility bias) may contaminate any index of proactive interference and, furthermore, if a latent factor is identified, it may be falsely assigned to a construct deemed to tap inhibition, when in fact, for older adults, failures in recollection may be at play.

Other research reported by Daniels et al. (2006) illustrated how multiple ECPs can be distinguished using the PDP. Research adopting the PDP explicitly supports the notion that successful execution of most complex tasks requires several ECPs, consistent with a "diversity" view of EF. More important, these can be estimated in elegant experiments designed to fractionate control processes specified a priori. The PDP offers to the field of EF and cognitive aging not only a technique with great potential to clarify aspects of ECP that are most vulnerable to, or spared from, the process of growing older, but also a formal model for conceptualizing the operationalizing of EF.

Mediation and Moderation in EF

The crux of ECPs is that they provide a mechanism for monitoring and regulating other cognitive processes. This modulation make take the form of EF mediating or moderating the relationship between age and a cognitive outcome, such as memory (Bryan & Luszcz, 2000a), as well as among executive cognitive processes and/or other cognitive processes (e.g., Head et al., 2008). Techniques to examine mediation and moderation explicitly address individual differences in EF and hence may demonstrate the nature and strength of their contribution to an outcome. Notwithstanding the debate about EF structure or component processes, we turn now to illustrative studies examining modulation of memory performance, impulsive behaviors, and goal setting by EF.

Work from our lab, based on data from the Australian Longitudinal Study of Ageing (ALSA), used three measures of fluency to index EF (Bryan & Luszcz, 2000b), along with measures of speed, verbal ability, and noncognitive individual differences to examine their meditation of age effects in incidental memory (Bryan & Luszcz, 2000a). Cross-sectional results provided small, but significant, evidence of EF mediation. In contrast, prospectively, over a six-year interval, once individual differences in baseline memory performance were taken into account further age-related variance in the memory measure on a second occasion could not be detected, precluding examination of its mediation by EF (Luszcz & Lane, 2008). However, individual differences in EF did predict change (across age) in memory. The contrast in cross-sectional and longitudinal findings bodes cautious interpretation of age differences from a single measurement occasion as indicative of developmental change.

Head et al. (2008, p. 491) wrote, that "mechanisms that mediate age-related declines in episodic memory are not well understood." Their study stands out as one that combined neuroanatomical (MRI regional volumes in prefrontal, caudate, hippocampus, and visual cortex) and cognitive mediators (processing speed, plus putative markers of EF: inhibitory control, working memory, temporal processing, and task switching) to examine age-related differences in episodic memory. Using a series of hierarchically nested path analyses, these variables completely mediated age-related differences in memory performance. Hippocampal shrinkage was the only region, and working memory, along with temporal processing, the only cognitive variables that directly affected episodic memory. Reductions in prefrontal regions affected inhibitory control which, along with processing speed, had their effects via working memory. Speed also had an indirect effect via temporal processing. These results illustrate the selectivity of neuroanatomical and EF effects, the complexity of their interface with each other and with processing speed, and the value of a multivariate approach to understanding brain-behavior relationships. A similar approach, done longitudinally, would shed light on how these neuroanatomical, executive- and non-executive cognitive processes capture change in episodic memory, as well as other varieties of memory.

Going beyond the cognitive domain, a few studies have begun to look at the role of ECPs in regulating impulses and goal setting. Social cognitive studies provide insight into situations where the role of EF mediates, or can be moderated by, social or motivational processes. Henry et al. (2009) postulated that executive deficits might contribute to socially inappropriate behaviors and disrupt social exchanges. Path analyses indicated that the effect of age on a composite measure of social functioning was completely eliminated when measures of EF (Trail Making and Fluency) and general ability were included in the model. As a further example, motivational influences were observed on controlled processing (inhibition of attention to distracting words) of text varying in relevance to participants (Germain & Hess, 2007). Both younger and older adults did better when text was judged to be more relevant to them, and the effect was especially strong for the older participants.

These studies are important in providing preliminary evidence for the importance of executive control in social settings. They also provide ecological validity for the ubiquity of ECPs in the daily lives of older people (see also Hess et al., 2009).

COGNITIVE NEUROSCIENCE AND PREFRONTAL INVOLVEMENT IN EF

Behavior is increasingly reported to map onto brain areas through activation patterns observed in neuroimaging and event-related potential (ERP) studies (Buckner, 2004; Park & Reuter-Lorenz, 2009; Wilson, 2008). Much has been written relating poorer executive functioning to differential brain atrophy localized to the frontal lobe, especially the PFC (Hogan, 2004; West, 1996). Until the turn of the century, however, research directly illustrating this relationship was scant and results were equivocal (Phillips & Henry, 2005; Tisserand & Jolles, 2003). Technological advances, neuroimaging techniques (see Hayes & Cabeza, 2008, for a review of techniques), and theories linking brain-behavior relationships in cognitive aging (Greenwood, 2007; Park & Reuter-Lorenz, 2009; Stern, 2009) are adding clarity to the field at an unprecedented rate. Theorizing has progressed from the descriptive level, characteristic of the frontal-executive hypothesis, to integrative theories of the aging mind, of which STAC (Park & Reuter-Lorenz, 2009) is exemplary. STAC proposes that pervasive age-related increased frontal activation is indicative of an adaptive brain, dynamically responding to challenges encountered in cognitive (or everyday) tasks, in the face of neurodegeneration. Scaffolding is a life-long process providing the mechanism for compensation for neurodegeneration.

The next section selectively reviews cognitive neuroscience approaches to identifying frontal involvement in executive functioning. A meta-analysis on brain activation (Spreng et al., 2010) in aging provides an extensive account, which is not possible here. Several chapters in this volume deal specifically with neurocognitive aging (especially Chapters 5 and 7).

Volumetric Work and a Specific Frontal Task

The first example draws on research using the WCST (Heaton, 1981), one of the most widely used neuropsychological indices of frontal function. Performance on the WCST has been shown to correlate with frontal lobe volume (e.g., Gunning-Dixon & Raz, 2003; Head et al., 2002) and has also been related to fluid ability. Thus the WCST requires recruitment of several ECP, notably shifting, monitoring, inhibiting of prepotent responses, and updating of working memory. Therefore it is likely that a combination of factors may contribute to performance. This is also true of fluid intelligence, which extends to, but is not isomorphic with, EF, and is also reliant on frontal integrity (see Duncan, 2005; Luszcz & Lane, 2008).

In a study including participants ranging in age from 20 to 92, Schretlen et al. (2000) demonstrated that fluid ability could be independently predicted not only by frontal integrity, but also by behavioral measures of EF (WCST), and speed. This suggests that neural substrates, along with ECPs and processing resources, combine additively to produce cognitive outcomes, consistent with the position of Wilson (2008) and Head et al. (2008).

Diffuse Brain Integrity and Frontal/Executive Function

An ambitious study by Rabbitt and colleagues (2007) addressed diffuse brain integrity and EF. Accepting that it is not "prudent" to link specific neurophysiological markers to specific cognitive processes, they tracked multiple markers of diffuse brain atrophy contemporaneously with administration of a large battery of cognitive and neuropsychological tasks in older adults (61–85 years). Magnetic resonance imaging brain scans, along with measures of cerebrospinal fluid (CSF) and carotid and basilar artery blood flow (CBF) were used together to construct a neurophysiological (NEURO) latent variable. The cognitive battery comprised multiple markers assessing each of five domains: frontal/executive function, fluid and crystallized intelligence, speed of processing, and memory. Structural equation modeling was implemented to examine direct and indirect effects of age and brain integrity measures on cognitive functioning. Because the role of speed in these relationships was also examined, this work marks an important step in addressing whether (1) neurophysiological effects are widespread and general or differentially salient for executive functioning and (2) whether they operate through processing resources to influence, for example, executive functioning.

A selection of findings most relevant to this chapter is highlighted. The NEURO measure had its strongest effect on speed and completely accounted for age-related variance in it. Furthermore, EF was more strongly predicted by the NEURO index than any of the remaining measures of cognition. Notably speed partially mediated the relationship between the NEURO index and executive functioning, with age continuing to contribute to executive functioning. Finally, fluid ability and EF were highly correlated and the effect of NEURO on executive tasks occurred partially through speed and intelligence.

The work of Rabbitt et al. (2007) showed that, if understanding of frontal/executive function is to be advanced, further research will be necessary to find ways to differentiate it from other cognitive constructs (Crawford & Henry, 2005; Luszcz & Lane, 2008). Secondly, while the array of NEURO markers was substantial, there are many other markers that could have been examined. Thirdly, there are wide individual differences in the patterns of change in both neurophysiological and cognitive systems (e.g., West et al., 2010), which make generalizations about the causal connections between them highly speculative. Finally, the results are silent concerning the frontal-executive hypothesis of cognitive aging: specific ECP and brain areas could not be linked in this study. Studies of frontal *activation* provide a way to do so, but they too have their limitations, particularly because they necessitate examining more circumscribed cognitive tasks.

Frontal Activation Patterns

A recent meta-analysis using activation likelihood estimation (ALE; Spreng et al., 2010) summarized results from brain areas from the "task-positive network" (TPN; see Toro et al., 2008) that are active during a wide range of externally driven cognitive tasks, including EF tasks, and the "default network," those areas active in response to internally driven cognitive processes or when people are at rest. Studies of frontal activation have shown that, compared to younger adults, *lower* activation occurs among older adults when they are at rest (Petit Taboué et al., 1998), encoding (Grady, 2002), or attending to information (Milham et al., 2002). On the other hand, there is evidence of *higher* levels of frontal activation on a range of externally driven tasks (Grady, 2002; Nielson et al., 2002). The TPN was active across age groups in the 80 studies in the meta-analysis; however, many areas showed age differences in activation levels and patterns. The frontal cortex featured prominently in distinguishing situations where age differences were, or were not, observed.

When performance of older and younger adults was equivalent (e.g., for spatial and temporal context retrieval, Rajah et al., 2010), older adults were more likely to activate the left dorsolateral prefrontal cortex (DLPFC), but young adults activated the left ventrolateral prefrontal cortex (VLPFC). Germaine to this chapter is that these two areas of frontal cortex are implicated in ECPs, such as holding of information in working memory (left VLPFC) and manipulation of information or strategic processing (left DLPFC).

When performance of older adults was poorer than that of younger adults (e.g., for relational encoding, Leshikar et al., 2010), it was the right PFC that distinguished the groups. EF tasks showed greater engagement of the rostrolateral prefrontal cortex (RLPFC), and activation increased with age. They concluded that "brain activity in young adults has a larger dynamic range than that of old adults" (DOI p. 10).

Bilaterality is another feature of activation that distinguishes older adults and younger adults. Older adults are more likely to demonstrate bilateral frontal activation, whereas younger adults' activation, for example, in memory encoding, is primarily in the left PFC, while retrieval activates the right (Nyberg et al., 1996). Decreases in left prefrontal activity in aging tend to be interpreted as indicative of neurocognitive decline, while increases in right prefrontal activity may reflect compensatory processes (Hayes & Cabeza, 2008) indicative of dysfunction (Spreng et al., 2010).

Cabeza and colleagues (2007) formalized these effects in the Posterior-Anterior Shift in Aging model (PASA; Dennis et al., 2007) and the Hemispheric Asymmetry Reduction in Older Adults model (HAROLD; Cabeza, 2002). Park and Reuter-Lorenz (2009) articulated how these patterns and compensatory scaffolding mediate the relationship between age and cognition.

Event-Related Potentials and Executive Functioning

Alongside the imaging work localizing activation associated with ECPs is research using ERPs to track in real time the occurrence and duration of these processes. Friedman et al. (2008) using a task-switching paradigm, showed that on switch trials ERP components relating to task-set attention, re-allocation of attention, and conflict monitoring/detection were elicited for younger, but not older adults. Rather, the older adults' data were more consistent with ongoing recruitment of executive processes when task demands did not require them to do so. They also interpreted their results in the context of selective breakdown of executive processes when resources required to implement them were over-taxed and compensation fails.

Other evidence from ERP studies can be seen early in filtering of irrelevant information (Zanto et al., 2010), related to inhibition, and later on for maintenance of multiple sets for task switching (Androver-Roig & Barceló, 2010). These results provided evidence of the unfolding of stages of processing indicative of EF tasks. West et al. (2010) examined EF in the oddball task, which requires monitoring of a series of stimuli for the occurrence of a low probability stimulus (i.e., the oddball) in the context of frequent (standard) or irrelevant (novel) stimuli. In these studies questions surrounded localization of the oddball effect to the frontal region or whether it was more distributed across other regions, determining if there were age differences in the expression of novelty, and how individual differences in EF might influence the effect of age. Neither age nor individual difference effects were observed in distinguishing the oddball from standard stimuli. For novel stimuli, in contrast, the expected posterior-anterior shift occurred and was stronger for older adults. The age effect interacted with individual differences in EF, with the novelty component revealed for both novel and oddball stimuli for older adults with lower EF, but only for novel stimuli in older adults with higher EF.

Interim Conclusion

In discussing neurological factors in cognitive aging, Wilson (2008) posited that the emerging picture is one of accumulation of neuropathological lesions resulting from genetic and experiential risk factors. Individual differences (e.g., Rabbitt et al., 2007; West et al., 2010) in rates and regions affected are widespread as well as evidence of loss of cognitive functioning or, depending on presence or absence of risk factors, maintenance of function. The best empirical example of the latter arises from the Religious Orders Study (Wilson et al., 2004, 2007).

That a frontal-executive hypothesis of cognitive aging is an oversimplification is the position of a number of writers (Daniels et al., 2006; Hayes & Cabeza, 2008; Hogan, 2004; Luszcz & Lane, 2008; Phillips & Henry, 2005; Rabbitt et al., 2007), but several recent theories have emerged that have elaborated on the involvement of the PFC in EF and its connectivity to other brain regions, and articulated how and when compensatory mechanisms are likely to maintain behavioral performance in older adults on par with younger adults. The diffuse and global nature of changes in the brain, and interrelations among white matter lesions, cell loss, and changes in cerebral blood flow suggest that no single area of the brain is responsible for particular cognitive changes and surely not all the age-related variance on a given cognitive task, executive or otherwise. Nonetheless, incremental progress is being made in the unveiling of brain-behavior relations in later life as indicated in other chapters in this handbook (eg., Chapters 5 and 7).

LOOKING FORWARD

On the one hand, the complexity of findings, differences in conceptualizations, interpretations, and implementation of EF research and a dynamic theoretical milieu auger well for the longevity of the field. On the other hand, EF skeptics have yet to be convinced that there is much theoretical traction to be gained by adding executive functions to the array of extant cognitive constructs with which they overlap. One way forward is to make more use of techniques like the PDP, elegant experimental designs, meta-analytic approaches, or integrative analysis of multiple datasets (Anstey et al., 2010) to distill the *essence* of EF. Utilization of more global frontal tasks will retain a place, particularly if their dominant subcomponents can be tied conceptually and methodologically to other more tractable domains of cognition.

Initial theoretical development relied on the somewhat amorphous frontal-executive hypothesis which posited that early and marked age-related changes localized to the frontal lobe were associated with deficient executive control processes. Theories like STAC, as well as notions of cognitive reserve and plasticity, have immense heuristic value not only in bringing together ideas about how brain aging and cognitive aging affect the aging mind, but also by putting meat on the conceptual bones of how compensation may occur when at the limits of cognitive challenge or environmental pressure. It goes without saying that as techniques advance for concomitant monitoring of brain and behavior, the subtleties of EF may be able to be mapped, and monitoring of them in real time and longitudinally will reveal more about the veracity of these hypotheses. Even more exciting is the potential that neuroimaging studies have for identifying age differences that are not apparent in behavioral measures (e.g., Rajah et al., 2010). However, at the construct level, there is much to be established about the behavioral side of ECPs to clarify just what is being mapped.

The interface of cognition, emotion, health, and social domains are waiting to be explored in relation to the aging of EF and warrant extensive further research. This suggestion arises not only because such investigations are in their infancy, but also because they contextualize the study of EF in situations where competence in their use is likely to be most critical for day-to-day functioning and quality of life. Initial work in this area is likely to stimulate much more along these lines.

The genetic work of Friedman et al. (2008) provided powerful evidence for the necessity to take individual differences in EF into account. Likewise more behavioral work (e.g., de Frias et al., 2009) and work combining behavioral and neurological measures (e.g., Head et al., 2008) to examine how individual differences in EF mediate age effects or cognitive outcomes is crucial. Across the board, the challenge remains to reconcile the unity and diversity of EF. Given their seeming ubiquity in the lab and when navigating life's dynamic transactions, the heuristic potential of the construct is immense.

CONCLUSIONS

The conflation of performance on executive tasks with underlying executive functions while not entirely helpful in advancing the field, has induced more careful consideration of the grain of analysis required to best understand EF it sparked the confluence of neuropsychology and cognitive psychology, which in turn highlighted brain-behavior relations, and, with the emergence of the cognitive neuroscience of aging, has focussed attention on the need for theory-based approaches to EF. One legacy from a neuropsychological approach, where executive assessments occur in the context of a frank or suspected acquired frontal neurological insult, has been to assume that processes underlying patients' performance and those of aging adults are the same. This conclusion is premature because disparities have been observed in both clinical samples (Andrés & Van der Linden, 2000; Burgess, 1997) and samples of "healthy" older adults (e.g., Salthouse et al., 2003) on tasks that purport to measure the same underlying construct.

The hodgepodge of tasks featured in the literature on executive functioning has led to much confusion and difficulty in clearly discerning the nature of the control processes underlying them (see Burgess et al., 2006 for excellent review and suggested solutions; Fuster, 2002 for an account of the morphological development of the PFC and its implications for cognition). This state of affairs can be attributed in large part to two interrelated practices characteristic of research on EF. One has to do with operationalizing the construct in terms of tasks, traditionally arising from neuropsychology, but more recently from cognitive psychology. Secondly, some researchers view the EF construct at a very general level (e.g., Duncan, 2005) while others have gone to great lengths to fractionate executive processes or varieties of it into smaller subcomponents (e.g., Kemper & McDowd, 2008).

Perhaps not since the advent of the general slowing hypothesis has the field of cognitive aging been captivated by the possibilities perceived in EF for advancing understanding of maintenance and loss of cognitive competence. Processing efficiency is a prerequisite for optimizing cognitive functioning, placing fundamental limits all along the information processing chain. Executive control processes provide mechanisms for flexibly adapting to cognitive demands. Fascination with these two constructs foreshadows continuation of a lively research agenda surrounding them, within and beyond the lab.

REFERENCES

Adrover-Roig, D., & Barceló, F. (2010). Individual differences in aging and cognitive control modulate the neural indexes of context updating and maintenance during task switching. *Cortex, 46*, 434–450.

Andrés, P., & Van der Linden, M. (2000). Age-related differences in supervisory attentional system functions. *Journals of Gerontology: Psychological Sciences, 55*, 373–380.

Anstey, K. J., Byles, J. E., Luszcz, M. A., Mitchell, P., Steel, D., Booth, H., et al. (2010). Cohort profile: The dynamic analyses to optimise ageing (DYNOPTA) project. *International Journal of Epidemiology, 39*(1), 44–51.

Anstey, K. J., Hofer, S. M., & Luszcz, M . A. (2003). Cross-sectional and longitudinal patterns of dedifferentiation in late-life cognitive and sensory function: The effects of age, ability, attrition and time of measurement. *Journal of Experimental Psychology: General, 132*, 470–487.

Atkinson, R. C., & Shiffrin, R. M. (1968). Human memory: A proposed system and its control processes. In K. Spence & J. Spence, (Eds.). *The psychology of learning and motivation*, (vol. 2, pp. 89–195). New York: Academic Press.

Band, G. P., Ridderinkhof, H., & Segalowitz, S. (2002). Explaining neurocognitive aging: Is one factor enough? *Brain and Cognition, 49*, 259–267.

Bryan, J., & Luszcz, M. A. (2000a). Measures of fluency as predictors of incidental memory among older adults. *Psychology and Aging, 15*, 483–489.

Bryan, J., & Luszcz, M. A. (2000b). The measurement of executive function: Considerations for detecting adult age differences.

Journal of Clinical and Experimental Neuropsychology, 22, 40–55.

Bryan, J., Luszcz, M. A., & Pointer, S. (1999). Executive function and processing resources as predictors of adult age differences in the implementation of encoding strategies. *Aging, Neuropsychology, and Cognition, 6*, 273–287.

Buckner, R. L. (2004). Memory and executive function in aging and AD: Multiple factors that cause decline and reserve factors that compensate. *Neuron, 44*(1), 195–208.

Burgess, P. W. (1997). Theory and methodology in executive function. In P. Rabbitt (Ed.), *Methodology of frontal and executive function* (pp. 81–116). Hove, England: Psychology Press.

Burgess, P. W., & Shallice, T. (1997). *The Hayling and Brixton Tests*. Thurston, England: Thames Valley Test.

Cabeza, R. (2002). Hemispheric asymmetry reduction in older adults: The HAROLD model. *Psychology and Aging, 17*, 85–100.

Carlson, M. C., Saczynski, J. S., Rebok, G. W., Seeman, T., Glass, T. A., McGill, S., et al. (2008). Exploring the effects of an "everyday" activity program on executive function and memory in older adults: Experience Corps. *The Gerontologist, 48*, 793–801.

Carstensen, L. L., Mikels, J. A., & Mather, M. (2006). Aging and the intersection of cognition, motivation, and emotion. In J. E. Birren & K. W. Schaie (Eds.), *Handbook of the psychology of aging* (6th ed.) (pp. 343–362). San Diego, CA: Academic Press.

Cohen, J. D. (2004). Cognitive control (executive functions): role of prefrontal cortex. In J. S. Neil & B. B. Paul (Eds.), *International Encyclopedia of the Social & Behavioral Sciences* (pp. 2089–2094). Oxford: Pergamon.

Crawford, J. R., Bryan, J., Luszcz, M. A., Obonsawin, M. C., & Stewart, L. (2000). Executive decline hypothesis of cognitive aging: do executive deficits qualify as differential deficits and do they mediate age-related memory decline?. *Aging, Neuropsychology, and Cognition, 7*, 9–31.

Crawford, J. R., & Henry, J. D. (2005). Assessment of executive deficits. In P. W. Halligan & N. Wade (Eds.), *The effectiveness of rehabilitation for cognitive deficits* (pp. 233–246). London: Oxford University Press.

Daniels, K., Toth, J., & Jacoby, L. (2006). The aging of executive functions. In E. Bialystock & F. I. M. Craik (Eds.), *Lifespan cognition: Mechanisms of change* (pp. 96–111). New York: Oxford University Press.

Darowski, E. S., Helder, E., Zacks, R. T., Hasher, L., & Hambrick, D. Z. (2008). Age-related differences in cognition: The role of distraction control. *Neuropsychology, 22*, 638–644.

Davis, S. W., Dennis, N. A., Daselaar, S. M., Fleck, M. S., & Cabeza, R. (2008). Que PASA? The posterior-anterior shift in aging. *Cerebral Cortex, 18*(5), 1201–1209.

de Frias, C. M., Dixon, R. F., & Strauss, E. (2006). Structure of four executive functioning tests in healthy older adults. *Neuropsychology, 20*, 206–214.

de Frias, C. M., Dixon, R . F., & Strauss, E. (2009). Characterizing executive functioning in older special populations: from cognitively elite to cognitively impaired. *Neuropsychology, 23*, 777–791.

Dennis, N. A., Daselaar, S., & Cabeza, R. (2006). Effects of aging on transient and sustained successful memory encoding activity. *Neurobiology of Aging, 28*, 1749–1758.

Dolcos, F., Rice, H. J., & Cabeza, R. (2002). Hemispheric asymmetry and aging: Right hemisphere decline on asymmetry reduction. *Neuroscience and Biobehavioral Reviews, 26*, 819–825.

Duncan, J. (2005). Frontal lobe function and general intelligence: Why it matters. *Cortex, 41*, 215–217.

Friedman, N. P., & Miyake, A. (2004). The relations among inhibition and interference control functions: A latent variable analysis. *Journal of Experimental Psychology: General, 133*, 101–135.

Friedman, N. P., Miyake, A., Young, S. E., DeFries, J. C., Corley, R. P., et al. (2008). Individual differences in executive functions are almost entirely genetic in origin. *Journal of Experimental Psychology: General, 137*, 201–225.

Friedman, D., Nessler, D., Johnson, R., Jr., Ritter, W., & Bersick, M. (2008). Age-related changes in executive function: An event-related potential (ERP) investigation of task-switching. *Aging, Neuropsychology, and Cognition, 15*, 95–128.

Fuster, J. M. (2002). Frontal lobe and cognitive development. *Journal of Neurocytology, 31*, 373–385.

Germain, C. M., & Hess, T. M. (2007). Motivational influences on controlled processing: Moderating distractibility in older adults. *Aging, Neuropsychology, and Cognition, 14*, 462–486.

Grady, C. L. (2002). Age-related differences in face processing: A meta-analysis of three functional neuroimaging experiments. *Canadian Journal of Experimental Psychology, 56*, 208–220.

Grady, C. L., Protzner, A. B., Kovacevic, N., Strother, S. C., Afshin-Pour, B., Wojtowicz, M. A., et al. (2010). A multivariate analysis of age-related differences in default mode and task positive networks across multiple cognitive domains. *Cerebral Cortex, 20*, 1423–1447.

Greenwood, P. M. (2007). Functional plasticity in cognitive aging: Review and hypothesis. *Neuropsychology, 21*, 657–673.

Gunning-Dixon, F., & Raz, N. (2003). Neuroanatomical correlates of selected executive functions in middle-aged and older adults: A prospective MRI study. *Neuropsychologia, 41*, 1929–1941.

Hasher, L., & Zacks, R. T. (1979). Automatic and effortful processes in memory. *Journal of Experimental Psychology: General, 108*(3), 356–388.

Hasher, L., & Zacks, R. T. (1988). Working memory, comprehension, and aging: A review and a new view. In G. H. Bower (Ed.), *The psychology of learning and motivation* (Vol. 22, pp. 193–225). Orlando, FL: Academic Press.

Hayes, S. M., & Cabeza, R. (2008). Imaging aging: Present and future. In S. M. Hofer & D. F. Alwin (Eds.), *The handbook of cognitive aging: Interdisciplinary perspectives* (pp. 308–326). Thousand Oaks, CA: Sage Publications.

Head, D., Buckner, R. L., Shimony, J. S., Girton, L. E., Akbudak, E., Conturo, T. E., et al. (2004). Differential vulnerability of anterior white matter in nondemented aging with minimal acceleration in dementia of the Alzheimer type. Evidence from diffusion tensor imaging. *Cerebral Cortex, 14*, 410–423.

Head, D., Raz, N., Gunning-Dixon, F., Williamson, A., & Acker, J. D. (2002). Age-related differences in the course of cognitive skill acquisition: The role of regional cortical shrinkage and cognitive resources. *Psychology and Aging, 17*, 72–84.

Head, D., Rodrigue, K. M., Kennedy, K. M., & Raz, N. (2008). Neuroanatomical and cognitive mediators of age-related differences in episodic memory. *Neuropsychology, 22*(4), 491–507.

Heaton, R. K. (1981). *A manual for the Wisconsin Card Sorting Test*. Odessa, FL: Psychological Assessment Resources.

Hedden, T., & Yoon, C. (2006). Individual differences in executive processing predict susceptibility to interference in verbal working memory. *Neuropsychology, 20*, 511–528.

Henry, J. D., & Phillips, L. H. (2006). Covariates of production and perseveration on tests of phonemic, semantic and alternating fluency in normal aging. *Aging, Neuropsychology, and Cognition, 13*, 529–551.

Henry, J. D., von Hippel, W., & Baynes, K. (2009). Social inappropriateness, executive control, and aging. *Psychology and Aging, 24*, 239–244.

Hess, T. M. (2006). Attitudes toward aging and their effects on behavior. In J. E. Birren & K. W. Schaie (Eds.), *Handbook of the psychology of aging* (6th ed.), (pp. 379–406). San Diego, CA: Academic Press.

Hess, T. M., Germain, C. M., Swaim, E. L., & Osowski, N. L. (2009). Aging and selective engagement: The moderating impact of motivation on older adults' resource utilization. *Journals of Gerontology: Psychological Sciences, 64B*, 447–456.

Hogan, M. J. (2004). The cerebellum in thought and action: A fronto-cerebellar aging hypothesis. *New Ideas in Psychology, 22*, 97–125.

Hull, R., Martin, R. C., Beier, M. E., Lane, D., & Hamilton, A. C. (2008). Executive function in older adults: A structural equation modeling approach. *Neuropsychology, 22*, 508–522.

Jackson, J. H. (1844). Croonian lectures on evolution and dissolution of the nervous system. *Lancet, 1, 555–558*(649–652), 739–744.

Jacoby, L. L. (1991). A process dissociation framework: Separating automatic from intentional uses of memory. *Journal of Memory and Language, 20*, 513–541.

Jacoby, L. L., Debner, J. A., & Hay, J. F. (2001). Proactive interference, accessibility bias, and process dissociations: Valid subjective reports of memory. *Journal of Experimental Psychology: Learning, Memory, and Cognition, 27*, 686–700.

Juardo, M. B., & Roselli, M. (2007). The elusive nature of executive functions: a review of our current understanding. *Neuropsychological Review, 17*, 213–233.

Kemper, S., & McDowd, J. (2008). Dimensions of cognitive aging: Executive function and verbal fluency. In S. M. Hofer & D. F. Alwin (Eds.), *The handbook of cognitive aging: Interdisciplinary perspectives* (pp. 181–192). Thousand Oaks, CA: Sage Publications.

Kray, J., Li, K. Z. H., & Lindenberger, U. (2002). Age-related changes in task-switching components: The role of task uncertainty. *Brain and cognition, 49*, 363–381.

Kray, J., & Lindenberger, U. (2000). Adult age differences in task switching. *Psychology and Aging, 15*, 126–147.

Leshikar, E. D., Gutchess, A. H., Hebrank, A. C., Sutton, B. P., & Park, D. C. (2010). The impact of increased relational encoding demands on frontal and hippocampal function in older adults. *Cortex, 46*(4), 507–521.

Lessov-Schlaggar, C. N., Swan, G. E., Reed, T., Wolf, P. A., & Carmelli, D. (2007). Longitudinal genetic analysis of executive function in elderly men. *Neurobiology of Aging, 28*(11), 1759–1768.

Luszcz, M. A., & Bryan, J. (1999). Toward understanding age-related memory loss in late adulthood. *Gerontology, 45*, 2–9.

Luszcz, M. A., & Lane, A. (2008). Executive function in cognitive, neuropsychological, and clinical aging. In S. M. Hofer & D. F. Alwin (Eds.), *The handbook of cognitive aging: Interdisciplinary perspectives* (pp. 193–206). Thousand Oaks: Sage Publications.

Male, S. J., Sheppard, D. M., & Bradsway, J. L. (2009). Aging extends the time required to switch cognitive set. *Aging, Neuropsychology , and Cognition, 16*, 589–606.

Milham, M. P., Erickson, K. I., Banich, M. T., Kramer, A. F., Webb, A., Wszalek, T., et al. (2002). Attentional control in the aging brain: Insights from an fMRI study of the Stroop task. *Brain and Cognition, 49*, 277–296.

Miyake, A., Friedman, N. P., Emerson, M. J., Witzkik, A. H., Howerter, A., & Wager, T. D. (2000). The unity and diversity of executive functions and their contributions to complex "frontal lobe" tasks: A latent variable analysis. *Cognitive Psychology, 41*, 49–100.

Nielson, K. A., Garavan, H., & Langenecker, S. A. (2002). Differences in the functional neuroanatomy of inhibitory control across the adult life span. *Psychology and Aging, 17*, 56–71.

Nyberg, L., Cabeza, R., & Tulving, E. (1996). Pet studies of encoding and retrieval: The HERA model. *Psychonomic Bulletin and Review, 3*, 135–148.

Park, D. C., & Reuter-Lorenz, P. (2009). The adaptive brain: Aging and neurocognitive scaffolding. *Annual Review of Psychology, 60*, 173–196.

Petit Taboué, M. C., Landeau, B., Desson, J. F., Desgranges, B., & Baron, J. C. (1998). Effects of healthy aging on the regional cerebral metabolic rate of glucose assessed with statistical parametric mapping. *Neuroimage, 7*, 176–184.

Phillips, L. H., & Andrés, P. (2010). The cognitive neuroscience of aging: New findings on compensation and connectivity. *Cortex, 46*(4), 421–424.

Phillips, L. H., & Henry, J. D. (2008). Adult aging and executive functioning. In V. Anderson, R. Jacobs, & P. J. Anderson (Eds.), *Executive functions and the frontal lobes: A lifespan perspective* (pp. 57–79). New York: Psychology Press.

Phillips, L. H., & Henry, J. D. (2005). An evaluation of the frontal lobe theory of cognitive aging. In J. Duncan, P. McLeod, & L . H. Phillips (Eds.), *Measuring the mind: Speed, control and age* (pp. 191–216). Oxford, UK: Oxford University Press.

Rabbitt, P. (1997). Introduction: Methodologies and models in the study of executive function. In P. Rabbitt (Ed.), *Methodology of frontal and executive function* (pp. 1–38). London: Psychology Press.

Rabbitt, P., Mogapi, O., Scott, M., Thacker, N., Lowe, C., Horan, M., et al. (2007). Effects of global atrophy, white matter lesions, and cerebral blood flow on age-related changes in speed, memory, intelligence, vocabulary, and frontal function. *Neuropsychology, 21*, 684–695.

Rajah, M. N., Languay, R., & Valiquette, L. (2010). Age-related changes in prefrontal cortex activity are associated with behavioural deficits in both temporal and spatial context memory retrieval in older adults. *Cortex, 46*(4), 535–549.

Raz, N. (2000). Aging of the brain and its impact on cognitive performance: Integration of structural and functional findings. In F. I. M. Craik & T. A. Salthouse (Eds.), *Handbook of aging and cognition* (pp. 1–90). Mahwah, NJ: Lawrence Erlbaum.

Royall, D. R., Lauterbach, E. C., Cummings, J. L., Reeve, A., Rummans, T. A., Kaufer, D. I., et al. (2002). Executive control function: A review of its promise and challenges for clinical research. *Journal of Neuropsychiatry and Clinical Neurosciences, 14*, 337–405.

Salthouse, T. A. (2000). Pressing issues in cognitive aging. In D. C. Park & N. Schwarz (Eds.), *Cognitive aging: A primer* (pp. 43–54). Philadelphia, PA: Psychology Press.

Salthouse, T. A. (2005). Relations between cognitive abilities and measures of executive functioning. *Neuropsychology, 19*, 532–545.

Salthouse, T. A., Atkinson, T. M., & Berish, D. E. (2003). Executive functioning as a potential mediator of age-related cognitive decline in normal adults. *Journal of Experimental Psychology: General, 132*, 566–594.

Salthouse, T. A., Toth, J. P., Hancock, H. E., & Woodard, J. L. (1997). Controlled and automatic forms of memory and attention: Process purity and the uniqueness of age-related influences. *Journals of Gerontology: Psychological Science, 52B*, P216–P228.

Schretlen, D., Pearlson, G. D., Anthony, J. C., Aylward, E. H., Augustine, A. M., Davis, A., et al. (2000). Elucidating the contributions of processing speed, executive ability, and frontal lobe volume to normal age-related differences in fluid intelligence. *Journal of the International Neuropsychological Society, 6*, 52–61.

Shiffrin, R. M., & Schneider, W. (1977). Controlled and automatic human information processing: II. Perceptual learning, automatic attending and a general theory. *Psychological Review, 84*, 127–190.

Spreng, R. N., Wojtowicz, M., & Grady, C. L. (2010). Reliable differences in brain activity between young and old adults: A quantitative meta-analysis across multiple cognitive domains. *Neuroscience & Biobehavioral Reviews*, in press.

Stern, Y. (2009). Cognitive reserve. *Neuropsychologia, 47*(10), 2015–2028.

Tisserand, D. J., & Jolles, J. (2003). On the involvement of prefrontal networks in cognitive aging. *Cortex, 39*, 1107–1128.

Toro, R., Fox, P. T., & Paus, T. (2008). Functional coactivation map of the human brain. *Cerebral Cortex, 18*, 2553–2559.

van Asselen, M., & Ridderinkhof, K. R. (2000). Shift costs of predictable and unexpected set shifting in young and older adults. *Psychologica Belgica, 40*, 259–273.

Verhaeghen, P., & Cerella, J. (2002). Aging, executive control, and attention: A review of meta-analyses. *Neuroscience and Biobehavioral Reviews, 26*, 849–857.

Verhaeghen, P., & Cerella, J. (2008). Everything we know about aging and response times: A meta-analytic integration. In S. M. Hofer & D. F. Alwin (Eds.), *The handbook of cognitive aging: Interdisciplinary perspectives* (pp. 134–150). Thousand Oaks, CA: Sage Publications.

West, R. L. (1996). An application of prefrontal cortex function theory to cognitive aging. *Psychological Bulletin, 120*, 272–292.

West, R., Schwarb, H., & Johnson, B. N. (2010). The influence of age and individual differences in executive function on stimulus processing in the oddball task. *Cortex, 446*, 550–563.

Wilson, R. L. (2008). Neurological factors in cognitive aging. In S. M. Hofer & D. F. Alwin (Eds.), *The handbook of cognitive aging: Interdisciplinary perspectives* (pp. 298–307). Thousand Oaks, CA: Sage Publications.

Wilson, R. S., Arnold, S. E., Schneider, J. A., Li, Y., & Bennett, D. A. (2007). Chronic distress, age-related neuropathology and late life dementia. *Psychosomatic Medicine, 69*, 47–53.

Wilson, R. S., Bienias, J. L., Evans, D. A., & Bennett, D. A. (2004). Religious Orders Study: Overview and change in cognitive motor speed. *Journal of Aging, Neuropsychology and Cognition, 11*, 281–303.

Witthöft, M., Sander, N., Sub, H. M., & Wittmann, W. (2009). Adult age differences in inhibitory processes and their predictive validity for fluid intelligence. *Aging, Neuropsychology, and Cognition, 16*(2), 133–163.

Zanto, T. P., Henning, K., Östberg, M., Clapp, W. C., & Gazzaley, A. (2010). Predictive knowledge of stimulus relevance does not influence top-down suppression of irrelevant information in older adults. *Cortex, 46*, 564–574.

Chapter | 5 |

The Cognitive Consequences of Structural Changes to the Aging Brain

Karen M. Rodrigue, Kristen M. Kennedy
School of Behavioral and Brain Sciences, University of Texas, Dallas, Texas, USA

CHAPTER CONTENTS

Introduction **73**
Volume of the Gray and White Matter **74**
Manual Morphometry to Study Brain Aging 74
Voxel-Based Morphometry 74
Studies of Regional Brain Volume and Cognitive Aging 75
Episodic Memory 75
Executive Function 75
Working Memory 76
Procedural Learning and Memory 76
Fluid Intelligence 76
Cortical Thinning to Study Brain Aging **76**
Studies of Regional Cortical Thickness and Cognitive Aging 77
Structure-Function Studies 77
Vascular Risk Modifies Structural Brain Aging 77
White Matter Integrity **77**
White Matter Hyperintensity Burden in Aging 77
Studies of WMH and Cognitive Aging 78
Executive Functioning 78
Working Memory 78
Fluid Intelligence 79
Episodic Memory 79
Processing Speed 79
Diffusion Tensor Imaging to Study Brain Aging **79**
DTI Studies of Cognitive Aging 80
Executive Functions 80
Working Memory 80
Episodic Memory 81
Processing Speed 81
Motor Performance 81
DTI and fMRI Integration Studies 81
Magnetization Transfer Imaging 82
Studies of MTR and Cognitive Aging 82
Beta-Amyloid Deposition **83**
Studies of Aβ Imaging and Cognitive Aging 83
Structure-Function Studies 83
Discussion **84**
Summary and Conclusions **84**
Acknowledgments **85**
References **85**

INTRODUCTION

Like all organs in the human body, the brain experiences wear and tear throughout the life span. Because the state of the brain's structure affects the quality of its function, the study of changes in brain structure has proven fruitful in understanding cognitive aging. In this chapter we briefly review the history of the morphometric research (changes to the size and shape of the brain's structure) on normal brain aging and examine in detail recently developed techniques for measuring the brain's structure and exploring structure-function association studies conducted within each neuroimaging modality in the context of aging. For comparison purposes, in this chapter we chose to review those studies whose participants included

DOI: 10.1016/B978-0-12-380882-0.00005-X

"normal" aging (excluding those who studied mild cognitive impairment or neurodegenerative disease) and whose methodology in each technique followed the most standard protocols. We conclude the chapter with a look toward needed future research directions with a particular focus on combined multimodality structure-function studies and a more careful selection and characterization of the health indices of the participants selected for cognitive aging studies.

VOLUME OF THE GRAY AND WHITE MATTER

Manual Morphometry to Study Brain Aging

Historically, measurement of brain structure (volume of the white matter, cerebral cortex, ventricular spaces) involved postmortem histology investigations (for review see Kemper, 1994), and with the advent of magnetic resonance imaging (MRI) progressed to digital 3D assessment of regional brain volume differences (as measured in cross-sectional studies) and changes (measured in longitudinal studies) with age (for review see Raz, 2000). Consistent with postmortem studies, in vivo MRI studies show significant negative correlations between age and overall brain tissue volume (e.g., $r = -0.41$ in Raz et al., 1997). However, because the last decades of research have established that brain aging is differential among its regions, this field of study has moved beyond simple whole brain, or whole gray or white matter measurements.

Most of what is known about aging of the brain's structure is based upon manual volumetry — a technique consisting of manually tracing individual brain regions of interest (ROIs) on each participant's high-resolution MRI scan and computing the total volume across the slices. Utilization of this "gold-standard" methodology has led to an understanding of the differential pattern of regional brain aging. This differential brain aging is reflected by the greatest age vulnerability in the association cortices, which are responsible for aggregating processing across modalities and for higher level cognitive processing. The primary sensory cortices — for example, primary visual cortex, primary motor, and somatosensory cortex — are less vulnerable to the aging process (for detailed reviews see Raz, 2000; Raz & Kennedy, 2009; Raz & Rodrigue, 2006). Regionally, the prefrontal cortex shows the highest associations with age ($r = -0.56$; Raz, 2004), temporal regions more moderate relations ($r = -0.37$), followed by smaller effects in parietal ($r = -0.20$) and occipital regions across studies ($r = -0.19$; Raz, 2004). For subcortical structures, volumes of the amygdala, hippocampus, cerebellum, and neostriatum (i.e., caudate and putamen) show a moderately negative age association (median correlations range between $r = -0.43$ and -0.30). In contrast, age-related differences observed in the globus pallidus ($r = -0.20$) and the thalamus ($r = -0.28$) have been minimal overall, and the pons appears resilient to aging, showing little to no volume reductions (median $r = 0.07$, Raz, 2004). These age associations tend to be linear in cortical gray matter regions, with the exception of the hippocampus, but tend to display an accelerated trajectory with age in the white matter volume. In fact, when examining the entire age span from infancy the white matter volume displays an inverted U-shaped function with growth until adolescence, a plateau in middle adulthood, and decline in older age (Bartzokis et al., 2001; Courchesne et al., 2000; Kennedy et al., 2009a; Raz et al., 2005).

Longitudinal studies of regional brain shrinkage (which measure true changes with aging) are rarer than cross-sectional studies of aging. However, the most frequent longitudinal studies use the manual volumetry approach. Fewer techniques discussed later in this chapter have been used in longitudinal studies to date, and thus the bulk of what we know about individual brain aging over time comes from the manual volumetry literature (reviewed in Raz & Kennedy, 2009). The consensus is that longitudinal studies show a similar pattern of regional decline to cross-sectional studies, with a tendency toward an *underestimation* of decline compared to true measurement of shrinkage (Raz & Kennedy, 2009; Raz et al., 2005), in contrast to the cross-sectional *overestimation* seen in cognitive aging studies (Sliwinski & Buschke, 1999). However, there also appears to be a great deal of temporal variability in regional volume as well, as evidenced by multiwave (i.e., greater than two time points) longitudinal studies (Raz et al., 2010). Many more longitudinal studies of regional brain volume change are needed, ideally with multiple time-point measures. However, this is difficult work to do and newer techniques are constantly evolving to allow the automation (or semi-automation) of brain structure measurement. The caveat is that these new methods are imperfect to varying degrees and must be used with caution and knowledge of neuroanatomy. We will discuss these new methods in turn in this chapter.

Voxel-Based Morphometry

Manual measurement of regional brain volume on MRI scans is vastly time-consuming work that needs to be conducted by trained personnel with a good knowledge of neuroanatomy and highly reproducible, reliable measurements. Thus, automated and semi-automated methods of estimating regional brain volume have been developed, one of which is voxel-based morphometry (VBM; Ashburner & Friston, 2000). VBM uses the intensity value of each voxel (3D pixel element) in the brain to assign it as gray, white, or cerebrospinal fluid (CSF) probability and after averaging all participants' brains in the study to a template coordinate space, can calculate group (e.g., age or disease) differences at each voxel. This technique became rapidly and widely popular in the last decade because of its ease of use. However, as validation studies and method comparisons began to be conducted it has been shown that VBM does not estimate true volume well (concordance between methods ranged from $r = 0.01$ to 0.56 across 15 regions tested; Kennedy et al., 2009a). This is likely because the method is based on intensity at each voxel instead of a more meaningful biological basis. Thus, VBM has come to be considered as a nonspecific measure of brain matter "density" and the technique is only recommended for hypothesis-generating exploratory studies to be followed up with specified regional analyses (Kennedy et al., 2009a; Tisserand et al., 2002).

Studies of Regional Brain Volume and Cognitive Aging

Given that the brain's function ostensibly relies on the brain's structural integrity, many studies have embarked on relating age differences (and changes) in regional volume to their putative underlying function. The resulting literature is mixed in its findings because the brain's volume fluctuates over decades (incorporating growth and shrinkage), and because middle and older aged adults are probably able to compensate for degradation to the brain's structure over time (Cabeza, 2002; Park & Reuter-Lorenz, 2009; Raz & Kennedy, 2009) or rely upon cognitive reserve resources to compensate for declines in structural integrity (Stern, 2002). Further, structure-cognition associations are not easily replicated and are sensitive to type of cognitive assessment and to sample composition. Below we summarize the volume-cognition studies by cognitive domain.

Episodic Memory

Probably the most investigated aspect of cognition is episodic memory. Several studies have examined regions of the temporal cortex for associations with memory performance. In general, smaller hippocampi volume in older adults is associated with poorer memory (e.g., Cardenas et al., 2009; Golomb et al., 1994; Raz et al., 1998; Walhovd et al., 2004; Ystad et al., 2009; Zimmerman et al., 2008), but overall these effect sizes are weak (Van Petten, 2004) and likely depend on a complex mixture of mediating factors (Head et al., 2008). Hackert et al. (2002) found in a large sample that selectively the anterior (head) of the hippocampus was associated with verbal memory performance. Others have found that not necessarily the hippocampus but the posterior portion of the parahippocampal gyrus volume is associated with memory decline over time (Burgmans et al., 2009). Still others have found that not hippocampal shrinkage (over five years) but entorhinal shrinkage in the oldest adults was associated with poorer memory performance (Rodrigue & Raz, 2004). In general, intact medial temporal (MTL) volume appears to be important in maintaining memory performance with aging, although the relative sensitivity of the precise MTL regions to cognitive decline is less clear. However, longitudinal evidence points to extra-hippocampal regions as the most sensitive to memory decline.

Executive Function

In total, it appears that the ability to successfully plan, organize, and execute cognitive output with age is dependent upon the availability of sufficiently intact volumes of prefrontal cortices (PFC). Better performance on some executive tasks (e.g., Wisconsin Card Sorting Test, WCST) is associated with larger PFC (Gunning-Dixon & Raz, 2003; Head et al., 2009; Raz et al., 1998). Multivariate analyses of brain volume and cognition reveal that age-related differences in volume exert effects on executive function via complex associations of mediating factors. For example, Head et al. (2009) found that age-related increase in perseveration on WCST is differentially dependent on the integrity of PFC but also on declines in selected cognitive processes such as processing speed, temporal order processing, working memory, and inhibition, which also depend upon this region. In old beagles, smaller PFC volume was associated with poorer inhibitory control and working memory performance (Tapp et al., 2004). Lateral frontal "volumes" significantly predicted performance on an executive function composite score in older adults in a VBM study (Zimmerman et al., 2006). In a deformation-based morphometry (DBM) study, which improves upon some of the problems in VBM, Cardenas et al. (2009) found that areas in the lateral posterior frontal gray matter and superior posterior cerebellum were associated with age-related changes in an executive function composite score. Finally, in a small sample of older adults, Elderkin-Thompson et al. (2008) found differential effects among the PFC subregions and differing aspects of executive function. In that study greater volume of the anterior cingulate was associated with Stroop interference and larger gyrus rectus volume was associated with inductive reasoning, whereas *smaller* orbitofrontal volume was associated with greater verbal fluency. Somewhat surprisingly, other studies have also found negative correlations between PFC volume and cognitive performance (Duarte et al., 2006; Salat et al., 2002; Van Petten et al., 2004), but these are usually found in truncated age-range samples. In sum, maintenance of executive functions with aging clearly depends upon an intact volume of the prefrontal cortex, and perhaps anterior cingulate and cerebellum as well.

Working Memory

The literature on neuroanatomical correlates of working memory is less clear. Salat et al. (2002) reported that better working memory was seen in older adults with *smaller* orbitofrontal volumes, and Gunning-Dixon & Raz (2003) did not find a significant association between working memory and either prefrontal or fusiform cortex volume. In a longitudinal study Raz et al. (2007) found that shrinkage of the fusiform gyrus over five years predicted working memory decline. While working memory is an interesting cognitive construct in its own right, most volume-cognition studies have used working memory performance as a mediating factor in predicting age-related differences in other domains of cognition. In an early study, Raz et al. (1998) found that secondary visual cortex volume, but not prefrontal volume, was associated with better nonverbal working memory, which in turn mediated age-related explicit memory performance. Similarly, age-related deficits in visuospatial mental imagery performance was selectively associated with smaller prefrontal cortex and age-related declines in working memory (Raz et al., 1999). Working memory has been found to be a significant mediator of episodic memory and perseverative errors, respectively, and in both cases working memory was mediated by PFC volume (Head et al., 2008, 2009). Working memory was also a salient mediator of implicit measures of priming and skill learning performance in many of our studies (e.g., Ghisletta et al., 2010; Kennedy & Raz, 2005; Kennedy et al., 2008; Kennedy et al., 2007; Kennedy et al., 2009c; Moffat et al., 2007; Raz et al., 2000). Thus, working memory likely depends upon intact volume in a wide variety of structures across the brain (mainly association cortices).

Procedural Learning and Memory

Volumes of specific brain regions have also been associated with age-related differences in procedural learning and memory tasks. Raz et al. (2000) found volume of the putamen and cerebellum (but not caudate or hippocampus) to be associated with a perceptual motor task (pursuit rotor) in early stages of learning, but only associated with cerebellar volume at later stages of learning. In a perceptual-motor skill-learning task with a more cognitive component (mirror drawing), larger caudate and prefrontal cortex volumes were associated with better accuracy and faster speed (Kennedy & Raz, 2005). In a visual-perceptual task (identification of fragmented pictures) Kennedy et al. (2009c) found that repetition priming was significantly associated with visual cortex volume, and skill learning on the same task was associated with PFC volume. Head et al. (2002), in a cognitive skill learning task (Tower of Hanoi), found that PFC volume was associated with early learning but not with performance at later trials. Finally, in a study of virtual spatial navigation, shorter distances to reach the end of the maze were associated with larger caudate, prefrontal gray and white matter volumes, and selectively for the younger adults, volume of the hippocampus (Moffat et al., 2007). Thus, it appears that procedural learning is independent of MTL structurally and depends upon prefrontal, neostriatal, and cerebellar regions of the brain (dependent on type of task). The importance of these regions shift with the transition from the earlier, more effortful phase to later more automatic processing.

Fluid Intelligence

Finally, a few studies have investigated the role of regional brain volumes in supporting fluid intelligence/reasoning abilities. In an early study, age-related declines in fluid intelligence were explained by smaller frontal lobe volume, executive ability, and processing speed (Schretlen et al., 2000). Raz et al. (2008) found in a five-year longitudinal study that lower levels of fluid intelligence were associated with smaller prefrontal and hippocampal volumes. Further, lower fluid intelligence scores were also linked to greater longitudinal shrinkage of the entorhinal cortex. When accounting for vascular risk factors, orbitofrontal cortex and the prefrontal white matter volumes as well as a five-year change in entorhinal volume predicted fluid intelligence level, whereas vascular risk was independently associated with smaller prefrontal volumes and lower fluid intelligence. In a VBM and stereology (i.e., point counting) study, Gong et al. (2005) found increased medial PFC gray matter VBM density to be associated with Cattell Culture Fair intelligence scores and with WAIS intelligence, but not verbal scores. They also found stereology correlations between dorsolateral prefrontal cortex volume and Cattell scores, all after controlling for age. Finally, Kennedy et al. (2009c) found that via prefrontal white matter volume, working memory and fluid intelligence mediated the age-related differences in perceptual repetition priming and skill learning. These results suggest that fluid intelligence is likely supported by intact prefrontal gray and white matter volume and is closely related to other domains of cognition such as working memory and processing speed.

CORTICAL THINNING TO STUDY BRAIN AGING

The majority of literature on brain structure and cognitive aging is focused on brain volume; however, there are two components to volume: surface area and thickness. Recently, (semi-) automated techniques have been developed to assess cortical thickness (e.g., FreeSurfer;

Fischl & Dale, 2000). This method generates the thickness of the outer gray matter cortical ribbon of the brain by measuring the distance between where the cortex begins at the surface of the brain (i.e., the pia mater lining) to where the gray matter meets the underlying white matter at each point along the entire cortical ribbon. This approach provides a great deal of spatial information across the brain, and (unlike VBM) offers the advantage of anatomically guided user correction of segmented images and the ability to generate regional volumes on the individual level in contrast to comparisons at the group level with VBM.

A few papers have amassed, characterizing the pattern of regional cortical thinning with normal aging. Salat et al. (2004) was the first to investigate normal aging and found the usual pattern of gray matter aging described previously with volume methods, with the exception of additionally finding age-related thinning of the primary motor and visual sensory cortices, regions that have been age-invariant using past methods of morphometry. Age-related thinning of primary sensory cortex, however, has yet to be consistently replicated (Fjell et al., 2009) and may depend on the health of the individuals sampled.

Studies of Regional Cortical Thickness and Cognitive Aging

Only a handful of cortical thinning and cognitive performance associations have been published to date, most of which are cross-sectional. Fjell et al. (2006) found that older adults who were aging cognitively better than average (on tests of fluid intelligence) had thicker cortex across the brain than the averagely performing old. Interestingly, the high functioning older adults had thicker posterior cingulate cortex than the young adults, suggesting that cortex may thicken and thin in a cyclic fashion across the duration of the adult life span. Dickerson et al. (2008) found in a small sample of older adults that verbal memory performance was associated with medial temporal cortical thickness, and Trail Making performance was associated with lateral parietal thickness. Attentional control assessed in a dichotic listening task was found to be correlated with cortical thickness estimates in posterior middle frontal cortex and in a posterior portion of the anterior cingulate (Andersson et al., 2009). Longitudinally, verbal recall after two to three months was better in individuals with thicker cortex in orbital and middle frontal, parietal regions, precuneus, and temporal regions (Walhovd et al., 2006).

Structure-Function Studies

In a structure-function association study, Fjell et al. (2007) demonstrated that for young adults, P3 amplitude during event-related potential recording from a visual oddball task was not associated with cortical thickness measures, whereas for older adults frontal, parietal, temporoparietal, and posterior cingulate thickness was associated with P3 potentials. Moreover, Braskie et al. (2009) found that those individuals with thicker left entorhinal cortex had increased activation in anterior cingulate and medial frontal cortex during associative verbal memory retrieval. These structure-behavioral association studies lend evidence for the integrity of the brain's structure giving rise to the quality of its functional capacity.

Vascular Risk Modifies Structural Brain Aging

Even within a tightly controlled sample of normal adults, both positive and negative modifiers can alter the trajectory of aging for each individual. Essential hypertension is a common age-related diagnosis that confers significant vascular risk to healthy neurocognitive aging (Marin & Rodriguez-Martinez, 1999). Chronic elevation of blood pressure increases the negative effects of aging on brain structure (e.g., de Leeuw et al., 2001). Untreated hypertension adversely affects performance on many cognitive tasks (e.g., Waldstein et al., 1991), but negative effects may be especially pronounced on tasks that tap executive functions, speed of processing, and memory (e.g., Harrington et al., 2000; Raz et al., 2003). A higher prevalence of white matter abnormalities and smaller volume of the PFC compared to demographically matched controls has been observed (Raz et al., 2003). Longitudinal research shows that age-related shrinkage of some brain regions (hippocampus, orbitofrontal cortex, prefrontal white matter) is accelerated by hypertension (Raz et al., 2005), and even regions considered impervious to structural aging, such as primary visual cortex, show mild age-related shrinkage (Raz et al., 2007). Consequently, what is perceived as healthy brain aging is confounded at least in part by vascular risk in most studies (see Raz & Rodrigue, 2006 for review). Because vascular health has such a significant effect on brain and cognitive measures, care should be taken to either screen for this risk factor, or explicitly examine it in future aging studies.

WHITE MATTER INTEGRITY

White Matter Hyperintensity Burden in Aging

A traditionally used indicator of white matter health is measurement of white matter hyperintensity (WMH) burden, so named because of the bright-appearing signal seen on T2-weighted and fluid attenuated inversion recovery (FLAIR) images. These

WMH occur around the borders of the ventricles (i.e., periventricular WMH) and deep in the subcortical white matter (i.e., deep WMH). Both qualitative and quantitative methods have been used to assess WMH burden. Qualitative methods generally use a point-counting system and quantitative methods measure the volumes of the WMH. It is generally accepted that the best measure of WMH burden is volume of WMH by lobe and by type — periventricular WMH or deep WMH (Yoshita et al., 2005). The pathogeneses of WMH lesions are multiple and varied and include decreased cerebral perfusion, subclinical ischemia, and axonal degeneration following neuronal loss (de Leeuw et al., 2001). WMH accumulation in the aging brain is believed to reflect insufficient perfusion to the brain as hypertension and reduced cerebral blood flow have been shown to increase risk of WMH (Raz et al., 2003; Tzourio et al., 2001) and hypertension is associated with increased progression of WMH over five years (Raz et al., 2007). Further, vascular impact on WMH may depend on the type of WMH; arterial stiffness has been associated with periventricular, but not deep WMH (Ohmine et al., 2008).

White matter hyperintensities are generally not present in healthy adults until about the age of 50 to 55 (Hopkins et al., 2006) at which point they begin to accumulate in prevalence and size. They also appear to be under strong genetic influence — the heritability rate is >70% (Carmelli et al., 1998). WMH burden is greatest in frontal and parietal white matter in healthy aging (Fazekas et al., 2005; Gootjes et al., 2004; Gunning-Dixon & Raz, 2000, 2003; Raz & Kennedy, 2009) and expands to occipital white matter in older adults with vascular risk (Raz et al., 2007).

Studies of WMH and Cognitive Aging

Given the importance of healthy functioning white matter in maintaining cognitive health, several studies have investigated the role of WMH burden on age-related declines in cognitive performance. An early meta-analysis found that WMH burden was most strongly associated with age-related declines in executive functions, processing speed, and memory (Gunning-Dixon & Raz, 2003). Others have reported that WMH burden is correlated with subjective cognitive complaints at an earlier stage than actual cognitive performance declines can be measured (Dufouil et al., 2005). It has also been proposed that WMH burden is a surrogate for reduced cerebral connectivity (Cook et al., 2002; Leuchter et al., 1994) and is responsible in part for age-related slowing of processing speed (Oosterman et al., 2004) and declines in frontally mediated cognitive functions (Bunce et al., 2007; DeCarli et al., 1995; Swan et al., 1998).

Executive Functioning

Because the distribution of WMH in normal aging is greatest in the frontal white matter, most studies have examined the effect of WMH burden on executive functioning. Many different aspects of executive functions have been examined, including perseveration (or mental inflexibility), set shifting, planning, task switching, verbal fluency, and inhibition. In the 2003 study by Gunning-Dixon & Raz, frontal lobe WMH (but not temporal lobe WMH) selectively predicted increased problems with perseveration, but not working memory. Similarly, in an independent sample Raz et al. (2003) found that individuals with hypertension had greater frontal WMH burden than normotensives, and hypertensives demonstrated increased perseveration problems compared to normotensive peers. However, others did not find an association between WMH and perseveration (Vannorsdall et al., 2009), perhaps because they did not measure WMH by region, and frontal WMH burden may play a selective role in perseverative behavior. Other studies examining WMH and executive functioning have reported a selective effect on the Trail Making Test (Cook et al., 2002) while others found no significant effect of WMH on that task of alternating sets (Oosterman et al., 2008). Verbal fluency has been investigated frequently as well with most studies finding increased WMH load associated with reduced fluency (Paul et al., 2005; Söderlund et al., 2006; Vannorsdall et al., 2009). Similarly, Oosterman et al. (2008) and Söderlund et al. (2006) found a significant relation between specifically periventricular WMH burden and Stroop interference, but Nebes et al. (2006) found no association between WMH and inhibition. Finally, further underscoring the heterogeneous nature of executive functions, one study found WMH to be correlated with maze navigation and set switching (Paul et al., 2005) and another found a significant association between WMH and planning (on a Tower of Hanoi type task) but not for set shifting (Oosterman et al., 2008).

Working Memory

Several studies have also investigated the role of WMH accumulation in working memory performance, a process that is posited to be distributed throughout brain regions, but with an important role of the frontal lobes. For example, in Raz et al. (2007) we found that five-year expansion of deep WMH was associated with declines in working memory span in the vascular risk group but not in the healthier group. Similarly, Gunning-Dixon & Raz (2003) did not find an association between frontal or temporal WMH and working memory in a healthy group of adults suggesting that for WMH to disrupt working memory performance, sufficient vascular risk must be present to induce greater WMH burden. Vannorsdall et al. (2009) found both periventricular and deep WMH burden associated with decreased working memory, but two other studies did not find an association (Nebes et al., 2006; Oosterman et al., 2008). Interestingly, in an fMRI study of verbal working memory and episodic memory, Nordahl et al. (2006) found that greater WMH burden in the prefrontal white matter was associated with decreased activation in the posterior parietal and anterior cingulate cortices, lending further support that WMH burden disrupts cognitive function because it degrades the transmittal of neural information not only in proximal but also in far distal brain regions.

Fluid Intelligence

Most studies of abstract reasoning and fluid intelligence have demonstrated a significant relation between WMH burden and these abilities. Longitudinal increase in WMH volume over five years was associated with longitudinal decline in fluid ability (Raz et al., 2007). Similarly, Garde et al. (2000) found in a cohort of 80 year olds who had been tested with the WAIS multiple times throughout their lives that both periventricular and deep WMH burden was associated with longitudinal decline in intelligence, primarily on tests that measure performance rather than verbal abilities, perhaps due to the motor and/or speeded nature of those tasks. In line with these findings, Vannorsdall et al. (2009) found periventricular WMH burden to be negatively associated with fluid, but not crystallized, intelligence scores. Cook et al. (2002) also found a significant association between lower abstract reasoning and increased WMH burden.

Episodic Memory

Of five studies that investigated episodic memory performance, three found a significant association of WMH burden (Nordahl et al., 2006; Petkov et al., 2004; van Petten et al., 2004) but the other two found no such association (Söderlund et al., 2006; Vannorsdall et al., 2009). Van Petten et al. (2004) found that a memory factor was predicted by subcortical WMH load, particularly visual paired associates, delayed cued recall of a word list, and logical memory for prose. In the Petkov et al. (2004) study WMH burden was the strongest predictor of delayed free-recall of all the structural brain measures. Söderlund et al. (2006) found no association for word list memory, and Vannorsdall et al. (2009) found no effect for verbal or visual memory. In their functional episodic memory study Nordahl et al. (2006) found that both global and frontal WMH burden predicted decreased PFC activity during episodic retrieval as well as decreased medial temporal and anterior cingulate activity, again underscoring the distributed effect of WMH on connectivity across the brain.

Processing Speed

Perhaps the most putatively relevant cognitive correlate of WMH burden would be speed of information processing that readily declines in even healthy aging. Indeed, WMH burden was found to be selectively related to processing speed (Nebes et al., 2006), with some evidence that periventricular WMH are more strongly associated with processing speed than deep WMH (Vannorsdall et al., 2009). When several domains of cognition are examined in one study, WMH correlate most strongly with processing speed tasks (Dufouil et al., 2003). Thus, these studies confirm that WMH are responsible in part for the slowing of motor and cognitive processing in the brain.

DIFFUSION TENSOR IMAGING TO STUDY BRAIN AGING

Whereas investigation of WMH provides a gauge of the state of the macrostructure of the white matter and its lesions, diffusion tensor imaging (DTI) provides a more microstructural index of white matter health. DTI is a relatively new neuroimaging technique (Pierpaoli & Basser, 1996) that gauges the microstructural integrity of the myelinated fibers in the brain at a level not detectable on T2-weighted or FLAIR images as WMH. DTI is based on the fact that water diffuses differently in different types of tissue: water diffuses almost at random in CSF, is more constrained in the gray matter, and highly constrained in white matter. As normal, healthy white matter tracts lose organization (i.e., with age or a disease process), the water diffuses in a less constrained fashion. Two measures that are commonly computed from DTI, fractional anisotropy (FA) and apparent diffusion coefficient (ADC), reflect integrity and directionality of the white matter microstructure (within a voxel) and the intactness of fiber tracts and water diffusibility across the fibers, respectively. FA is a scalar measure that ranges from 0 to 1, with higher numbers reflecting greater anisotropy, or more directionally constrained fibers. ADC is a measure of the speed of diffusion (mm^2/s) across the tissue. More recently, the eigenvalues of the tensor have been used to describe more specific components of diffusion. The eigenvalues of the principle axis of diffusion (along the axon) is termed axial or longitudinal diffusivity, whereas the average of the other two eigenvalues, termed radial or transverse diffusivity, is an index of diffusion across the axon. It is believed, then, that reduced axial diffusivity reflects axonal damage, whereas reduced radial diffusivity reflects myelin-specific damage. Further animal work needs to be done to confirm these relations, but thus far this finer distinction of diffusivity seems to hold promise for specifying the type of white matter damage measured by DTI.

Early DTI studies used histogram analyses or voxel-based measures to investigate the whole brain white matter compartment and therefore are unable to speak to regional, anatomically specific age differences in white matter integrity. However, many studies reported regional variability in the age-related FA declines and ADC increases, thus suggesting that white matter vulnerability to aging may be selective and differential (e.g., Hugenschmidt et al., 2008; Kennedy & Raz, 2009a; Pfefferbaum et al., 2000; Pfefferbaum & Sullivan, 2003; Salat et al., 2005; Sullivan et al., 2001). Among the studies that focused on regional diffusion properties of the cerebral white matter, most agree upon a decrease in FA and increase in ADC in the centrum semiovale, corona radiata, pericallosal frontal and parietal areas, and periventricular regions. Less consistent patterns of results have been found in other regions, such as the limbs of the internal capsule and the splenium. According to some studies, the effect of age is greater in the anterior than posterior regions of the brain (e.g., Head et al., 2004; Kochunov et al., 2007; Madden et al., 2007; O'Sullivan et al., 2001; Pfefferbaum et al., 2000; Salat et al., 2005; Sullivan et al., 2001; Sullivan & Pfefferbaum, 2006). However, age-related declines in the splenium of the corpus callosum and the occipital white matter have been reported as well (e.g., Abe et al., 2002; Head et al., 2004; Kennedy & Raz, 2009a; Pfefferbaum et al., 2000, 2005; Sullivan et al., 2006). More important, these posterior aging findings may be selectively due to vascular (Kennedy & Raz, 2009a) and/or genetic effects (Kennedy et al., 2009b). In fact, the splenium of the corpus callosum has a threefold higher heritability rate than the genu of the callosum (Pfefferbaum et al., 2001).

Fiber-tracking analysis of DTI data showed that the most prominent age-related deterioration of the white matter is observed in association fibers (Stadlbauer et al., 2008), which connect the regions that are the last to complete myelination in the course of development (Flechsig, 1901). In fact, Raz (2000) and Raz & Kennedy (2009) reported a strong correspondence between the developmental order of myelination and the magnitude of volume decline with age. Regression of regional age effect measures and annualized shrinkage rates on Flechsig's myelination precedence ranks revealed that regions late to myelinate were those that demonstrated the strongest age-related shrinkage (inferior temporal, dorsolateral prefrontal, inferior parietal, orbitofrontal cortices). Myelination order accounts for 36% of the variance in age differences in regional cortical volumes, and 38% of the variance in regional cortical shrinkage in a 5-year period (Raz & Kennedy, 2009).

DTI Studies of Cognitive Aging

Executive Functions

In the earliest study that examined white matter integrity effects on cognitive performance in aging, O'Sullivan et al. (2001) found that increased diffusivity in the anterior third of the brain correlated 0.61 with poorer performance on an executive function test (Trail Making Test, but not on WCST) and FA in the "middle" third correlated 0.61 with verbal fluency in 17 older adults. These findings led the authors to put forth the results as evidence for cortical disconnection as a mechanism of age-related cognitive decline. Since then, executive functions have been the most widely examined domain of cognition using DTI. Reduced verbal fluency has been associated with increased frontal, occipital, and deep white matter diffusivity (Shenken et al., 2005). Further, Deary et al. (2006) additionally found in a group of 83 year olds that decreased frontal white matter integrity was associated with poorer choice reaction time, Letter/Number sequencing, and verbal fluency. Perry et al. (2009) reported significant associations of FA from fiber tracking in the inferior fronto-occipital white matter and Trail Making test performance. Increased task switching costs have been associated with decreased integrity of frontoparietal white matter (Gold et al., 2010) integrity of prefrontal, anterior corpus callosum, superior/posterior parietal, and occipital white matter (Kennedy & Raz, 2009b), and the genu and in splenium-parietal fibers of the corpus callosum (Madden et al., 2009). In a small fiber tracking study (Sullivan et al., 2006) regional corpus callosum fiber properties correlated moderately with reading speed on color-word Stroop task (but not in the interference scores), and Kennedy and Raz (2009b) found an association between reduced anisotropy of the posterior white matter (parietal, splenium, and occipital) and higher Stroop interference cost. Interestingly, although several studies have examined WCST perseveration, no direct associations with regional or global indices of white matter integrity have been found (Charlton et al., 2008; Kennedy & Raz, 2009b; O'Sullivan et al., 2001). Grieve et al. (2007) examined voxel-wise (and lobar) FA and age-related performance on several tasks and found only performance on an executive maze to be correlated with frontal FA voxel clusters. Davis et al. (2009), comparing fiber tracking in younger and older adults, found that higher FA in anterior regions was associated with better executive functioning and higher FA in posterior regions was associated with better visual functioning.

Working Memory

The extant DTI studies suggest that working memory performance depends on white matter integrity in a widespread network of regions, more so than other cognitive processes. In a neuropsychological battery of several tests of executive function, working memory, and processing speed, Charlton et al. (2006, 2008) found only working memory (composite of WAIS Digit Symbol and Letter/Number sequencing) significantly correlated with DTI indices beyond the effects of age in large segments of white matter (anterior ($r = -0.24$), middle ($r = -0.21$), and posterior white matter ($r = -0.26$). In a structural equation model of the same data, average ADC from 10 axial slices again predicted only working memory (Charlton et al., 2008). In a careful region of interest study, Kennedy & Raz (2009b) found that age reductions in working memory were related to age-related declines in widespread networks ranging from anterior (prefrontal, anterior callosum, and internal capsule) to posterior (posterior internal capsule, temporal and occipital white matter) reflecting the importance of intact white matter across the brain for working memory performance. Zahr et al. (2009) found age differences in working memory and problem solving were associated with lesser integrity of the corpus callosum genu and the fornix. These DTI findings bolster the understanding that working memory is a multidimensional construct that reflects the state of a wide range of neural substrates encompassing most of the deep cerebral white matter, which may also explain why working memory is so often seen as a mediator of other cognitive performance declines in aging.

Episodic Memory

Few studies have investigated white matter integrity and age-related memory performance. Kennedy & Raz (2009b) found that age-related reductions in white matter microstructure in the internal capsule, temporal stem, and superior/parietal regions were associated with reduced performance on several memory tasks. Hence, intact white matter across temporoparietal network may underlie better memory in older adults. Other studies failed to find correlates of mnemonic performance (Deary et al., 2006; Grieve et al., 2007; Shenkin et al., 2005); however, those studies examined coarse sections of the white matter and the regions that Kennedy & Raz (2009b) found associated with memory were not measured.

Processing Speed

The literature on white matter substrates of age differences in processing speed is inconsistent. In older adults, reaction time measured on simple tasks is related to global indices of white matter integrity in some (Deary et al., 2006) but not other (Charlton et al., 2006, 2008; Grieve et al., 2007) samples. Kennedy & Raz (2009b) found that slowed speed of cognitive processing was related to reduced integrity of primarily anterior (and frontoparietal) white matter regions. Reaction times from other cognitive processes have also been associated with white matter integrity as links between regional anisotropy and visual detection speed (Madden et al., 2004) as well as the magnitude of speed influence on episodic retrieval (Bucur et al., 2008) have been reported. Taken together, these studies indicate that quick cognitive processing depends on the integrity of at least the prefrontal and anterior callosum fibers, and, as suggested by some studies, also the frontoparietal fibers, which are the networks considered to be the neural substrate of executive controlled processes. In classic theories of disconnection syndromes, a breakdown of transmission in the white matter connective fiber bundles disrupts or slows the mode of cognition that relies on the joined regions (see Catani & ffytche, 2005). Thus, the DTI literature supports the idea that slowing stems from degraded neural transmission along the axons of the aging brain.

Motor Performance

Regional white matter integrity is to also sensitive to motor performance differences; scores from the finger-tapping test correlated with FA in the parietal pericallosal region and splenium. Gait and balance also correlated with white matter FA (Sullivan et al., 2001). FA along several different white matter tracts (Sullivan et al., 2010) was also associated with perceptual-motor speed (e.g., corpus callosum, internal and external capsules), fine finger movements (internal and external capsules), and balance (e.g., frontal forceps) and Zahr et al. (2009) found age differences in motor performance to be associated with the genu and splenium of the callosum, fornix, and uncinate fasciculus (a white matter bundle connecting the frontal and temporal lobes).

Together, these studies stand in support of a disconnection hypothesis of cognitive aging that white matter degradation along the major association pathways may lead to a sufficient disconnection that hampers transmission between cortical regions that provide neural support for different aspects of cognition. If maintenance of optimal cognitive performance in older adults depends upon compensatory "rerouting" of the information flow, then such a process is significantly jeopardized by reduced anisotropy and increased diffusivity in these regions. Further tests of this hypothesis will come from studies that combine DTI and fMRI in older adults.

DTI and fMRI Integration Studies

A few recent investigations have embarked on this task (Li et al., 2009; Madden et al., 2004, 2007; Persson et al., 2006). In two studies, Madden and colleagues investigated the role of regional white matter integrity in visual search response times using groups of young and older adults. In both groups, slower responses in the visual task were associated with lower FA in the cerebral white matter. They observed an interesting pattern of age differences where younger adults showed an association of response time with splenium FA, whereas older adults evidenced this association with FA in the anterior limb of the internal capsule (Madden et al., 2004). In a follow-up fMRI experiment (Madden et al., 2007), older and younger adults again displayed different patterns of regional brain effects, this time in cortical activation pattern. Whereas top-down guided visual search yielded activation in fusiform cortex for the young, frontoparietal activation was necessary for the older adults. This recruitment of frontal regions in older adults to support cognitive processing is a highly replicated pattern (Cabeza, 2002). Madden et al. (2007) did not find FA in any region to mediate this cortical activation, however. In a third study, Bucur et al. (2008) found age-reduced FA in frontal and genu selectively mediated the relation between perceptual speed and episodic retrieval speed. In a study that combined DTI, fMRI, and hippocampal volume measures to predict memory decline, Persson et al. (2006) chose two groups of older adults (aged 49 to 74 years) based on memory stability or decline over 10 years. Hippocampal volume and FA in the genu of the corpus callosum were both reduced in the memory decliner group. In the incidental encoding task (abstract vs. concrete word categorization), both older adult groups displayed the typical pattern of increased frontal activation, but the highest memory decliners also showed additional recruitment of right prefrontal cortex, which was correlated with FA in the genu $r = -0.39$. Finally Li et al. (2009) examined in 11 young and 15 older women whether DTI-derived measures of connectivity originating from bilateral prefrontal regions of interest were associated with verbal working memory activation differences in the older adults. This preliminary study found a moderate correlation ($r = 0.55$, $p = 0.05$) between DTI laterality index and activation bilaterality.

Together, these studies provide preliminary evidence that decreased cognitive performance, whether behaviorally, or expressed as differential cortical activation patterns, is likely due in part to lesser integrity of the white matter structural connectivity in the brains of older adults, and lends support to a disconnection syndrome in aging. Further, the white matter seems to be especially vulnerable to vascular processes.

Magnetization Transfer Imaging

In addition to DTI methods, another neuroimaging method used to index white matter (and gray matter) integrity is Magnetization Transfer Ratio (MTR). Magnetization transfer imaging (MTI) shares properties with DTI in that it capitalizes on the ability to measure water content in brain tissue; however, MTR is a measure of macromolecular integrity. In this type of MRI sequence, two scans are acquired (one with and one without a radio-frequency pulse) and the difference between the tissue signal intensity between the two scans reflects properties of the tissue, generally with a focus on white matter (Wolff & Balaban, 1989). The resulting magnetization transfer image contains lower intensity regions reflecting less constrained water, and higher intensity regions reflecting restricted water movement, usually in myelinated axons. MTI has gained popularity because it can add specificity to potential mechanisms underlying decreased FA and increased diffusivity seen in DTI studies of aging and diseases involving white matter pathology such as multiple sclerosis, because lower MTR is thought to be specifically sensitive to myelin loss (Wozniak & Lim, 2006). Both MTR and DTI FA (but not DTI diffusivity) correlate strongly with axon and myelin properties measured in postmortem tissue (Mottershead et al., 2003). MTR is more sensitive than DTI measures in detecting damage to myelinated axons and lower MTR is found in regions of WMH (Bastin et al., 2009; Fazekas et al., 2005; Mezzapesa et al., 2003).

A few studies have examined MTR differences in younger and older adults with conflicting results. Most studies find that MTR decreases in the white matter with age (Rovaris et al., 2003; Silver et al., 1997), perhaps at an accelerated rate (Ge et al., 2002). However some studies did not find age decline in MTR (Armstrong et al., 2004; Benedetti et al., 2006; Mehta et al., 1995). The extant studies suggested that the anterior-to-posterior gradient of brain aging observed in other neuroimaging modalities holds for MTR (Gunning-Dixon et al., 2009; Spilt et al., 2005).

Studies of MTR and Cognitive Aging

Only a handful of studies have examined cognitive associations with MT imaging. In a study of older adults (some of which scored at cognitive impairment levels), Lee et al. (2004) found significant correlations between whole brain MTR histogram peak and tests of naming, memory, and verbal fluency, but not on attention/working memory. Notably, MTR was a better predictor of cognition than total brain or WMH volume. Three other studies, however, found no significant association with multiple measures of cognitive performance (Deary et al., 2006; Fazekas et al., 2005; van der Hiele et al., 2007), although the Fazekas et al. (2005) study found a marginal effect of frontal MTR on fine motor dexterity. Finally, Schiavone et al. (2009) compared whole brain MTR with WMH and DTI indices in their ability to predict cognitive performance. They found a mild association between whole brain MTR and processing speed, executive function, and episodic memory, but MTR was less sensitive to detect these associations than either DTI or WMH. Thus far it appears that MTI may be a sensitive predictor of age-related differences in cognition. However, these few findings cannot be definitively interpreted and more investigations of MTI correlates of cognitive aging are needed, especially studies that take care to reliably measure specific regions of interest rather than using global whole brain indices of integrity. A further consideration is that the neuroimaging sequences collected to measure WMH and DTI are simpler to implement than the sequence to measure MTR, as it requires subtraction of two images.

As an example of multimodality imaging using MTR, in three studies, Düzel and colleagues examined MTR in the substantia nigra/ventral tegmentum nuclei (SN/VTA), which is the primary site of dopamine projections, and the association with emotional attention (Bunzeck et al., 2007) and memory (Düzel et al., 2008, 2010). Düzel et al. (2008) reported a positive correlation between MTR in the SN/VTA and frontal white matter with verbal learning performance in the older adults, but a negative correlation in the younger adults, perhaps reflecting different developmental mechanisms. In contrast, Düzel et al. (2010) did not find an association of verbal learning and MTR in the SN/VTA; however, they did find a significant association between this cognitive measure and MTR in the nucleus basalis (the primary site of acetylcholine projections). Finally, in an fMRI study of emotional attention, Bunzeck et al. (2007) found that novelty activation in SN/VTA correlated positively with MTR in SN/VTA and the hippocampus. Combining different imaging modalities in this manner in the future will allow more sophisticated and specific questions to be asked about how structure and function interact to affect cognitive performance with aging.

BETA-AMYLOID DEPOSITION

More recently there have been advances in the ability to image in vivo the accumulation of beta-amyloid (Aβ) plaques in the human brain (for a broader review see Rodrigue et al., 2009). Aβ is a protein fragment that is deposited on the brain in the form of sticky, starch-like plaques, more so in persons with Alzheimer's disease (AD) than in healthier older adults. However, it has recently been suggested that 20 to 30% of cognitively normal older adults have Aβ deposition at the level of those adults with AD. What this means for the aging of the brain's structure is still under investigation, but it appears that amyloid deposition may be an early event that begins a cascade of events that lead to atrophy and eventual cognitive impairment or dementia (Jack et al., 2009). In fact, in aged beagles smaller prefrontal cortex volume was significantly associated with greater Aβ load at autopsy and those dogs with smaller frontal volume performed significantly worse on executive function tasks and those with amyloid performed poorer on visual discrimination learning (Head et al., 1998; Tapp et al., 2004).

Aβ is measured in vivo using a radiolabeled tracer (either Carbon-11 or Fluorine-18) and positron emission tomography (PET) scanning to measure the magnitude and distribution of Aβ plaques in the brain as these ligands bind to the aggregated fibrillar form of Aβ (Jagust, 2009). Prior to this method, Aβ burden was only measurable postmortem, where it was impossible to study its effect on cognition. Amyloid imaging studies with normal aging samples have generally found that Aβ accumulates in the frontal, parietal, precuneus, and cingulate cortices of approximately 20 to 30% of older adults (Rodrigue et al., 2009).

Studies of Aβ Imaging and Cognitive Aging

While still early, the extant Aβ imaging studies of cognitive performance in normal older adults show inconsistent associations. The mechanisms through which Aβ has its effects, however, are still under investigation. It may be that cognitive decline is an indirect effect of Aβ accumulation via a cascade of processes involving cortical atrophy and reduced structural and functional connectivity (Rodrigue et al., 2009). Thus, studies examining Aβ deposition and cognition cross-sectionally in age-restricted samples of older adults may be unable to detect an association. Some studies failed to find associations between Aβ deposition and memory in normal elderly (Aizenstein et al., 2008; Jack et al., 2008), but others found a relation between memory performance and Aβ binding in healthy older adults ($r = -0.38$, Pike et al., 2007), as well as an association between higher Aβ binding in frontal and parietal cortex and poorer cognitive performance (Braskie et al., 2008). Evidence (Mormino et al., 2009) showed that the relation between memory performance and Aβ deposition is mediated by hippocampal volume, suggesting a temporal order for the cascade of events that build to affect memory decline. Longitudinally, healthy elderly who declined clinically showed a significant association of memory performance and amyloid deposition (Fripp et al., 2008). Thus, the effect of Aβ deposition on cognition in normal aging is unclear and longitudinal studies with a broader age sample are needed to understand these multivariate and time-dependent relationships.

Structure-Function Studies

There have recently been a few investigations of Aβ deposition on brain function, mostly the default network. Several studies have examined the effects of Aβ deposition on the default network, a set of brain regions that are active when the brain is at rest (for review see Buckner et al., 2008) including the ventromedial and dorsomedial prefrontal, posterior cingulate/retrosplenial, inferior parietal, and lateral temporal cortices. Older adults display difficulty shifting out of the default mode to task-relevant modes when confronted with a cognitive task, and several studies have shown that greater Aβ deposition is associated with deactivation in the default network (Buckner et al., 2005, 2009; Sheline et al., 2010; Sperling et al., 2009) especially in the precuneus and posterior cingulate cortex. However, the samples in these early studies are small and thus far these associations do not always correlate with cognitive performance. One fMRI study of task activation (Nelissen et al., 2007) found that persons with AD showed lesser activation than normal older adults in the superior temporal cortex, and this activation was associated with greater Aβ load in the same region. However, in the contralateral hemisphere the pattern was reversed with greater activation in the patients than controls, and this contralateral recruitment was positively correlated with cognitive performance, demonstrating that at least in early stage AD, functional reorganization can help overcome negative effects of Aβ deposition. It seems likely that Aβ deposition has its effects on cognitive performance indirectly through atrophy of hippocampus and cortical regions and disruption of functional connectivity. Resolving the nature of these associations will be a major goal of future research in the areas of both normal cognitive aging and in AD.

DISCUSSION

Several techniques exist to gauge age-related alterations to the brain's structure. For gray matter measurement, while manual regional tracing remains the gold standard, it is effortful and becomes less practical as neuroimaging sample sizes increase and as multiple time points are added. Weighing the limitations of the available techniques, we strongly favor semi-automated user interactive measures (such as FreeSurfer to measure cortical thinning and volume) over fully automated techniques that are not based on neuroanatomical information (such as VBM). For white matter evaluation, diffusion-based measures (such as DTI) seem more sensitive to cognitive differences than more macromolecular measures (such as WMH).

After reviewing the large body of literature on the cognitive correlates of aging effects on the brain's structure we conclude that while mixed in their findings, decrements to the brain's physical structure appear to yield decrements to cognitive performance. However, more longitudinal studies of these associations are sorely needed to better understand these complex relations. For example, because the brain is able to adapt (both structurally and functionally) to these age-associated structural changes, compensatory processes may mask some effects of brain shrinkage on performance as suggested by the Scaffolding Theory of Aging and Cognition (STAC) by Park & Reuter-Lorenz (2009). It also appears that the more microstructural neuroimaging investigations of aging cognition (e.g., DTI investigations) are more sensitive to detecting changes in cognition compared to macrostructural techniques, perhaps because they are detecting structural degradation at an earlier stage. It is also at this more microstructural level that the brain is the most plastic and able to benefit from compensatory mechanisms such as scaffolding. Future research, in addition to focusing on longitudinal designs, needs to incorporate multiple measures of brain structure and function and to begin to pay better attention to sample composition in terms of health modifiers of age-associated changes to structure, function, and cognitive performance.

Another promising future direction for cognitive neuroscience of aging research is the incorporation of modifiers of health in normally aging adults (see Raz & Kennedy, 2009 and Raz & Rodrigue, 2006 for more thorough reviews). These new directions should incorporate the effects of genetic risk on the brain and cognition (e.g., as in Kennedy et al., 2009b; Moffat et al., 2000; Raz et al., 2008; Raz et al., 2009a,b; Raz & Kennedy, 2009) and on commonly found conditions that occur with advancing age, especially changes to the vascular system such as hypertension and other vascular risks (e.g., as in Burgmans et al., 2010; Kennedy & Raz, 2009a; Kennedy et al., 2009a; Raz & Kennedy, 2009; Raz et al., 2003, 2005, 2007, 2008). Ideally, cognitive aging studies in the future will acquire sufficient sample sizes so that the interactions among these modifiers can be evaluated. Lastly, health factors that have the potential to convey neuroprotection to aging adults also warrant significant study such as the positive effects of hormone replacement therapy in women (Erickson et al., 2005; Raz et al., 2004) and perhaps in men (Moffat, 2005), as well as the beneficial effects of exercise on the brain and cognition (Fabel & Kempermann, 2008; Hillman et al., 2008).

SUMMARY AND CONCLUSIONS

1. The regions of the human brain age in a differential fashion, with some areas quite vulnerable to the aging process (association cortices) and others relatively resistant (primary sensory). Therefore, future studies need to use regional, rather than whole brain or whole tissue types of measurements.
2. The different tissue components, which have a different cellular make up, also age differentially. The cortical gray matter appears to follow a steady linear decline across the life span, whereas white matter shrinkage appears to accelerate in late middle age.
3. Longitudinal investigations of aging brain structure are scarce in most imaging modalities, and nonexistent in others. However, based on volumetric research it appears that cross-sectional studies underestimate true longitudinal shrinkage.

4. Many neuroimaging techniques exist to examine aging of brain structure. For measuring volume, manual volumetry remains the gold standard, with VBM not recommended for use (except in exploratory studies to suggest regions for manual follow up). Semi-automated measures of cortical thickness and volume (e.g., FreeSurfer) are better measures than VBM and are faster and easier to implement than manual methods, but need to be carefully implemented with anatomical corrections by the user. For white matter structure measurement, moving from macromolecular (e.g., WMH) to microstructural (e.g., DTI) indices appears to yield more sensitivity to aging and cognitive associations.
5. The structural techniques most sensitive to detecting age-related cognitive decline are unclear, but appear to vary by cognitive domain. For some domains, a multimodal approach will likely be most fruitful, whereas for other domains of cognition there appears to be specific neuroanatomical substrates. For example, gray matter measures appear to be more sensitive to memory performance, whereas speed of processing seems most strongly associated with white matter integrity. Further, some aspects of cognition may be more functionally located (e.g., memory), while others depend on widespread connectivity (e.g., working memory).
6. Vascular health risk factors such as hypertension, appear to accelerate structural brain aging. Cognitive aging studies of normal adults with vascular risk report a less differentiated pattern of cortical and subcortical aging, with decreased volume apparent in more posterior brain regions and stronger age influence in white matter volume and integrity compared to the effects in healthy adults.
7. Cognitive aging and its neural substrates is highly influenced by modifiers of health, for example functioning of the vascular system and likely, Aβ plaque deposition. Much more research is necessary in these areas to distinguish healthy from pathological aging. It is also becoming clear that brain and cognitive aging are under at least partial genetic control, and genetic risk interacts with vascular risk to produce cognitive decline. Further studies of the lifestyle variables under our control (e.g., nutrition, exercise, hypertension, hypercholesterolemia, hormone replacement, etc.) and their effects on cognitive performance in middle-aged and older adults are needed.
8. Finally, to supplement the rich history of investigating the effects of brain structure on cognitive performance using behavioral measures, we now need to examine the role of brain structure in brain and cognitive function using functional imaging techniques. These studies are just beginning to emerge and show promise for elucidating how changes to the brain's structure with age affects the brain's function to determine cognitive outcomes. It is through these studies that we are likely to understand the ways in which the brain is plastic and undergoes reorganization to maintain healthy, functional cognitive performance into old age.

ACKNOWLEDGMENTS

Preparation of this chapter was supported by National Institutes of Health grant 5 R37 AG-006265-25 to Denise C. Park.

REFERENCES

Abe, O., Aoki, S., Hayashi, N., Yamada, H., Kunimatsu, A., Mori, H., et al. (2002). Normal aging in the central nervous system: Quantitative MR diffusion-tensor analysis. *Neurobiology of Aging, 23*, 433–441.

Aizenstein, H. J., Nebes, R. D., Saxton, J. A., Price, J. C., Mathis, C. A., Tsopelas, N. D., et al. (2008). Frequent amyloid deposition without significant cognitive impairment among the elderly. *Archives of Neurology, 65*, 1509–1517.

Andersson, M., Ystad, M., Lundervold, A., & Lundervold, A. J. (2009). Correlations between measures of executive attention and cortical thickness of left posterior middle frontal gyrus — a dichotic listening study. *Behavioral and Brain Functions, 5*, 41.

Armstrong, C. L., Traipe, E., Hunter, J. V., Haselgrove, J. C., Ledakis, G. E., Tallent, E. M., et al. (2004). Age-related, regional, hemispheric, and medial-lateral differences in myelin integrity in vivo in the normal adult brain. *American Journal of Neuroradiology, 25*, 977–984.

Ashburner, J . A., & Friston, K. J. (2000). Voxel-based morphometry — the methods. *Neuroimage, 11*, 805–821.

Bartzokis, G., Beckson, M., Lu, P. H., Nuechterlein, K. H., Edwards, N., & Mintz, J. (2001). Age-related changes in frontal and temporal volume in men: A magnetic resonance imaging study. *Archives of General Psychiatry, 58*, 461–465.

Bastin, M. E., Clayden, J. D., Pattie, A., Gerrish, I. F., Wardlaw, J. M., & Deary, I. J. (2009). Diffusion tensor and magnetization transfer MRI measurements of periventricular white matter hyperintensities in old age. *Neurobiology of Aging, 30*, 125–136.

Benedetti, B., Charil, A., Rovaris, M., Judica, E., Valsasina, P., Sormani, M. P., et al. (2006). Influence of aging on brain gray and white matter changes assessed by conventional, MT, and DT MRI. *Neurology, 66*, 535–539.

Braskie, M. N., Klunder, A. D., Hayashi, K. M., Protas, H., Kepe, V., Miller, K. J., et al. (2008). Plaque and tangle imaging and cognition in normal aging and Alzheimer's disease. *Neurobiology of Aging*. [Epub ahead of print].

Braskie, M. N., Small, G. W., & Bookheimer, S. Y. (2009). Entorhinal cortex structure and functional MRI response during an associative verbal memory task. *Human Brain Mapping*.

Buckner, R. L., Andrews-Hanna, J. R., & Schacter, D. L. (2008). The brain's default network: anatomy, function, and relevance to disease. *Annals of New York Academy of Sciences, 1124*, 1–38.

Buckner, R. L., Sepulcre, J., Talukdar, T., Krienen, F. M., Liu, H., Hedden, T., et al. (2009). Cortical hubs revealed by intrinsic functional connectivity: Mapping, assessment of stability, and relation to Alzheimer's disease. *Journal of Neuroscience, 29*, 1860–1873.

Buckner, R. L., Snyder, A. Z., Shannon, B. J., LaRossa, G., Sachs, R., Fotenos, A. F., et al. (2005). Molecular, structural, and functional characterization of Alzheimer's disease: Evidence for a relationship between default activity, amyloid, and memory. *Journal of Neuroscience, 25*, 7709–7717.

Bucur, B., Madden, D. J., Spaniol, J., Provenzale, J. M., Cabeza, R., White, L. E., et al. (2008). Age-related slowing of memory retrieval: Contributions of perceptual speed and cerebral white matter integrity. *Neurobiology of Aging, 7*, 1070–1079.

Bunce, D., Anstey, K. J., Christensen, H., Dear, K., Wen, W., & Sachdev, P. (2007). White matter hyperintensities and within-person variability in community-dwelling adults aged 60–64 years. *Neuropsychologia, 45*, 2009–2015.

Bunzeck, N., Schütze, H., Stallforth, S., Kaufmann, J., Düzel, S., Heinze, H. J., et al. (2007). Mesolimbic novelty processing in older adults. *Cerebral Cortex, 17*, 2940–2948.

Burgmans, S., van Boxtel, M. P., van den Berg, K. E., Gronenschild, E. H., Jacobs, H. I., Jolles, J., et al. (2009). The posterior parahippocampal gyrus is preferentially affected in age-related memory decline. *Neurobiology of Aging* [Epub ahead of print].

Burgmans, S., van Boxtel, M. P. J., Gronenschild, E. H. B. M., Vuurman, E. F. P. M., Hofman, P., Uylings, H. B. M., et al. (2010). Multiple indicators of age-related differences in cerebral white matter and the modifying effects of hypertension. *Neuroimage, 49*, 2083–2093.

Cabeza, R. (2002). Hemispheric asymmetry reduction in older adults: The HAROLD model. *Psychology and Aging, 17*, 85–100.

Cardenas, V. A., Chao, L. L., Studholme, C., Yaffe, K., Miller, B. L., Madison, C., et al. (2009). Brain atrophy associated with baseline and longitudinal measures of cognition. *Neurobiology of Aging* [Epub ahead of print].

Carmelli, D., DeCarli, C., Swan, G. E., Jack, L. M., Reed, T., Wolf, P. A., et al. (1998). Evidence for genetic variance in white matter hyperintensity volume in normal elderly male twins. *Stroke, 29*, 1177–1181.

Charlton, R. A., Barrick, T. R., McIntyre, D. J., Shen, Y., O'Sullivan, M., Howe, F. A., et al. (2006). White matter damage on diffusion tensor imaging correlates with age-related cognitive decline. *Neurology, 66*, 217–222.

Catani, M., & Hytche, D. H. (2005). The rises and falls of disconnection syndromes. *Brain, 128*, 2224–2239.

Charlton, R. A., Landau, S., Schiavone, F., Barrick, T. R., Clark, C. A., Markus, H. S., et al. (2008). A structural equation modeling investigation of age-related variance in executive function and DTI measured white matter damage. *Neurobiology of Aging, 29*, 1547–1555.

Cook, I. A., Leuchter, A. F., Morgan, M. L., Conlee, E. W., David, S., Lufkin, R., et al. (2002). Cognitive and physiologic correlates of subclinical structural brain disease in elderly healthy control subjects. *Archives of Neurology, 59*, 1612–1620.

Courchesne, E., Chisum, H. J., Townsend, J., Cowles, A., Covington, J., Egaas, B., et al. (2000). Normal brain development and aging: Quantitative analysis at in vivo MR imaging in healthy volunteers. *Radiology, 216*, 672–682.

Davis, S. W., Dennis, N. A., Buchler, N. G., White, L. E., Madden, D. J., & Cabeza, R. (2009). Assessing the effects of age on long white matter tracts using diffusion tensor tractography. *Neuroimage, 46*, 530–541.

Deary, I. J., Bastin, M. E., Pattie, A., Clayden, J. D., Whalley, L. J., Starr, J. M., et al. (2006). White matter integrity and cognition in childhood and old age. *Neurology, 66*, 505–512.

DeCarli, C., Murphy, D. G., Tranh, M., Grady, C. L., Haxby, J. V., Gillette, J. A., et al. (1995). The effect of white matter hyperintensity volume on brain structure, cognitive performance, and cerebral metabolism of glucose in 51 healthy adults. *Neurology, 45*, 2077–2084.

de Leeuw, F. E., de Groot, J. C., Achten, E., Oudkerk, M., Ramos, L. M., Heijboer, R., et al. (2001). Prevalence of cerebral white matter lesions in elderly people: A population based magnetic resonance imaging study. The Rotterdam Scan Study. *Journal of Neurological Neurosurgical Psychiatry, 70*, 9–14.

Dickerson, B. C., Fenstermacher, E., Salat, D. H., Wolk, D. A., Maguire, R. P., Desikan, R., et al. (2008). Detection of cortical thickness correlates of cognitive performance: Reliability across MRI scan sessions, scanners, and field strengths. *Neuroimage, 39*, 10–18.

Duarte, A., Hayasaka, S., Du, A., Schuff, N., Jahng, G. H., Kramer, J., et al. (2006). Volumetric correlates of memory and executive function in normal elderly, mild cognitive impairment and Alzheimer's disease. *Neuroscience Letters, 406*, 60–65.

Dufouil, C., Alpérovitch, A., & Tzourio, C. (2003). Influence of education on the relationship between white matter lesions and cognition. *Neurology, 60*, 831–836.

Dufouil, C., Fuhrer, R., & Alpérovitch, A. (2005). Subjective cognitive complaints and cognitive decline: Consequence or predictor? The epidemiology of vascular aging study. *Journal of the American Geriatric Society, 53*, 616–621.

Düzel, S., Schütze, H., Stallforth, S., Kaufmann, J., Bodammer, N., Bunzeck, N., et al. (2008). A close relationship between verbal memory and SN/VTA integrity in young and older adults. *Neuropsychologia, 46*, 3042–3052.

Düzel, S., Münte, T. F., Lindenberger, U., Bunzeck, N., Schütze, H., Heinze, H. J., et al. (2010). Basal forebrain integrity and cognitive memory profile in healthy aging. *Brain Research, 1308*, 124–136.

Elderkin-Thompson, V., Ballmaier, M., Hellemann, G., Pham, D., & Kumar, A. (2008). Executive function and MRI prefrontal volumes among healthy older adults. *Neuropsychology, 22*, 626–637.

Erickson, K. I., Colcombe, S. J., Raz, N., Korol, D. L., Scalf, P., Webb, A., et al. (2005). Selective sparing of brain tissue in postmenopausal women receiving hormone replacement therapy. *Neurobiology of Aging, 26*, 1205–1213.

Fabel, K., & Kempermann, G. (2008). Physical activity and the regulation of neurogenesis in the adult and aging brain. *Neuromolecular Medicine, 10*, 59–66.

Fazekas, F., Ropele, S., Enzinger, C., Gorani, F., Seewann, A., Petrovic, K., et al. (2005). MTI of white matter hyperintensities. *Brain, 128*, 2926–2932.

Fischl, B., & Dale, A. M. (2000). Measuring the thickness of the human cerebral cortex from magnetic resonance images. *Proceedings of the National Academies of Science USA, 97*, 11050–11055.

Fjell, A. M., Westlye, L. T., Amlien, I., Espeseth, T., Reinvany, I., Raz, N., et al. (2009). High consistency of regional cortical thinning in aging across multiple samples. *Cerebral Cortex, 19*, 2001–2012.

Fjell, A. M., Walhovd, K. B., Reinvang, I., Lundervold, A., Salat, D., Quinn, B. T., et al. (2006). Selective increase of cortical thickness in high-performing elderly — structural indices of optimal cognitive aging. *Neuroimage, 29*, 984–994.

Fjell, A. M., Walhovd, K. B., Fischl, B., & Reinvang, I. (2007). Cognitive function, P3a/P3b brain potentials, and cortical thickness in aging. *Human Brain Mapping, 28*, 1098–1116.

Flechsig, P. (1901). Developmental myelogenetic localisation of the cerebral cortex in the human subject. *The Lancet*, October 19, 1027–1029.

Fripp, J., Bourgeat, P., Acosta, O., Raniga, P., Modat, M., Pike, K. E., et al. (2008). Appearance modeling of 11C PiB PET images: characterizing amyloid deposition in Alzheimer's disease, mild cognitive impairment and healthy aging. *Neuroimage, 43*, 430–439.

Garde, E., Mortensen, E. L., Krabbe, K., Rostrup, E., & Larsson, H. B. (2000). Relation between age-related decline in intelligence and cerebral white-matter hyperintensities in healthy octogenarians: A longitudinal study. *Lancet, 356*, 628–634.

Ge, Y., Grossman, R. I., Babb, J. S., Rabin, M. L., Mannon, L. J., & Kolson, D. L. (2002). Age-related total gray matter and white matter changes in normal adult brain. Part II: quantitative magnetization transfer ratio histogram analysis. *American Journal of Neuroradiology, 23*, 1334–1341.

Ghisletta, P., Kennedy, K. M., Rodrigue, K. M., Lindenberger, U., & Raz, N. (2010). Adult Age Differences and cognitive resources in perceptual-motor skill acquisition: Application of a multilevel exponential model. *Journals of Gerontology: Psychological Sciences, 65B*, 163–173.

Gold, B. T., Powell, D. K., Xuan, L., Jicha, G. A., & Smith, C. D. (2010). Age-related slowing of task switching is associated with decreased integrity of frontoparietal white matter. *Neurobiology of Aging, 31*, 512–522.

Golomb, J., Kluger, A., de Leon, M. J., Ferris, S. H., Convit, A., Mittelman, M. S., et al. (1994). Hippocampal formation size in normal human aging: A correlate of delayed secondary memory performance. *Learning and Memory, 1*, 45–54.

Gong, Q. Y., Sluming, V., Mayes, A., Keller, S., Barrick, T., Cezayirli, E., et al. (2005). Voxel-based morphometry and stereology provide convergent evidence of the importance of medial prefrontal cortex for fluid intelligence in healthy adults. *Neuroimage, 25*, 1175–1186.

Gootjes, L., Teipel, S. J., Zebuhr, Y., Schwarz, R., Leinsinger, G., Scheltens, P., et al. (2004). Regional distribution of white matter hyperintensities in vascular dementia, Alzheimer's disease and healthy aging. *Dementia and Geriatric Cognitive Disorders, 18*, 180–188.

Grieve, S. M., Williams, L. M., Paul, R. H., Clark, C. R., & Gordon, E. (2007). Cognitive aging, executive function, and fractional anisotropy: A diffusion tensor MR imaging study. *American Journal of Neuroradiology, 28*, 226–235.

Gunning-Dixon, F. M., & Raz, N. (2000). The cognitive correlates of white matter abnormalities in normal aging: A quantitative review. *Neuropsychology, 14*, 224–232.

Gunning-Dixon, F. M., & Raz, N. (2003). Neuroanatomical correlates of selected executive functions in middle-aged and older adults: A prospective MRI study. *Neuropsychologia, 41*, 1929–1941.

Gunning-Dixon, F. M., Brickman, A. M., Cheng, J. C., & Alexopoulos, G. S. (2009). Aging of cerebral white matter: A review of MRI findings. *International Journal of Geriatric Psychiatry, 24*, 109–117.

Hackert, V. H., den Heijer, T., Oudkerk, M., Koudstaal, P. J., Hofman, A., & Breteler, M. M. (2002). Hippocampal head size associated with verbal memory performance in nondemented elderly. *Neuroimage, 17*, 1365–1372.

Harrington, F., Saxby, B. K., McKeith, I. G., Wesnes, K., & Ford, G. A. (2000). Cognitive performance in hypertensive and normotensive older subjects. *Hypertension, 36*, 1079–1082.

Head, D., Raz, N., Gunning-Dixon, F., Williamson, A., & Acker, J. D. (2002). Age-related differences in the course of cognitive skill acquisition: The role of regional cortical shrinkage and cognitive resources. *Psychology & Aging, 17*, 72–84.

Head, D., Buckner, R. L., Shimony, J. S., Girton, L. E., Akbudak, E., Conturo, T. E., et al. (2004). Differential vulnerability of anterior white matter in nondemented aging with minimal acceleration in dementia of the Alzheimer type: Evidence from diffusion tensor imaging. *Cerebral Cortex, 14*, 410–423.

Head, D., Rodrigue, K. M., Kennedy, K. M., & Raz, N. (2008). Neuroanatomical and cognitive mediators of age-related differences in episodic memory. *Neuropsychology, 22*(4), 491–507.

Head, D., Kennedy, K. M., Rodrigue, K. M., & Raz, N. (2009). Age-differences in perseveration: Cognitive and neuroanatomical mediators of performance on the Wisconsin Card Sorting Test. *Neuropsychologia, 47*(4), 1200–1203.

Head, E., Callahan, H., Muggenburg, B. A., Cotman, C. W., & Milgram, N. W. (1998). Visual-discrimination learning ability and beta-amyloid accumulation in the dog. *Neurobiology of Aging, 19*, 415–425.

Hillman, C. H., Erickson, K. I., & Kramer, A. F. (2008). Be smart, exercise your heart: Exercise effects on brain and cognition. *Nature Reviews Neuroscience, 9*, 58–65.

Hopkins, R. O., Beck, C. J., Burnett, D. L., Weaver, L. K., Victoroff, J., & Bigler, E. D. (2006). Prevalence of white matter hyperintensities in a young healthy population. *Journal of Neuroimaging, 16*, 243–251.

Hugenschmidt, C. E., Peiffer, A. M., Kraft, R. A., Casanova, R., Deibler, A. R., Burdette, J. H., et al. (2008). Relating imaging indices of white matter integrity and volume in healthy older adults. *Cerebral Cortex, 18*, 433–442.

Jack, C. R., Lowe, V. J., Senjem, M. L., Weigand, S. D., Kemp, B. J., Shiung, M. M., et al. (2008). 11C PiB and structural MRI provide complementary information in imaging of Alzheimer's disease and amnestic mild cognitive impairment. *Brain, 131*, 665–680.

Jack, C. R., Jr., Lowe, V. J., Weigand, S. D., Wiste, H. J., Senjem, M. L., Knopman, D. S., et al. (2009). Serial PIB and MRI in normal, mild cognitive impairment and Alzheimer's disease: Implications for sequence of pathological events in Alzheimer's disease. *Brain, 132*, 1355–1365.

Jagust, W. (2009). Mapping brain beta-amyloid. *Current Opinion in Neurology, 22*, 356–361.

Kemper, T. L. (1994). Neuroanatomical and neuropathological changes during aging and in dementia. In M. L. Albert & E. J. E. Knoepfel (Eds.), *Clinical Neurology of Aging* (2nd ed.) (pp. 3–67). New York: Oxford University Press.

Kennedy, K. M., & Raz, N. (2005). Age, sex, and regional brain volumes predict perceptual-motor skill acquisition in healthy adults. *Cortex, Special Issue: Cognition and the Ageing Brain, 41*(4), 560–569.

Kennedy, K. M., & Raz, N. (2009a). Pattern of normal age-related regional differences in white matter microstructure is modified by vascular risk. *Brain Research, 1297*, 41–56.

Kennedy, K. M., & Raz, N. (2009b). Aging white matter and cognition: differential effects of regional variations in diffusion properties on memory, executive functions, and speed. *Neuropsychologia, 47*, 916–927.

Kennedy, K. M., Rodrigue, K. M., & Raz, N. (2007). Fragmented pictures revisited: Long-term changes in repetition priming, relation to skill learning, and the role of cognitive resources. *Gerontology, 53*(3), 148–158.

Kennedy, K. M., Partridge, T., & Raz, N. (2008). Age-related differences in acquisition of perceptual-motor skills: Working memory as a mediator. *Aging, Neuropsychology and Cognition, 15*(2), 165–183.

Kennedy, K. M., Erickson, K. I., Rodrigue, K. M., Voss, M. W., Colcombe, S. J., Kramer, A. F., et al. (2009a). Age-related differences in regional brain volumes: A comparison of optimized voxel-based morphometry to manual volumetry. *Neurobiology of Aging, 30*(10), 1657–1676.

Kennedy, K. M., Rodrigue, K. M., Land, S. J., & Raz, N. (2009b). BDNF Val66Met polymorphism influences age differences in microstructure of the corpus callosum. *Frontiers in Human Neuroscience, 3*, 19.

Kennedy, K. M., Rodrigue, K. M., Head, D., Gunning-Dixon, F., & Raz, N. (2009c). Neuroanatomical and cognitive mediators of age-related differences in perceptual priming and learning. *Neuropsychology, 23*(4), 475–491.

Kochunov, P., Thompson, P. M., Lancaster, J. L., Bartzokis, G., Smith, S., Coyle, T., et al. (2007). Relationship between white matter fractional anisotropy and other indices of cerebral health in normal aging: Tract-based spatial statistics study of aging. *Neuroimage, 35*, 478–487.

Lee, K. Y., Kim, T. K., Park, M., Ko, S., Song, I. C., & Cho, I. H. (2004). Age-related changes in conventional and magnetization transfer MR imaging in elderly people: comparison with neurocognitive performance. *Korean Journal of Radiology, 5*, 96–101.

Leuchter, A. F., Dunkin, J. J., Lufkin, R. B., Anzai, Y., Cook, I. A., & Newton, T. F. (1994). Effect of white matter disease on functional connections in the aging brain. *Journal of Neurology, Neurosurgery, and Psychiatry, 57*, 1347–1354.

Li, Z., Moore, A. B., Tyner, C., & Hu, X. (2009). Asymmetric connectivity reduction and its relationship to "HAROLD" in aging brain. *Brain Research, 1295*, 149–158.

Madden, D. J., Whiting, W. L., Huettel, S. A., White, L. E., MacFall, J. R., & Provenzale, J. M. (2004). Diffusion tensor imaging of adult age differences in cerebral white matter: Relation to response time. *Neuroimage, 21*, 1174–1181.

Madden, D. J., Spaniol, J., Whiting, W. L., Bucur, B., Provenzale, J. M., Cabeza, R., et al. (2007). Adult age differences in the functional neuroanatomy of visual attention: A combined fMRI and DTI study. *Neurobiology of Aging, 28*, 459–476.

Madden, D. J., Spaniol, J., Costello, M. C., Bucur, B., White, L. E.,

Cabeza, R., et al. (2009). Cerebral white matter integrity mediates adult age differences in cognitive performance. *Journal of Cognitive Neuroscience, 21*, 289–302.

Marin, J., & Rodriguez-Martinez, M. A. (1999). Age-related changes in vascular responses. *Experimental Gerontology, 34*, 503–512.

Mehta, R. C., Pike, G. B., & Enzmann, D. R. (1995). Magnetization transfer MR of the normal adult brain. *American Journal of Neuroradiology, 16*, 2085–2091.

Mezzapesa, D. M., Rocca, M. A., Pagani, E., Comi, G., & Filippi, M. (2003). Evidence of subtle gray-matter pathologic changes in healthy elderly individuals with nonspecific white-matter hyperintensities. *Archives of Neurology, 60*, 1109–1112.

Moffat, S. D. (2005). Effects of testosterone on cognitive and brain aging in elderly men. *Annals of New York Academy of Sciences, 1055*, 80–92.

Moffat, S. D., Szekely, C. A., Zonderman, A. B., Kabani, N. J., & Resnick, S. M. (2000). Longitudinal change in hippocampal volume as a function of apolipoprotein E genotype. *Neurology, 55*, 134–136.

Moffat, S. D., Kennedy, K. M., Rodrigue, K. M., & Raz, N. (2007). Extra-hippocampal contributions to age differences in human spatial navigation. *Cerebral Cortex, 17*, 1274–1282.

Mormino, E. C., Kluth, J. T., Madison, C. M., Rabinovici, G. D., Baker, S. L., Miller, B. L., et al. (2009). Episodic memory loss is related to hippocampal-mediated {beta}-amyloid deposition in elderly subjects. *Brain, 132*, 1310–1323.

Mottershead, J. P., Schmierer, K., Clemence, M., Thornton, J. S., Scaravilli, F., Barker, G. J., et al. (2003). High field MRI correlates of myelin content and axonal density in multiple sclerosis – a post-mortem study of the spinal cord. *Journal of Neurology, 250*, 1293–1301.

Nebes, R. D., Meltzer, C. C., Whyte, E. M., Scanlon, J. M., Halligan, E. M., Saxton, J. A., et al. (2006). The relation of white matter hyperintensities to cognitive performance in the normal old: Education matters. *Aging Neuropsychology and Cognition, 13*, 326–340.

Nelissen, N., Vandenbulcke, M., Fannes, K., Verbruggen, A., Peeters, R., Dupont, P., et al. (2007). A beta amyloid deposition in the language system and how the brain responds. *Brain, 130*, 2055–2069.

Nordahl, C. W., Ranganath, C., Yonelinas, A. P., DeCarli, C., Fletcher, E., & Jagust, W. J. (2006). White matter changes compromise prefrontal cortex function in healthy elderly individuals. *Journal of Cognitive Neuroscience, 18*, 418–429.

O'Sullivan, M., Jones, D. K., Summers, P. E., Morris, R. G., Williams, S. C. R., & Markus, H. S. (2001). Evidence for cortical 'disconnection' as a mechanism of age-related cognitive decline. *Neurology, 57*, 632–638.

Ohmine, T., Miwa, Y., Yao, H., Yuzuriha, T., Takashima, Y., Uchino, A., et al. (2008). Association between arterial stiffness and cerebral white matter lesions in community-dwelling elderly subjects. *Hypertension Research, 31*, 75–81.

Oosterman, J. M., Sergeant, J. A., Weinstein, H. C., & Scherder, E. J. (2004). Timed executive functions and white matter in aging with and without cardiovascular risk factors. *Reviews in the Neurosciences, 15*, 439–462.

Oosterman, J. M., Vogels, R. L., van Harten, B., Gouw, A. A., Scheltens, P., Poggesi, A., et al. (2008). The role of white matter hyperintensities and medial temporal lobe atrophy in age-related executive dysfunctioning. *Brain and Cognition, 68*, 128–133.

Park, D. C., & Reuter-Lorenz, P. (2009). The adaptive brain: Aging and neurocognitive scaffolding. *Annual Review of Psychology, 60*, 173–196.

Paul, R. H., Haque, O., Gunstad, J., Tate, D. F., Grieve, S. M., Hoth, K., et al. (2005). Subcortical hyperintensities impact cognitive function among a select subset of healthy elderly. *Archives of Clinical Neuropsychology, 20*, 697–704.

Perry, M. E., McDonald, C. R., Hagler, D. J., Jr., Gharapetian, L., Kuperman, J. M., Koyama, A. K., et al. (2009). White matter tracts associated with set-shifting in healthy aging. *Neuropsychologia, 47*, 2835–2842.

Persson, J., Nyberg, L., Lind, J., Larsson, A., Nilsson, L.-G., Ingvar, M., et al. (2006). Structure–function correlates of cognitive decline in aging. *Cerebral Cortex, 16*, 907–915.

Petkov, C. I., Wu, C. C., Eberling, J. L., Mungas, D., Zrelak, P. A., Yonelinas, A. P., et al. (2004). Correlates of memory function in community-dwelling elderly: The importance of white matter hyperintensities. *Journal of the International Neuropsychological Society, 10*, 371–381.

Pfefferbaum, A., & Sullivan, E. V. (2003). Increased brain white matter diffusivity in normal adult aging: Relationship to anisotropy and partial voluming. *Magnetic Resonance in Medicine, 49*, 953–961.

Pfefferbaum, A., Adalsteinsson, E., & Sullivan, E. V. (2005). Frontal circuitry degradation marks healthy adult aging: Evidence from diffusion tensor imaging. *Neuroimage, 26*, 891–899.

Pfefferbaum, A., Sullivan, E. V., Hedehus, M., Lim, K. O., Adalsteinsson, E., & Moseley, M. (2000). Age-related decline in brain white matter anisotropy measured with spatially corrected echo-planar diffusion tensor imaging. *Magnetic Resonance in Medicine, 44*, 259–268.

Pfefferbaum, A., Sullivan, E. V., & Carmelli, D. (2001). Genetic regulation of regional microstructure of the corpus callosum in late life. *Neuroreport, 12*, 1677–1681.

Pierpaoli, C., & Basser, P. J. (1996). Toward a quantitative assessment of diffusion anisotropy. *Magnetic Resonance in Medicine, 36*, 893–906.

Pike, K. E., Savage, G., Villemagne, V. L., Ng, S., Moss, S. A., Maruff, P., et al. (2007). Beta-amyloid imaging and memory in non-demented individuals: Evidence for preclinical Alzheimer's disease. *Brain, 130*, 2837–2844.

Raz, N. (2000). Aging of the brain and its impact on cognitive performance: Integration of structural and functional findings. In F. I. M. Craik, &

T. A. Salthouse (Eds.), *Handbook of aging and cognition: Vol. II* (pp. 1–90). Mahwah, NJ: Erlbaum.

Raz, N. (2004). The aging brain observed in vivo: Differential changes and their modifiers. In R. Cabeza, L. Nyberg, & D. C. Park (Eds.), *Cognitive neuroscience of aging: Linking cognitive and cerebral aging* (pp. 17–55). New York: Oxford University Press.

Raz, N., Briggs, S. D., Marks, W., & Acker, J. D. (1999). Age-related deficits in generation and manipulation of mental images: II. The role of dorsolateral prefrontal cortex. *Psychology and Aging, 14*, 436–444.

Raz, N., Dahle, C. L., Rodrigue, K. M., Kennedy, K. M., & Land, S. (2009b). Effects of age, genes and pulse pressure on executive functions in healthy adults. *Neurobiology of Aging*. Epub ahead of print.

Raz, N., Ghisletta, P., Rodrigue, K. M., Kennedy, K. M., & Lindenberger, U. (2010). Trajectones of brain aging in middle-aged and older adults: regional and individual differences. *Neuroimage, 51*, 501–511.

Raz, N., Gunning, F. M., Head, D., Dupuis, J. H., McQuain, J. M., Briggs, S. D., et al. (1997). Selective aging of human cerebral cortex observed in vivo: Differential vulnerability of the prefrontal gray matter. *Cerebral Cortex, 7*, 268–282.

Raz, N., Gunning-Dixon, F. M., Head, D., Dupuis, J. H., & Acker, J. D. (1998). Neuroanatomical correlates of cognitive aging: Evidence from structural magnetic resonance imaging. *Neuropsychology, 12*, 95–114.

Raz, N., & Kennedy, K. M. (2009). A systems approach to age-related change: Neuroanatomical changes, their modifiers, and cognitive correlates (Chap. 4). In W. Jagust & M. D'Esposito (Eds.), *Imaging the aging brain* (pp. 43–70). New York: Oxford University Press.

Raz, N., Lindenberger, U., Ghisletta, P., Rodrigue, K. M., Kennedy, K. M., & Acker, J. D. (2008). Neuroanatomical correlates of fluid intelligence in healthy adults and persons with vascular risk factors. *Cerebral Cortex, 18*, 718–726.

Raz, N., Lindenberger, U., Rodrigue, K. M., Kennedy, K. M., Head, D., Williamson, A., et al. (2005). Regional brain changes in aging healthy adults: General trends, individual differences, and modifiers. *Cerebral Cortex, 15*(11), 1676–1689.

Raz, N., & Rodrigue, K. M. (2006). Differential aging of the brain: Patterns, cognitive correlates and modifiers. *Neuroscience and Biobehavioral Reviews, 30*, 730–748.

Raz, N., Rodrigue, K. M., & Acker, J. D. (2003). Hypertension and the brain: Vulnerability of the prefrontal regions and executive functions. *Behavioral Neuroscience, 17*, 1169–1180.

Raz, N., Rodrigue, K. M., Kennedy, K. M., & Acker, J. D. (2007). Vascular health and longitudinal changes in brain and cognition in middle-aged and older adults. *Neuropsychology, 21*, 149–157.

Raz, N., Rodrigue, K. M., Kennedy, K. M., & Acker, J. D. (2004). Hormone replacement therapy and age-related brain shrinkage: Regional effects. *NeuroReport, 15*(16), 2531–2534.

Raz, N., Rodrigue, K. M., Kennedy, K. M., & Land, S. (2009a). Genetic and vascular modifiers of age-sensitive cognitive skills: Effects of COMT, BDNF, APoE and Hyper-tension. *Neuropsychology, 23*, 105–116.

Raz, N., Williamson, A., Gunning-Dixon, F., Head, D., & Acker, J. D (2000). Neuroanatomical and cognitive correlates of adult age differences in acquisition of a perceptual-motor skill. *Microscopy Research and Techniques, 51*, 85–93.

Rodrigue, K. M., & Raz, N. (2004). Shrinkage of the entorhinal cortex over five years predicts memory performance in healthy adults. *Journal of Neuroscience, 24*, 956–963.

Rodrigue, K. M., Kennedy, K. M., & Park, D. C. (2009). Beta-amyloid deposition and the aging brain. *Neuropsychology Review, 19*, 436–450.

Rovaris, M., Iannucci, G., Cercignani, M., Sormani, M. P., De Stefano, N., Gerevini, S., et al. (2003). Age-related changes in conventional, magnetization transfer, and diffusion-tensor MR imaging findings: Study with whole-brain tissue histogram analysis. *Radiology, 227*, 731–738.

Salat, D. H., Kaye, J. A., & Janowsky, J. S. (2002). Greater orbital prefrontal volume selectively predicts worse working memory performance in older adults. *Cerebral Cortex, 12*, 494–505.

Salat, D. H., Buckner, R. L., Snyder, A. Z., Greve, D. N., Desikan, R. S., Busa, E., et al. (2004). Thinning of the cerebral cortex in aging. *Cerebral Cortex, 14*, 721–730.

Salat, D. H., Tuch, D. S., Greve, D. N., van der Kouwe, A. J. W., Hevelone, N. D., Zaleta, A. K., et al. (2005). Age-related alterations in white matter microstructure measured by diffusion tensor imaging. *Neurobiology of Aging, 26*, 1215–1227.

Schiavone, F., Charlton, R. A., Barrick, T. R., Morris, R. G., & Markus, H. S. (2009). Imaging age-related cognitive decline: A comparison of diffusion tensor and magnetization transfer MRI. *Journal of Magnetic Resonance in Imaging, 29*, 23–30.

Schretlen, D., Pearlson, G. D., Anthony, J. C., Aylward, E. H., Augustine, A. M., Davis, A., et al. (2000). Elucidating the contributions of processing speed, executive ability, and frontal lobe volume to normal age-related differences in fluid intelligence. *Journal of the International Neuropsychological Society, 6*, 52–61.

Sheline, Y. I., Raichle, M. E., Snyder, A. Z., Morris, J. C., Head, D., Wang, S., & et al. (2010). Amyloid plaques disrupt resting state default mode network connectivity in cognitively normal elderly. *Biological Psychiatry, 67*, 584–58.

Shenkin, S. D., Bastin, M. E., Macgillivray, T. J., Deary, I. J., Starr, J. M., Rivers, C. S., et al. (2005). Cognitive correlates of cerebral white matter lesions and water diffusion tensor parameters in community-dwelling older people. *Cerebrovascular Disease, 20*, 310–318.

Silver, N. C., Barker, G. J., MacManus, D. G., Tofts, P. S., & Miller, D. H. (1997). Magnetisation transfer ratio of normal brain white matter: a normative database spanning four decades of life. *Journal of Neurology, Neurosurgery, & Psychiatry, 62*, 223–228.

Sliwinski, M., & Buschke, H. (1999). Cross-sectional and longitudinal relationships among age, cognition, and processing speed. *Psychology and Aging, 14*, 8–33.

Söderlund, H., Nilsson, L. G., Berger, K., Breteler, M. M., Dufouil, C., Fuhrer, R., et al. (2006). Cerebral changes on MRI and cognitive function: the CASCADE study. *Neurobiology of Aging, 27*, 16–23.

Sperling, R. A., Laviolette, P. S., O'Keefe, K., O'Brien, J., Rentz, D. M., Pihlajamaki, M., et al. (2009). Amyloid deposition is associated with impaired default network function in older persons without dementia. *Neuron, 63*, 178–188.

Spilt, A., Geeraedts, T., de Craen, A. J., Westendorp, R. G., Blauw, G. J., & van Buchem, M. A. (2005). Age-related changes in normal-appearing brain tissue and white matter hyperintensities: More of the same or something else? *American Journal of Neuroradiology, 26*, 725–729.

Stadlbauer, A., Salomonowitz, E., Strunk, G., Hammen, T., & Ganslandt, O. (2008). Age-related degradation in the central nervous system: assessment with diffusion-tensor imaging and quantitative fiber tracking. *Radiology, 247*, 179–188.

Stern, Y. (2002). What is cognitive reserve? Theory and research application of the reserve concept. *Journal of the International Neuropsychological Society, 8*, 448–460.

Sullivan, E. V., & Pfefferbaum, A. (2006). Diffusion tensor imaging and aging. *Neuroscience and Biobehavioral Reviews, 30*, 749–761.

Sullivan, E. V., Adalsteinsson, E., Hedehus, M., Ju, C., Moseley, M., Lim, K. O., et al. (2001). Equivalent disruption of regional white matter microstructure in ageing healthy men and women. *Neuroreport, 12*, 99–104.

Sullivan, E. V., Adalsteinsson, E., & Pfefferbaum, A. (2010). Selective age-related degradation of anterior callosal fiber bundles quantified in vivo with fiber tracking. *Cerebral Cortex, 16*, 1030–1039.

Sullivan, E. V., Rohlfing, T., & Pfefferbaum, A. (2010). Quantitative fiber tracking of lateral and interhemispheric white matter systems in normal aging: Relations to timed performance. *Neurobiology of Aging, 31*, 464–481.

Swan, G. E., DeCarli, C., Miller, B. L., Reed, T., Wolf, P. A., Jack, L. M., et al. (1998). Association of midlife blood pressure to late-life cognitive decline and brain morphology. *Neurology, 51*, 986–993.

Tapp, P. D., Siwak, C. T., Gao, F. Q., Chiou, J. Y., Black, S. E., Head, E., et al. (2004). Frontal lobe volume, function, and beta-amyloid pathology in a canine model of aging. *Journal of Neuroscience, 24*, 8205–8213.

Tisserand, D. J., Pruessner, J. C., Sanz Arigita, E. J., van Boxtel, M. P., Evans, A. C., Jolles, J., et al. (2002). Regional frontal cortical volumes decrease differentially in aging: An MRI study to compare volumetric approaches and voxel-based morphometry. *Neuroimage, 17*, 657–669.

Tzourio, C., Lévy, C., Dufouil, C., Touboul, P. J., Ducimetière, P., & Alpérovitch, A. (2001). Low cerebral blood flow velocity and risk of white matter hyperintensities. *Annals of Neurology, 49*, 411–414.

van der Hiele, K., Vein, A. A., van der Welle, A., van der Grond, J., Westendorp, R. G., Bollen, E. L., et al. (2007). EEG and MRI correlates of mild cognitive impairment and Alzheimer's disease. *Neurobiology of Aging, 28*, 1322–1329.

Van Petten, C., Plante, E., Davidson, P. S., Kuo, T. Y., Bajuscak, L., & Glisky, E. L. (2004). Memory and executive function in older adults: Relationships with temporal and prefrontal gray matter volumes and white matter hyperintensities. *Neuropsychologia, 42*, 1313–1335.

Van Petten, C. (2004). Relationship between hippocampal volume and memory ability in healthy individuals across the lifespan: Review and meta-analysis. *Neuropsychologia, 42*, 1394–1413.

Vannorsdall, T. D., Waldstein, S. R., Kraut, M., Pearlson, G. D., & Schretlen, D. J. (2009). White matter abnormalities and cognition in a community sample. *Archives of Clinical Neuropsychology, 24*, 209–217.

Waldstein, S. R., Manuck, S. B., Ryan, C. M., & Muldoon, M. F. (1991). Neuropsychological correlates of hypertension: Review and methodologic considerations. *Psychological Bulletin, 110*, 451–468.

Walhovd, K. B., Fjell, A. M., Reinvang, I., Lundervold, A., Fischl, B., Quinn, B. T., et al. (2004). Size does matter in the long run: Hippocampal and cortical volume predict recall across weeks. *Neurology, 63*, 1193–1197.

Walhovd, K. B., Fjell, A. M., Dale, A. M., Fischl, B., Quinn, B. T., Makris, N., et al. (2006). Regional cortical thickness matters in recall after months more than minutes. *Neuroimage, 31*, 1343–1351.

Wolff, S. D., & Balaban, R. S. (1989). Magnetization transfer contrast (MTC) and tissue water proton relaxation in vivo. *Magnetic Resonance in Medicine, 10*, 135–144.

Wozniak, J. R., & Lim, K. O. (2006). Advances in white matter imaging: A review of in vivo magnetic resonance methodologies and their applicability to the study of development and aging. *Neuroscience and Biobehavioral Review, 30*, 762–774.

Yoshita, M., Fletcher, E., & DeCarli, C. (2005). Current concepts of analysis of cerebral white matter hyperintensities on magnetic resonance imaging. *Topics in Magnetic Resonance Imaging, 16*, 399–407.

Ystad, M. A., Lundervold, A. J., Wehling, E., Espeseth, T., Rootwelt, H., Westlye, L. T., et al. (2009). Hippocampal volumes are important predictors for memory function in elderly women. *BMC Medical Imaging, 9*, 17.

Zahr, N. M., Rohlfing, T., Pfefferbaum, A., & Sullivan, E. V. (2009). Problem solving, working memory, and motor correlates of association and commissural fiber bundles in normal aging: A quantitative fiber tracking study. *Neuroimage, 44*, 1050–1062.

Zimmerman, M. E., Brickman, A. M., Paul, R. H., Grieve, S. M., Tate, D. F., Gunstad, J., et al. (2006). The relationship between frontal gray matter volume and cognition varies across the healthy adult lifespan. *American Journal of Geriatric Psychiatry, 14*, 823–833.

Zimmerman, M. E., Pan, J. W., Hetherington, H. P., Katz, M. J., Verghese, J., Buschke, H., et al. (2008). Hippocampal neurochemistry, neuromorphometry, and verbal memory in nondemented older adults. *Neurology, 70*, 1594–1600.

Chapter | 6 |

Behavior Genetics of Aging

William S. Kremen[1], Michael J. Lyons[2]

[1]Department of Psychiatry, Center for Behavioral Genomics, University of California, San Diego, La Jolla, CA; VA San Diego Healthcare System, La Jolla, CA

[2]Department of Psychology, Boston University, Boston, MA; Harvard Institute of Psychiatric Epidemiology and Genetics, Boston, MA

CHAPTER CONTENTS

Introduction 93
Quantitative Approaches 94
Twin Studies of Aging 95
Findings from Twin Studies of Aging 96
Molecular Genetics 98
Genotyping and Genetic Association Studies 98
Candidate Gene and Genome-Wide Association Studies 98
Copy Number Variants 98
Epigenetics 99
Replication and Interaction 99
Genes that may be Important for Cognitive and Brain Aging 99
Stress Responsivity 100
Other Neuroendocrine Factors 100
Integrating Twin and Molecular Genetic Approaches 102
The Problem of Phenotype Definition 102
The Construct-Measurement Fallacy: Is the Phenotype Heritable? 102
Broad versus Narrow Phenotypes 103
Summary 104
Acknowledgments 104
References 104

INTRODUCTION

Genetic factors influence a very wide range of physical and psychological characteristics. A complete understanding of the aging process will necessarily include recognition of the role that genes play in both normative and pathological aging. A number of dimensions apply to the behavior genetics of aging. Broadly speaking, genetic methodologies can be divided into quantitative and molecular approaches. Prior *Handbook* chapters on behavior genetics have focused almost exclusively on the former (McClearn & Foch, 1985; McClearn & Vogler, 2001; Omenn, 1977; Pedersen, 1996; Plomin & McClearn, 1990; Vogler, 2006). Given the exponential growth of molecular approaches in recent years, we have increased the coverage of these methods in this chapter, and we address some ways in which the two approaches may complement one another.

Another important dimension is the nature of the phenotype to be examined. Obviously, in examining the psychology of aging, the focus is on behavioral phenotypes (and the biological structures and functions that underlie them). The primary behavioral phenotypes that are relevant to aging are cognitive phenotypes such as memory and intelligence, personality phenotypes, psychosocial phenotypes, and pathologies such as depression and dementia. Throughout this chapter, key terms in genetics are italicized.

Several basic developmental questions can be asked about genetic influences during the aging process: (1) What is the relative influence of genetic and environmental factors over time? (2) To what degree are change and stability influenced by genetic and environmental factors? (3) Do the same or different genetic and environmental factors operate at different developmental stages? The extent to which genetic influences change at different ages is not well understood for most traits. Because an individual's genotype is fixed at conception, it is tempting to think of the influence of genetic factors as a stable, static phenomenon. However, while the individual's genotype does not change during the life span, different genes may be expressed or "switched on" at different

DOI: 10.1016/B978-0-12-380882-0.00006-1

developmental periods (Vogler, 2006). Over the course of development very different sets of genes might express themselves in a given characteristic, while the relative magnitude of genetic influences, that is, heritability, remained constant.

The process of aging reflects not only the unfolding of genetically regulated developmental programs over time, but also the exposure over time of the individual (and his or her genotype) to the environment. Given that both genes and environment contribute to virtually all human characteristics, one could say that all behavior is the result of the interaction of genes and environment. Although this statement is true on a descriptive level, it is not necessarily always true in the formal statistical sense. A true *gene x environment interaction* refers to a phenomenon by which genetic factors moderate the relationship between an environmental influence and a phenotypic outcome. Shanahan and Hofer (2005) utilized existing examples of gene x environment interactions to identify four putative mechanisms by which the environment may moderate genetic influences: (1) the social environment can trigger a genetic diathesis, (2) the social environment can compensate for a genetic diathesis, (3) the social environment can act as a control to prevent behaviors for which there is a genetic predisposition, and (4) the social environment can enhance adaptation through proximal processes.

Gene-environment correlation refers to a phenomenon by which genetic factors influence exposure to the environment. For example, there is substantial evidence that genetic factors play a major role in tobacco use and tobacco use disorders (Li & Burmeister, 2009). Tobacco use is a significant environmental exposure for a number of health outcomes that typically manifest themselves as individuals age. To have a comprehensive understanding of the relationship between genetic factors and, for example, lung cancer, it would be important to include the role that genetic factors play in influencing the individual's exposure to the primary risk factor for lung cancer (i.e., smoking). Numerous environmental factors relevant to aging in addition to smoking such as diet, alcohol consumption, and exercise are significantly influenced by genetic factors. Almost certainly, aspects of the social environment, such as social networks and the type of cognitive activities in which an individual participates are influenced, at least to some extent, by genetic factors. For example, although life events are, by definition, part of the "environment," Saudino and colleagues (1997) found that for women, controllable, desirable, and undesirable life events were significantly influenced by genetic factors. In other words, one's genetic endowment plays a significant role in determining to which aspects of the environment the individual is exposed.

Evolution operates through a process by which certain genetically mediated characteristics are more likely to be passed on to subsequent generations and certain characteristics less likely. This process "selects" traits that promote the survival of the individual's genes. After the individual completes his or her reproductive period, natural selection for adaptive traits may no longer operate because the individual is no longer competing to pass along his or her genes. In this view, evolution is indifferent to the fate of organisms in their post-reproductive years. However, alternative views have been suggested. Ekman and colleagues (2003) suggested that findings on the psychology of aging are consistent with the operations of evolutionary pressures during later life. They point out that the most significant cognitive loss associated with aging is new learning, while integrated knowledge of the world increases with age. They argued that improvements in socioemotional regulation associated with aging increases investment in emotionally meaningful others, particularly kin, and these late-life psychological characteristics contribute to the reproductive success of those with whom the individual shares his or her genes (i.e., kin). Flatt and Schmidt (2009) argued that progress in understanding the molecular genetics of aging will be facilitated by integrating evolutionary approaches (e.g., addressing whether longevity genes are under selection in natural populations).

QUANTITATIVE APPROACHES

The three traditional methodologies utilized in quantitative genetic studies are family, twin, and adoption studies. The traditional family study examines the degree of similarity in whatever traits are studied among related individuals. Resemblance among family members reflects genetic influences and shared environmental influences. There have been, and continue to be, genetically informative studies of aging that utilize families, but the large majority use molecular genetic approaches and/or address nonpsychological characteristics. A notable exception is the Seattle Longitudinal Study (Schaie, 1983). The primary focus of the study is not genetic, but the structure of the extensive data that have been collected permits genetic questions to be addressed. Family studies cannot unambiguously distinguish between genetic factors and shared environmental factors as the sources of family resemblance, but as Schaie et al. (1993) have pointed out, it may be reasonable to assume that the influence of the shared environment on cognitive abilities during adulthood is quite modest. Schaie and colleagues examined sibling resemblance and parent–offspring resemblance in a broad range of intellectual abilities and the dimension of social responsibility (Schaie, 2005; Schaie et al., 1992; Schaie et al., 1993; Schaie & Zuo, 2001). Significant heritability was observed for measures of verbal meaning, spatial orientation, reasoning, numeric ability, word fluency, cognitive flexibility, and psychomotor speed. Only the dimension of social responsibility and perceptual speed did not appear to be heritable. Moreover, results suggested that, in general, genetically influenced familial similarity is stable and maintained throughout adult life. However, the magnitude of the family resemblance varied somewhat in relation to the sex of the individuals in the dyads and for parent–offspring versus sibling dyads.

Adoption studies capitalize on a naturally occurring experiment in which some individuals are given their genes by one family and given their environment by another family. This is a powerful approach for disentangling the effects of genes from the effects of the family environment. However, with the very notable exception of the Swedish Adoption/Twin Study of Aging (SATSA), the adoption design has rarely been utilized to study aging. The twin design is the other traditional approach in quantitative genetic research, and it has been used extensively in research on the psychology of aging.

The twin method capitalizes on the existence of two types of twins: monozygotic (MZ) twins who share 100% of their genes and dizygotic (DZ) twins who share 50% of their genes on average. The most basic application compares the degree of similarity of MZ twins to that of DZ twins. If MZ twins are significantly more similar than DZ twins, then the trait studied is influenced, at least to some extent, by genetic factors, that is, it is heritable. Heritability is the proportion of variance accounted for by genetic influences. In this method, the total genetic plus environmental variance can be decomposed into the following proportions: (1) *genetic variance* (heritability), (2) *shared environmental variance* (environmental factors making twins similar), and 3) *unique environmental variance* (environmental factors making twins different).

Through the use of biometrical modeling, it is also possible to distinguish between additive genetic influences (in which a trait is influenced by numerous genes, each presumed to be of relatively small influence, acting additively) and nonadditive genetic influences (which reflect either the presence of a single gene of large effect or a gene x gene interaction, known as *epistasis*). Multivariate versions of the twin design make it possible to determine the extent to which two or more phenotypes have genetic and/or environmental determinants in common.

Twin Studies of Aging

Here we briefly describe several of the largest and most prominent twin studies of aging. SATSA is a longitudinal project with several waves of data collection (Pedersen et al., 1984). It has provided numerous findings in areas such as cognition, personality, coping, psychiatric and medical disorders, and physical functioning. The Finnish Twin Study on Aging (FITSA) is a study of genetic and environmental effects on the disablement process in older female twins. The participants were recruited from the Finnish Twin Cohort Study, the older cohort of which has been used to investigate genetic and environmental determinants of common, complex diseases, and their behavioral risk factors. The Norwegian Twin Registers include several sets of population-based subregisters. In 1990 the entire register became available in computerized form and a number of twin studies have utilized different parts of the register.

The Danish Twin Registry, the oldest national twin register in the world, was started in 1954. The Longitudinal Study of Aging Danish Twins (LSADT; K. Christensen et al., 1999; McGue & Christensen, 2007) includes a sample derived from the older cohorts of the Danish Twin Registry (Skytthe et al., 2002). This registry now comprises 127 birth cohorts of twins. It supports studies of genetic influence on aging and age-related health problems, normal variation in clinical parameters associated with the metabolic syndrome and cardiovascular diseases, and clinical studies of specific diseases. The Minnesota Twin Study of Adult Development (MTSADA; Finkel & McGue, 1993) is a population-based sample drawn from state birth records. The research primarily utilizes questionnaires assessing personality, occupational interests, demographics, and leisure-time activities.

There are several twin studies of aging that utilize U.S. military veterans. The Vietnam Era Twin Study of Aging (VETSA) focuses primarily on cognitive and brain aging and related processes from middle to later adulthood (Kremen et al., 2006). The National Academy of Sciences — National Research Council Twin Registry includes twins who served in the U.S. military mostly during World War II. It includes studies of dementia, Parkinson's disease, age-related physical diseases, and cognitive and structural brain changes with age.

The Older Australian Twins Study (OATS) was developed to study genetic and environmental factors in healthy brain aging and aging-related neurocognitive disorders. It utilizes a longitudinal design and links with a brain donor program. The Osaka University Aged Twin Registry (OUATR) is Japan's largest adult twin registry (Hayakawa et al., 2006). It has investigated environmental and genetic influences on physical and cognitive aging, longevity, and aging-dependent diseases in later adulthood. There are also important twin studies of aging that focus on samples selected for particular characteristics such as the OCTO-Twin study (McClearn et al., 1997) that examined twins over the age of 80 years and the Carolina African American Twin Study on Aging (CAATSA; Whitfield et al., 2009).

Findings from Twin Studies of Aging

Twin studies of aging have addressed a very wide array of psychological phenotypes. A review of all relevant phenotypes is beyond the scope of this chapter. In this section we will briefly review findings on general cognitive ability and personality which exemplify the research of this type. The area of cognition has been a particular focus of genetic research on psychological aspects of aging. Here we will briefly review relevant findings concerning general cognitive ability. The issue of how genetic factors influence general cognitive ability during aging is significant in its own right, but it also exemplifies how various issues related to aging have been addressed.

A number of genetically uninformative studies have demonstrated very substantial stability for general cognitive ability from youth through middle to later adulthood. After reviewing the extant research findings, Deary et al. (2000) concluded that "the genetic and environmental sources of this remarkable stability of individual differences in human intelligence must be sought" (p. 54). Bouchard and McGue (2003) reviewed genetic research on cognition and concluded — based primarily on cross-sectional results — that the relative strength of genetic and environmental influences on intelligence varies with age. Haworth et al. (2009) examined general intellectual ability in 11,000 child and adolescent twin pairs. The data were combined from cross-sectional studies using different cognitive measures. Results were consistent with the conclusion of Bouchard and McGue (2003). In 2003 Bouchard and McGue noted the "extreme paucity" of genetic studies of intelligence in adult twins and suggested that studies of young twins "swamp the database." Nearly two decades later, it is still true that the large majority of developmentally oriented studies of cognitive ability have examined children and adolescents. Interestingly, Schaie (1975) had already addressed some of these issues 35 years ago. He pointed out that differences observed between age groups in cross-sectional studies may be due to either age differences or cohort differences (or both). Observations of no differences in age groups could reflect age and cohort effects that operate in opposite directions. To resolve this type of problem, he described study design options that optimize the ability to draw inferences from developmental behavior genetics research.

Studies that have addressed the issue of possible changes in the relative magnitude of genetic and environmental influences during adulthood have used primarily cross-sectional methods. In a study of individuals from the SATSA with an average age of 65, Pedersen et al. (2002) found a heritability of 0.81 for the first principal component of their cognitive measures. Although their data were cross-sectional, they utilized a hierarchical multiple regression approach and reported that heritability did not differ significantly as a function of age over the age range they studied (50 to 84 years). Finkel et al. (1998) used a cohort sequential design to study cognitive ability with three measurement occasions separated by three-year intervals in another examination of the SATSA sample. They found a significant decrease in the genetic variance for the principal component representing general cognitive ability. The heritability of their measure of general cognitive ability fell from approximately 0.80 for their three younger cohorts to approximately 0.60 for the three older cohorts. In their study the longest longitudinal interval was six years.

Finkel et al. (1995) reported results of cross-sectional analyses in which they combined samples from the SATSA and the MTSADA. They divided the samples into three age groups: (younger adults 27 to 50 years; middle-aged 50 to 65 years; and older 65 to 88 years). They found a heritability of 0.80 for all three age groupings of the MTSADA twins and the two younger SATSA cohorts and 0.56 for the older Swedish twins. The data from MTSADA suggest no change in the heritability of cognitive ability across age cohorts, whereas the Swedish sample was consistent with stability during the first two age groups and a possible decline in heritability in late adulthood. Using cross-sectional data from an extended twin design, Posthuma et al. (2001) reported results of intelligence testing in two cohorts (mean ages 26.2 years and 50.4 years) of Dutch twins. For Verbal IQ and Performance IQ, heritabilities were 85% and 69%, respectively. The two age cohorts did not differ in heritability.

Using a cohort sequential design, McGue and Christensen (2002) examined a sample of Danish twins over age 70 (most were considerably older than 70) on a battery of brief cognitive measures. They used a cohort sequential design covering eight years with two-year intervals. The mean age at the first assessment was 75.7 years and the mean age at the fourth and last assessment was 85.6 years. They observed little systematic difference in genetic variance across the four measurement occasions with a heritability of about 0.50. In a longitudinal study, Plomin et al. (1994) assessed a sample of older twins on two occasions spanning three years (mean ages 64 and 67) and observed a heritability of approximately 0.80 for general cognitive ability at both times. Reynolds et al. (2005), in a study using SATSA with longitudinal assessments spanning 30 years (at ages 50, 60, 70, and 80), found an inverted U-shaped pattern for genetic variance; that is, genetic variance increased somewhat from age 50 to 60 years and then decreased. In a longitudinal study covering a 35-year period, the VETSA observed a heritability of 0.49 for general cognitive ability around age 20 years and a heritability of 0.57 at age 55 (Lyons et al., 2009). Combined with the child and adolescent data, it appears that the pattern is one of increasing genetic influences from childhood through adolescence, a leveling off through late middle age, and then a decrease from later middle to older age. It has been suggested that increased genetic influences through adolescence is due to gene-environment correlation such that people with greater intellectual ability tend to seek out environments that further develop their intellectual capacity (Haworth et al., 2009). The greater frequency of serious medical conditions might be a reason for the decrease in genetic influences in later life.

Only longitudinal twin data permit the determination of the extent to which the same or different genetic factors are operating during different developmental periods. There have been a number of studies that addressed this issue during childhood and adolescence (e.g., Haworth et al., 2009). However, the VETSA is the only study of which we are aware that addressed this issue in adulthood. That study found a genetic correlation of 1.0 for general cognitive ability from early adulthood to late middle age, indicating that the same genes were operating at both times (Lyons et al., 2009).

Several studies have examined the extent to which genetic factors contribute to stability and change of cognitive ability over time. McGue and Christensen (2002) found a heritability of 0.76 for the mean score on the cognitive measures, but a heritability of 0.06 for the linear change in cognitive scores over four testing occasions spanning six years. Plomin et al. (1994) observed a phenotypic stability of 0.92 over a three-year test/retest interval and found that genetic factors accounted for nearly 90% of the stability. Reynolds et al. (2005) found that the heritability of linear change in their first principal cognitive component was 0.01, while the nonshared environment explained 0.99 of the variance. The quadratic trend (acceleration of cognitive change over time or "change in the change") had a heritability of 0.43 and a contribution from the nonshared environment of 0.57. DeFries et al. (1987) found that the genetic contribution to the cognitive stability observed between age 4 and adulthood was 0.28. In the VETSA, it was found that stability in general cognitive ability primarily reflects genetic and shared environmental influences: 71.3% of the correlation between age 20 and age 55 was due to genetic factors, 22.4% due to shared environmental factors, and 6.3% due to nonshared environments. Changes were overwhelmingly (83.1%) due to aspects of the environment that were not shared by twins (Lyons et al., 2009).

There have been a number of genetic studies that have examined personality and related constructs in later life. Mosing and colleagues (2009) examined the relationship among optimism and mental and physical health in a large sample of Australian twins over age 50. Each of the three phenotypes was moderately heritable (heritabilities from 34 to 46%) with no influence from the shared environment. Significant genetic covariance among the variables indicated that genes predisposing to high optimism also predispose to good mental and physical health among older adults. Johnson et al. (2005) conducted a longitudinal study of aging in which twins from the MTSADA were assessed twice, averaging 59.4 years of age at first and 64.4 years of age at second testing (average retest interval 5.0 years). They observed extremely high stability for both means and standard deviations of scale scores and results from the two occasions were highly correlated (average $r = 0.76$ across scales). The genetic influences on most scales were almost perfectly correlated over time with somewhat lower, but still substantial, correlations between nonshared environmental influences. The high stability of personality traits in later adulthood reflected a very strong genetic foundation, supplemented by stable environmental influences.

Kato and Pedersen (2005) utilized the SATSA sample to investigate the relationship of personality to coping among older adults. They found that genetic influences on coping scales were partly due to genetic factors that also influenced personality traits. This finding suggests that the relationship of personality to coping style in part reflects genetic influences that are common to both. Heiman et al. (2003) studied women from the American Association of Retired Persons twin sample. They compared younger (age 50–65) and older (age 66+) groups (based on a median split) and found moderate heritability estimates for the four included personality dimensions (novelty seeking, harm avoidance, reward dependence, and persistence). There were no significant age differences in the proportion of genetic and environmental influences on the personality traits.

McCartney and colleagues (1990) carried out a meta-analysis of twin studies that included a number of personality variables, along with cognitive variables. Among a number of interesting findings, they observed that there was striking homogeneity among the effect sizes (in this case intraclass correlations for MZ twins and DZ twins) for the personality dimensions that they included (activity–impulsivity, aggression, anxiety, dominance, emotionality, masculinity–femininity, sociability, and task orientation). Intraclass correlations for intelligence were consistently larger than for personality variables. McCartney et al. (1990) found that as there was increasing dissimilarity within both MZ and DZ pairs as age increased, confirming the "growing up and growing apart" hypothesis with which they had started their investigation. However, the oldest age of subjects for whom personality data were available was 50 years, so their meta-analysis does not address the issue of genetic and environmental influences on personality during the later parts of the life span.

Pedersen and Reynolds (1998) utilized four waves of personality data collected from the SATSA sample. They observed stability of means in neuroticism, extraversion, and openness to experience. Very substantial genetic stability was observed across time while environmental effects were primarily responsible for new variance. The shared environment demonstrated little influence on the included personality traits. Individuals' rate of change in personality indicated that variability increased with age, especially for openness to experience. Genetic influences that operated at one time were generally still operating at subsequent times, however, environmental influences were less stable and new environmental influences appeared over time. No time-specific genetic influences were observed after age 30, but new nonshared environmental influences were found at each assessment, demonstrating that genetic influences are substantially more stable than environmental influences.

Viken et al. (1994) utilized a cohort-sequential design with Finnish twins between the ages of 18 and 59. The stability of genetic and environmental influences over a six-year interval was evaluated. Extraversion and neuroticism demonstrated moderate heritabilities with decreasing magnitude of genetic influence across age. However, there was no evidence for significant new genetic influences after 29 years of age with age-to-age genetic correlations of unity. New environmental influences were observed at each age and time point.

Thus, the stability of both general intellectual ability and personality traits appears to be largely due to genetic influences. The heritability of general intellectual ability tends to be higher than it is for personality characteristics. It is also worth noting that the pattern observed for personality traits contrasts with the increasing genetic influences on general intellectual ability through the same age period.

MOLECULAR GENETICS

In contrast to the twin method, in which genetic influences are latent constructs and the specific genes that account for a particular aging-related trait are anonymous, molecular genetics refers to methods that attempt to identify specific genetic variations that underlie the trait of interest. At this time, the workhorse approach is the genetic association study.

Genotyping and Genetic Association Studies

Association studies do not require related individuals. This approach tests for the association of particular polymorphisms (inherited DNA sequence variations or genotypes) with a particular phenotype, most commonly via interrogation of *single nucleotide polymorphisms* (SNPs). SNPs occur when a single nucleotide differs across individuals at a particular position on a gene. An SNP is composed of one of the four bases (A, C, G, or T) plus a sugar and a phosphate molecule. To be considered an SNP, a variant must generally be present in at least one percent of the population. The variant may be a substitution, deletion, or insertion. If an SNP is associated with a trait of interest, it suggests that it is causally related to the trait or that it is in linkage disequilibrium with a locus that is causally related to the trait. *Linkage disequilibrium* refers to the fact that the SNP is likely to be close to the locus responsible for the trait, and thus tends to go together with that locus.

It is now common to have microarray gene chips with 1 million SNPs to provide excellent coverage of the genome. With an estimated 20,000 to 30,000 genes in the human genome, these chips include multiple SNPs within a given gene. Only about one or two percent of SNPs appear to be functional. Functional change refers to amino acid changes in the process of translation. *Translation* refers to the production of proteins after DNA has been transcribed into RNA; this is how the genetic information in the DNA becomes expressed.

Although genetic association studies provide quantitative results, they do not provide direct information about biological function. Also, environmental factors are not excluded from observed associations. As in twin studies, associations with a particular SNP reflect how much the genetic variance "stands out" over the total genetic and environmental variance (Kendler, 2005). The difference is that the association study involves the identification of specific genes.

Candidate Gene and Genome-Wide Association Studies

The candidate gene approach is a hypothesis-testing approach based on a priori selection of genes or SNPs on the basis of presumed biological plausibility and empirical evidence. In genome-wide association studies (GWAS), one attempts to search as much of the genome as possible in a hypothesis-generation approach. GWAS takes the problem of multiple statistical tests to its highest level. Adjusting alpha levels to control the false discovery rates for hundreds of thousands of statistical tests will require large effect sizes. However, most psychological aging phenomena are likely to be polygenic; that is, determined by multiple genetic and environmental factors, each likely to be of small effect). It might seem that the solution to this problem is to generate a priori hypotheses and use a candidate gene approach. Unfortunately, this approach has not always been successful, indicating that our understanding of underlying genetic processes is incomplete.

Copy Number Variants

Copy number variants (CNVs) are large DNA segments for which differences in copy numbers among individuals have been demonstrated. Thus, in addition to differences in the coding sequence, gene dosage is also a source of genetic diversity. CNVs may be inherited or occur de novo (in germ cells of either parent) or at later developmental stages. Most CNV research has used dichotomous, disease phenotypes. For example, CNVs appear to play a central role in the pathogenesis of Alzheimer's and Parkinson's disease (Lee & Lupski, 2006). Furthermore, CNVs may account for more human variation than SNPs, including significant variation in cognitive, behavioral, and psychological characteristics (Lee & Lupski, 2006; Lupski, 2007). Bruder et al. (2008) demonstrated CNV differences in a small sample of MZ twins. Consistent with the notion that CNVs may account for normal variation, differences were observed even in healthy pairs.

Epigenetics

Epigenetics refers to functional differences, that is, changes by non-genetic factors that result in alternations in the expression (activation or inhibition) of genes, but not the basic structure or sequence of the DNA. *Gene expression* refers to the process of genetic information being turned into a functional gene product via transcription and translation. *Transcription* is the process by which DNA is read and re-copied into messenger RNA (mRNA). In the process of translation, information in the RNA is translated into enzymes and other proteins. The genetic blueprint or genetic information in the DNA thus becomes expressed in the production of specific enzymes which, in turn, leads to modifications in the phenotype.

DNA methylation refers to the chemical modification of DNA by the addition of a methyl group. This process happens in *dinucleotides* (cytosine and guanine separated by a phosphate), and it is the mechanism by which gene expression takes place. Methylation not only alters gene expression, but it can be inherited via cell division even though such changes are not passed on to offspring through the germ line. DNA methylation is important with respect to aging for several reasons. It is associated with longevity (Gravina & Vijg, 2009). Normal aging is associated with declines in DNA methylation throughout the brain, and it has been suggested that this DNA methylation is associated with memory function (Gravina & Vijg, 2009; Liu et al., 2009). Stress experienced early in life may also cause lasting changes in DNA methylation that may affect gene expression and behavior throughout the life course. For example, severe early adversity was associated with widespread differences in brain DNA methylation in the glucocorticoid receptor gene in adults (McGowan et al., 2009).

The epigenome differs from the structural genome in two major ways: DNA methylation and gene expression are both dynamic and tissue-specific processes. Thus, although MZ twins have identical genotypes, they can differ in terms of gene expression or DNA methylation. However, not all epigenetic processes are a reflection of environmental influences. Individual differences in the degree of DNA methylation or gene expression are also under varying degrees of genetic control; that is, they are heritable and their heritability may vary for different CpG sites (Heijmans et al., 2007). Some of these epigenetic processes may also change with age. (B. C. Christensen et al., 2009). Factors that contribute to methylation changes are also factors important for aging; these include carcinogen exposure (including tobacco and alcohol), inflammation, diet, and stress (B. C. Christensen et al., 2009; McGowan et al., 2009).

Replication and Interaction

Many of the problems noted for genotyping studies apply to the study of CNVs and epigenetics as well. At this time, adequate solutions have not been developed and failures to replicate are common. However, there is even serious debate about the meaning of failures to replicate. One notion is that such failures reflect *genetic heterogeneity;* that is, different genetic variants may be responsible for similar phenotypic outcomes. Alternatively, it has been suggested that with complex polygenic phenomena, gene-gene interactions are likely to be the norm rather than the exception (Moore, 2003). Moreover, lack of replication of gene association is likely to indicate that epitasis is present rather than indicating that the original finding was a false positive as shown by Moore (2003). Complicating this issue is the fact that, with the number of SNPs in a GWAS, there are an astronomical number of potential interactions.

There is also a question of how specific a replication must be. It is likely that redundancies are built into the system so that damage to any single gene does not have to be catastrophic. It may be that associations with different genes that are in the same pathway (gene ontology) are meaningful, even if the replication is not found for the same specific single gene.

Genes that may be Important for Cognitive and Brain Aging

Several areas of focus are common to studies of cognitive and brain aging because they examine phenomena that directly or indirectly influence these aging processes. Direct measures are, of course, cognitive assessment and neuroimaging. An example of indirect measures would be indicators of cardiovascular function. Hypertension, for example, has been associated with subtly poorer cognitive performance and with increased white matter abnormalities and smaller prefrontal cortex (DeCarli et al., 1999; Raz et al., 2003).

Genes that may have an impact on cognitive aging have been summarized in reviews by Deary et al.

(2004) and Mattay et al. (2008), and they have been organized largely around some of these common categories. These include genes associated with the following:

Dementia. Examples include: APOE (apolipoprotein E), APP (amyloid precursor protein), PSEN1, PSEN2 (presenelin 1 and 2), SORL1 (sortilin-related receptor).

Cognitive function. These include genes associated with general intellectual ability, or specific processes such as working memory or episodic memory. Examples include: COMT (catechol-*O*-methyl transferase), 5HT2a (serotonin 2a receptor), 5HTTLPR (serotonin transporter), BDNF (brain-derived neurotrophic factor), KIBRA, GRM3 (glutamate receptor metabotropic).

Cardiovascular function. Examples include: ACE (angiotensin 1 converting enzyme), MTHFR (methyl-tetrahydrofolate reductase).

Inflammatory processes. Proinflammatory cytokines may affect brain function via neurodegenerative, excitotoxic, and other processes. Examples include: IL-1β, IL-2, IL-6, IL-8 (interleukin 1β, 2, 6, and 8), and TNF-α (tumor necrosis factor alpha).

Oxidative stress. The brain is particularly vulnerable to oxidative stress from free radicals. Examples include: KLOTHO, PRNP (prion protein gene), IGF (insulin-like growth factor), DAPK1 (death-associated protein kinase 1).

Other processes that we would add include genes associated with the following.

Stress Responsivity

The hypothalamic-pituitary-adrenal (HPA) axis is a major stress response system. Alterations in cortisol regulation and responsivity (a key HPA component) have been associated with age-related conditions such as hypertension, diabetes, central obesity, and depression, as well as differences in cognition and brain structure. Prefrontal cortex and hippocampus — brain regions manifesting important age-related changes — have high concentrations of glucocorticoid receptors. Thus, genes involved in regulating the stress response system may play a role in modulating cognitive and brain aging. Possible candidates include: CRF, CRF1 (corticotropin-releasing factor), NR3C1 GR promoter (glucorticoid receptor [nuclear receptor subfamily 3, group C, member 1]), and FKBP5. Note also that these categories are not necessarily mutually exclusive; for example, inflammatory processes also reflect stress responsivity.

Other Neuroendocrine Factors

Other hormones such as testosterone, estrogen, and DHEA may also play modulatory roles that impact cognitive and brain aging (Ferrari & Magri, 2008). For example, androgen receptors are highly expressed in the hippocampus, frontal cortex, and hypothalamus (Beyenburg et al., 2000; Pike et al., 2008; Raber et al., 2002). Functional polymorphisms of the androgen receptor gene have been associated with episodic memory, even in women (Kovacs et al., 2009). DHEA and testosterone both have opposing actions to cortisol such that these androgens may offset or protect against the deleterious effects of elevated cortisol (Oettel et al., 2003; Wolkowitz & Reus, 2003). Circulating levels of both DHEA and testosterone also decrease with age (Oettel et al., 2003; Tenover, 1997; Wolkowitz & Reus, 2003). Differences in the rate of testosterone decline with age, and thus could have an impact on cortisol and its effects on brain and cognition. Therefore, genes regulating these hormones, such as the androgen receptor (AR) gene, may play a role in regulating cognitive and brain aging.

The most solid genetic association finding in cognitive and brain aging research is the association of ε4 allele of the APOE gene and risk for Alzheimer's disease. There are three alleles for the biallelic APOE gene (ε2, ε3, and ε4). Inheriting one ε4 allele increases the risk of developing Alzheimer's disease, and inheriting two results in still greater risk; possessing an ε2 allele may be protective (Farrer et al., 1997). Given the replicated association with Alzheimer's disease, it is not surprising that APOE has been studied extensively with regard to episodic memory performance and hippocampal volume. A meta-analysis has also shown that possessing an ε4 allele is associated with subtle cognitive deficits in healthy aging; this effect is small and has been observed primarily in general cognitive ability, episodic memory, and executive function (Small et al., 2004).

A natural consequence of this work is the question of how early APOE-related abnormalities manifest themselves and whether they are associated with age-related cognitive decline in general. This work is of obvious importance for the basic understanding of cognitive and brain aging, but it is also important for the possible development of strategies for prevention or early intervention. In contrast to results for Alzheimer's disease, the findings of associations between APOE genotype and cognitive or brain abnormalities in relatively younger individuals who have not developed dementia have been mixed.

IQ differences were not found between ε4+ and ε4− individuals in two samples of school-aged children (Deary et al., 2003; Turic et al., 2001). In 19- to 21-year-old women, full scale IQ was not significantly different in ε4+ and ε4− individuals, but performance IQ was significantly higher in ε4 carriers (Yu et al., 2000). Even though full scale IQ was not significantly different in this study, it was higher in ε4 carriers and the effect size was 0.34. Results from another study of school-aged children and one of individuals ranging in age from 6 to 65 both found evidence of cognitive advantages in people with an ε4 allele (Alexander et al., 2007; Bloss et al., 2008). The latter two studies suggested that antagonistic pleiotropy might be at work. Antagonistic pleiotropy is a phenomenon in which a gene with harmful effects at a later stage in life might confer some benefits earlier in life (G. C. Williams, 1957). At this time, it is uncertain whether the APOE genotype is truly an example of antagonistic pleiotropy and whether having an ε4 is associated with subtle cognitive or brain abnormalities in relatively younger, nondemented individuals.

Family history of Alzheimer's disease could be a factor that interacts with APOE genotype, but it appears that these two factors may have independent and additive (not interactive) effects on cognitive decline (Hayden et al., 2009). However, it should be noted that this conclusion came from a study in which cognition was assessed with only a screening instrument (Modified Mini-Mental Status Examination). A full understanding of the impact of the APOE genotype on cognitive and brain aging will likely require more extensive study of its interaction with other genes or biological factors. An example comes from animal studies that suggest androgen receptors may moderate the deleterious effects of the APOE-ε4 allele. Indeed, Raber (2008) proposed that different APOE genotypes differentially regulate androgen receptors. As we have already noted, there are high concentrations of androgen receptors in both prefrontal cortex and hippocampus, there are consistent age-related changes in androgens (e.g., lowering of testosterone levels) that might influence the number or the efficiency of androgen receptors in the brain, and cortisol levels tend to remain the same or increase with age. Sex differences in APOE effects have also been reported. Taken together, these data suggest that it is likely to be important to consider interactions between APOE genotype and genes that are involved in the regulation of androgens (e.g., AR gene) or other non-genetic indicators such as testosterone or cortisol levels. For example, there is some evidence that having both an ε4 allele and a low level of circulating testosterone increases the risk for Alzheimer's disease (Hogervorst et al., 2002).

COMT and BDNF are two of the most extensively studied genes with respect to cognition. COMT is often presented as a gene that is important for executive function and working memory, whereas BDNF is often presented as a gene that is important for episodic memory. Although there is some validity to this characterization, a close look at the literature indicates that their effects are often pleiotropic. Thus, simplistic notions of "one gene-one specific cognitive ability" should be avoided. Moreover, there is growing evidence for the importance of their interaction with other genes.

As shown in several twin studies, genetic influences may change with age. Lindenberger and colleagues (2008; Nagel et al., 2008) have articulated a compelling theory to account for age-related differences in the effects of genes on cognitive function. They observed that cognitive differences associated with COMT polymorphisms have been studied mostly in younger adults and that findings have been inconsistent. They also point out that variability in cognitive performance is increased in older adults (Bäckman et al., 1999). They hypothesized that brain resources modulate the effects of genetic variant on cognitive function, and that the relationship between brain resources and cognition is nonlinear. This nonlinear relationship means that a reduction in brain resources with normal aging results in larger effects on cognition. Thus, genetic differences are more likely to be associated with cognitive function differences in older than in younger adults.

The relationship between dopamine activity and cognitive function fits an inverted U-shaped function (G. V. Williams & Goldman-Rakic, 1995). Because frontal dopamine signaling is lower in older adults, they are on a steeper portion of the curve compared with younger adults; that is, they are presumed to be shifted to the leftward side of the inverted U. Consequently, Val/Val versus Met/Met COMT genotypes in older adults may differ in dopamine signaling strength by similar amounts as their younger counterparts. But, by being on the steeper part of the curve, older adults may manifest greater cognitive differences as a function of COMT genotype (Nagel et al., 2008). Interestingly, this result was shown, in part, with the Wisconsin Card Sorting Test (WCST); performance differences according to COMT genotype were found only in older, not younger, adults. This result appears to contradict findings that the WCST is not heritable. However, the heritability studies were on children and younger adults. Therefore, it is possible that the WCST may be heritable in much older adults. A similar pattern was found for BDNF genotypes, but only for WCST reaction time and not errors. Thus, the BDNF results may be relevant to processing speed rather than executive function or working memory per se. Nevertheless, both findings are consistent with hypotheses about reduced brain resources with aging leading to increased genetic effects on cognitive performance.

Nagel et al. (2008) also found an interaction between COMT and BDNF. Another gene-gene interaction was observed between COMT and DAT with respect to reward processing (Yacubian et al., 2007). In addition to putative links to executive function and working memory, there have been associations reported between COMT and processing speed and attention (Bilder et al., 2002), reward processing (Yacubian et al., 2007), and response to aversive stimuli (Smolka et al., 2007). COMT has also been associated with visuospatial ability in middle-aged adults (de Frias et al., 2005), and episodic memory in older adults (de Frias et al., 2004). Bilder et al. (2004)

attempted to integrate the literature on the neurobehavioral significance of COMT by theorizing that it plays a key role in the balance between tonic and phasic dopamine activity, which may have fairly wide-ranging neurobehavioral effects. As noted, other studies point to age-related differences in the behavioral manifestations of COMT (de Frias et al., 2004, 2005; Lindenberger et al., 2008; Nagel et al., 2008). These findings serve to highlight the potential importance of gene-gene interactions, pleiotropic effects, use of different phenotype definitions, and age effects. A general rule of thumb for genetic association studies is, of course, that results need to be replicated. We suggest that a corollary to this rule might be that gene associations should also be followed up with tests of related phenotypes to determine the broadness or narrowness of the phenotype, and additional age groups to determine whether a genetic association is specific to a particular developmental period.

INTEGRATING TWIN AND MOLECULAR GENETIC APPROACHES

Integrating twin and gene association methods is a powerful approach that can advance the progress of genetic association studies. Twin methods can be used in a variety of ways to optimize both cross-sectional and longitudinal phenotypes for genetic association studies. As such, twin studies can inform genetic association studies of aging in important ways, including generating predictions.

The Problem of Phenotype Definition

Despite all of the technological advances in high-throughput techniques that allow for the identification of hundreds of thousands of SNPs, it has still been difficult to identify the genes for aging-related or other behavioral and psychological characteristics that are likely to be polygenic. Phenotype definition is probably one of the major rate-limiting factors in genetic association studies. One key factor may be that our traditional cognitive measures were not developed with genetics in mind, and may, thus, be less than optimal for use in genetic studies (Goldberg & Weinberger, 2004). The same can be said of most other behavioral or psychological measures. Technological advances that make it possible to interrogate larger numbers of genes or SNPs will not obviate the need for appropriately defined phenotypes. Yet it seems safe to say that not enough attention has been paid to the goal of developing phenotypes that are optimal for genetic studies.

The Construct-Measurement Fallacy: Is the Phenotype Heritable?

The most basic requirement for any phenotype for genetic studies is that it must be heritable. This point is obvious, yet fairly often overlooked. We suspect that there are at least two reasons for this. One is that heritability data were simply not available for the particular measure of interest. The other is what we refer to as the "construct-measurement fallacy." This is the unstated assumption that if a construct is heritable, any measure within that substantive domain will be heritable. For example, meta-analysis indicates that broadly defined memory is moderately heritable (0.48) averaged across multiple studies with different instruments and different age groups (Bouchard & McGue, 2003). The tendency is to assume that any memory measure must, therefore, be heritable. However, it is still possible that a particular memory measure might not be heritable, even though the underlying construct is indeed influenced by genes.

In addition, memory is not a unitary construct. Behavior genetic studies have not often appreciated the need to separate the different components of memory as is the practice within a cognitive neuroscience framework. The result might be a lack of differentiation between short-term/working memory and episodic memory, or lack of differentiation within either of these domains. For example, episodic memory performance includes encoding, storage, and retrieval. It is an empirical question that is far from fully answered whether these different component processes are influenced by the same or different genes. If it turns out that they are influenced by different genes, it would then suggest that findings in genetic studies could be obscured if researchers do not separate those components when studying memory phenotypes. For example, no association was found between memory scores and APOE genotype in over 6500 nondemented adults ages 20–64 (Jorm et al., 2007). The memory measure in this study was trial 1 of the California Verbal Learning Test (CVLT; Delis et al., 1987). Despite the fact that the APOE-ε4 allele is a well-known risk factor for Alzheimer's disease, these results suggest that memory deficits are not manifest in APOE-ε4 carriers this early in life. That conclusion is, in part, dependent on CVLT trial 1 being heritable. If it were not, then one would predict the result that was obtained; that is, test scores for a measure that is not heritable should not vary according to genetic differences (i.e., one's genotype). We have estimated the heritability of multiple CVLT measures in over 1200 middle-aged male twins (unpublished data). Many CVLT scores were heritable, but trial 1 scores were not. Therefore, it appears that these results cannot fully address the question of whether ε4 carriers manifest memory deficits prior to age 65.

The WCST, a widely used and well-validated measure of executive function and working memory, serves as another example. Despite its use in many genetic association studies, four of five twin studies have shown that its heritability is at or near zero (Chou et al., 2009; Kremen et al., 2007). Consequently, genetic associations with the WCST are likely to be inconsistent at best. Of course, this does not mean that genes play no role in executive functions. On the contrary, many studies indicate that they do. Inferring from these findings that executive function and working memory are not influenced by genetic factors would constitute the construct-measurement fallacy in reverse. It simply suggests that the WCST is not an efficient way to measure these cognitive abilities for genetic studies. In this case, we have suggested that the problem may be due to the fact that the WCST is a relatively complex and multidetermined phenotype that involves multiple component cognitive processes (Kremen et al., 2007). The processes that account for deficits may be quite different in different individuals. If a test score reflects different processes for different people, it could obscure the genetic signal of each of those processes; perhaps in this case, canceling each other out and resulting in zero heritability.

Broad versus Narrow Phenotypes

Another key question for phenotype definition is whether it is better to have broad or narrow phenotypes. Broad phenotypes tend to have higher heritability than narrow phenotypes (Hasler et al., 2006). IQ or *g*, for example, tends to have higher heritability than specific cognitive abilities (Bouchard & McGue, 2003). Although heritability carries no information regarding how many genes are involved or how powerful the effect of any individual gene may be on a given phenotype (Plomin et al., 2001), higher heritability still provides greater confidence in the importance of genetic factors. On the other hand, a potential drawback of broader phenotypes is that they may really be a composite of different processes or abilities, as in the example of the WCST. This notion also applies to IQ because two people with the same full scale IQ may have rather different profiles of cognitive strengths and weaknesses. We refer to these traditional, relatively complex and multidetermined tests as "broad-brush-stroke" cognitive tests.

Unlike the WCST, however, IQ is a highly heritable broad-brushstroke test. It seems clear then that the only way to gauge the heritability of a measure is to test it empirically. In the case of IQ, even though it is highly heritable, its inherent broad-brushstroke nature may limit its utility as a phenotype for genetic studies of cognitive aging because it may limit precision. Knowing, for example, that the overall test is heritable is not necessarily informative about the heritability of the specific component processes that are thought to be most relevant to cognitive aging.

One solution to this problem is to delineate narrower phenotypes by parsing the components of a broader measure. Twin studies are an ideal vehicle for accomplishing this goal. In the context of multivariate twin analysis, it is not only possible to parse the components of a broader measure but one can also parse the genetic and environmental influences on the different components. As such, this approach integrates cognitive neuroscience and behavioral genetic approaches. Multivariate twin analysis is also capable of separating common and specific genetic influences. The heritability of particular components is likely to be lower than the heritability of the broader construct, but if the multivariate twin analysis shows that a component has specific genetic influences (i.e., genes that influence a particular component and are independent of the genes that influence other components of the test), the component with specific genetic influences may be a more optimal phenotype for genetic association studies. In other words, a narrower phenotype may have lower heritability but greater genetic specificity because it would reduce the chances of the genetic "signal" being obscured by genetic "noise." A broader phenotype is more likely to be influenced by additional genes that are not relevant to the key construct or process of interest.

Note that although we used cognition as an example, the same logic applies to phenotypes in any psychological or behavioral domain. An example of this concept comes from the examination of cortical thickness and cortical surface area in a magnetic resonance imaging study of 474 middle-aged twins (Panizzon et al., 2009). How age-related structural brain changes are associated with age-related cognitive changes is an issue of importance to many cognitive aging researchers. Volume is the most commonly assessed brain structure phenotype, but cortical volume is the product of cortical thickness and surface area. The twin analysis showed that these two components of cortical volume are genetically independent, a finding that is consistent with the radial unit hypothesis of cortical development (Rakic, 2007). Thus, volume measures may obscure the presence of two essentially independent sets of genes. Support for this distinction comes from recent studies in which SNPs of the genes MECP2, CDK5RAP2, MCPH1, and ASPM were found to be associated with cortical surface area, but not with cortical thickness (Joyner et al., 2009; Rimol et al., 2010). Determining when narrower (parsed) measures or broader (composite) measures make better phenotypes for genetic studies remains an empirical question that requires evaluation on a case-by-case basis. A key point here is the importance of efforts to more fully understand a phenotype from a genetic perspective before proceeding with genetic association studies of aging. Put differently, the advent of high-throughput techniques and sequencing of the human genome have not made the twin study approach obsolete or unnecessary. In fact, aging researchers should benefit from more efforts to integrate twin and molecular genetic approaches.

SUMMARY

Early optimism about applying sophisticated new molecular and statistical techniques to discover individual genes with substantial effects on behavioral aging have given way to a much more modest and pragmatic approach. The likelihood that numerous genes and environmental factors contribute to many, if not most, human characteristics and that there are likely to be complex interactions among genes and environmental factors suggests that achieving a full understanding of how genes affect the psychology of aging will be a slow, painstaking process. Advances in high-throughput techniques have paved the way for major advances in molecular genetics. These include the study of individual differences based on genotype, CNV, and epigenetics. However, for the study of cognitive, behavioral, and other psychological phenomena, definition of the phenotype remains a major rate-limiting factor. Use of twin methods as a complement to molecular genetic approaches is suggested as a way to refine behavioral genetic research on aging. Although genes have been implicated in cognitive and other aging processes, more attention needs to be paid to replication of findings and to the additive or multiplicative effects of genes. More attention also needs to be paid to pleiotropic and differential effects of genes at different points in the aging process. Finally, those of us who are interested in behavior genetics must be cautious about overemphasizing genetic influences at the expense of environmental factors. It is hoped that the growth of epigenetics will reinvigorate the study of gene-environment interaction and gene-environment correlation as they impact the aging process.

ACKNOWLEDGMENTS

Preparation of this chapter was supported by grants from the National Institute on Aging to William Kremen (AG022381, AG018384, and AG022982) and Michael Lyons (AG018386), and by the Center of Excellence for Stress and Mental Health at the VA San Diego Healthcare System. The authors gratefully acknowledge the assistance of Molly Franz in reviewing research literature for this chapter.

REFERENCES

Alexander, D. M., Williams, L. M., Gatt, J. M., Dobson-Stone, C., Kuan, S. A., Todd, E. G., et al. (2007). The contribution of apolipoprotein E alleles on cognitive performance and dynamic neural activity over six decades. *Biological Psychology, 75*, 229–238.

Bäckman, L., Small, B. J., Wahlin, A., & Larsson, A. (1999). Cognitive functioning in very old age. In F. I. Craik, & T. A. Salthouse (Eds.), *Handbook of aging and cognition: Vol. 2* (pp. 499–588). Mahwah, NJ: Erlbaum.

Beyenburg, S., Watzka, M., Clusmann, H., Blumcke, I., Bidlingmaier, F., Elger, C. E., et al. (2000). Androgen receptor mRNA expression in the human hippocampus. *Neuroscience Letters, 294*, 25–28.

Bilder, R. M., Volavka, J., Czobor, P., Malhotra, A. K., Kennedy, J. L., Ni, X., et al. (2002). Neurocognitive correlates of the COMT Val^{158}Met Polymorphism in chronic schizophrenia. *Biological Psychiatry, 52*, 701–707.

Bilder, R. M., Volavka, J., Lachman, H. M., & Grace, A. A. (2004). The catechol-O-methyltransferase polymorphism: relations to the tonic-phasic dopamine hypothesis and neuropsychiatric phenotypes. *Neuropsychopharmacology, 29*, 1943–1961.

Bloss, C. S., Delis, D. C., Salmon, D. P., & Bondi, M. W. (2008). APOE genotype is associated with left-handedness and visuospatial skills in children. *Neurobiology of Aging* [Epub ahead of print].

Bouchard, T. J., Jr., & McGue, M. (2003). Genetic and environmental influences on human psychological differences. *Journal of Neurobiology, 54*, 4–45.

Bruder, C. E., Piotrowski, A., Gijsbers, A. A., Andersson, R., Erickson, S., de Stahl, T. D., et al. (2008). Phenotypically concordant and discordant monozygotic twins display different DNA copy-number-variation profiles. *American Journal of Human Genetics, 82*, 763–771.

Chou, L. N., Kuo, P. H., Lin, C. C., & Chen, W. J. (2009). Genetic and environmental influences on the Wisconsin Card Sorting Test performance in healthy adolescents: A twin/sibling study. *Behavior Genetics* [Epub ahead of print].

Christensen, B. C., Houseman, E. A., Marsit, C. J., Zheng, S., Wrensch, M. R., Wiemels, J. L., et al. (2009). Aging and environmental exposures alter tissue-specific DNA methylation dependent upon CpG island context. *PLoS Genetics, 5*, e1000602.

Christensen, K., Holm, N. V., McGue, M., Corder, L., & Vaupel, J. W. (1999). A Danish population-based twin study on general health in the elderly. *Journal of Aging and Health, 11*, 49–64.

de Frias, C. M., Annerbrink, K., Westberg, L., Eriksson, E., Adolfsson, R., & Nilsson, L. G. (2004). COMT gene polymorphism is associated with declarative memory in adulthood and old age. *Behavior Genetics, 34*, 533–539.

de Frias, C. M., Annerbrink, K., Westberg, L., Eriksson, E., Adolfsson, R., & Nilsson, L. G. (2005). Catechol O-methyltransferase Val158Met polymorphism is associated with cognitive performance in nondemented adults. *Journal of Cognitive Neuroscience, 17*, 1018–1025.

Deary, I. J., Whalley, L. J., Lemmon, H., Crawford, J. R., & Starr, J. M. (2000). The stability of individual differences in mental ability from childhood to old age: Follow-up of the 1932 Scottish mental survey. *Intelligence, 28*, 49–55.

Deary, I. J., Whalley, L. J., St., Clair, D., Breen, G., Leaper, S., Lemmon, H., et al. (2003). The influence of the e4 allele of the apolipoprotein E gene on childhood IQ, nonverbal reasoning in old age, and lifetime cognitive change. *Intelligence, 31*, 85–92.

Deary, I. J., Wright, A. F., Harris, S. E., Whalley, L. J., & Starr, J. M. (2004). Searching for genetic influences on normal cognitive ageing. *Trends in Cognitive Sciences, 8*, 178–184.

DeCarli, C., Miller, B. L., Swan, G. E., Reed, T., Wolf, P. A., Garner, J., et al. (1999). Predictors of brain morphology for the men of the NHLBI twin study. *Stroke, 30*, 529–536.

DeFries, J. C., Plomin, R., & Labuda, M. C. (1987). Genetic stability of cognitive development from childhood to adulthood. *Developmental Psychology, 23*, 4–12.

Delis, D., Kramer, J., Kaplan, E., & Ober, B. (1987). *The California Verbal Learning Test*. San Antonio: Psychological Corporation.

Ekman, P., Campos, J. J., Davidson, R. J., & DeWaal, F. B. M. (2003). *Emotions inside out: 130 years after Darwin's The Expression of the Emotions in Man and Animals: Vol. 1000*. New York: Annals of the New York Academy of Sciences.

Farrer, L. A., Cupples, L. A., Haines, J. L., Hyman, B., Kukull, W. A., Mayeux, R., et al. (1997). Effects of age, sex, and ethnicity on the association between apolipoprotein E genotype and Alzheimer disease. A meta-analysis. APOE and Alzheimer Disease Meta Analysis Consortium. *Journal of the American Medical Association, 278*, 1349–1356.

Ferrari, E., & Magri, F. (2008). Role of neuroendocrine pathways in cognitive decline during aging. *Ageing Research Reviews, 7*(3), 225–233.

Finkel, D., Pedersen, N., Plonin, R., & McClearn, G. E. (1998). Longitudinal and cross-sectional twin data on cognitive abilites in adulthood. The Swedish adoption/twin study of aging. *Developmental Psychology, 34*(6), 1400–1413.

Finkel, D., & McGue, M. (1993). 25-year follow-up of child-rearing practices: Reliability of retrospective data. *Personality and Individual Differences, 15*, 147–154.

Finkel, D., Pedersen, N. L., McGue, M., & McClearn, G. E. (1995). Heritability of cognitive abilities in adult twins: Comparison of Minnesota and Swedish data. *Behavior Genetics, 25*, 421–431.

Flatt, T., & Schmidt, P. S. (2009). Integrating evolutionary and molecular genetics of aging. *Biochimica et Biophysica Acta, 1790*, 951–962.

Goldberg, T. E., & Weinberger, D. R. (2004). Genes and the parsing of cognitive processes. *Trends in Cognitive Sciences, 8*, 325–335.

Gravina, S., & Vijg, J. (2009). Epigenetic factors in aging and longevity. *European Journal of Physiology, 459*(2), 247–258.

Hasler, G., Drevets, W. C., Gould, T. D., Gottesman, I. I., & Manji, H. K. (2006). Toward constructing an endophenotype strategy for bipolar disorders. *Biological Psychiatry, 60*, 93–105.

Haworth, C. M., Wright, M. J., Luciano, M., Martin, N. G., de Geus, E. J., van Beijsterveldt, C. E., et al. (2009). The heritability of general cognitive ability increases linearly from childhood to young adulthood. *Molecular Psychiatry* [Epub ahead of print].

Hayakawa, K., Kato, K., Onoi, M., Yang-Ping, C., Kanamori, M., Doi, S., et al. (2006). The Osaka University Aged Twin Registry: Epigenetics and identical twins discordant for aging-dependent diseases. *Twin Research and Human Genetics, 9*, 808–810.

Hayden, K. M., Zandi, P. P., West, N. A., Tschanz, J. T., Norton, M. C., Corcoran, C., et al. (2009). Effects of family history and apolipoprotein E epsilon4 status on cognitive decline in the absence of Alzheimer dementia: The Cache County Study. *Archives of Neurology, 66*, 1378–1383.

Heijmans, B. T., Kremer, D., Tobi, E. W., Boomsma, D. I., & Slagboom, P. E. (2007). Heritable rather than age-related environmental and stochastic factors dominate variation in DNA methylation of the human IGF2/H19 locus. *Human Molecular Genetics, 16*, 547–554.

Heiman, N., Stallings, M. C., Hofer, S. M., & Hewitt, J. K. (2003). Investigating age differences in the genetic and environmental structure of the tridimensional personality questionnaire in later adulthood. *Behavior Genetics, 33*, 171–180.

Hogervorst, E., Lehmann, D. J., Warden, D. R., McBroom, J., & Smith, A. D. (2002). Apolipoprotein E epsilon4 and testosterone interact in the risk of Alzheimer's disease in men. *International Journal of Geriatric Psychiatry, 17*, 938–940.

Johnson, W., McGue, M., & Krueger, R. F. (2005). Personality stability in late adulthood: A behavioral genetic analysis. *Journal of Personality, 73*, 523–552.

Jorm, A. F., Mather, K. A., Butterworth, P., Anstey, K. J., Christensen, H., & Easteal, S. (2007). APOE genotype and cognitive functioning in a large age-stratified population sample. *Neuropsychology, 21*, 1–8.

Joyner, A. H., Roddey, C., Dale, A. M., Andreassen, O. A., Schork, N. J., Bloss, C. S., et al. (2009). *MECP2 variants associate with measures of brain size and IQ*. Paper presented at the Presented at the fifth International Imaging Genetics Conference.

Kato, K., & Pedersen, N. L. (2005). Personality and coping: A study of twins reared apart and twins reared together. *Behavior Genetics, 35*, 147–158.

Kendler, K. S. (2005). Introduction. In K. S. Kendler & L. J. Eaves (Eds.), *Psychiatric Genetics* (pp. 1–17). Washington, DC: American Psychiatric Publishing.

Kovacs, D., Vassos, E., Liu, X., Sun, X., Hu, J., Breen, G., et al. (2009). The androgen receptor gene polyglycine repeat polymorphism is associated with memory performance in healthy Chinese individuals. *Psychoneuroendocrinology, 34*, 947–952.

Kremen, W. S., Eisen, S. A., Tsuang, M. T., & Lyons, M. J. (2007). Is the Wisconsin Card Sorting Test a useful neurocognitive endophenotype? *American Journal Medical Genetics (Neuropsychiatric Genetics), 144B*, 403–406.

Kremen, W. S., Thompson-Brenner, H., Leung, Y. J., Grant, M. D., Franz, C. E., Eisen, S. A., et al. (2006). Genes, environment, and time: The Vietnam Era Twin Study of Aging (VETSA). *Twin Research and Human Genetics, 9*, 1009–1022.

Lee, J. A., & Lupski, J. R. (2006). Genomic rearrangements and gene copy-number alterations as a cause of nervous system disorders. *Neuron, 52*, 103–121.

Li, M. D., & Burmeister, M. (2009). New insigts into the genetics of addiction. *Nature Reviews Genetics, 10*(4), 225–231.

Lindenberger, U., Nagel, I. E., Chicherio, C., Li, S. C., Heekeren, H. R., & Backman, L. (2008). Age-related decline in brain resources modulates genetic effects on cognitive functioning. *Frontiers in Neuroscience, 2*, 234–244.

Liu, L., van Groen, T., Kadish, I., & Tollefsbol, T. O. (2009). DNA methylation impacts on learning and memory in aging. *Neurobiology of Aging, 30*, 549–560.

Lupski, J. R. (2007). Structural variation in the human genome. *New England Journal of Medicine, 356*, 1169–1171.

Lyons, M. J., York, T. P., Franz, C. E., Grant, M. D., Eaves, L. J., Jacobson, K. C., et al. (2009). Genes determine stability and environment determines change in cognitive ability during 35 years of adulthood. *Psychological Science, 11*, 1146–1152.

Mattay, V. S., Goldberg, T. E., Sambataro, F., & Weinberger, D. R. (2008). Neurobiology of cognitive aging: Insights from imaging genetics. *Biological Psychology, 79*, 9–22.

McCartney, K., Harris, M., & Bernieri, F. (1990). Growing up and growing apart: A developmental meta-analysis of twin studies. *Psychological Bulletin, 107*, 226–237.

McClearn, G. E., & Foch, T. (1985). Behavior genetics. In J. E. Birren & K. W. Schaie (Eds.), *Handbook of the psychology of aging* (2nd ed.) (pp. 113–143). New York: Van Nostrand Reinhold.

McClearn, G. E., Johansson, B., Berg, S., Pedersen, N. L., Ahern, F., Petrill, S. A., et al. (1997). Substantial genetic influence on cognitive abilities in twins 80 or more years old. *Science, 276*, 1560–1563.

McClearn, G. E., & Vogler, G. P. (2001). The genetics of behavioral aging. In J. E. Birren & K. W. Schaie (Eds.), *Handbook of the pyschology of aging* (5th ed.). San Diego, CA: Academic Press.

McGowan, P. O., Sasaki, A., D'Alessio, A. C., Dymov, S., Labonte, B., Szyf, M., et al. (2009). Epigenetic regulation of the glucocorticoid receptor in human brain associates with childhood abuse. *Nature Neuroscience, 12*, 342–348.

McGue, M., & Christensen, K. (2002). The heritability of level and rate-of-change in cognitive functioning in Danish twins aged 70 years and older. *Experimental Aging Research, 28*, 435–451.

McGue, M., & Christensen, K. (2007). Social activity and healthy aging: A study of aging Danish twins. *Twin Research and Human Genetics, 10*, 255–265.

Moore, J. H. (2003). The ubiquitous nature of epistasis in determining susceptibility to common human diseases. *Human Heredity, 56*, 73–82.

Mosing, M. A., Zietsch, B. P., Shekar, S. N., Wright, M. J., & Martin, N. G. (2009). Genetic and environmental influences on optimism and its relationship to mental and self-rated health: A study of aging twins. *Behavior Genetics, 39*, 597–604.

Nagel, I. E., Chicherio, C., Li, S. C., von Oertzen, T., Sander, T., Villringer, A., et al. (2008). Human aging magnifies genetic effects on executive functioning and working memory. *Frontiers in Human Neuroscience, 2*, 1–8.

Oettel, M., Hubler, D., & Patchev, V. (2003). Selected aspects of endocrine pharmacology of the aging male. *Experimental Gerontology, 38*, 189–198.

Omenn, G. S. (1977). Behavior genetics. In J. E. Birren & K. W. Schaie (Eds.), *Handbook of the psychology of aging* (pp. 190–280). New York: Van Nostrand Reinhold.

Panizzon, M. S., Fennema-Notestine, C., Eyler, L. T., Jernigan, T. L., Prom-Wormley, E., Neale, M. C., et al. (2009). Distinct genetic influences on cortical surface area and cortical thickness. *Cerebral Cortex, 19*, 2728–2735.

Pedersen, N. L. (1996). Gerontological behavior genetics. In J. E. Birren & K. W. Schaie (Eds.), *Handbook of the psychology of aging* (4th ed.) (pp. 59–77). San Diego, CA: Academic Press.

Pedersen, N. L., Friberg, L., Floderus-Myrhed, B., McClearn, G. E., & Plomin, R. (1984). Swedish early separated twins: Identification and characterization. *Acta Geneticae Medicae et Gemellologiae (Roma), 33*, 243–250.

Pedersen, N. L., Lichtenstein, P., & Svedberg, P. (2002). The Swedish Twin Registry in the third millennium. *Twin Research, 5*, 427–432.

Pedersen, N. L., & Reynolds, C. A. (1998). Stability and change in adult personality: Genetic and environmental components. *European Journal of Personality, 12*, 338–365.

Pike, C. J., Nguyen, T. V., Ramsden, M., Yao, M., Murphy, M. P., & Rosario, E. R. (2008). Androgen cell signaling pathways involved in neuroprotective actions. *Hormones and Behavior, 53*, 693–705.

Plomin, R., DeFries, J. C., McClearn, G. E., & McGuffin, P. (2001). *Behavioral genetics* (4th ed.). New York: Worth.

Plomin, R., & McClearn, G. E. (1990). Human behavior genetics of aging. In J. E. Birren & K. W. Schaie (Eds.), *Handbook of the psychology of aging* (3rd ed.) (pp. 67–79). San Diego, CA: Academic Press.

Plomin, R., Pedersen, N. L., Lichtenstein, P., & McClearn, G. E. (1994). Variability and stability in cognitive abilities are largely genetic later in life. *Behavior Genetics, 24*, 207–215.

Posthuma, D., de Geus, E. J., & Boomsma, D. I. (2001). Perceptual speed and IQ are associated through common genetic factors. *Behavior Genetics, 31*, 593–602.

Raber, J. (2008). AR, apoE, and cognitive function. *Hormones and Behavior, 53*, 706–715.

Raber, J., Bongers, G., LeFevour, A., Buttini, M., & Mucke, L. (2002). Androgens protect against apolipoprotein E4-induced cognitive deficits. *Journal of Neuroscience, 22*, 5204–5209.

Rakic, P. (2007). The radial edifice of cortical architecture: From neuronal silhouettes to genetic engineering. *Brain Research Review, 55*, 204–219.

Raz, N., Rodrigue, K. M., & Acker, J. D. (2003). Hypertension and the brain: Vulnerability of the prefrontal regions and executive functions. *Behavioral Neuroscience, 117*, 1169–1180.

Reynolds, C. A., Finkel, D., McArdle, J. J., Gatz, M., Berg, S., & Pedersen, N. L. (2005). Quantitative genetic analysis of latent growth curve models of cognitive abilities in adulthood. *Developmental Psychology, 41*, 3–16.

Rimol, L. M., Agartz, I., Djurovic, S., Brown, A. A., Roddey, J. C., Kähler, A. K., et al. (2010). Sex-dependent association of common variants of microcephaly genes with brain structure. *Proceedings of the National Academy of Sciences U.S.A*, 107(1), 384–388.

Saudino, K. J., Pedersen, N. L., Lichtenstein, P., McClearn, G. E., & Plomin, R. (1997). Can personality explain genetic influences on life events? *Journal of Personality and Social Pyschology, 72*, 196–206.

Schaie, K. W. (1975). Research strategy in the development of human behavior genetics. In K. W. Schaie, E. V. Anderson, G. E. McClearn, & J. Money (Eds.), *Developmental human behavior genetics* (pp. 205–220). Lexington, MA: D.C. Heath.

Schaie, K. W. (1983). The Seattle Longitudinal Study: A twenty-one year exploration of psychometric intelligence in adulthood. In K. W. Schaie (Ed.), *Longitudinal studies of adult psychological development* (pp. 64–135). New York: Guilford.

Schaie, K. W. (2005). Influences of family environment on cognition. In K. W. Schaie (Ed.), *Developmental influences on adult intelligence: The Seattle Longitudinal Study* (pp. 367–394). New York: Oxford University Press.

Schaie, K. W., Plomin, R., Willis, S. L., Gruber-Baldini, A., & Dutta, R. (1992). Natural cohorts: Family similarity in adult cognition. In T. Sonderegger (Series Ed.) & *Psychology and aging. Nebraska Symposium on Motivation, 1991* (pp. 205–243). Lincoln: University of Nebraska Press.

Schaie, K. W., Plomin, R., Willis, S. L., Gruber-Baldini, A., Dutta, R., & Bayan, U. (1993). Longitudinal studies of family similarity in intellectual abilities. In J. J. Schroots & J. E. Birren (Eds.), *The next generation of longitudinal studies of health and aging* (pp. 183–198). Amsterdam: Elsevier.

Schaie, K. W., & Zuo, Y. L. (2001). Family environments and cognitive functioning. In R. J. Sternbeg & E. Grigorenko (Eds.), *Cognitive development in context* (pp. 337–361). Hillside, NJ: Erlbaum.

Shanahan, M. J., & Hofer, S. M. (2005). Social context in gene-environment interactions: Retrospect and prospect. *Journals of Gerontology B. Psychological Sciences and Social Sciences, 60 Spec No, 1*, 65–76.

Skytthe, A., Kyvik, K., Holm, N. V., Vaupel, J. W., & Christensen, K. (2002). The Danish Twin Registry: 127 birth cohorts of twins. *Twin Research, 5*, 352–357.

Small, B. J., Rosnick, C. B., Fratiglioni, L., & Backman, L. (2004). Apolipoprotein E and cognitive performance: A meta-analysis. *Psychology and Aging, 19*, 592–600.

Smolka, M. N., Buhler, M., Schumann, G., Klein, S., Hu, X. Z., Moayer, M., et al. (2007). Gene-gene effects on central processing of aversive stimuli. *Molecular Psychiatry, 12*, 307–317.

Tenover, J. (1997). Testosterone and the aging male. *Journal of Andrology, 18*, 103–106.

Turic, D., Fisher, P. J., Plomin, R., & Owen, M. J. (2001). No association between apolipoprotein E polymorphisms and general cognitive ability in children. *Neuroscience Letters, 299*, 97–100.

Viken, R. J., Rose, R. J., Kaprio, J., & Koskenvuo, M. (1994). A developmental genetic analysis of adult personality: Extraversion and neuroticism from 18 to 59 years of age. *Journal of Personality and Social Psychology, 66*, 722–730.

Vogler, G. P. (2006). Behavior genetics and aging. In J. E. Birren & K. W. Schaie (Eds.), *Handbook of the psychology of aging* (6th ed.) (pp. 41–55). San Diego, CA: Elsevier.

Whitfield, K. E., Kiddoe, J., Gamaldo, A., Andel, R., & Edwards, C. L. (2009). Concordance rates for cognitive impairment among older African American twins. *Alzheimer's and Dementia, 5*, 276–279.

Williams, G. C. (1957). Pleiotropy, natural selection and the evolution of senescence. *Evolution, 11*, 398–411.

Williams, G. V., & Goldman-Rakic, P. S. (1995). Modulation of memory fields by dopamine D1 receptors in prefrontal cortex. *Nature, 376*, 572–575.

Wolkowitz, O. M., & Reus, V. I. (2003). Dehydroepiandrosterone in psychoneuroendocrinology. In O. M. Wolkowitz & A. J. Rothschild (Eds.), *Psychoneuroendocrinology: The Scientific Basis of Clinical Practice* (pp. 205–241). Washington, DC: APA Press.

Yacubian, J., Sommer, T., Schroeder, K., Glascher, J., Kalisch, R., Leuenberger, B., et al. (2007). Gene-gene interaction associated with neural reward sensitivity. *Proceedings of the National Academy of Sciences USA, 104*, 8125–8130.

Yu, Y. W., Lin, C. H., Chen, S. P., Hong, C. J., & Tsai, S. J. (2000). Intelligence and event-related potentials for young female human volunteer apolipoprotein E epsilon4 and non-epsilon4 carriers. *Neuroscience Letters, 294*, 179–181.

Chapter | 7 |

Neuroplasticity, Aging, and Cognitive Function

Denise C. Park, Gérard N. Bischof
The Center for Vital Longevity, University of Texas, Dallas, Texas, USA

CHAPTER CONTENTS

Introduction 109
Overview of Age-Related Changes in Brain and Behavior 110
The Scaffolding Theory of Aging and Cognition 112
Evidence for Experience-Based Changes in Neural Function in Older Adults 113
Expert Behaviors 114
Neural Correlates of Long-Term Memory Training 114
Neural Correlates of Training Executive Function 114
Experimental Studies of Engagement 115
Fitness Training as a Cognitive Intervention 116
Conclusions 116
Acknowledgments 117
References 117

INTRODUCTION

In the past five years, there has been a marked societal concern about what can be done to maintain "mental sharpness" as people age. A burgeoning industry has developed with an array of products available that claim to purportedly improve mental function. Many of these products utilize a software-based approach to "train the brain" and decrease one's mental age from an older to a younger age. Much of the software is based on an adaptation of neuropsychological tests such as the Stroop task (Stroop, 1935) and Digit-Symbol task (Wechsler, 1997) to a more game-based approach, where the user, after initial performance on a set of tasks, is provided with his or her "mental age." After more practice or training on these tasks, the mental age is recalculated, with the outcome being that "brain age" has typically decreased to a younger and more desirable age. Implicit in the marketing of brain training software is the notion that the brain can be fundamentally changed in some fashion with training, much as one develops increased muscle, aerobic capacity, and physical endurance with exercise training. Despite the public's enthusiasm and optimism about the role of mental exercise in maintaining brain function, the evidence to support this belief is actually quite limited. A recent study examined the impact of cognitive training on over 11,000 participants who were recruited to train online on cognitive tasks (Owen et al., 2010). Although the authors found evidence that participants improved on the specific tasks on which they trained, there was no evidence for a general "sharpening" of abilities, as no improvement was observed for transfer of skill increases to untrained tasks. In the same month this study was published, the National Institutes of Health (NIH) convened a "State-of-the Science Conference" to assess evidence for factors that might play a role in preventing Alzheimer's disease (AD) and explicitly considered the role of brain training and experience in preventing or delaying the onset of AD. They concluded that there was very limited evidence to support the possibility that cognitive engagement and cognitive training delays cognitive decline, but also concluded that there was at least preliminary evidence to suggest that there is a "beneficial association of physical activity and a range of leisure activities…with the preservation of cognitive function" (NIH State-of-the-Science Conference Preventing Alzheimer's Disease and Cognitive Decline, Final Statement, p. 6).

DOI: 10.1016/B978-0-12-380882-0.00007-3

Implicit in the controversy about whether there are interventions that delay age-related cognitive decline or the onset of AD is the requirement that, for interventions to be effective, the brain, as it ages, must retain plasticity. By plasticity, we mean that the brain retains the ability to change and develop as a result of experiences. In this chapter, we address the relatively narrow question of what evidence exists to indicate that cognitive interventions change neural function or structure of the brain. The related issue of whether interventions change cognitive behavior is ably addressed by Chapter 10 in the present volume. We also note that other excellent and recent comprehensive reviews of training effects in older adults are available (Hertzog et al., 2009; Lustig et al., 2009; Noack et al., 2009). Our goal with this chapter, then, is to provide a brief overview of neural changes that occur in the brain with age, a theoretical model for understanding the relationship between neural changes with age and the role that interventions might play in heightening plasticity, and then review extant evidence that addresses the relationship between neurocognitive function and cognitive interventions. We conclude with unresolved questions and recommendations for future research in this important domain that has clearly captivated the interest of both scientists and the public, as well as marketing executives and software companies.

OVERVIEW OF AGE-RELATED CHANGES IN BRAIN AND BEHAVIOR

It is clear that as people age, they show declines in tasks that are markers of fluid intelligence such as speed of processing, working memory function, long-term memory, and reasoning. At the same time as changes in cognitive hardware occurs, there is preservation, if not growth, in markers of crystallized ability such as vocabulary and general knowledge. Figure 7.1 shows results from a large, cross-sectional study of highly selected adults (Park et al., 2002). It demonstrates reliable differences in speed of processing, working memory, and long-term memory as a function of age, while showing age invariance in measures of knowledge. Although differences in the trajectory of age-related decline are observed across different studies, Figure 7.1 is representative of the cognitive aging literature, which demonstrates that even very healthy adults experience some decline in fluid abilities with advancing age, although the age at which deflection occurs is variable (e.g., Schaie, 2005).

The advent of the neuroimaging era has vastly expanded our knowledge of the aging mind. Initial work in aging focused on imaging the brain structure or brain volume of different cortical regions, providing reliable evidence that some cortical areas of the brain show shrinkage in volume with age, whereas volume is maintained in other structures. A very thorough and comprehensive treatment of age differences in neural structure is presented in this volume by Karen Rodrigue and Kristen Kennedy, and the interested reader is referred to Chapter 5. Briefly, the evidence indicates that the frontal cortex of the brain is most susceptible to age-related shrinkage in volume (e.g., Raz, 2005) followed by medial temporal areas, particularly the hippocampus (e.g., Raz & Rodrigue, 2006). The occipital regions are largely protected from volumetric shrinkage with age. Along with these volumetric changes, there is also a decrease in the structural integrity of the white matter (Head et al.,

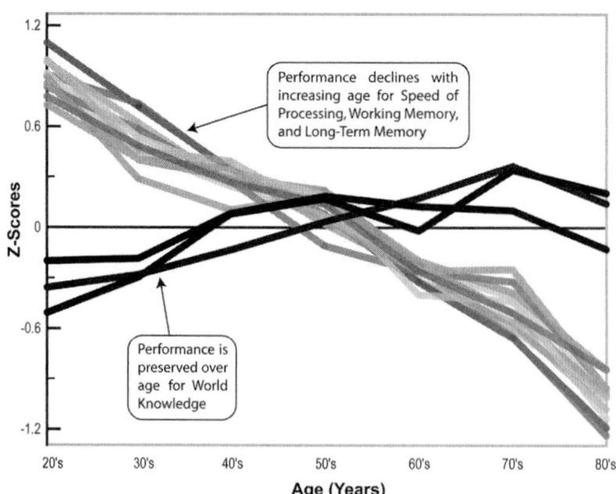

Figure 7.1 Cross-sectional aging data adapted from Park et al. (2002) showing behavioral performance on measures of speed of processing (i.e., Digit Symbol, Letter Comparison, Pattern Comparison), working memory (i.e., Letter Rotation, Line Span, Computation Span, Reading Span), Long-Term Memory (i.e., Benton, Rey, Cued Recall, Free Recall), and world knowledge (i.e., Shipley Vocabulary, Antonym Vocabulary, Synonym Vocabulary). Almost all measures of cognitive function show negative effects with age, except world knowledge, which even show positive age effects.

2004; Kennedy & Raz, 2009), an increase in small white matter lesions evidenced by hyperintensities in structural brain images (e.g., Gunning-Dixon et al., 2009), and a dysregulation and depletion in dopaminergic receptors (e.g., Kaasinen et al., 2000). Most recently, techniques have become available that permit researchers to measure amyloid deposition on neural structures by injecting radiotracers (Pittsburgh Compound B, 18F-labeled tracer FDDNP or AV-45, Avid Pharmaceuticals) that bind with amyloid, a protein that deposits in the brain in some individuals with age. PET scanning of the injected individual provides a detailed assessment of the amount of amyloid as well as distribution of it in the brain. Amyloid deposition is a characteristic feature of virtually all patients with AD. However, it is also present in many normal adults (Rowe et al., 2010; see Rodrigue et al., 2009 for a review) and it is often a harbinger of conversion to AD (e.g., Andreasen et al., 1999; Diniz et al., 2008; Jack et al., 2008).

Functional imaging data, in contrast to behavioral and structural data, reveal evidence for increasing activation with age, rather than presenting a pattern of decline like the structural and cognitive data do. There is clear evidence that with age, older adults show more activation in prefrontal cortex than young adults on verbal memory tasks (see Figure 7.2). Figure 7.2 demonstrates that both young and old evidence focal, left prefrontal activity when confronted with a verbal processing task, but old show additional activation relative to young in the right hemisphere (Cabeza et al., 2002; Reuter-Lorenz et al., 2000). There is growing evidence that this additional contralateral recruitment is indeed functional and supportive of cognition in older adults. First, the tendency for older adults to engage both hemispheres compared to younger adults has been associated with higher performance in older adults (Cabeza et al., 2002; Reuter-Lorenz et al., 2000; Rypma & D'Esposito, 2001). Second, overactivation of prefrontal regions at encoding has been specifically linked to improved memory in older adults (Gutchess et al., 2005; Morcom et al., 2003). Third, older individuals who showed the most shrinkage in hippocampal volume over a 10-year period had poorer memories, but also showed the greatest additional activation in the right prefrontal cortex (Persson et al., 2006). Hence, individuals who endured the greatest neural insults and memory decline also showed the greatest extra prefrontal activation. Finally, Rossi et al. (2004) conducted a study using repetitive transcranial magnetic stimulation (rTMS), which allows the experimenter to create a focal and temporary "brain lesion." Rossi et al. (2004) reported that young adults' memory retrieval accuracy was primarily disrupted when the rTMS was applied to the left compared to the right hemisphere. In contrast, older adults' retrieval was equally affected by the rTMS, whether it was applied to left or right, suggesting that the activations in both hemispheres were useful for performing the recognition task for older adults.

In addition to the ubiquitous finding of increased frontal recruitment with age, there is growing evidence that older adults show less neural specificity in face, place, and object-recognition areas of the brain (Chee et al., 2006; Goh et al., 2010; Park et al., 2004). Activation patterns are less selective to different categories in old compared to young, providing a neural equivalent to the behavioral measures of dedifferentiation described by Lindenberger & Baltes (1994). There is also evidence of overall, decreased activation in sensory areas in the brain of old compared to

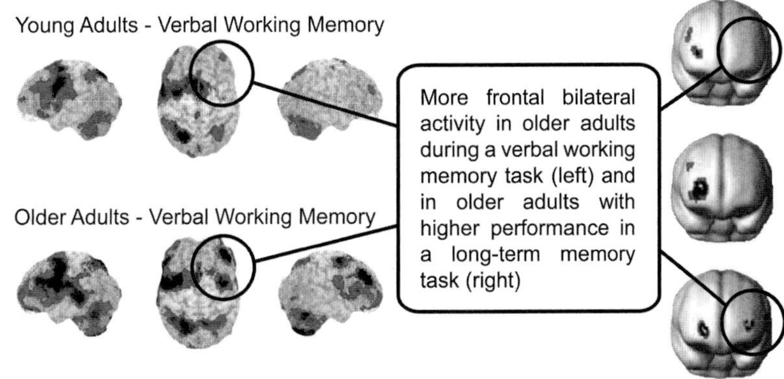

Figure 7.2 Frontal bilaterality is increased with age. (Left side). Left lateralized frontal engagement in young adults during a verbal working memory task; in older adults, an additional right frontal engagement is observed (adapted from Reuter-Lorenz et al., 2000). (Right side) *(adapted from Cabeza et al., 2002)*. Right lateralized engagement in young adults and low-performing older adults during a long-term memory task, and bilateral frontal engagement in high-performing older adults.

young adults (Cabeza et al., 2004; Davis et al., 2007) with the suggestion that some of the frontal activation is compensatory for decreased sensory function.

The other major functional imaging finding with respect to age involves the default network — sites that are activated during the baseline interval when the brain is supposedly at "rest" – which includes sites across frontal, parietal, medial temporal and visual areas (Raichle et al., 2001). Perhaps the most notable aspect of the default network is that it is suppressed when the brain shifts to a demanding cognitive task (Greicius et al., 2003). However, there is clear evidence that old adults show significantly less suppression of the default network than young adults (Grady et al., 2006; Park et al., 2010; Persson et al., 2007) with evidence that the failure to suppress is actively related to lower performance on some cognitive tasks (Damoiseaux et al., 2007; Park et al., 2010; Persson et al., 2007). It seems plausible that another reason increased frontal activity may occur in older adults is due to a failure to shift out of this relaxation or default state into more active modes of cognitive processing (Reuter-Lorenz & Lustig, 2005; Reuter-Lorenz & Cappell, 2008). There is also clear evidence that older adults show less connectivity at resting state (i.e., less synchronization of activity across different sites of the default network) among the default sites (Andrews-Hanna et al., 2007; Grady et al., 2010; Park et al., 2010) when compared to young adults.

THE SCAFFOLDING THEORY OF AGING AND COGNITION

The Scaffolding Theory of Aging and Cognition (STAC; Park & Reuter-Lorenz, 2009) provides an integrated view of the many changes that occur in the neurocognitive system with age (behaviorally, structurally, and functionally), and relates these changes to neuroplasticity. The STAC model is portrayed in Figure 7.3. Figure 7.3 indicates that aging is accompanied by deterioration of both neural structures and neural function. Declines in neural structure are represented as "neural challenges" and these are evidenced by volumetric shrinkage, white matter changes, cortical thinning, dopamine depletion, and amyloid deposition that increases with age. Deterioration in neural function occurs in direct response to the magnitude of neural challenge the aging brain faces and is marked by neural dedifferentiation, decreased hippocampal recruitment, and poor structural connectivity and disruption of the default network. The STAC model also postulates that the brain responds to this functional and structural degradation by reorganizing or creating neural scaffolds that serve as supportive structures that preserve cognitive function. The ability to form neural scaffolding in response to age-related neural insults is an index of neural plasticity. According to the STAC model, compensatory frontal recruitment, more distributed neural processing, and growth of new neurons (i.e., neurogenesis) are all mechanisms that are forms of neural scaffolding or protective reorganization. The degree of neural burden the brain faces, combined with the ability to engage in compensatory scaffolding, ultimately predicts cognitive function. Particularly noteworthy in the present discussion is the "scaffolding enhancement" component of the model, which allows for the possibility that individuals vary in their exposure to experiences that may enhance their ability to scaffold or create neuroprotective structures. This is the most speculative component of the STAC model as it posits that scaffolding can be enhanced by external experiences such as new learning, social and cognitive engagement, exercise, and cognitive training. Thus, the STAC model predicts that the aging brain can be induced to compensate more effectively for neural deterioration by external experiences

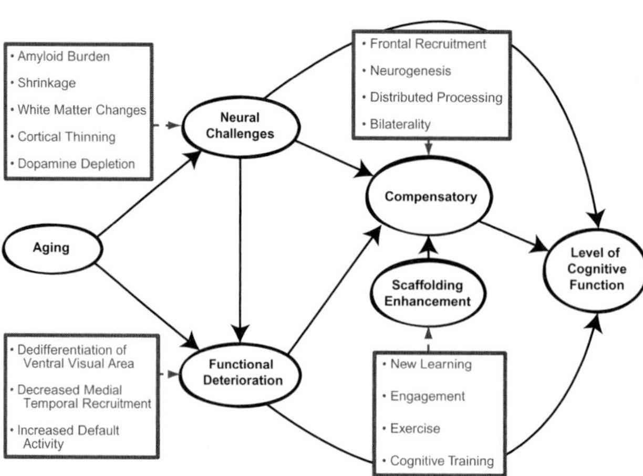

Figure 7.3 A conceptual model of the scaffolding theory of aging and cognition (STAC).

that lead to increased brain volume (e.g., neurogenesis) and more effective neural recruitment. The remainder of this chapter will focus on studies that have attempted to change neural circuitry or neural structures with interventions and assess their success. We should also note that the construct of scaffolding is in some ways similar to the construct of cognitive reserve postulated by Stern and colleagues (2002). Cognitive reserve has been hypothesized to be a latent pool of neural resources that allows individuals to evidence normal cognitive function in the face of a high pathology burden (e.g., amyloid deposition, white matter deterioration, etc.). The instantiation of cognitive reserve has been relatively fuzzy and typically equated with high education, as there is growing evidence that educated individuals dement at older ages (Hall et al., 2007) and are more likely to have a high amyloid burden while evidencing normal cognition (Fotenos et al., 2008). The STAC model makes more explicit the neural mechanisms that could conceivably account for cognitive reserve by suggesting that more scaffolding is a direct consequence of learning experience, fitness, and training and that scaffolding confers protection from some of the cognitive decline that would typically be associated with structural and functional degradation.

EVIDENCE FOR EXPERIENCE-BASED CHANGES IN NEURAL FUNCTION IN OLDER ADULTS

There are three lines of evidence (outside of the human experimental training literature that we will review) that suggest that older adults retain considerable neural plasticity and thus the ability to enhance neural function as a result of specific experiences. First, older animals subjected to enriched environments show increases in brain weight and even neurogenesis in hippocampal regions (Kempermann et al., 1997; Nilsson et al., 1999; Rosenzweig & Bennett, 1996), which provides some basis to consider it plausible that intellectual enrichment in humans might have a parallel effect. Second, older adults who suffer limb amputation show evidence for reorganization of neural tissue that is associated with the use of the limb (Ramachandran & Hirstein, 1998), a finding that has also been demonstrated for macular degeneration and reorganization of visual cortex (Baker et al., 2005; Schumacher et al., 2008). Similarly, older adults who suffer strokes show evidence for neural reorganization within new brain areas when they are forced to try to use or move a hand affected by stroke when the intact, contralateral hand has been restrained (Taub et al., 2002). All of these findings suggest that there is potential for the brain to change in middle to old age. A third line of evidence comes from studies that relate lifestyle variables to cognitive function in late adulthood or to age of onset of dementia. Hertzog et al. (2009) reviewed this literature at length and noted that there are a series of longitudinal studies that relate self-report of engagement in intellectually stimulating activities such as reading and attending cultural events to a consistently reduced rate of cognitive decline in late adulthood and/or a later onset of dementia. Nevertheless, alternative explanations for these relationships are possible, particularly the possibility that activity levels decline in a prodromal Alzheimer's state, making it difficult to conclude definitively that a cognitively engaged lifestyle is protective of cognitive function in late adulthood. Taken together, these three divergent lines of research do suggest that there should be ways to develop interventions that will delay onset of AD or increase mental acuity in late adulthood.

Expert Behaviors

There is a growing literature that demonstrates sustained engagement in a domain of expertise sculpts the structure or function of the brain in areas that are selectively engaged by the expert behavior. For example, musicians who spend long hours over a period of many years engaging in highly specific coordinated sensorimotor behaviors have subtle differences in brain structure relative to non-musicians. Moreover, the specificity of the effects is quite striking. For example, piano players have an enlarged left and right precentral gyrus whereas string players show enlargement only on the right side, reflecting the bimanual versus unimanual component of piano playing versus string performance (Bangert & Schlaug, 2006). There is also evidence for greater diffusivity of white matter in musicians (reflecting greater white matter integrity) in the corticospinal tract compared to non-musicians, reflecting a more efficient development of this tract which conveys sensorimotor information (Imfeld et al., 2009). Evidence that these effects are the result of experience is found when one considers that effects for both gray and white matter are more pronounced with earlier onset of musical training, suggesting the observed effects reflect training-induced neural changes rather than individual differences in brain structures that lead to a proclivity to obtain musical training. Similar to musical expertise is evidence regarding the relationship between spatial navigation abilities and hippocampal volume. Maguire et al. (2000) studied the hippocampal volume (a structure used for wayfinding) in London taxicab drivers relative to non-taxicab drivers. Not only did they find that cab drivers had greater hippocampal volume, the relative difference between drivers and non-drivers increased with age and experience, suggesting that it was experience that increased hippocampal volume, rather than hippocampal volume that led to the selection of cab driving as a profession.

These studies of experts provide evidence that experiences across the life span play an important role in shaping specific neural structures, suggesting that continuous shaping of neural organization occurs across the life span, but they do not provide direct evidence for neural scaffolding or plasticity in late adulthood. One approach that does directly address the issue of neural plasticity at different ages would involve developing a rigorous experimental training paradigm that trains expertise into young and old adults in a domain where specific neural effects might be expected and then, following training, assessing the magnitude of such training effects in the different age groups. The only domain where a study of this type has been done that includes neuroimaging data pre and post involves a study focused on juggling. In an initial study, Draganski et al. (2004) demonstrated that three months of training in juggling by inexperienced young adult volunteers yielded evidence for increase in volume in the mid-temporal and left parietal areas. Non-jugglers showed no such changes. It is important to note that the changes they observed in the jugglers were transient; that is, when participants were imaged again after they ceased to juggle for three months, the increases in neural tissue were no longer evident. In a second study, Boyke et al. (2008) applied this approach to older adults, utilizing the same procedure as in the juggling study of young adults. They reported a similar increase in gray matter volume in old adults in the mid-temporal region, as well as in the hippocampus and the nucleus accumbens. When the data from the two experiments were entered into a single analysis, Boyke et al. (2008) reported a slightly smaller increase in gray matter volume in older adults compared to young adults. To summarize these important findings, the authors, across the two studies, reported clear evidence for experience-based plasticity in both old and young adults, with evidence for slightly more plasticity in the young. The fact that the increases in structural volume were transient suggests that the old adage of "use it or lose it" appears to have some merit. Much more work is needed in a broad range of domains to understand both the potential and limits of neural plasticity in older adults. Of particular importance is whether experience-induced changes can result in lasting increases in neural structure or function, or whether all experience-induced changes are transient in nature and quickly disappear when the expert behavior is no longer practiced.

Neural Correlates of Long-Term Memory Training

We are aware of only one published study in the literature that trained young and old on a memory task and utilized pre- and posttest neuroimaging, although there are many more behavioral studies. Before discussing the neural study, we would like to mention one classic study utilizing only behavioral methods that was conducted by Kliegl et al. (1990). They trained young and older adults in the method of loci over a prolonged period. The method of loci is a memory training technique that involves memorizing a series of locations at training and then later utilizing these locations to learn a list of words. The individual attaches each word in the presented list to a specific location using interactive imagery and then later retrieves the words by reviewing the locations. Although young and old participants were trained to have equivalent memory for the locations, the results nevertheless demonstrated that older adults could not achieve the same level of proficiency as young adults in list learning even after weeks of training. In fact the best performing older adult never achieved the performance level of the worst performing young adult. These data suggest that older adults have less behavioral plasticity than young adults. Moreover, one might have expected, if neuroimaging techniques would have been available at the time, researchers would have observed more pronounced gains in structural thickness of neural regions associated with memory or encoding, or more pronounced and focal activations in the young adults in these areas, reflecting their greater neural plasticity.

The first neuroimaging study to examine memory training effects was conducted by Nyberg et al. (2003). They reported that after acquisition training in the method of loci, young adults showed increased activation in frontal and *occipitoparietal regions*. Older adults did not show increased frontal activation after the training. Moreover, only older adults who actually profited from the training showed the increase in occipitoparietal regions. The lack of frontal activation increase was interpreted to suggest a general decrease in overall processing capacity of older adults. The older adults who failed to show improvement and also failed to show increase of activation in occipitoparietal areas were suggested to be deficient in task-relevant operations. Finally, in a later analysis, Jones et al. (2006) reported that the young subjects as well as old subjects who profited from the training showed an increase in medial temporal activations, and suggested that this was related to training of effective binding operations, which are typically associated with the hippocampus (Cohen et al., 1999).

Neural Correlates of Training Executive Function

Executive function can be thought of as the control operations needed to maintain cognitive function and include the ability to shift, update, and inhibit information (Miyake et al., 2000). Dahlin et al. (2008b) conducted a behavioral study where they attempted to train the updating function in young and old adults across a series of tasks. In the training task, subjects listened to a stream of letters and were required to report the last four letters that they heard whenever a probe occurred. To perform accurately they had to continually update the four items held in memory. Although old adults performed more poorly than young adults on the updating task at training, the magnitude of improvement across weeks of training was the same for old and young. When transfer to other cognitive functions was assessed from the training, there were no general transfer effects for the old adults but young adults exhibited improved performance on a three-back working memory task, which had a substantial updating component as well as an additional short-term memory component. Importantly, when subjects were tested 18 months later on an updating task, gains were maintained relative to a control group for both old and young. This suggested maintenance of trained task-specific improvement in executive function in old and young adults.

The same group (Dahlin et al., 2008a) examined the neural underpinnings associated with the effects observed on the updating task, testing the hypothesis that transfer effects in young to the three-back task were mediated by the striatum. This hypothesis was confirmed by a series of findings. First, young adults showed transfer to the three-back task but not to the Stroop task. Second, the training task and the three-back task shared activations in the striatal region, whereas the Stroop task did not share these activations with the training task. Also of interest was a third finding that indicated old adults did not activate the striatal region during the training task and simultaneously did not show transfer to the three-back task. Based on these findings the authors concluded that transfer effects observed in young from the updating task to the three-back task occurred because the training task and a transfer task engaged similar processes and brain systems. They suggested that such shared neural activation is the basis for transfer of training effects.

In a very recent study on training of executive function, Mozolic et al. (2010) trained older adults to suppress distraction in a visual and auditory attention task. They reported that the training resulted in an increase in cerebral blood flow to prefrontal cortex. They were unable to find differences in gray matter volume, but suggested that a combination of attentional training with physical fitness training might lead to such structural changes.

Finally, Erickson et al. (2006) conducted a dual-task training study in young and old adults, examining the impact of two weeks of training on performance on two attentional tasks. Training improved performance and yielded evidence in old adults for decreased bilaterality in dorsal and ventral prefrontal cortex, while control subjects showed no change in neural recruitment patterns. The decreased bilaterality was interpreted as evidence for cortical plasticity in neural function with age. There was also an increase in the left ventral prefrontal cortex, possibly due to adaptation of an inner speech strategy.

Experimental Studies of Engagement

We are aware of only two experimental studies of lifestyle engagement and its impact on cognition and neural function. One effort, the Synapse Study, conducted in our lab at the Center for Vital Longevity, evaluates the effect of older adults' engagement in novel activities by using a controlled experimental study design, and relates engagement to neural correlates of brain structure and brain function. Our older participants engage in learning new activities, such as learning to quilt or learning digital photography over a period of 14 weeks, with a minimum participation of 15 hours a week. We chose quilting and digital photography, because we anticipated that those activities are both sensitive to observe changes in neural and cognitive function compared to a social control group (volunteers engaging in activities such as game playing and field trips but who do not acquire a new skill), a placebo control (participants are listening to educational programs or classical music at home or play simple computer games), and a no treatment control group. We also compare the effects of engagement alone to fitness training as well as to a condition that involves both exercise and engagement. We developed a detailed cognitive and psychosocial battery as well as a comprehensive neuroimaging protocol to assess volunteers prior to the enrollment and after the intervention period to examine whether providing a rich cognitive environment that challenges multiple aspects of cognition actually changes cognitive functioning, brain structure, or patterns of neural recruitment (for further details see Goh & Park, 2009).

Another major project that examines the impact of engagement on cognitive function is the Experience Corps (EC) Program. This is an innovative program that utilizes the experience and skill set of older adults (55 and older) to assist teachers in kindergarten through third grade to promote children's educational outcomes and improve children's literacy (Carlson et al., 2009). Recently Carlson and colleagues (2009) examined possible neural correlates of the EC program in 8 female volunteers who participated for 15 weeks during the academic year. Participants were African American females with relatively low levels of education and low income and average Mini-Mental-State Examination (MMSE) Scores of 24. Given that the average MMSE scores of the participants were relatively low, the authors suggested that the volunteers were at-risk for accelerated development of cognitive impairment. They compared brain activity elicited during an executive control task to patterns of brain activation in age-matched, non-active controls before participating in EC and after. During the executive control task no reliable differences between the groups were found at baseline. However, after the EC intervention, the EC group showed significantly more activity in the anterior cingulate gyrus and left prefrontal cortex compared to control participants as well as better performance in executive function. Whereas some limitations (e.g., small sample size and only females from one ethnicity) of this study constrain its interpretation, these findings nevertheless provide promising evidence of potential benefits of post-retirement lifestyle activities that are embedded in a context of cognitive and social complexity. In addition the usage of neuroimaging tools provide a powerful way to examine mechanisms and effects of use-dependent neural plasticity and will provide future insights into the malleability and potential of the aging mind.

FITNESS TRAINING AS A COGNITIVE INTERVENTION

There is a growing body of research that suggests fitness training in older adults enhances both neural structure and function. Colcombe et al. (2003), investigated the effects of cardiovascular fitness and age on both gray and white matter volumes using voxel-based morphometry (VBM) in 55 older adults. Cardiovascular fitness was measured using estimates of maximal oxygen uptake (VO_2max). They found that increased fitness was related to decreased age-related brain atrophy, particularly in areas most affected by aging. In a subsequent study utilizing a more direct approach to assess the effect of fitness as a cognitive intervention, Colcombe et al. (2006) assigned healthy, sedentary older adult participants to an aerobic training group or to a toning and stretching control group for a 6-month period. The authors estimated gray and white matter volume pre- and post-fitness training and reported fitness training resulted in a significant increase in volume in prefrontal and temporal cortex areas as a function of aerobic fitness training, but not for older adults who participated in the toning and stretching control group. Further research by the same group (Erickson et al., 2009) with an even larger sample demonstrated that fitness training increased hippocampal volume and that increase mediated performance on a spatial memory task. Finally, Voelcker-Rehage et al. (2010) examined differential effects of motor fitness (i.e., balance, agility, and flexibility) and physical fitness (muscle strength and cardiovascular fitness) on cognitive performance and brain activation patterns in a sample of 72 older adults. Consistent with prior research, physical fitness (i.e., as measured with grip force and spiroergometry, a measurement of oxygen consumption) had a positive effect on executive function. In addition motor fitness (i.e., as measured with a heterogeneous battery of motor fitness tasks including hand tapping, feet tapping, one-leg-stand with eyes open and eyes closed, and a fine coordination task) was associated with both executive control task and processing speed. Interestingly, participants with higher physical and motor fitness showed reduced task activation in frontal, temporal, and occipital areas, perhaps indicative of more efficient neural processing. Furthermore, the two different dimensions of fitness had differential effects on activated brain areas. Whereas high physical fitness was associated with activation in frontal and temporal brain areas, high motor fitness was selectively related to activation in parietal areas.

CONCLUSIONS

Generally, studies that yield increases in volume of brain structures as a result of experience, such as the expertise research, provide good evidence for plasticity of neural function with age. Similarly, the fitness research provides convincing evidence that there are modest gains to be realized in cognitive function by maintaining a moderate to high level of fitness at older ages. The evidence with respect to training and engagement studies is less clear, and the absolute number of studies available are very limited. We note that training studies that yield evidence for task-specific changes as a result of sustained experience with the training task provide a great deal of important evidence about the neural processes that underlie behavioral change, but do not necessarily demonstrate brain plasticity. Studies that show improvement only on a training task may be confounding evidence for plasticity with evidence for strategy change. It is possible that training induces a change in strategy that is accompanied by a change in activation patterns. It is not clear that such a strategic change reflects a fundamental change in the way the brain functions or a strengthening of brain function, which is the defining aspect of neural plasticity. We suggest that the gold standard for demonstration of plasticity is evidence that the newly trained circuitry is deployed on another task that shares a process with the trained task, but is nevertheless different. This pattern was demonstrated in the Dahlin et al. (2008) study for young but not old adults. Whether older adults will demonstrate changes in neural recruitment patterns that are flexibly deployed across a range of relevant situations (general transfer) remains to be determined. Our guess is that it is likely that findings of this sort will emerge, but at present this has proven to be an elusive goal. Our review of the training studies to date suggests that there is little scientific evidence that brain training software will delay the onset of age-related cognitive decline. Despite these caveats, we nevertheless recognize that training studies in combination with neuroimaging represent a daunting logistical and resource-intensive challenge that are well worth the investment, as they will yield fundamental evidence about the potential and limits of the aging human brain.

ACKNOWLEDGMENTS

This work was supported by grants from the National Institute on Aging 5R37AG006265-24 and RO1AG026589 whose support is gratefully acknowledged. Additionally, the authors thank Blair Flicker for his assistance in preparing this chapter.

REFERENCES

Andreasen, N., Minthon, L., Vanmechelen, E., Vanderstichele, H., Davidsson, P., Winblad, B., et al. (1999). Cerebrospinal fluid tau and Abeta42 as predictors of development of Alzheimer's disease in patients with mild cognitive impairment. *Neuroscience Letters, 273*, 5–8.

Andrews-Hanna, J. R., Snyder, A. Z., Vincent, J. L., Lustig, C., Head, D., Raichle, M. E., et al. (2007). Disruption of large-scale brain systems in advanced aging. *Neuron, 56*, 924–935.

Baker, C. I., Peli, E., Knouf, N., & Kanwisher, N. G. (2005). Reorganization of visual processing in macular degeneration. *Journal of Neuroscience, 25*, 614–618.

Bangert, M., & Schlaug, G. (2006). Specialization of the specialized in features of external human brain morphology. *European Journal of Neuroscience, 24*, 1832–1834.

Boyke, J., Driemeyer, J., Gaser, C., Büchel, C., & May, A. (2008). Training-induced brain structure changes in the elderly. *Journal of Neuroscience, 28*(28), 7031–7035.

Cabeza, R., Anderson, N. D., Locantore, J. K., & McIntosh, A. R. (2002). Aging gracefully: compensatory brain activity in high-performing older adults. *Neuroimage, 17*(3), 1394–1402.

Cabeza, R., Daselaar, S. M., Dolcos, F., Prince, S. E., Budde, M., & Nyberg, L. (2004). Task-independent and task-specific age effects on brain activity during working memory, visual attention and episodic retrieval. *Cerebral Cortex, 14*(4), 364–375.

Carlson, M. C., Erickson, K. I., Kramer, A. F., Voss, M. W., Bolea, N., Mielke, M., et al. (2009). Evidence for neurocognitive plasticity in at-risk older adults: the experience corps program. *Journals of Gerontology Series A: Biological Sciences and Medical Sciences, 64*(12), 1275–1282.

Chee, M. W., Goh, J. O., Venkatraman, V., Tan, J. C., Gutchess, A., Sutton, B., et al. (2006). Age-related changes in object processing and contextual binding revealed using fMR adaptation. *Journal of Cognitive Neuroscience, 18*, 495–507.

Cohen, N. J., Ryan, J., Hunt, C., Romine, L., Wszalek, T., & Nash, C. (1999). Hippocampal system and declarative (relational) memory: summarizing the data from functional neuroimaging studies. *Hippocampus, 9*, 83–98.

Colcombe, S. J., Erickson, K. I., Raz, N., Webb, A. G., Cohen, N. J., McAuley, E., et al. (2003). Aerobic fitness reduces brain tissue loss in aging humans. *Journals of Gerontology Series A: Biological Sciences and Medical Sciences, 62*(1), 32–44.

Colcombe, S. J., Erickson, K. I., Scalf, P. E., Kim, J. S., Prakash, R., McAuley, E., et al. (2006). Aerobic exercise training increases brain volume in aging humans. *Journals of Gerontology: Medical Sciences, 61*(11), 1166–1170.

Dahlin, E., Neely, A. S., Larsson, A., Bäckman, L., & Nyberg, L. (2008a). Transfer of learning after updating training mediated by the striatum. *Science, 320*(5882), 1510–1512.

Dahlin, E., Nyberg, L., Bäckman, L., & Neely, A. S. (2008b). Plasticity of executive functioning in young and older adults: Immediate training gains, transfer and long-term maintenance. *Psychology and Aging, 23*(4), 720–730.

Damoiseaux, J. S., Beckmann, C. F., Arigita, E. J., Barkhof, F., Scheltens, P., et al. (2007). Reduced resting-state brain activity in the "default network" in normal aging. *Cerebral Cortex, 18*(8), 1856–1864.

Davis, S. W., Dennis, N. A., Daselaar, S. M., Fleck, M. S., & Cabeza, R. (2007). Que PASA? The posterior anterior shift in aging. *Cerebral Cortex, 18*(5), 1201–1209.

Diniz, B. S., Pinto, J. A., & Forlenza, O. V. (2008). Do CSF total tau, phosphorylated tau, and beta-amyloid 42 help to predict progression of mild cognitive impairment to Alzheimer's disease? A systematic review and meta-analysis of the literature. *World Journal of Biological Psychiatry, 9*, 172–182.

Draganski, B., Gaser, C., Busch, V., Schuierer, G., Bogdahn, U., & May, A. (2004). Neuroplasticity: Changes in grey matter induced by training. *Nature, 427*, 311–312.

Erickson, K. I., Prakash, R. S., Voss, M. W., Chaddock, L., Hu, L., Morris, K. S., et al. (2009). Aerobic fitness is associated with hippocampal volume in elderly humans. *Hippocampus, 19*(10), 1030–1039.

Erickson, K. I., Colcombe, S. J., Wadhwa, R., Bherer, L., Peterson, M. S., Scalf, P. E., et al. (2006). Training-induced plasticity in older adults: Effects of training on hemispheric asymmetry. *Neurobiology of Aging, 28*, 272–283.

Fotenos, A. F., Mintun, M. A., Snyder, A. Z., Morris, J. C., & Buckner, R. L. (2008). Brain volume decline in aging: evidence for a relation between socioeconomic status, preclinical Alzheimer disease, and reserve. *Archives of Neurology, 65*, 113–120.

Goh, J. O, Suzuki, A., & Park, D. C. (2010). Reduced neural selectivity increases fMRI adaptation with age during face discrimination. *Neuroimage, 51*, 336–344.

Goh, J. O., & Park, D. C. (2009). Neuroplasticity and cognitive aging: The scaffolding theory of aging and cognition. *Restorative Neurology and Neuroscience, 27*, 391–403.

Grady, C. L., Protzner, A. B., Kovacevic, N., Strother, S. C., Afshin-Pour, B., Wojtowicz, M., et al. (2010). A multivariate analysis of age-related differences in default mode and task-positive networks across multiple cognitive domains. *Cerebral Cortex, 20*(6), 1432–1447.

Grady, C. L., Springer, M. V., Hongwanishkul, D., McIntosh, A. R., & Winocur, G. (2006). Age-related changes in brain activity across the adult lifespan. *Journal of Cognitive Neuroscience, 18*(2), 227–241.

Greicius, M. D., Krasnow, B., Reiss, A. L., & Menon, V. (2003). Functional connectivity in the resting brain: A network analysis of the default mode hypothesis. *Proceedings of the National Academy of Sciences of the United States of America, 100*(1), 253–258.

Gunning-Dixon, F., Brickman, A., Cheng, J., & Alexopoulos, G. (2009). Aging of cerebral white matter: A review of MRI findings. *International Journal of Geriatric Psychiatry, 24*, 109–117.

Gutchess, A. H., Welsh, R. C., Hedden, T., Bangert, A., Minear, M., Liu, L. L., et al. (2005). Aging and the neural correlates of successful picture encoding: Frontal activations compensate for decreased medial-temporal activity. *Journal of Cognitive Neuroscience, 17*, 84–96.

Hall, C. B., Derby, C., LeValley, A., Katz, M. J., Verghese, J., & Lipton, R. B. (2007). Education delays accelerated decline on a memory test in persons who develop dementia. *Neurology, 69*(17), 1657–1664.

Head, D., Buckner, R. L., Shimony, J. S., Girton, L. E., Akbudak, E., Conturo, T. E., et al. (2004). Differential vulnerability of anterior white matter in nondemented aging with minimal acceleration in dementia of the Alzheimer type: Evidence from diffusion tensor imaging. *Cerebral Cortex, 14*, 410–423.

Hertzog, C., Kramer, A. F., Wilson, R. S., & Lindenberger, U. (2009). Enrichment effects on adult cognitive development. *Psychological Science in the Public Interest, 9*, 1–65.

Imfeld, A., Oechslin, M. S., Meyer, M., Loenneker, T., & Jancke, L. (2009, Jul 1). White matter plasticity in the corticospinal tract of musicians: A diffusion tensor imaging study. *Neuroimage, 46*(3), 600–607.

Jack, C. R., Lowe, V. J., Senjem, M. L., Weigand, S. D., Kemp, B. J., Shiung, M. M., et al. (2008). 11C PiB and structural MRI provide complementary information in imaging of Alzheimer's disease and amnestic mild cognitive impairment. *Brain, 131*, 665–680.

Jones, S., Nyberg, L., Sandblom, J., Neely, A. S., Ingvar, M., Petersson, K. M., et al. (2006). Cognitive and neural plasticity in aging: General and task-specific limitations. *Neuroscience and Biobehavioral Reviews, 30*, 864–871.

Kaasinen, V., Vilkman, H., Hietala, J., Någren, K., Helenius, H., Olsson, H., et al. (2000). Age-related dopamine D2/D3 receptor loss in extrastriatal regions of the human brain. *Neurobiology of Aging, 21*(5), 683–688.

Kempermann, G., Kuhn, H. G., & Gage, F. H. (1997). More hippocampal neurons in adult mice living in an enriched environment. *Nature, 386*(6624), 493–495.

Kennedy, K. M., & Raz, N. (2009). Pattern of normal age-related regional differences in white matter microstructure is modified by vascular risk. *Brain Research, 1297*, 41–56.

Kliegl, R., Smith, J., & Baltes, P. B. (1990). On the locus and process of magnification of age differences during mnemonic training. *Developmental Psychology, 26*(1990), 894–904.

Lindenberger, U., & Baltes, P. B. (1994). Sensory functioning and intelligence in old age: A strong connection. *Psychology and Aging, 9*(3), 339–355.

Lustig, C., Shah, P., Seidler, R., & Reuter-Lorenz, P. (2009). Aging, training, and the brain and future directions. *Neuropsychological Review, 19*, 504–522.

Maguire, E. A., Gadian, D. G., Johnsrude, I. S., Good, C. D., Ashburner, J., Frackowiak, R. S., et al. (2000). Navigation-related structural change in the hippocampi of taxi drivers. *Proceedings of the National Academy of Sciences of the United States of America, 97*(8), 4398–4403.

Miyake, A., Friedman, N. P., Emerson, M. J., Witzki, A. H., Howerter, A., & Wager, T. D. (2000). The unity and diversity of executive functions and their contributions to complex "Frontal Lobe" tasks: A latent variable analysis. *Cognitive Psychology, 41*(1), 49–100.

Morcom, A. M., Good, C. D., Frackowiak, R. S., & Rugg, M. D. (2003). Age effects on the neural correlates of successful memory encoding. *Brain, 126*, 213–229.

Mozolic, J. L., Hayasaka, S., & Laurienti, P. J. (2010). A cognitive training intervention increases cerebral blood flow in healthy older adults improvement in adulthood and aging. *Frontiers in Human Neuroscience, 12*(4), 16.

NIH State-of-the-Science Conference Preventing Alzheiner's Disease and Cognitive Decline. Retreived from http://consensus.nih.gov/2010/docs/alz/ALZ_Final_Statement.pdf (1-19).

Nilsson, M., Perfilieva, E., Johansson, U., Orwar, O., & Eriksson, P. S. (1999). Enriched environment increases neurogenesis in the adult rat dentate gyrus and improves spatial memory. *Journal of Neurobiology, 39*(4), 569–578.

Noack, H., Lövdén, M., Schmiedek, F., & Lindenberger, U. (2009). Cognitive plasticity in adulthood and old age: Gauging the generality of cognitive intervention effects. *Restorative Neurology and Neuroscience, 27*(5), 435–453.

Nyberg, L., Sandblom, J., Jones, S., Neely, A. S., Petersson, K. M., Ingvar, M., et al. (2003). Neural correlates of training-related memory improvement in adulthood and aging. *Proceedings of the National Academy of Sciences of the United States of America, 100*(23), 13728–13733.

Owen, A. M., Hampshire, A., Grahn, J. A., Stenton, R., Dajani, S., Burns, A. S., et al. (2010). Putting brain training to the test. *Nature*. 2010 Apr 20 [Epub ahead of print].

Park, D. C., Lautenschlager, G., Hedden, T., Davidson, N. S., Smith, A. D., & Smith, P. K. (2002). Models of visuospatial and verbal memory across the adult life span. *Psychology and Aging, 17*, 299–320.

Park, D. C., & Reuter-Lorenz, P. A. (2009). The adaptive brain: Aging and neurocognitive scaffolding. *Annual Review of Psychology, 60*, 173–196.

Park, D. C., Polk, T. A., Hebrank, A. C., & Jenkins, L. J. (2010). Age differences in default mode activity on easy and difficult spatial judgment tasks. *Frontiers in Human Neuroscience, 3*, 75.

Park, D. C., Polk, T. A., Park, R., Minear, M., Savage, A., & Smith, M. R. (2004). Aging reduces neural specialization in ventral visual cortex. *Proceedings of the National Academy of Sciences of the United States of America, 101*, 13091–13095.

Persson, J., Lustig, C., Nelson, J. K., & Reuter-Lorenz, P. A. (2007). Age differences in deactivation: a link to cognitive control? *Journal of Cognitive Neuroscience, 19*(6), 1021–1032.

Persson, J., Nyberg, L., Lind, J., Larsson, A., Nilsson, L. G., et al. (2006). Structure-function correlates of cognitive decline in aging. *Cerebral Cortex, 16*(7), 907–915.

Raichle, M. E., MacLeod, A. M., Snyder, A. Z., Powers, W. J., Gusnard, D. A., & Shulman, G. L. (2001). A default mode of brain function. *Proceedings of the National Academy of Sciences of the United States of America, 98*(2), 676–682.

Ramachandran, V. S., & Hirstein, W. (1998). The perception of phantom limbs. *Brain, 121*(9), 1603–1630.

Raz, N. (2005). The aging brain observed in vivo: Differential changes and their modifiers. In R. Cabeza, L. Nyberg, & D. C. Park (Eds.), *Cognitive neuroscience of aging: Linking cognitive and cerebral aging* (pp. 17–55). New York: Oxford University Press.

Raz, N., & Rodrigue, K. M. (2006). Differential aging of the brain: patterns, cognitive correlates and modifiers. *Neuroscience and Biobehavioral Reviews, 30*, 730–748.

Reuter-Lorenz, P. A., & Cappell, K. (2008). Neurocognitive aging and the compensation hypothesis. *Current Direction in Psychological Science, 17*(3), 177–182.

Reuter-Lorenz, P. A., Jonides, J., Smith, E. E., Hartley, A., Miller, A., et al. (2000). Age differences in the frontal lateralization of verbal and spatial working memory revealed by PET. *Journal of Cognitive Neuroscience, 12*(1), 174–187.

Reuter-Lorenz, P. A., & Lustig, C. (2005). Brain aging: reorganizing discoveries about the aging mind. *Current Opinion in Neurobiology., 15*(2), 245–251.

Rodrigue, K. M., Kennedy, K. M., & Park, D. C. (2009). Beta-amyloid deposition and the aging brain. *Neuropsychology Review, 19*, 436–450.

Rosenzweig, M. R., & Bennett, E. L. (1996). Psychobiology of plasticity: Effects of training and experience on brain and behavior. *Behavioural Brain Research, 78*, 57–65.

Rossi, S., Miniussi, C., Pasqualetti, P., Babiloni, C., Rossini, P. M., & Cappa, S. F. (2004). Age-related functional changes of prefrontal cortex in long-term memory: a repetitive transcranial magnetic stimulation study. *Journal of Neuroscience, 24*(36), 7939–7944.

Rowe, C. C., Ellis, K. A., Rimajova, M., Bourgeat, P., Pike, K. E., Jones, G., et al. (2010). Amyloid imaging results from the Australian Imaging, Biomarkers and Lifestyle (AIBL) study of aging. *Neurobiology of Aging* [Epub ahead of print].

Rypma, B., & D'Esposito, M. (2001). Age-related changes in brain-behaviour relationships: Evidence from event related functional MRI studies. *European Journal of Cognitive Psychology, 13*(1–2), 235–256.

Schaie, K. W. (2005). *Developmental influences on adult intelligence: The Seattle Longitudinal Study*. New York: Oxford University Press.

Schumacher, E. H., Jacko, J. A., Primo, S. A., Main, K. L., Moloney, K. P., Kinzel, E. N., et al. (2008). Reorganization of visual processing is related to eccentric viewing in patients with macular degeneration. *Restorative Neurology and Neuroscience, 26*, 391–402.

Stern, Y. (2002). What is cognitive reserve? Theory and research application of the reserve concept. *Journal of the International Neuropsychological Society, 8*, 448–460.

Stroop, J. R. (1935). Studies of interference in serial verbal reactions. *Journal of Experimental Psychology, 18*, 643–662.

Taub, E., Uswatte, G., & Elbert, T. (2002). New treatments in neurorehabilitation founded on basic research. *Nature Reviews Neuroscience, 3*(3), 228–236.

Voelcker-Rehage, C., Godde, B., & Staudinger, U. M. (2010). Physical and motor fitness are both related to cognition in old-age. *European Journal of Neuroscience, 1*, 167–176.

Chapter | 8 |

Memory Changes and the Aging Brain: A Multimodal Imaging Approach

Lars Nyberg[1], *Lars Bäckman*[2]

[1]*Departments of Integrative Medical Biology and Radiation Sciences, Umeå University, Umeå, Sweden;* [2]*Aging Research Center, Karolinska Institute, Stockholm, Sweden*

CHAPTER CONTENTS

Introduction	**121**
Memory Changes in Aging	**121**
Linking Memory Changes in Aging to Brain Changes	**122**
Multimodal Appoaches to the Cognition-Brain Relation in Aging	**123**
Structure-Function Interactions	125
Interactions between Neurotransmission and Functional Brain Activity	127
Conclusions and Future Prospects	**128**
Acknowledgments	**129**
References	**129**

INTRODUCTION

Cognitive aging is a very broad research topic that spans age-related changes in higher order abilities, such as learning and memory, thinking, planning, and problem solving. Cognitive changes fundamentally affect the life quality of individuals, and much research is currently directed toward furthering our understanding of the brain on the bases of these changes (see Cabeza et al., 2005). Modern brain imaging techniques play a key role in this regard (Jagust & D'Esposito, 2009). In this chapter, age-related memory changes will be discussed from a cognitive neuroscience perspective. In particular, the idea will be developed that progress requires consideration and *integration* of findings obtained with different imaging modalities, as these provide unique and complementary information. Thus, the current review is quite focused, and for more comprehensive reviews of the neural underpinnings of age-related memory changes the reader is referred to other excellent contributions (e.g., Buckner, 2004; Cabeza, 2002; Hedden & Gabrieli, 2004; Park & Reuter-Lorenz, 2008).

MEMORY CHANGES IN AGING

Memory changes in advanced aging are well documented. However, simply stating that memory fails in older age is clearly an oversimplification. This is for a number of reasons, including the following three.

First, numerous studies have shown that different memory systems and processes are not uniformly affected by aging. First, at a very general level, there is much evidence for a relative sparing of implicit, nondeclarative long-term memory compared to declarative long-term memory and working memory (Bäckman et al., 2001; Gabrieli, 2000). Moreover, within the domain of declarative long-term memory, episodic memory is more affected than semantic memory in old age, and age-related impairments are more apparent on episodic recall tasks than on recognition tasks (Craik & McDowd, 1987; Nyberg et al., 2003). Thus, aging does not affect all memory systems and processes in a uniform manner (for additional examples, see Bäckman et al., 2001).

Second, although the bulk of empirical studies has been concerned with mean trends, there are ample demonstrations of substantial inter-individual variability within the aging population. One illustration comes from a multivariate analysis of age-related changes in memory and cognition in a large sample (N = 1963) of individuals aged 55 to 85 years

DOI: 10.1016/B978-0-12-380882-0.00008-5

(Habib et al., 2007). Whereas most of the individuals who fell within the upper level of the performance distribution were from the younger age cohorts, a subsample of individuals aged 70 years and above performed at or above the level of middle-age individuals.

Third, even when it comes to mean-level changes in older age relative to middle or younger age, there is still no consensus on how to best characterize age-related changes. This is particularly evident in the case of episodic memory, which is typically conceived as the most age-sensitive, long-term memory system. However, whereas some authors have argued that episodic memory starts to decline already in the 20 to 30 years age range (Park et al., 2003; Salthouse, 2009), others have suggested a much later onset of age-related memory impairment (Rönnlund et al., 2005; Schaie, 1994; Zelinski & Burnight, 1997). One major source of variability in this context is the type of design used to estimate how aging influences performance across the life span. Although still a topic of intense debate (see e.g., Salthouse, 2009 with commentary by Nilsson et al., 2009), it seems as if studies that provide evidence for a very early onset of decline tend to use a cross-sectional design, whereas studies based on a longitudinal design support a later onset of memory decline. A main factor contributing to greater age differences in cross-sectional studies is age-related differences in level of education (Rönnlund et al., 2005). Such differences magnify the (true) performance advantage of younger adults in cross-sectional comparisons.

LINKING MEMORY CHANGES IN AGING TO BRAIN CHANGES

The difference in findings between cross-sectional and longitudinal designs is illustrative of the many questions that still remain with regard to the characterization of memory changes in aging. This impression holds, and is even magnified, when one attempts to link cognitive changes in aging to associated brain changes. We wish to make several points about some of the most important issues related to linking memory changes to brain changes.

The first point concerns differential age-cognition relations for distinct systems and processes. In functional neuroimaging studies in general, and in age-comparative functional-imaging studies in particular, it is rarely the case that multiple tasks are compared. However, the available evidence indicates that consideration of differential effects of aging on diverse processes is highly relevant. For example, Rypma and D'Esposito (2000) used fMRI and found evidence that age-related working-memory deficits are more related to retrieval than encoding or maintenance processes, and that retrieval processes mediated by the dorsolateral prefrontal cortex (PFC) are more affected than those subserved by ventrolateral PFC. In addition to highlighting the importance of careful consideration of processes, the Rypma and D'Esposito study indicated alternative ways of conceptualizing the mapping of the age-cognition-brain link than what may be derived from standard taxonomies (Squire et al., 1993; Tulving & Schacter, 1990). Specifically, regardless of whether they are taxing implicit or explicit memory, one might predict that tasks that draw on dorsolateral PFC (DLPFC) will be age sensitive. A similar "brain inspired" taxonomy of cognitive functions has been proposed in studies with younger adults (e.g., Cabeza & Nyberg, 2000; Nyberg et al., 2002).

Turning to the second point regarding the linkage of memory changes to brain changes, inter-individual variability, this topic has received attention in studies of brain functioning (Lupien & Wan, 2004) and "cognitive reserve" (Stern, 2009). One issue, in particular, has been highlighted in age-comparative functional imaging studies; namely the apparent overactivation of some brain regions, notably the PFC, during task performance in some elderly individuals (see Persson & Nyberg, 2006). Such overactivation has occasionally been observed for high-functioning elderly persons (e.g., Cabeza et al., 2002) and interpreted in terms of compensation for age-related brain changes (Cabeza, 2002; Grady, 2009; Park & Reuter-Lorenz, 2008).

Critically, however, it has also been reported that overactivation in aging is associated with declining cognitive performance. One example comes from the Betula study and involved separating middle-aged individuals into those who showed a stable level of episodic memory performance over a decade preceding the imaging session from those who showed marked decline over the same time period (Persson et al., 2006). Analyses of volumetric changes showed that memory decline went along with hippocampal atrophy, and analyses of diffusion tensor imaging (DTI) data revealed frontal white-matter changes for those with declining cognition. In addition to these structural changes, cognitive decline was associated with altered frontal activity. Specifically, both groups showed comparable activation of left inferior frontal regions during a verbal categorization task that served as incidental encoding, but the declining participants also showed significant recruitment of the homologous right inferior frontal region.

Thus, the Persson et al. study (2006) suggested that overactivation may be a sign of "dysfunction," and recent evidence supports this position by showing that high-performing elderly adults showed a "youth-like" load-dependent modulation of the fMRI BOLD signal during spatial white matter performance (Nagel et al., 2010). Given the great interest in understanding the meaning of age-related overactivation during cognitive performance, it is important to keep in mind that (a) additional recruitment in old age routinely comes with underactivation of task-relevant brain regions recruited by young adults; and (b) underactivation in aging during, for example, working memory and episodic memory is considerably more common than overactivation (see e.g., Persson & Nyberg, 2006). More generally, in recent years, brain imaging studies tend to include larger samples, which opens up for more detailed examination of individual differences in brain structure and function and how these factors relate to individual differences in memory performance.

The third qualifying point, the nature of the design (cross-sectional vs. longitudinal), is as relevant in the context of imaging studies as in behavioral studies. This point was underscored by Jagust and D'Esposito (2009, p. 7), who in an introduction to a recent volume on imaging the aging brain wrote: "There is a growing consensus that we have over-relied on cross-sectional as opposed to longitudinal studies." This impression is most obvious in case of analyses of age-related structural brain changes. As recently shown in a review by Raz and Kennedy (2009), cross-sectional studies have focused on the PFC as the most vulnerable region of the aging brain. This is supported by results from the relatively few longitudinal studies that are available (e.g., Raz et al., 2005). In addition, however, the longitudinal type of studies show larger age-related structural changes than what might be expected from cross-sectional evidence in many other regions as well (such as the inferior parietal cortex, the hippocampus, and the cerebellum). Longitudinal analyses of age-related functional brain changes as measured with PET or fMRI are even scarcer. Analyses of eight-year changes in task-induced activation changes measured with PET revealed large-scale changes that were most pronounced in frontal and temporal areas (Beason-Held et al., 2008a, b). Preliminary results from a study examining six-year changes in fMRI BOLD signal during a categorization task showed that longitudinal changes were much larger and more widespread than corresponding changes from cross-sectional analyses (Nyberg, 2010). This observation is in good agreement with the pattern seen in studies of structural changes, but additional studies are needed before firm conclusions can be drawn. This is equally true for studies of age-related changes in neurotransmitter systems, such as dopamine. PET-based measures of both pre- and post-synaptic dopaminergic transmission show pronounced age-related changes, and these changes account for substantial portions of the age-related variance in cognitive measures (see Bäckman et al., 2006). For quite some time it has been speculated that a common neurobiological basis for decline in working memory and strategic long-term memory in normal aging and Parkinson's disease may be a deficient frontostriatal dopaminergic system (Gabrieli, 1996; Nyberg & Bäckman, 2004). However, with no exception, the existing data on normal aging are based on cross-sectional studies.

The fact that longitudinal studies of brain aging may reveal greater age-related decline compared to cross-sectional estimates (Nyberg, 2010; Raz et al., 2005; Raz & Kennedy, 2009) is intriguing because it runs counter to the bulk of age-comparative cognitive-behavioral studies (Rönnlund et al., 2005; Schaie, 1996). The fact that cross-sectional cognitive studies typically show larger age differences than the decline observed in longitudinal studies has multiple origins, including (a) generational effects favoring later-born cohorts, and (b) practice effects reducing within-person changes in performance. Magnification of degree of brain aging in longitudinal research is also likely to stem from several sources, including (a) positive selection of older adults in cross-sectional studies, and (b) individual differences (e.g., genetics, exposure) that are minimized in longitudinal studies. In particular, positive selection should be a key issue since many age-comparative studies involve extensive screening of the participants to exclude individuals with various forms of brain insults that might influence the results. While this strategy has its merits, it also means that the examined older adults often will be "super-elderly" who may not be representative for their cohorts.

Finally, in the context of the apparent difference in direction of how the design influences cognitive and brain-imaging studies (i.e. toward later vs. earlier onset of age differences), it should be stressed that longitudinal analyses of (i) memory performance (Rönnlund et al., 2005), (ii) structural brain changes (Raz et al., 2005), and (iii) functional brain-activity differences (Nyberg, 2010) converge on changes around age 60. Structural changes appear to precede cognitive and functional brain changes, thus indicating a potential causal cascade of events where structural changes lead to impaired cognition and associated alterations in functional brain-activity patterns. However, the issue of how various forms of measurements of brain structure/function relate remains a largely unexplored topic. In the remainder of this chapter we will present some initial attempts at bridging different methodological approaches to examining the aging mind/brain.

MULTIMODAL APPOACHES TO THE COGNITION-BRAIN RELATION IN AGING

Despite the fact that several methodological challenges remain, as summarized above, there is evidence for pronounced age-related changes in certain memory tasks, such as demanding episodic- and working-memory tasks. In addition, age-comparative studies have revealed neural correlates (task-induced increases as well as decreases) of such age-related cognitive changes, notably in the PFC. Furthermore, advanced aging is associated with structural changes in several regions including the hippocampus and DLPFC (Raz et al., 2005), and with changes in dopaminergic neurotransmission (Bäckman et al., 2006) that may reflect dysfunctional frontostriatal functioning. A working model of how these observations hang together is schematically illustrated in Figure 8.1 (cf. Buckner, 2004; Kaye, 2009).

Figure 8.1 outlines how genetic and environmental factors induce changes in brain structure and neurotransmitter systems. In turn, these changes affect metabolic and hemodynamic signals and translate into compromised functional systems along with lowered performance on select cognitive tasks. More specifically, in the upper row of the figure, the double helix and the graduation picture represent genetic and environmental factors. Such factors have influences on brain integrity (e.g., as measured by structural MRI) and neurotransmission (as measured by PET). This is indicated in the figure by the arrow pointing from the upper to the middle row. The middle row shows a coronal slice from a structural MRI scan and a horizontal scan from a PET study of striatal dopamine binding. With regard to genetic factors, it has, for example, been demonstrated that carriers of the ε4 allele of apolipoprotein ε gene (ApoE) have elevated risk for dementia and smaller hippocampal volume (e.g., Lind et al., 2006a). At the same time, there is compelling evidence that genetic risk can be modulated by certain environmental factors, such as participating in physical and social activities (Fratiglioni et al., 2004). Recent evidence indicates that ApoE ε4 carriers may be particularly supported by lifestyle

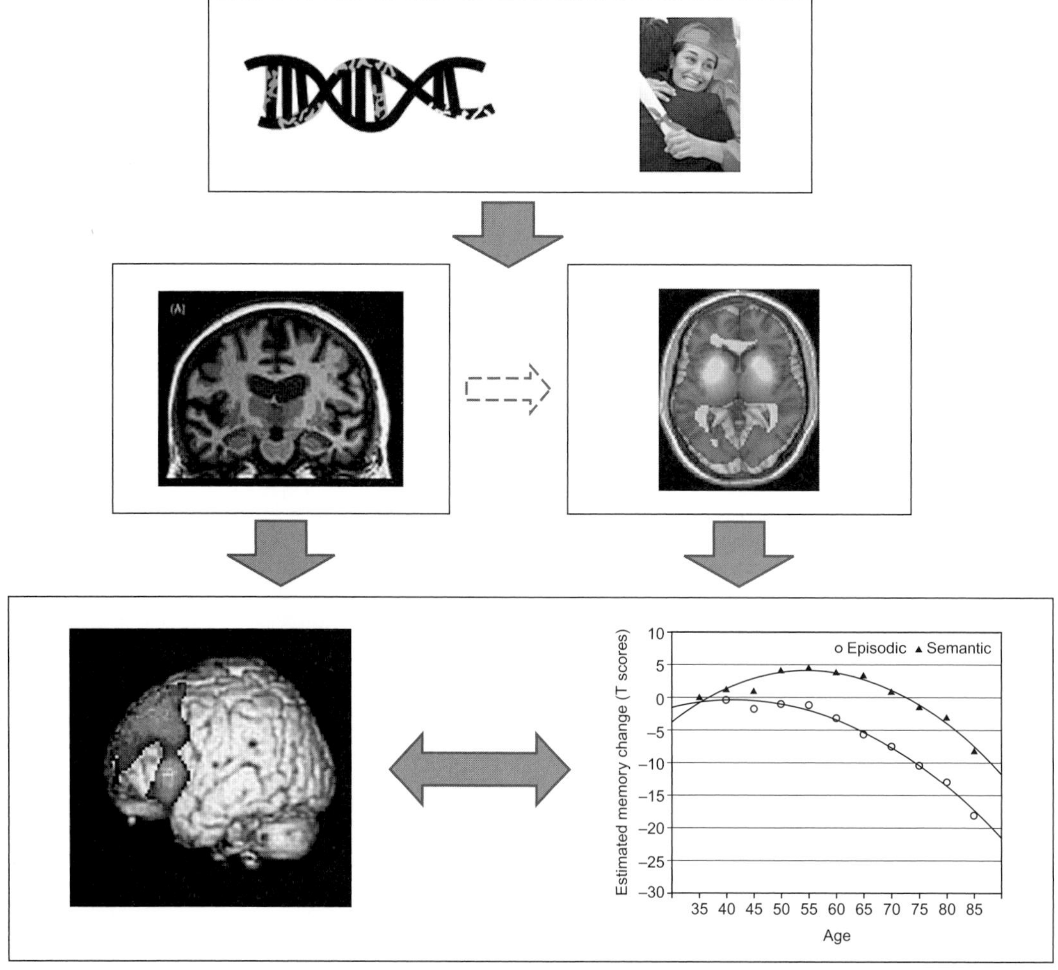

Figure 8.1 Schematic illustration of how genetic and environmental factors induce changes in brain structure and neurotransmission, which in turn affect age-related memory changes and corresponding changes in functional brain activity. The dashed arrow reflects interactions between brain structure and measures of neurotransmission.
The data on age-related memory changes are from Rönnlund et al. (2005)

factors (Niti et al., 2008). These and many other examples indicate that genetic and environmental influences interact to affect brain structure and neurotransmission. In turn, the integrity of brain structure and neurotransmission is constraining memory performance and associated task-induced functional brain-activity patterns. This is illustrated in the bottom row by a cortical map of task-induced frontal activity, and the graph to the right that outlines age-related changes of episodic and semantic memory across the adult life span (cf. the section above on age-related changes in memory). The bi-directional arrow between the functional brain map and the performance curve highlights the reciprocal relation between functional activity and performance, such that the task you are engaged in will influence the pattern of brain activity and how well you actually perform the task will be reflected in differential brain activity.

By combining different imaging techniques, various predictions derived from the model in Figure 8.1 can be tested. Specifically, one can examine whether at least some age-related alterations of the phenotype of main interest in this chapter (i.e., task-induced changes in brain activity) might be accounted for in terms of age-related changes in brain structure or neurotransmission (although not of primary concern here, it should be noted that the model also accommodates other complex relations, such as the potential influence of atrophy on PET-based measures of neurotransmission; cf. the dashed arrow in the middle row).

The combination of different techniques, *multimodal imaging*, offers great promise for understanding mechanisms of age-related cognitive decline (cf. Bäckman et al., 2006; Jagust & D'Esposito, 2009; Li et al., 2009; for a discussion of different imaging techniques, see Albert & Killiany, 2001). For example, multimodal imaging might involve integrating findings about brain volume with functional activation patterns (i.e., interrelating two types of MRI-derived measures). Multimodal imaging might also involve integration of different kinds of imaging measures, such as fMRI and PET/SPECT measures (e.g., Bäckman et al., 2010; Nyberg et al., 2009) or fMRI and EEG/ERP data (e.g., Kompus et al., 2010).

Next, we will present results from a few relevant multimodal imaging studies. It should be noted that the number of published studies in which different kinds of imaging data are formally integrated is still very limited, which at least in part is likely due to the many technical challenges that multimodal imaging raises — not least when it comes to integrating different kinds of data in the same analytic space. We focus on studies of "normal aging"; that is, older adults without (diagnosed) diseases such as dementia, but when available we will also consider findings from samples with increased risk for pathology. At least for structural data, there is evidence that brain-cognition associations are stronger in such samples (Raz & Kennedy, 2009).

Structure-function interactions can take many different forms, including age-related increases in functional brain activity along with structural alterations (e.g., Brassen et al., 2009; Persson et al., 2006). Here we will focus on whether age-related decreases in regional brain activity can be accounted for, fully or in part, by (i) age-related changes in the gray- or white matter of corresponding brain regions, and (ii) biomarkers of dopaminergic neurotransmission. Age-related decreases (i.e., BOLD signal reductions) have been observed in virtually all brain areas in response to various functional challenges. However, at least in working memory and strategic episodic long-term memory, the most consistent age-related reductions have been seen in frontal and medial-temporal regions (see e.g., Persson & Nyberg, 2006). These regions will also be of main concern in the context of multimodal imaging findings.

Structure-Function Interactions

Age-related frontal and hippocampal functional changes are noteworthy in view of the fact that prefrontal association cortex and the hippocampus are among the regions that show most age-related atrophy, and age-related white-matter changes are most consistently observed in anterior brain regions such as the genu of the corpus callosum (e.g., Head et al., 2004; see Raz & Kennedy, 2009). Such between-studies comparisons of age-related structure-function changes indicate that there exists a relation between structural changes in the hippocampus and PFC and corresponding age-related functional changes. As already noted, the number of studies that have directly examined the relation is still limited, but some interesting findings have emerged.

Nordahl and colleagues (2006) related white-matter degeneration, measured as MRI white matter hyperintensities (WMH), to the magnitude of task-induced prefrontal activity in a group of elderly individuals; such WMHs are typically observed in cognitively normal older persons (e.g., Söderlund et al., 2003). Nordahl et al. considered both the *local* relation between WMH in dorsolateral frontal cortex and PFC functional activity, as well as *distant* relations between PFC hyperintensities and anatomically and functionally connected regions outside the PFC. The functional imaging protocol consisted of a verbal working memory task and an episodic retrieval task. A region of interest (ROI) statistical approach was used to examine correlations between frontal WMHs and functional activity. The results revealed considerable inter-individual variability in WMHs, with some individuals having a substantial portion of WMHs relative to their total cranial volume (see Figure 8.2A, left panel). Analyses of fMRI BOLD activity showed that both tasks elicited

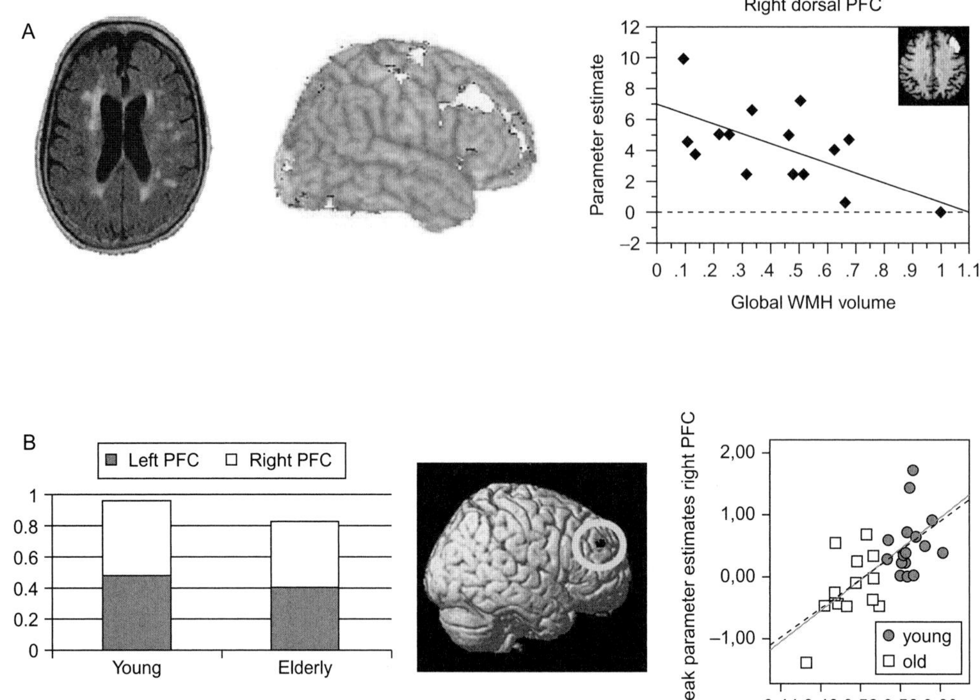

Figure 8.2 Structure-function interactions. (A) Empirical example of how white-matter changes account for age-related changes in task-induced frontal brain activity. Data from Nordahl et al. (2006). (B) Empirical example of how frontal gray-matter atrophy accounts for age-related changes in task-induced frontal brain activity.
Data from Brassen et al. (2009)

robust activation of prefrontal regions, as exemplified in Figure 8.2A (middle panel) during the working-memory task. Finally and most critically, analyses of interrelations between WMHs and regional BOLD changes revealed significant correlations, both locally and distally. Figure 8.2A (right panel) shows the association between global WMH volume and right dorsal PFC activity during the working-memory task. As can be seen, there was a strong negative correlation, such that more white-matter degeneration was associated with lower functional activity during the working memory task. Subsequent analyses of regional dorsal PFC WMHs in relation to functional activity also revealed negative distal relationships (e.g., BOLD signal changes in the parietal cortex). A similar pattern was seen for the episodic retrieval task, including significant distal correlations between frontal WMH and BOLD changes in the medial temporal cortex. Taken together, these findings provide evidence that disruption of white-matter integrity may be one mechanism for the PFC dysfunction seen in many older individuals, manifested as lowered functional brain activity and reduced working- and episodic-memory performance.

Brassen et al. (2009) assessed gray matter density of the PFC and MTL in a sample of younger and older individuals using an automated voxel-based morphometry (VBM) procedure. As illustrated in Figure 8.2B (left panel), there was a significant age effect on the volume estimates. Next, the authors used the density estimates as structural covariates in analyses of fMRI data from an episodic retrieval task. It was found that the contrast between correct and incorrect responses was associated with differentially stronger right PFC activation in the young compared to the old (Figure 8.2B, middle panel). Across young and old subjects, gray-matter density was associated with degree of right PFC activity in all examined regions. This is illustrated in Figure 8.2B (right panel) for averaged density in right and left PFC and MTL. Thus, similar to what was found in the study by Nordahl et al. (2006), the findings of Brassen and colleagues (2009) indicated both local and distal structure-function interactions and suggest that age-related decreases in task-induced PFC activity may not only be a consequence of local (i.e., frontal) loss of brain integrity but also of a more general structural disruption in aging (cf. Persson et al., 2006).

Dickerson et al. (2004) examined memory-associated MTL activation in 32 elderly persons with mild cognitive impairment. The participants performed a visual encoding task during scanning and were then given an episodic retrieval task at a post-scanning

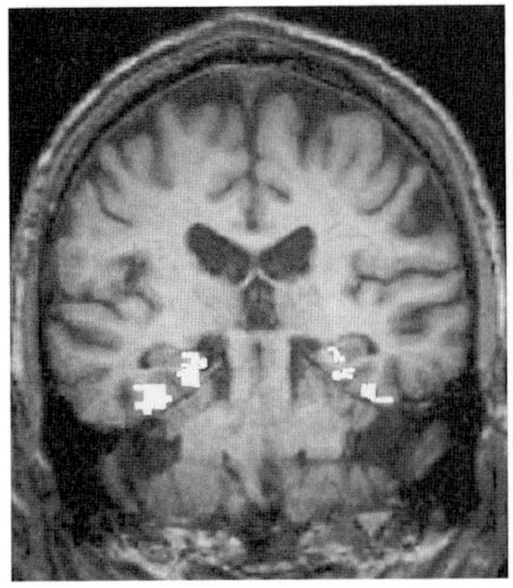
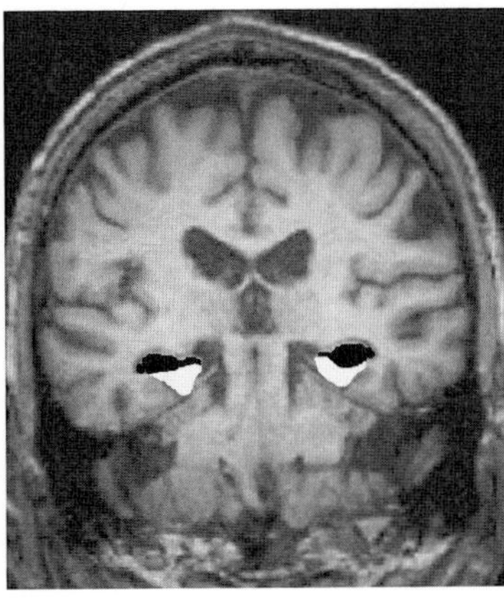

Figure 8.3 Medial temporal lobe regions where the extent of functional brain activity (left) and brain volume (right) was significantly correlated with subsequent memory performance. *Data from Dickerson et al. (2004)*

session. It was found that the extent of MTL activity, including the right hippocampus, was significantly correlated with subsequent memory performance (Figure 8.3, left panel). It was further observed that the volume of the right hippocampal formation (Figure 8.3, right panel) was also correlated with subsequent memory performance. When the fMRI activation response was volume adjusted, its correlation with subsequent performance was no longer statistically significant. As such, the findings by Dickerson and colleagues (2004) provided additional evidence for structure-function interactions, such that consideration of inter-individual differences in brain volume can account for functional changes and their relation to memory performance.

Interactions between Neurotransmission and Functional Brain Activity

Dopamine (DA) has traditionally been considered in relation to motor rather than cognitive functions, but there is converging evidence from animal work, clinical and pharmacological studies, gene-association studies, and computational modeling for a role of DA in higher order cognitive functions such as working memory and strategic episodic long-term memory (Bäckman et al., 2006; Li et al., 2009). There is also accumulating evidence that DA systems undergo substantial decline during the course of normal aging, with sizeable changes in striatal, frontal, and hippocampal brain regions (see Li et al., 2009). Bäckman and colleagues (2006) focused on the similarities between age-related cognitive and DA changes and proposed "the correlative triad" among DA, cognition, and aging. By this view, age-related changes in DA functioning (cf. Karlsson et al., 2009) are seen as a key underlying factor of age-related cognitive changes as well as associated age-related reductions in functional brain activity. This view receives some support from the findings in studies of age-homogenous samples, showing a relation between PET- or SPECT-based measures of DA markers and functional brain activity (Landau et al., 2009; Nyberg et al., 2009). Stronger support was obtained in a recent multimodal (PET-MRI) brain-imaging study by Bäckman and colleagues (2010).

Bäckman et al. (2010) used PET to measure D1 receptor binding in the caudate and DLPFC in groups of younger and older adults. As expected, an age reduction in D1 binding was observed for both regions (the loss of D1 binding potential per decade was estimated to be 8% in caudate and 14% in DLPFC). In addition, fMRI was used to assess brain activity during a spatial working-memory task (comparison of low- and high-memory load). In keeping with findings from many previous studies (Mattay et al., 2006; Nagel et al., 2009; Nyberg et al., 2009), a load-dependent modulation of working-memory activity was observed in frontoparietal cortex for younger adults (Figure 8.4A). For older adults, the corresponding modulation was much weaker and nonsignificant. To test whether this diminished BOLD response to increased working memory load could be accounted for by age-related changes in D1 binding, a regression approach was used to estimate the association between chronological age and the variation in regional BOLD response "in isolation" as well as after controlling for individual differences in D1 binding. Critically, it was found that DA completely accounted for the age effect in left frontal cortex, such that age no longer significantly predicted BOLD (Figure 8.4A). A substantial reduction was also seen for the left parietal cortex, with an attenuation of approximately 50%. These findings provided novel evidence that age-related changes in DA systems mediate age-related differences in task-induced brain activity.

In an accompanying study (Fischer et al., 2010), based on the same fMRI conditions as in the Bäckman et al. (2010) study, pharmacological fMRI was used to "simulate cognitive aging," comparing young adults

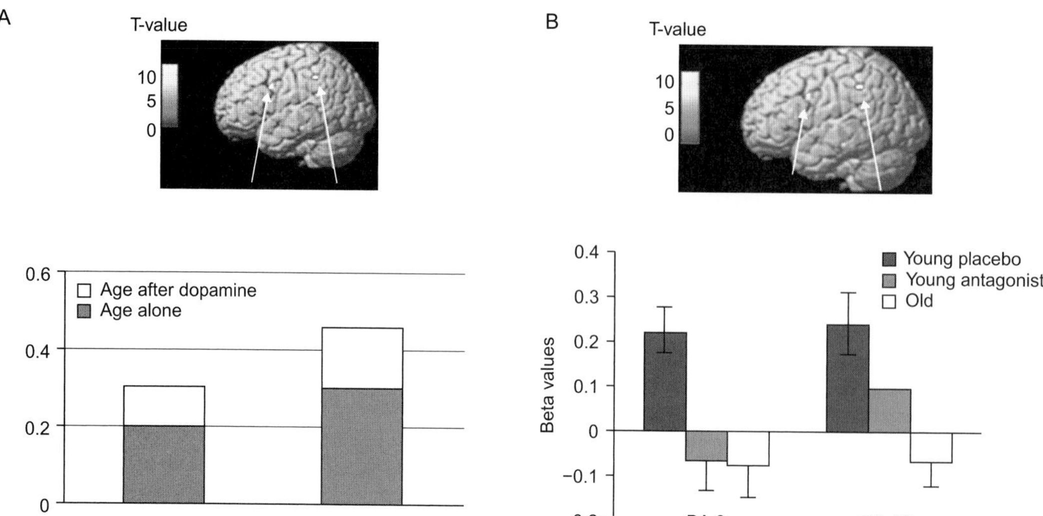

Figure 8.4 Interactions between Neurotransmission and Functional Brain Activity. (A) Age differences in BOLD signal in frontoparietal cortex were largely accounted for by statistical control of age-related changes in dopaminergic neurotransmission. Data from Bäckman et al. (2010). (B) Pharmacological blockage of approximately 50 % of D1 receptors in younger adults resulted in a lowering of working-memory performance along with a diminished load-sensitive frontoparietal response that resembled that of older adults.
Data from Fischer et al. (2010)

under placebo and drug conditions to old adults under placebo conditions regarding working-memory performance and associated functional brain activity. A D1 receptor antagonist was used to pharmacologically block approximately 50% of D1 receptors in the young sample. This resulted in a lowering of working-memory performance along with a diminished load-sensitive frontoparietal response, mimicking the nonresponsive BOLD signal seen in old adults under placebo conditions (Figure 8.4B). These findings support and extend the observation that statistical control of age-related differences in D1 binding accounts for age-related differences in functional brain activity. Thus, DA depletion leads to altered brain-behavior responses, whether caused ontogenetically or pharmacologically.

CONCLUSIONS AND FUTURE PROSPECTS

In the first half of this chapter we addressed three issues in the cognitive neuroscience of aging. With the first issue we noted that all memory systems and processes are not uniformly affected by aging. Cognitive studies have shown that episodic recall and demanding working-memory tasks are highly age sensitive, and brain-imaging studies have demonstrated that increased cognitive demands and associated recruitment of DLPFC will magnify the effects of aging. The second issue concerned inter-individual variability in aging. Although many 70- to 80-year-old adults show evidence of age-related decline, some continue to maintain very high levels of cognitive performance. Preserved cognitive functioning tends to be associated with a "youth-like" brain-activity pattern. The third issue concerned the issue of when aging, at the mean level, has a significant effect on memory performance. Longitudinal cognitive and functional brain-imaging studies converge on a fairly late-onset of decline, starting around the age of 60 years.

The point of departure in the second and main part of the chapter was evidence that structural brain changes appear to precede cognitive and functional brain changes, indicating a potential causal of events where structural changes lead to impaired cognition and associated alterations in functional brain-activity patterns. To address this issue, we reviewed multimodal imaging studies that examined whether age-related decreases in regional brain activity can be accounted for, fully or in part, by age-related changes in the gray or white matter of corresponding brain regions and/or biomarkers of dopaminergic neurotransmission. The reviewed studies support the model outlined in Figure 8.1 by showing that consideration of inter-individual differences in brain structure and in the integrity of neurotransmitter systems have a substantial influence on age-related functional-brain activity differences and associated cognitive deficits in aging. Future studies should attempt to integrate additional imaging measures to see how this influences age-related changes, such as electromagnetic and hemodynamic measures

(Balsters et al., 2010) and PET-based measures of amyloid load (Nordberg, 2004). A more complete understanding of structure-function interactions in aging will also require consideration of additional factors, such as the aging neurovascular system (D'Esposito et al., 2009) and age differences in resting-state brain networks (e.g., Lustig et al., 2003).

Needless to say, the kind of integrated approach that has been introduced in this chapter is still in its infancy and many challenges remain. These include methodological issues. For example, most studies to date have used a regions-of-interest approach when relating different kinds of imaging results. Whole-brain voxel-by-voxel comparisons may yield additional information, including novel data on unexpected distal relations. Such an approach is critically dependent on developments in pre- and post-processing aspects of imaging analysis, such as integration of data into a common anatomical space and multivariate analysis of different kinds of imaging data (see e.g., Chen et al., 2009).

A challenge for the future will also be to examine in detail how genetic and environmental factors, portrayed at the top of the model in Figure 8.1, influence age-related brain and cognitive changes. There is by now agreement that specific genes have a large influence on brain structure and function. Some candidate genes (e.g., ApoE, COMT, BDNF) have been examined already in the context of cognitive aging (e.g., Li et al., 2010; Lind et al., 2006b; Nagel et al., 2008), and future studies will no doubt reveal additional genes as well as complex gene-structure-function interactions that shape cognitive performance across the adult life span. Similarly, with regard to environmental factors, cardiovascular, stress-related, and fitness-related factors have been highlighted (Raz & Kennedy, 2009). There is, for example, evidence that more physically fit elderly persons have better preserved brain structure (Colcombe et al., 2006) and a task-induced activation pattern that mimics that of younger adults (e.g., Kramer & Erickson, 2007).

Finally, it should be noted that not all age-related reductions in functional brain activity may have a structural origin. For example, there is evidence that age-related underactivation of frontal regions during episodic encoding may be reversed if task conditions become more supportive (Logan et al., 2002). That type of regional underactivation cannot be easily accounted for in terms of age-related changes in brain structure. However, the pattern might reflect a less responsive dopamine system (cf. Karlsson et al., 2009). Specifically, elderly persons may have difficulties engaging adequate functional systems under conditions that pose strong demands on self-initiated processing, because of faulty neuromodulation. Future studies will help to define the boundary conditions for a structure/neurotransmission account of age-related reductions in task-induced brain activity and cognitive performance.

ACKNOWLEDGMENTS

LN & LB are supported by the Swedish Science Council. The assistance in preparing this chapter from Dr. Gregoria Kalpouzos and Alireza Salami is greatly acknowledged.

REFERENCES

Albert, M., & Killiany, R. J. (2001). Age-related cognitive change and brain–behavior relationships. In J. E. Birren & K. W. Schaie (Eds.), *Handbook of the psychology of aging* (5th ed.) (pp. 161–185). San Diego, CA: Academic Press.

Bäckman, L., Small, B. J., & Wahlin, A. (2001). Aging and memory: cognitive and biological perspectives. In J. E. Birren & K. W. Schaie (Eds.), *Handbook of the psychology of aging* (5th ed.) (pp. 349–377). San Diego, CA: Academic Press.

Bäckman, L., Karlsson, S., Fischer, H., Karlsson, P., Brehmer, Y., Rieckmann, A., et al. (2010). Dopamine D(1) receptors and age differences in brain activation during working memory. Neurobiology of Aging, in press.

Bäckman, L., Nyberg, L., Lindenberger, U., Li, S.-C., & Farde, L. (2006). The correlative triad among aging, dopamine, and cognition: Current status and future prospects. *Neuroscience and Biobehavioral Reviews, 30*, 791–807.

Balsters, J. H., O´Connell, R. G., Campbell, W., Bodke, A., Upton, N., & Robertson, I. H. (2010, March). *Simultaneous ERP/fMRI highlights fronto-parietal interactions in aging*. Poster presented at the 20th Annual Rotman Research Institute Conference on The Frontal Lobes, Toronto, Canada.

Beason-Held, L. L., Kraut, M. A., & Resnick, S. M. (2008a). Longitudinal changes in aging brain function. *Neurobiology of Aging, 29*, 483–496.

Beason-Held, L. L., Kraut, M. A., & Resnick, S. M. (2008b). Temporal patterns of longitudinal change in aging brain function. *Neurobiology of Aging, 29*, 497–513.

Brassen, S., Buchel, C., Weber-Fahr, W., Lehmbeck, J. T., Sommer, T., & Braus, D. F. (2009). Structure-function interactions of correct retrieval in healthy elderly women. *Neurobiology of Aging, 30*, 1147–1156.

Buckner, R. L. (2004). Memory and executive function in aging and AD: Multiple factors that cause decline and reserve factors that compensate. *Neuron, 44*, 195–208.

Cabeza, R. (2002). Hemispheric asymmetry reduction in old adults: The HAROLD Model. *Psychology & Aging, 17*, 85–100.

Cabeza, R., Anderson, N. D., Locantore, J. K., & McIntosh, A. R. (2002). Aging gracefully: compensatory brain activity in high-performing older adults. *Neuroimage, 17*, 1394–1402.

Cabeza, R., & Nyberg, L. (2000). Neural bases of learning and memory: functional neuroimaging evidence. *Current Opinion in Neurology, 13*, 415–421.

Cabeza, R., Nyberg, L., & Park, D. (2005). *Cognitive neuroscience of aging: Linking cognitive and cerebral aging*. New York: Oxford University Press.

Chen, K. W., Reiman, E. M., Huan, Z. D., Caselli, R. J., Bandy, D., Ayutyanont, N., et al. (2009). Linking functional and structural brain images with multivariate network analyses: a novel application of the partial least square method. *Neuroimage, 47*, 602–610.

Colcombe, S. J., Erickson, K. I., Scalf, P. E., Kim, J. S., Prakash, R., McAuley, E., et al. (2006). Aerobic exercise training increases brain volume in aging humans. *Journals of Gerontology: Biological and Medical Sciences, 61*, 1166–1170.

Craik, F. I., & McDowd, J. M. (1987). Age differences in recall and recognition. *Journal of Experimental Psychology: Learning, Memory, and Cognition, 13*, 474–479.

D'Esposito, M., Jagust, W., & Gazzaley, A. (2009). Methodological and conceptual issues in the study of the aging brain. In M. D'Esposito & W. Jagust (Eds.), *Imaging the aging brain*. Oxford, UK: Oxford University Press.

Dickerson, B. C., Salat, D. H., Bates, J. F., Atiya, M., Killiany, R. J., Greve, D. N., et al. (2004). Medial temporal lobe function and structure in mild cognitive impairment. *Annals of Neurology, 56*, 27–35.

Fischer, H., Nyberg, L., Karlsson, S., Karlsson, P., Brehmer, Y., Rieckmann, A., et al. (2010). Simulating neurocognitive aging. Effects of a dopaminergic antagonist on brain activity during working memory. *Biological Psychiatry, 67*, 575–580.

Fratiglioni, L., Paillard-Borg, S., & Winblad, B. (2004). An active and socially integrated lifestyle in late life might protect against dementia. *Lancet Neurology, 3*, 343–353.

Gabrieli, J. D. E. (1996). Memory systems analyses of mnemonic disorders in aging and age-related diseases. *Proceedings of the National Academy of Science, 93*, 13534–13540.

Grady, C. L. (2009). *Compensatory reorganization of brain networks in older adultsImaging the Aging Brain*. New York: Oxford University Press Oxford Scholarship Online. Oxford University Press. 26 March 2010.

Habib, R., Nyberg, L., & Nilsson, L.-G. (2007). Cognitive and non-cognitive factors contributing to the longitudinal identification of successful older adults in the *Betula* study. *Aging, Neuropsychology, and Cognition, 14*, 257–273.

Head, D., Buckner, R. L., Shimony, J. S., Williams, L. E., Akbudak, E., Conturo, T. E., et al. (2004). Differential vulnerability of anterior white matter in nondemented aging with minimal acceleration in dementia of the Alzheimer type: evidence from diffusion tensor imaging. *Cerebral Cortex, 14*, 410–423.

Hedden, T., & Gabrieli, J. D. (2004). Insights into the ageing mind: A view from cognitive neuroscience. *National Review of Neuroscience, 5*, 7–96.

Jagust, W., & D'Esposito, M. (2009). *Imaging the Aging Brain*. New York: Oxford University Press Oxford Scholarship Online. Oxford University Press. 26 March 2010.

Karlsson, S., Nyberg, L., Karlsson, P., Fischer, H., Thilers, P., Macdonald, S., et al. (2009). Modulation of striatal dopamine D1 binding by cognitive processing. *Neuroimage, 48*, 398–404.

Kaye, J. (2009). *Imaging cognitive decline in aging: Predicting decline with structural imagingImaging the Aging Brain*. New York: Oxford University Press Oxford Scholarship Online. Oxford University Press. 26 March 2010.

Kompus, K., Eichele., T., Hugdahl, K., & Nyberg, L. (2010). Multimodal imaging of incidental retrieval: The low route to memory. *Journal of Cognitive Neuroscience*

Kramer, A. F., & Erickson, K. I. (2007). Capitalizing on cortical plasticity: Influence of physical activity on cognition and brain function. *Trends in Cognitive Neuroscience, 11*, 342–348.

Landau, S. M., Lal, R., O'Neil, J. P., Baker, S., & Jagust, W. J. (2009). Striatal dopamine and working memory. *Cerebral Cortex, 19*, 445–454.

Li, S.-C., Chicherio, C., Nyberg, L., von Oertzen, T., Nagel, I. E., Papenberg, G., et al. (2010). Ebbinghaus revisited: Influences of the BDNF Val66Met polymorphism on backward serial recall are modulated by human aging. *Journal of Cognitive Neuroscience, 22*, 2164–2173.

Li, S. C., Lindenberger, U., Nyberg, L., Heekeren, H. R., & Bäckman, L. (2009). *Dopaminergic modulation of cognition in human gingImaging the Aging Brain*. New York: Oxford University Press Oxford Scholarship Online. Oxford University Press. 26 March 2010.

Lind, J., Larsson, A., Persson, J., Ingvar, M., Nilsson, L.-G., Bäckman, L., et al. (2006a). Reduced hippocampal volume in non-demented carriers of the apolipoprotein E ε4: Relation to chronological age and recognition memory. *Neuroscience Letters, 396*, 23–27.

Lind, J., Persson, J., Ingvar, M., Larsson, A., Cruts, M., Van Broeckhoven, C., et al. (2006b). Reduced functional brain activity response in cognitively intact apolipoprotein E ε4 carriers. *Brain, 129*, 1240–1248.

Logan, J. M, Sanders, A. L, Snyder, A. Z, Morris, J. C., & Buckner, R. L. (2002). Under-recruitment and non-selective recruitment: dissociable neural mechanisms associated with aging. *Neuron, 33*, 827–840.

Lupien, S. J., & Wan, N. (2004). Successful aging: from cell to self. *Philosophical Transactions of the Royal Society of London, Series B, 359*, 1413–1426.

Lustig, C., Snyder, A. Z., Bhakta, M., et al. (2003). Functional deactivation: Change with age and dementia of the Alzheimer type. *Proceedings of the National Academy of Science, 100*, 14505–14509.

Mattay, V. S., Fera, F., Tessitore, A., Hariri, A. R., Berman, K. F., Das., S., et al. (2006). Neurophysiological correlates of age-related changes in WM capacity. *Neuroscience Letter, 392*, 32–37.

Nagel, I. E., Chicherio, C., Li, S.-C., von Oertzen, T., Sander, T., Villringer, A., et al. (2008). Human aging magnifies genetic effects on executive functioning and working memory. *Frontiers in Human Neuroscience, 2*, 1–8.

Nagel, I. E., Preuschhof, C., Li, S.-C., Nyberg, L., Bäckman, L., Lindenberger, U., et al. (2009). Performance level modulates adult age differences in brain activation during spatial working memory. *Proceedings of the National Academy of Science, 106*, 22552–22557.

Nilsson, L.-G., Sternäng, O., Rönnlund, M., & Nyberg, L. (2009). Challenging the notion of an early-onset of cognitive decline. *Neurobiology of Aging, 30*, 521–524.

Niti, M., Yap, K. B., Kua, E. H., et al. (2008). Physical, social and productive leisure activities, cognitive decline and interaction with APOE-epsilon 4 genotype in Chinese older adults. *International Psychogeriatrics, 20*, 237–251.

Nordahl, C. W., Ranganath, C., Yonelinas, A. P., DeCarli, C., Fletcher, E., & Jagust, W. J. (2006). White matter changes compromise prefrontal cortex function in healthy elderly individuals. *Journal of Cognitive Neuroscience, 18*, 418–429.

Nordberg, A. (2004). PET imaging of amyloid in Alzheimer's disease. *Lancet Neurology, 3*, 519–527.

Nyberg, L. (2010, January). *Longitudinal changes in memory-related fMRI-activity: Data from the Betula project*. Invited presentation at the 1st Dallas-ACC conference, Dallas, TX.

Nyberg, L., Andersson, M., Forsgren, L., Jakobsson-Mo, S., Larsson, A., Nilsson, L.-G., et al. (2009). Striatal dopamine D2 binding is related to frontal BOLD response during updating of long-term memory representations. *Neuroimage, 46*, 1194–1199.

Nyberg, L., Dahlin, E., Stigsdotter Neely, A., & Bäckman, L. (2009). Neural correlates of variable working memory load across adult age and skill: Dissociative patterns within the fronto-parietal network. *Scandinavian Journal of Psychology, 50*, 41–46.

Nyberg, L., Petersson, K. M., Cabeza, R., Forkstam, C., & Ingvar, M. (2002). Brain imaging of human memory systems: Between-systems similarities and within-system differences. *Cognitive Brain Research, 13*, 281–292.

Nyberg, L., & Bäckman, L. (2004). Cognitive aging: A view from brain imaging. In R. Dixon, L. Bäckman, & L.-G. Nilsson (Eds.), *New frontiers in cognitive aging* (pp. 135–160). New York: Oxford University Press.

Nyberg, L., Maitland, S. B., Rönnlund, M., Bäckman, L., Dixon, R. A., Wahlin, Å., et al. (2003). Selective adult age differences in an age-invariant multi-factor model of declarative memory. *Psychology and Aging, 18*, 149–160.

Park, D. C., & Reuter-Lorenz, P. (2008). The adaptive brain: aging and neurocognitive scaffolding. *Annual Review of Psychology, 60*, 173–196.

Park, D. C., Welsh, R. C., Marshuetz, C., Gutchess, A. H., Mikels, J., Polk, T. A., et al. (2003). Working memory for complex scenes: age differences in frontal and hippocampal activations. *Journal of Cognitive Neuroscience, 15*, 1122–1134.

Persson, J., & Nyberg, L. (2006). *Altered brain activity in healthy seniors: What does it mean?* Progress in Brain Research (Vol. 157). Elsevier, pp. 45–56.

Persson, J., Nyberg, L., Lind, J., Larsson, A., Nilsson, L.-G., Ingvar, M., et al. (2006). Structure-Function Correlates of Cognitive Decline in Aging. *Cerebral Cortex, 16*, 907–915.

Prull, M. W., Gabrieli, J. D . E., & Bunge, S. A. (2000). Age-related changes in memory: A cognitive neuroscience perspective. In F. I. M. Craik & T. A. Salthouse (Eds.), *Handbook of aging and cognition* (2nd ed.) (pp. 91–154). Mahwah, NJ: Lawrence Erlbaum Associates.

Raz, N., & Kennedy, K. M. (2009). *A systems approach to the aging brain: Neuroanatomic changes, their modifiers, and cognitive correlates in imaging the aging brain Imaging the Aging Brain*. New York: Oxford University Press Oxford Scholarship Online. Oxford University Press. 26 March 2010.

Raz, N., Lindenberger, U., Rodrigue, K. M., Kennedy, K. M., Head, D., Williamson, A., et al. (2005). Regional brain changes in aging healthy adults: general trends, individual differences and modifiers. *Cerebral Cortex, 15*, 1676–1689.

Rönnlund, M., Nyberg, L., Bäckman, L., & Nilsson, L.-G. (2005). Stability, growth, and decline in adult life span development of declarative memory: Cross-sectional and longitudinal data from a population-based study. *Psychology and Aging, 20*, 3–18.

Rypma, B., & D'Esposito, M. (2000). Isolating the neural mechanisms of age-related changes in human working memory. *Nature Neuroscience, 3*, 509–515.

Salthouse, T. A. (2009). When does age-related cognitive decline begin? *Neurobiology of Aging, 30*, 507–514.

Schaie, K. W. (1994). The course of adult intellectual development. *American Psychologist, 49*, 304–313.

Schaie, K. W. (1996). *Adult intellectual development: The Seattle Longitudinal Study*. New York: Cambridge University Press.

Söderlund, H., Nyberg, L., Nilsson, L.-G., & Launer, L. J. (2003). High prevalence of white matter lesions in normal aging: Relation to blood pressure and cognition. *Cortex, 39*, 1093–1105.

Squire, L. R., Knowlton, B., & Musen, G. (1993). The structure and organization of memory. *Annual Review of Psychology, 44*, 453–495.

Stern, Y. (2009). *Cognitive reserve and agingImaging the Aging Brain*. New York: Oxford University Press Oxford Scholarship Online. Oxford University Press. 26 March 2010.

Tulving, E., & Schacter, D. L. (1990). Priming and human memory systems. *Science, 247*(4940), 301–306.

Zelinski, E. M., & Burnight, K. P. (1997). Sixteen-year longitudinal and time lag changes in memory and cognition in older adults. *Psychology and Aging, 12*, 503–513.

Chapter | 9 |

Age Differences in Complex Decision Making

Ellen Peters[1], Nathan F. Dieckmann[2], Joshua Weller[2]

[1]Department of Psychology, The Ohio State University, Columbus, Ohio, USA; [2]Decision Research, Eugene, Oregon, USA

CHAPTER CONTENTS

Introduction 133

The Construction of Preferences in Older-Adult Decisions 134

Less Preference Construction in Familiar Decisions 135

Thinking and Feeling Our Way Through A Complex World 135

The Affect Revolution and Age-Related Differences in the Influence of Affect 136

Increased Influence of Affective Information 137

Endowment Effects 137

Risky-Choice Framing Effects 137

Affective Learning 138

Time Preferences 138

Incidental Affect 139

The Positivity Effect 139

Risky-Choice Framing Effects 140

Pre-Choice Information Processing 140

Age Declines in Deliberative Abilities and their Influence on Decision Making 141

Perceptions of Covariation 142

Other Decision Tasks that Require Deliberation 142

Query Theory 143

Numeracy 143

Selectivity and Motivated Use of Deliberative Processes 144

Limitations 144

Summary and Conclusions 145

Acknowledgments 146

References 146

INTRODUCTION

The psychological study of complex decision making examines the mechanisms underlying people's choices and judgments and attempts to discover how to improve decision-making processes. Although many of the same cognitive processes underlying judgments and decisions have been studied in other fields of psychology (e.g., problem solving), the field of judgment and decision making has tended to focus more on how people process information (e.g., the use of heuristics, the balance between emotional and nonemotional ways of understanding), how they understand uncertainty and risk, and how they choose between alternative courses of action in an uncertain world. Decision research developed out of economic theory and, as a result of this rationalistic origin, concentrated at first on calculation-based explanations for how people make decisions and form judgments (Kahneman & Tversky, 1979). The implicit assumption that good decision making is a conscious, deliberative process has been one of the field's most enduring themes. More recent research, however, has examined the role of affect and intuition in decisions. In both cases (the study of deliberative and affective/intuitive processes), a major underlying theme has been the construction of preferences. Its central idea is that in many situations we do not really know what we prefer, and, as a result, we construct our preferences "on the spot" based on internal and external cues available at the moment. "Virtually every current theory in decision making can be considered a theory of preference construction" (Lichtenstein & Slovic, 2006, p. 3). Such judgments underlie preferences that decision makers form and decisions that they make.

In this chapter we cover research and theories, in a necessarily abbreviated form, that address some of the issues that older adults (generally defined as 65 years

DOI: 10.1016/B978-0-12-380882-0.00009-7

and older) face in making everyday judgments and decisions. A decision, of course, is a choice between two or more options or alternatives (e.g., choosing a car). One of those options could be the status quo (e.g., doing nothing or making no change). A judgment, in contrast, is the psychological appraisal or evaluation of information. It is an understanding of a situation or an individual (e.g., I'm having some stomach distress. How likely is it to be due to my new medication?). Due to limited longitudinal research on age and decision making (see Limitations section on cohort effects), we generally discuss age differences rather than age changes in decision making.

THE CONSTRUCTION OF PREFERENCES IN OLDER-ADULT DECISIONS

Preference construction depends on how decision makers process available information. This processing can be altered by aspects of the situation and by characteristics of the individual decision maker. For example, in terms of situational aspects, preference construction can be influenced by how the decision is presented (e.g., framing effects), how it is asked (e.g., asking a decision maker to choose between two options can result in a different decision than asking her to reject an option; Shafir et al., 1993), and by the availability of logically irrelevant information (see many examples in Lichtenstein & Slovic, 2006). Individual differences also influence constructive processes because they can mark differences in what information a decision maker attends to and how he or she processes this information (e.g., emotional reactivity, memory, and numeracy). Decisions are not always constructed in the same manner, and some differences in constructive processes likely map on to age differences in information processing. As a result, we focus here on age as one particularly important individual difference.

Research suggests that preferences will more likely be constructed when decisions are (1) unfamiliar, (2) complex (including too much information and conflicting goals), or (3) familiar but not often experienced personally (Payne et al., 1999). Preference construction also may be more likely when (4) the decision maker's values are clear, but how to make trade-offs between values is not (this may be particularly true with emotionally difficult trade-offs (Luce, 2005); and (5) decision makers lack an affective response to decision options, have difficulty translating feelings on to a numerical scale (e.g., fresh local produce tastes great; how much more am I willing to pay for it?) or have different affective responses depending on how options are presented (Peters et al., 2006).

These conditions imply that preferences are likely to be constructed in many consequential health, financial, and other life decisions that older adults face (moving to a retirement home, complicated and numerous medical treatments, retirement-income choices). A decision to give up driving, for example, is unfamiliar, complex, and involves emotionally difficult trade-offs as the older adult balances safety concerns with concerns about personal freedom and convenience. Decisions involving numeric information, such as indicators of hospital quality or characteristics of health insurance plans, may be particularly susceptible to preference construction because processing numeric information is difficult and people are not always proficient with numbers (Dehaene, 1997; Paulos, 1988). As a result, individuals will not always use numeric information in meaningful ways (Peters et al., 2009). The emerging view in the decision literature is that, in many situations, preference measurement is best considered as architecture (building a set of preferences) rather than as archaeology (uncovering existing preferences; Gregory et al., 1993; Payne et al., 1999; Slovic, 1995). These constructive processes can lead to preference instability, which is considered a sign of less competent decision making (Bruine de Bruin et al., 2007; Finucane et al., 2002). Understanding and harnessing the power of constructed preferences, however, can also lead to better decisions (see the Summary and Conclusions section and Epstein & Peters, 2009).

In this chapter we explore whether older adults might show less preference construction than younger adults in situations that take advantage of their greater experience (and therefore more stable values). They may, however, show greater or different preference construction in less familiar decisions because they process information in ways that are different from younger adults. These age-related differences in information processing include declines in deliberative efficiency, motivated selectivity in the use of deliberative capacity, and changes in the use of affective information. We cover a diversity of decision topics throughout this chapter including the use of heuristics; the influence of gains, losses, and probabilities; mood effects; pre-choice information processing; memory effects; and numeracy among others. Although the stereotype of older adults appears to include an inability to make good decisions, we suggest that the quality of older-adult decisions will sometimes be better and other times will be worse, than that of younger adults. This difference will depend on preference-construction processes and, specifically, on how older adults process information compared to younger adults. In addition, it will depend on diagnosing the decision situation and whether there is a match between the information processing that takes place and what information processing will produce better decisions in that given situation (see also Yoon et al., 2009).

LESS PREFERENCE CONSTRUCTION IN FAMILIAR DECISIONS

Some studies have emphasized the importance of experience – and its associated knowledge – as a moderator of age differences in the quality of judgments and decisions. If preferences are more stable in familiar situations and older adults, by dint of more years of experience, have greater familiarity with and knowledge in common decision situations, then they should demonstrate less preference construction in them. In fact, Tentori et al. (2001) demonstrated that older adults were less likely to let situational information (e.g., the attractiveness of a discount in comparison to other available discounts) influence their decision when its choice would require a larger minimum purchase than their usual budget. Tentori et al. (2001) argued that older adults' everyday life experience with the grocery-store context is advantageous because they have knowledge of the situational variables that may influence their judgments and can discount irrelevant information (see also Kim & Hasher, 2005, for similar results).

Other studies also have demonstrated older adults drawing on their life experiences. In an example in the domain of health, Meyer et al. (1995) studied a group of women diagnosed with breast cancer and found that the older women behaved more like experts by seeking out less information, making decisions faster, and arriving at decision outcomes equivalent to those of younger women. In a follow-up study, Meyer and Pollard (2004) suggested that the effect was due to the availability of specific information about breast cancer. Consistent with an expertise-based explanation, the presence of relevant information in the problem domain facilitated decision making in older women. Fisk and Rogers (2000) also reviewed evidence that decisions in well-learned environments (e.g., driving) are preserved with age. Finally, Bruine de Bruin et al. (2009) demonstrated that older adults had preserved decision-making ability on tasks that involve skills learned through experience (e.g., recognizing social norms and resistance to sunk costs; see also Strough et al., 2008). The association between age and performance on tasks that required experiential skills remained after controlling for fluid cognitive ability. Like the Tentori et al. (2001) study, these studies supported older adults' ability to use their life experiences when considering contextual variables and to prevent this context from influencing judgments and decisions.

Older adults' life experiences may allow them to develop both specific and general expertise in ways that benefit judgment and decision making. For example, Mata et al. (2007, 2009) found that both younger and older adults appeared to adapt to the demands of current decision environments. Although older adults have fewer cognitive resources upon which to draw and such deliberative declines could result in less ability to adjust to decision environments, both age groups adjusted information search and strategy selection as needed. Pachur et al. (2009) also found adaptive use of recognition as a simple heuristic strategy in decision making among younger and older adults faced with environments in which the use of recognition was a valid cue (e.g., population of American cities is well estimated by the recognizability of the city name) and a less valid cue (disease mortality statistics). Older adults, however, were somewhat more likely to (incorrectly) use the recognition heuristic when it was a less valid cue, suggesting that older adults may not adapt their use of the recognition heuristic as effectively as younger adults. Further research would be useful to uncover whether the strategies used by older adults might be based on their greater life experience with decisions, whereas that of younger adults might be based on more effortful strategies.

Although early research pointed toward improvements in everyday problem solving with age (Cornelius & Caspi, 1987), a more recent meta-analysis of studies of everyday problem solving found that age declines in everyday problem solving exist and are likely due to age-related cognitive declines (Thornton & Dumke, 2005). However, young and middle-aged adults did not differ in problem-solving ability, presumably because the benefits of accumulated experience outweighed deliberative decline. In addition, although older adults (mean age of 70 years) showed worse performance, this difference was attenuated when the problem content was interpersonal (involving other people) rather than instrumental (involving something one is trying to accomplish, achieve, or get better at) in focus, suggesting an important motivational component to older-adult problem solving (Blanchard-Fields et al., 1995, 2007; Thornton & Dumke, 2005).

THINKING AND FEELING OUR WAY THROUGH A COMPLEX WORLD

Information in decision making appears to be processed using two different modes of thinking: an affective/experiential mode and a deliberative one (S. Epstein, 1994; Loewenstein et al., 2001; Reyna, 2004; Sloman, 1996; these modes are sometimes called System 1 and 2, respectively – see Kahneman, 2003 and Stanovich & West, 2002). Both modes of thought are important to forming decisions. The experiential mode produces thoughts and feelings in a relatively effortless and spontaneous manner. The operations of this mode are implicit, intuitive, automatic, associative, and fast and appear to be based primarily on affective (emotional) feelings. As shown in a number of studies, affect provides information about the goodness or badness of an option that might warrant further consideration and can directly motivate a behavioral tendency in choice processes (Damasio, 1994; Osgood et al., 1957; Peters, 2006). The effects of preference stability in familiar decisions have been linked to affective processes. One of a large number of dual-process theorists, Seymour Epstein (1994, p. 716) observed:

> ***The experiential system is assumed to be intimately associated with the experience of affect, … which refer[s] to subtle feelings of which people are often unaware. When a person responds to an emotionally significant event … the experiential system automatically searches its memory banks for related events, including their emotional accompaniments… If the activated feelings are pleasant, they motivate actions and thoughts anticipated to reproduce the feelings. If the feelings are unpleasant, they motivate actions and thoughts anticipated to avoid the feelings.***

The deliberative mode, in contrast, is conscious, analytical, reason-based, verbal, and relatively slow. It is the deliberative mode of thinking that is more flexible and provides effortful control over more spontaneous experiential processes. Kahneman (2003) suggested that one of the functions of the deliberative mode is to monitor the quality of the information processing emerging from the experiential mode and its impact on behavior. Both modes of thinking are important and some researchers claim that good choices are most likely to emerge when affective and deliberative modes work in concert and decision makers think as well as feel their way through judgments and decisions (e.g., Damasio, 1994).

Some disagreement exists as to whether these influences on decision making are due to dual processes, a single process, or many interdependent processes. For example, deliberation about reasons for choice can distract decision makers from their feelings and have a negative effect on some decision processes (e.g., Wilson et al., 1989). Research has also demonstrated that affect may have a relatively greater influence when deliberative capacity is lower, suggesting that, at least in some cases, these two modes could exist on a single continuum (Hammond, 1996; Kruglanski et al., 2003; Peters & Slovic, 2007). Shiv and Fedorikhin (1999), for example, demonstrated that decision makers were more likely to choose an affect-rich option (and make a decision of the heart) when deliberative capacity was diminished by cognitive load. Finucane et al. (2000) also found that the inverse relation between risks and benefits (linked to affect by Alhakami & Slovic, 1994) was enhanced under time pressure; reducing the time for deliberation appeared to increase the use of affect. A balance between affect and deliberation could explain some age differences in information processing and decision making, with declining resources leading to greater affective input in decisions. As reviewed later, cognitive-aging research is more consistent with the existence of both modes of processing and understanding them (including their interactions) may ultimately enrich what we know about how information is processed in decisions across the life span.

THE AFFECT REVOLUTION AND AGE-RELATED DIFFERENCES IN THE INFLUENCE OF AFFECT

Two dominant perspectives exist on the influence of affective considerations on cognitive performance (e.g., memory, judgment processes, decision making). The first is a motivational perspective that is focused on aging-related chronic activation of emotion-regulation goals and an associated motivation to process affective information, as typified in socioemotional selectivity theory (Carstensen, 1993, 2006). This theory posits that changes in time perspective result in emotional goals becoming increasingly important as the end of life nears, which in turn results in greater monitoring of affective information. Because older adults are, by virtue of age, closer to the end of life, age should be associated with an increased importance of emotional goals that allow for the optimization of emotional experience. Thus, the increased importance of emotional goals results in two separate predictions: (1) an age-related increase in attention to emotional content and choices that allow for the regulation of emotional experiences; and (2) a positivity effect, with either an increased focus on positive information and/or a decreased focus on negative information. These predictions have potentially great relevance to the impact of affect and emotions in judgment and decision making.

Novak and Mather (2007), for example, explored variety seeking in younger and older adults. They presented participants with choices among jellybeans and different types of music. Older adults showed less variety seeking when choosing what to use at a later time as compared to immediate consumption. Younger adults engaged in the same amount of variety seeking when choosing what to use immediately and what to use at a later time. The authors relate this finding to the tendency for older adults to focus more on regulating future emotional experiences. Novak and Mather (2007) argued that this regulatory process results in older adults choosing reliably satisfactory products for future consumption so as not to take the emotional risks associated with variety seeking for future consumption.

The second perspective is more cognitive in nature and focuses on the impact of changing cognitive skills on the relative influence of affective processes on performance. This perspective is typified by theories such as the dynamic integration theory by Labouvie-Vief (2003, 2005) and by neuropsychological approaches that focus on the differential impact of aging on normative changes in cortical systems underlying affective and deliberative processes. Research suggests that neural structures associated with affective processing (e.g., amygdala) undergo less normative functional change with aging relative to those areas underlying executive or deliberative functions (e.g., the dorsolateral prefrontal cortex; e.g., Bechara, 2005; Chow & Cummings, 2000; Moscovitch & Winocur, 1995). This relative-preservation view is supported by research demonstrating that adult age differences in performance are less on those tasks thought to be supported by affective-processing systems (e.g., Kensinger et al., 2002; MacPherson et al., 2002; Mikels et al., 2005) compared to those associated with executive functions (for reviews, see Grady, 2000; West, 1996). Its primary prediction overlaps with the prediction of the socioemotional selectivity theory of an age-related relative increase in the influence of affective information. The cognitive-decline perspective presumably requires the effect, however, to be stronger for older adults with fewer cognitive resources; this second prediction has received scant attention.

In the next two sections, we review whether existing evidence supports an increased influence of affective information in older-adult decisions and a positivity effect in decision processes.

Increased Influence of Affective Information

Recent empirical work has shown that aging is associated with an increase in attention to emotional content. For example, Fung and Carstensen (2003) found that, relative to younger adults, older adults exhibited greater preference and superior memory for emotional advertisements than for nonemotional ones. Several effects on judgments and decisions might be observed if this is the case. First, more affective sources of information such as anecdotal or hedonic information may receive greater weight (Dhar & Wertenbroch, 2000; Strange & Leung, 1999). Consistent with this notion, Blanchard-Fields et al. (1997) found that older adults focus more than younger adults on emotional aspects of everyday problems. Second, losses may loom equally large or larger for older adults than for younger adults if both positive and negative information are accentuated. Decision paradigms, such as endowment studies and risky-choice framing studies, often involve positive and negative information and can be used to examine these age-difference hypotheses.

Endowment Effects

Different processing of negative and positive information is used to explain effects such as the "endowment effect." In endowment-effect studies, subjects are either (1) endowed with a product such as a coffee mug and asked the minimum amount for which they would sell it, or (2) they are not endowed with the products and are asked the maximum amount for which they would be willing to buy it. Sellers tend to require much more money than buyers are willing to pay (Thaler, 1980). The effect has been linked to affective processes, with losses looming larger than gains (also called loss aversion or a negativity bias) and appears to be larger when subjects have stronger affective reactions (Knutson et al., 2008; Lerner et al., 2004; Peters et al., 2003). Older adults, if they generally rely more on feelings, should therefore exhibit a stronger endowment effect. In support, Johnson et al. (2006) demonstrated greater endowment effects with increasing age in a large sample of auto buyers. Kovalchik et al. (2005), on the other hand, found no endowment effect for older or younger adults, but their task appeared to maximize the amount of deliberation in the task and therefore may have minimized the role of feelings found to be important to this effect (Peters et al., 2003). No other age-difference studies of the endowment effect could be located.

Risky-Choice Framing Effects

A similar prediction can be tested within the domain of framing effects, in which the same decision problem is framed or described in a positive or negative format. One of the most well-known findings in the decision-making literature concerns risky-choice framing effects (Tversky & Kahneman, 1981). In the classic "Asian Disease" problem, individuals presented with options described in a gain frame (the number of lives saved) tend to be risk averse, choosing an option that saves a guaranteed number of lives over an option with a possibility of saving all lives. In contrast, decision makers presented with options described in a loss frame (the number of lives lost) tend to be risk seeking, choosing an option with a possibility of not losing any lives rather than losing a certain number of lives. Although gain and loss options are numerically equivalent, different affective reactions are elicited from the separate frames.

If a general affective bias is evident, then the negativity bias should be enhanced and older adults should produce stronger framing effects relative to younger adults, leaving them more vulnerable to possible manipulation through intentional or nonintentional framing. In support of this interpretation, framing effects were larger for undergraduate participants low in need for cognition (Smith & Levin, 1997). In addition, Bennett (2001) linked larger framing effects to the addition of emotion-laden visual portrayals. Multiple studies concerning age differences in framing effects have found that older adults demonstrated significantly stronger framing effects (Kim et al., 2005;

Lauriola & Levin, 2001; Weber et al., 2004; Weller et al., 2010). Three remaining studies, however, found no age difference in the effect of frames (Holliday, 1988; Mayhorn et al., 2002; Rönnlund et al., 2005), and one study found weaker framing effects with age (Mikels & Reed, 2009). In particular, Weller et al. (2010) reported that the degree to which individuals displayed the classic "preference shift" in risk taking (i.e., with risk taking to avoid losses being greater than risk taking to achieve gains; see Levin et al., 1998) increased as a function of age, and reached an asymptote around 45 years. The bulk of the evidence demonstrates stronger effects of frame for older than younger adults, consistent with the affective bias posited both by socioemotional selectivity theory and the cognitive-decline perspective (although note that not all study results are consistent). In a later section, we review existing evidence for The Positivity Effect in these and other studies.

Affective Learning

Hess et al. (1996) also examined adult age differences in the ability to learn about a prototypical group member from descriptions of group members and nonmembers. Despite the claim by Fisk and Warr (1998, p. 112) that "it is well established that older people tend to learn more slowly than do younger ones," older adults performed better than younger adults in abstracting a prototype based on affective information, providing support for an overweighting of emotional information. Hess et al. (1996) argued that the greater controlled-processing abilities of younger adults interfered with their ability to abstract the affective information.

These findings suggest that in choice tasks that involve learning through experience, affective information should be particularly salient to older adults, thus improving their ability to abstract and use it in their choices despite cognitive declines. Evidence in favor of such an explanation comes from studies examining performance in the Iowa Gambling Task (IGT) and other similar tasks (Damasio, 1994) in which age differences are sometimes observed to be absent (e.g., Denburg et al., 2005; Kovalchik et al., 2005; MacPherson et al., 2002; Zamarian et al., 2008). Denburg et al. (2005) found, however, that a subset of older adults made particularly poor choices, but none of the cognitive measures used could explain the difference between older adults who made good choices and those who made bad choices. This research was consistent with similar, independent investigations (Denburg et al., 2009; Fein et al., 2007; Zamarian et al., 2008), demonstrating age-related declines in IGT performance.

Prior research has shown that performance on this task is based in part on affective processes, as scores on self-report measures of affective reactivity were associated with choices made by college-student participants in the original and modified versions of the task (Peters & Slovic, 2000). Wood et al. (2005) also found that older and younger adults performed equally well on the original version of the gambling task. Using a cognitive model for this task that provides a theoretical decomposition of performance into learning, motivational, and response components, they were able to demonstrate different processes used by younger and older adults. Specifically, younger adults relied more on memory processes whereas older adults relied more on an accurate representation of gains and losses in the task. This suggests that the relative preservation of affective processes in older adults could enable them to compensate for losses in deliberative processes.

At this point, the mixed results make it unclear what age differences may exist in performance on the IGT and similar risky-choice tasks. The conflicting results may be due in part to age differences in responses to ambiguity as opposed to risk per se (Zamarian et al., 2008). Alternatively, individual difference variables (not yet identified) may be differentially associated with performance across different age groups, and perhaps across the various samples that have been used (e.g., Denburg et al., 2009). It is clear, however, that older adults perform less well than younger adults when payoff structures change unexpectedly, perhaps because of the flexibility of overwriting a learned concept based on working-memory processes as opposed to affective processes (Mell et al., 2005).

Recent research has also suggested that, under some circumstances, performance in complex decisions can be better when individuals do not engage in extensive deliberation (Dijksterhuis & Nordgren, 2006). Although the validity and generalizability of the theory of unconscious thought are still open issues, parallels exist between their effects and the age differences we address. Older adults may rely more on affective and intuitive processes in their everyday decisions (a general affective bias) and they may actively deliberate less in those decisions due to cognitive limitations. Whether the Dijksterhuis et al. (2006) findings are based on these same kinds of processes is an open question. However, Queen and Hess (2010) demonstrated that older adult decision making was relatively preserved on an affective (unconscious thought processing) task, whereas they showed the typical declines on a separate deliberative (conscious thought processing) task as compared to younger adults.

Time Preferences

Finally, socioemotional selectivity theory suggests that in old age, when time is perceived as limited, short-term benefits should become relatively more important (Lang & Carstensen, 2002). In terms of time preferences, it implies that older adults will value future money relatively less and, thus, would show a relative preference for a smaller immediate reward over a larger later reward. Economic theory and results thus far are mostly consistent with this suggestion (Lee et al., 2008; Read & Read, 2004; Sozou & Seymour, 2003; Trostel & Taylor, 2001). A simpler explanation is that older adults may perceive the likelihood of cashing in later as being lower due to shorter expected life span or shorter expected healthy life span. Although the short time spans used in most of these studies makes this explanation somewhat less tenable, we could say with greater assurance that the effect was due to chronically activated emotional goals if such effects were shown by older adults more for affective options over less affective options.

Incidental Affect

A large body of research findings suggests that incidental sources of affect (mood states, affective primes, or conditioned responses that are normatively irrelevant to a decision) influence people's evaluations, judgments, motivation, and information processing (for a review see Forgas, 1995). We predict that incidental affect may particularly influence older adults' judgments for two reasons: (a) incidental mood states are more frequent, intense, and salient among older adults (Lawton, 2001); and (b) older adults may lack the capability of discounting or correcting for the influence of mood in judgments and decisions, a cognitive process that younger adults are capable of performing under normal conditions (Schwarz & Clore, 1983).

Results from several studies partially support this hypothesis with incidental sources of affect influencing both younger and older adults. This influence, however, tends to be similar between the two age groups with older adults perhaps showing the effect in a more robust way across studies. For example, in looking at mood-congruency effects, individuals induced to a positive mood tended to respond more to positive items than negative ones, whereas those induced to a negative mood showed the opposite pattern (Ferraro et al., 2003; Knight et al., 2002). Knight et al. (2002) did demonstrate more robust effects with older than younger adults across multiple tasks. Using a different source of incidental affect, Hess et al. (2000) examined the effects of affective primes on likeability judgments about Japanese Kanji characters. Presentation of each of these characters was preceded by a positively or negatively valenced word that was presented either above or below the participant's perceptual threshold. Consistent with previous research by Murphy and Zajonc (1993), likeability judgments tended to be consistent with the valence of the prime word when participants were unaware of the prime word. It appeared that individuals misattributed the primed affective response to the Kanji characters when they were unaware of the source. In contrast, when participants could consciously perceive the prime, only older adults exhibited priming effects, suggesting that younger adults could correct for the prime's influence whereas older adults could not.

Results from a modest number of studies have generally supported the hypothesis that affective information has a relatively greater influence on older adults than on younger adults. These results are consistent with both socioemotional selectivity theory and cognitive-decline perspectives. The cognitive-decline perspective also predicts that the increased influence of affect would be even greater for those older individuals with fewer cognitive resources, but this additional hypothesis has received little attention.

The Positivity Effect

Socioemotional selectivity theory also predicts, for motivational reasons, a specific focus on positive over negative information in later life as older adults seek to optimize emotional experience. The dynamic integration theory of adult development by Labouvie-Vief (2003) suggested a similar positivity effect arising out of qualitative differences in the processing of affect across ages that is based in aging-related changes in the dynamic balance between processes of affect optimization (of happiness) and affect differentiation (the ability to tolerate negativity to maintain objective representations). Her prediction of a positivity bias, however, is based on age-related limitations in cognitive resources that result in an adaptive shift to less resource-demanding positive affect (Gross et al., 1997). In her view, older adults' declining cognitive resources may lead to a gating out of negative information and other sources of negative emotion. However, the results of memory studies by Mather and Knight (2005) do not support this cognitive-decline hypothesis as positivity effects were shown only by older adults with access to greater cognitive resources, leaving socioemotional selectivity theory with greater support thus far.

Leaving aside whether positivity effects shown in attention and memory studies are due to cognitive decline or motivational goals, the possible existence of a positivity effect has marked implications for judgments and decision making. Older adults who focus relatively more on positive information may process gain versus loss information in decisions differently than their younger counterparts who do not share this same focus. Robust findings with younger adults (illustrated by the S-shaped value function of prospect theory) indicate that losses tend to loom larger than gains (Kahneman & Tversky, 1979). If a positivity effect exists among older adults, then losses may not loom as large for them as for younger adults.

Decision paradigms originally conducted with younger adults show some inconsistent support for the positivity effect and are used to examine whether the effect is due to a greater focus on positive information, a lesser focus on negative information, or both. For example, the IGT, described earlier, can also be used to examine the negativity bias because decision makers face both gains and losses in that task. Wood et al. (2005) examined model parameters from their theoretical decomposition and concluded that older adults, unlike the younger college students, did not show a negativity bias, providing some support for the positivity effect. However, as discussed in the next section, results are equivocal in risky-choice framing studies.

Risky-Choice Framing Effects

If age differences exist such that older adults weigh positive outcomes more, then they should show greater risk aversion in gains compared to younger adults. This prediction is because, if older adults weigh positive information more than younger adults, then the value function should be steeper near the origin in the domain of gains for older adults than for younger adults. Thus, the smaller number for sure should be valued higher for them. While there may also be an age difference in value between that smaller amount and the larger one, presumably that difference will be smaller than the age difference in value for the smaller amount due to diminishing marginal returns. This conjecture is based on the assumption that the value function curves for each age group converge at a higher outcome level. However, if older adults weigh negative outcomes less, less risk seeking in losses should be found; and if they weigh affective information more in general, then they should show greater risk seeking in losses and greater risk aversion in gains relative to their younger counterparts. Five relevant studies have been conducted and show age results that are largely inconsistent with the positivity effect, and more so, even with each other. First and consistent with one interpretation of the positivity effect, Weller et al. (2010) found that risk aversion in gains increased consistently across the life span (as if positive information was weighed more), whereas for loss-related decision making, risk seeking was relatively constant across ages. Their study included a large sample of individuals ranging from 5 to 85 years of age. Consistent with a different interpretation of the positivity effect, Mikels and Reed (2009) found that older adults demonstrated less risk seeking in the loss frame compared to younger adults (as if negative outcomes were weighed less) but similar choices in the gain domain; their study may not have been sufficiently powered due to small sample sizes.

Other risky-choice framing studies have not supported the positivity effect, however. Lauriola and Levin (2001) found results consistent with a greater weighing of both positive and negative information (a more general emotion bias as suggested in the last section). Specifically, older adults demonstrated both greater risk aversion in gains and greater risk seeking in losses. Weber et al. (2004) conducted a meta-analysis of studies and found that increasing age (age ranges were not specified in their paper) was associated with greater risk seeking in losses (more choices of a gamble over a sure thing) as if older adults weighed negative information more; no significant link existed between increasing age and risk aversion in gains (more choices of a sure thing over a gamble) — suggesting no age-related changes in the domain of gains. Finally, Holliday (1988) found no age differences from 20 to 76 years old in choices between gambles and sure things for gains or losses.

Findings from framing studies highlight two important points. First, they support the idea that decision making for risky gains and losses may follow different developmental paths. Findings that older adults may choose to take similar risks as younger adults when faced with losses (Weller et al., 2010) are consistent with the notion that risk taking to avoid losses is an early learned, reflexive strategy (Reyna, 2004) and are consistent with the findings of Mather and Knight (2006) that threat detection (i.e., recognition of angry faces) are not impaired in older adults. Due to conflicting findings across studies, however, it is not yet clear whether the propensity to take risks to avoid certain losses may develop early and may be less affected by age-related cognitive declines. Second, and perhaps most important, inconsistency across framing studies points toward the possible existence of as yet undiscovered but important moderating or mediating variables. It may be, for example, that heterogeneity exists across individuals, age groups, and specific paradigms used in what is considered negative and positive information (if I don't win money, do I consider it a loss?; if I don't lose money, do I consider that a gain?).

Pre-Choice Information Processing

Support for the positivity effect is more robust when pre-choice information processing is considered. Löckenhoff and Carstensen (2007, 2008), for example, have examined how older and younger adults use and recall valenced information in a context-rich healthcare decision-making task. Participants were presented with computer-based healthcare scenarios that had positive, negative, and neutral information about different doctors and healthcare plans. When making choices, older adults were found to examine and recall a greater proportion of positive information as compared to younger adults. They replicated this finding in a second study (Löckenhoff & Carstensen, 2008), but also found that the effect was only present when older adults made choices for themselves or for someone else of similar age. When older adults were asked to choose for a person considerably younger, they did not show an increased focus on positive information. Younger adults did not show any differences in information use or recall when asked to choose for themselves, someone the same age, or someone considerably older.

Pre-choice information processing was also considered by Kim et al. (2008), who had younger and older adults make choices between products. In one condition, they were asked to explicitly evaluate the options, whereas in the other condition they were not. In the evaluation condition, older adults listed more positive than negative attributes of the options prior to choosing, and they were more satisfied with their choices than younger adults. These evaluation-condition findings are consistent with post-choice findings of Mather and Johnson (2000), who found that older adults were more likely than young adults to remember positive features over negative features of selected options but remembered negative features more than positive features of unselected options, even when overall level of memory performance was controlled. Importantly, in the study by Mather and Johnson (2000), younger adults were found to exhibit a similar bias when asked to focus on the emotional content of their choices. Kim et al. (2008) also found, however, that the positivity effect for older adults was dependent on whether they were asked to explicitly evaluate the options in a choice task. There were no differences between younger and older adults in the no-evaluation condition.

Of interest, the positivity effect among older adults requires greater deliberative input rather than compensating for declines in deliberation (Mather & Knight, 2005). This research implies that the relatively greater influence of positive than negative information on older-adult decisions will occur only for those older adults who have the resources necessary (due to ability, motivation, or time) to meet the motivational goals hypothesized in socioemotional selectivity theory. It is suggestive of another explanation for the mixed findings in this literature such that, across studies, populations may differ in deliberative abilities, and minor changes in decision paradigms may alter the degree of deliberative effort required. Interestingly, the findings of Mather and Knight (2005) also support the existence of dual processes rather than a single continuum, with greater deliberative capacity associated with greater affective input. However, we are not aware of any published research directly examining this possibility in decision making.

To summarize, the results of findings on the positivity effect have been somewhat supportive (particularly for pre-choice information processing) at the same time as it has been difficult to pin down whether the positivity effect emerges due to an age-related positivity bias (greater weighing of positive information) or an age-related lack of a negativity bias (lesser weighing of negative information). Research has demarcated some boundary conditions for the positivity effect – the effect appears to emerge only when older adults are evaluating information for themselves or a similar aged adult and may exist only when older adults have sufficient cognitive capacity to enact their motivational goals (Mather & Knight, 2005). Importantly, the effect is also shown by younger adults asked to focus on the emotional content of their choices, supporting the underlying motivational and emotional basis of the effect.

AGE DECLINES IN DELIBERATIVE ABILITIES AND THEIR INFLUENCE ON DECISION MAKING

Although older adults do show improvements or at least resilience in experience-based and affective processes, several lines of research support declines in the controlled processes of the deliberative system that may have negative impacts on decisions (see also Chapter 4, this volume). First, because older adults process information less quickly than younger adults do (e.g., Salthouse, 1992, 1994), their deliberative abilities may suffer due to less efficient processing of perceived information. Salthouse (1996) has hypothesized that the products of older adults' early processing may be lost by the time later processing occurs and/or that later processing might not occur because early processing required so much time. Second, the evidence indicates age-related deficits in explicit memory, explicit learning, and other executive functions (Cohen, 1996; Kausler, 1990; Salthouse et al., 1999). In particular, working memory and executive functions (e.g., the control and regulation of cognition) associated with the prefrontal cortex deteriorate with normal aging (e.g., Amieva et al., 2003). In the past decade, a rapidly expanding body of evidence from the field of geriatric neuropsychology has provided support for the "frontal lobe hypothesis" of cognitive aging, which states that the frontal lobes are the first brain areas to show functional decline over the life span (Brown & Park, 2003; West, 1996). This theory is supported by both longitudinal and cross-sectional neuroanatomical data that show age-related structural declines in the prefrontal cortex, particularly the orbitofrontal and lateral prefrontal cortices (Good et al., 2001; Kennedy et al., 2008; Raz et al., 2005; Resnick et al., 2003). Older adults have been found to perform more poorly than their younger counterparts on executive function tasks, which are presumably related to frontal lobe function, while performing comparably on tasks that are not dependent on frontal lobe function. Finally, Hasher and Zacks (1988) argued that aging is associated with a decrease in the ability to inhibit false and irrelevant information. If good decisions depend on such deliberative skills (and deliberation is often considered the hallmark of good decision making), then judgments and decisions will generally suffer as we age (although see Healey & Hasher, 2009 for an interesting analysis of how deliberative declines may sometimes improve decisions).

Perceptions of Covariation

Several studies have identified biases on judgment processes that increase with age and were linked with deliberative processes such as working memory. For example, Mutter (2000) and Mutter and Pliske (1994) examined the impact of illusory correlation on performance. (In an illusory correlation, people perceive that two variables covary consistently with their prior expectations even though no actual relation exists.) They found that older adults' judgments were more influenced by prior expectancies than were those of younger adults, particularly under distraction conditions. This finding is important because we often judge whether one action produces a particular outcome or not (e.g., will taking an aspirin reduce my headache?).

Older adults were also less likely to correct their judgments when accurate information regarding the co-occurrence of events was made salient. Interestingly, Mutter (2000) found that age differences were more evident for memory-based judgments than for on-line judgments, suggesting that age differences in illusory-correlation biases may be based in part on the declining ability to encode and retrieve veridical information from episodic memory. Such a conclusion is bolstered by other research that examined age differences in the ability to detect covariation between two events when there were no strong prior expectancies regarding contingencies between the events (Mutter & Pliske, 1996; Mutter & Williams, 2004). In this research, aging-related declines in the ability to accurately judge covariation were eliminated when performance was adjusted to take into account memory errors. Finally, age differences were greater when accurate performance depended upon construction of a rule rather than just retrieval of cue–outcome associations. Such findings suggest that some declines in judgments and decisions in later adulthood may be tied to age-related reductions in cognitive resources.

Other Decision Tasks that Require Deliberation

Consistent with this, older adults are less able than younger adults to control the impact of automatic processing on their judgments (Hess et al., 1998, 2000). Note, however, that Healey and Hasher (2009) argued that an inability to inhibit irrelevant information may sometimes produce better decisions when irrelevant information is remembered and later becomes relevant to the next decision. Compared with younger adults, older adults also may be less consciously aware of factors that influence their judgments and decisions (Lopatto et al., 1998). They are less accurate in estimating absolute numeric frequencies (Mutter & Goedert, 1997) and may be more overconfident in their judgments (Crawford & Stankov, 1996). In a recent study, Hansson et al. (2008) predicted and found that older age resulted in more overconfidence when reporting confidence through a confidence interval, but not when reporting confidence through a probability assessment (see similar probability results in Bruine de Bruin et al., 2007). Their prediction was based on a process model in which generating confidence intervals requires more working memory and executive processing capacity than probability estimation. These effects were, indeed, mediated by a general cognitive ability factor suggesting that the decreased executive processing capacity of the older adults was responsible for the greater overconfidence in the interval estimation task. In a similar manner, Bruine de Bruin et al. (2009) demonstrated that older adults show declines on specific decision-making tasks that involve fluid cognitive ability (e.g., resistance to framing, applying decision rules). The relation between age and performance on these tasks was mediated by fluid cognitive ability.

Research by Chen (2002, 2004; Chen & Blanchard-Fields, 2000) has also suggested that aging-related declines in deliberative processes negatively influence judgment processes. In these studies, participants were presented with information about an individual, some of which was identified as true and some as false (and thus to be ignored); then they were asked to make judgments based upon this information. Chen found that the judgments of older adults were more likely to be influenced by the false information than were those of younger adults. In addition, younger adults in a divided-attention condition performed similarly to older adults under full attention. These findings suggest that older adults may have more difficulty controlling attention and monitoring the accuracy of information in memory, which in turn makes judgments more prone to error based upon irrelevant information. In a related study, Skurnik et al. (2005) found that repeatedly identifying a (false) consumer claim as false assisted older adults short-term in remembering that it was false. Longer term, however, the repetition caused them to misremember it as true. A pragmatic implication of these studies is that information providers need to take care to not provide older adults with a "fact" and then state that it is a myth. This and similar tactics are surprisingly common (e.g., the U.S. Food and Drug Administration's "Facts about Generic Drugs" poses a question such as "Are brand-name drugs made in better factories than generic drugs?" and then answers "No.").

Evidence exists also that, when making decisions, older adults use less complex strategies and consider fewer pieces of information than younger adults do. In a series of studies, Johnson and colleagues (Johnson, 1990, 1993; Johnson & Drungle, 2000; Riggle & Johnson, 1996) examined decision-making strategies by different-aged adults using an information matrix that contained specific features (shown in rows) for different product choices (shown in columns). Participants were allowed to view only one cell of the matrix at a time, but they could view as many cells as they wished for as long as necessary before making a product decision. A relatively consistent finding in this research, across different types of products (e.g., cars, apartments, over-the-counter drugs), was that older adults spent a longer time studying each cell but sampled fewer pieces of information than did younger adults before making their decisions. Similar results were obtained by Streufert et al. (1990) in a study of decision making in managers, and by Hershey et al. (1990) in a financial-planning task.

Query Theory

A recent addition to the decision literature, Query Theory, may be extended at some point to account for some age differences in decision making due to memory declines. According to Query Theory (Johnson et al., 2007; Weber et al., 2007), questions that the decision maker asks him or herself during the decision process prompt the decision maker to serially reflect on specific memories about choice alternatives. The first query generally makes the strongest impression, due to a temporary decrease in the accessibility for other competing options (i.e., retrieval interference). Query Theory, for example, can account for endowment effects in the sense that buyers and sellers base their valuation on different queries. Buyers first consider why they might not enter into the transaction (resulting in more thoughts about why the good is not worth much), whereas sellers consider why they might enter the transaction first (resulting in value-increasing thoughts about the good). Such differential ordering of queries leads to disparities in object valuation. However, by simply switching the order of the query for one party, the endowment effect diminishes in younger adults (Johnson et al., 2007). Although not yet tested with older adults, one might expect older adults to show a greater effect of query order because they are less able to avoid retroactive interference (e.g., Hedden & Park, 2001) and show less ability in directed forgetting tasks (Zacks et al., 1996). Thus, Query Theory would predict that some decision effects, such as preferences for immediate rewards (time preference effects) and endowment effects, would be greater among older adults. Query Theory also points toward prescriptive solutions for undesired effects; simply directing decision makers to change the order of the queries they ask themselves appears to attenuate these effects.

Numeracy

Many choices that individuals make involve numeric information that generally requires deliberative capacity to process; comprehension and use of such information appears to decline with age. For example, results from health plan choice studies support these age declines in comprehension of numeric information and suggest that elderly decision makers do not always comprehend even fairly simple information. Hibbard et al. (2001) presented employed-aged adults (18–64 years old; $n = 239$) and older adults (65–94 years old; $n = 253$) with 33 decision tasks that involved interpretation of numbers from tables and graphs. In one task, participants were asked to identify the health insurance plan with the lowest copayment from a table that included four plans with information about monthly premiums and copayments. A comprehension index reflected the total number of errors made across the 33 tasks. The youngest participants (aged 18–35) averaged 8% errors; the oldest participants (aged 85–94) averaged 40% errors; the correlation between age and the number of errors was 0.31 ($p < 0.001$). Higher education was somewhat protective of these age declines. Age declines in numeric ability have been demonstrated across age cohorts as well as longitudinally (Peters, 2008; Reyna et al., 2009; Schaie & Zanjani, 2006). More research is needed to uncover age versus cohort differences in the wide range of abilities with numbers that could influence older adult decisions (e.g., reading tables and figures, addition/subtraction, understanding of risk including probabilities).

Less numerate individuals, whether young or old, do not necessarily perceive themselves as "at risk" in their lives due to limited skills; however, research shows that having inadequate numeric skills is associated with lower comprehension and use of numeric information. In particular, inadequate numeracy may be an important barrier to individuals' understanding and use of health, financial, and other risks. Further study is required to discover formats to provide numeric information that will facilitate processing even in less numerate older adults (Peters et al., 2007). Formats that highlight the affective meaning of numbers may be particularly appropriate for them (Peters et al., 2009).

Given the age-related declines in deliberative processes, it is not surprising that older adults may sometimes prefer less choice for themselves (Reed et al., 2008). For example, a majority of older adults feel that the current Medicare Prescription Drug Benefit is too complex and provides too many choices (Cummings et al., 2009). Hanoch et al. (2009) found that, indeed, older age was associated with more errors in choosing the best Medicare prescription drug plan. In another study by the same group, however, older age was not a significant predictor of decision-making performance in a task modeled after Medicare Part D, although numeracy and speed of processing did affect performance (Tanius et al., 2009).

In sum, the pattern of observed performance in these studies appears to be consistent with what might be expected with a decline in deliberative processes with aging. In fact, research has demonstrated that younger adults adopt a strategy similar to that observed in older adults when task demands are increased. It may be that information load interacting with limited cognitive resources in later adulthood results in the adoption of strategies that minimize demands on deliberative processes (e.g., eliminating alternatives, satisficing, etc.).

There are several findings from these studies, however, that might temper interpretation of the observed age differences in terms of declining resources. First is the observation that age differences in decision outcomes were not always observed in these studies. Thus, even though older adults tended to sample less information and to do so occasionally in a less systematic fashion than younger adults, the chosen option did not vary with age (e.g., Meyer et al., 1995). Second, it was also found that experience-based factors moderated searches. For example, in examining decisions about over-the-counter drugs, Johnson and Drungle (2000) found that older adults were more likely to focus on active ingredients than were younger adults and were also more systematic in their information searches, presumably reflecting their greater experience with using these drugs. Stephens and Johnson (2000) also found that older adults were more likely to focus on side effects and drug interactions than young adults. Such information is of obvious relevance to older adults, who are more likely than the young to be taking multiple prescription drugs at any one time.

SELECTIVITY AND MOTIVATED USE OF DELIBERATIVE PROCESSES

Older adults, in fact, also may adapt to real or perceived declines in cognitive resources by becoming increasingly selective about where they spend effort (Hess, 2000). They may be more careful than younger adults in how and when they allocate their more limited cognitive resources. According to Hess, this aging-related resource conservation should be most apparent in situations of low relevance or meaningfulness to the individual, with fewer age differences as relevance and meaningfulness increase.

In support of this hypothesis, Hess et al. (2005) examined the extent to which attitudes toward proposed legislation were influenced by irrelevant affective information (i.e., the likeability of the lawmaker proposing the legislation). When the personal relevance of the legislation was low, older adults exhibited attitudes that were consistent with how much they liked the lawmaker, whereas younger adults' attitudes were unaffected by this information. In contrast, when the legislation was rated high in personal relevance, neither the younger or older adults were influenced by the irrelevant affective information. Related findings were reported by Chen (2004), who observed that increasing personal accountability had a disproportionate benefit on older adults' source memory relative to the effects on younger adults' performance. Aging appears to be associated with increased selectivity in engagement of deliberative processes, with older adults' selective engagement dependent on the availability of and motivation to use limited cognitive resources. Situations may occur in which older adults are capable of completing cognitive tasks but lack the motivation to do so.

LIMITATIONS

The study of age-related changes in decision making is quite new, with only a smattering of different decision paradigms in use and at most a handful of studies in any one area. Thus, many opportunities exist for future research. Most published studies have also used only small samples of older and younger adults and some question exists as to whether they are adequately powered. Inconsistency of the comparison age groups also exists across studies. Although research is becoming increasingly sensitive to this issue, results may vary as a function of comparison group. Some research has used age groups as young as 18 years old, generally undergraduates, as a comparison group with a community sample of older individuals. All efforts should be made to collect data from a large spectrum of ages, if possible. A further complication of cross-sectional designs is, of course, cohort effects. The wider the age difference between groups, the greater potential exists for contamination of cohort effects. Individuals from different cohorts have grown up in different time periods, and each generation may possess a different perspective toward and expertise in approaching decisions. Although costly and time-intensive to conduct, use of accelerated longitudinal designs (Aber & McArdle, 1991) that enable researchers to study individual development over a longer interval of the life course by gathering data during a comparatively short interval of time would be ideal. Most important, such designs also allow one to separate developmental effects from cohort and period effects. Currently, however, even traditional longitudinal studies are the exception, rather than the rule.

SUMMARY AND CONCLUSIONS

Life-span theories are used fruitfully to provide predictions about age differences in judgment and decision making. Thus far, research to date has begun to attempt replications of well-known decision phenomenon examined initially in younger-adult studies with older-age samples (e.g., heuristics, risky choices, negativity biases). One of the main findings is that this literature is small but growing rapidly and offers sometimes opposing results. As a result, it also offers many opportunities for research that can illuminate both life-span and decision theories. In many areas of decision making, few, if any, published age-difference studies exist. In general, older adults appear to rely more on affective information when making judgments and decisions, and they appear to show a positivity effect at least in pre-choice information processing. Older adults' stereotypical less efficient judgment and decision-making processes are evident, but, among healthy older adults, such declines in decision making may be found mostly in unfamiliar situations devoid of affective significance to the decision maker.

Life-span theories also point toward phenomena in decision making that have been little studied. The role of arousal in decision making is one example. Based on dynamic integration theory, Wurm et al. (2004) proposed that age-related cognitive declines could be used to explain an age-related increase in the disruptive influence of emotionally arousing stimuli and thus increased attention to emotional content and other automated processes. In particular, they point toward arousal as the key mechanism, however, rather than valence (although they predict a positivity effect, their prediction is based on positive information being less arousing than negative information). Arousal has been little studied in decision making up to this point, but seems likely to be a key construct with respect to older-adult decision making in particular. Additional research is needed to clarify theoretical propositions linking affect, arousal, and cognitive resources in information processes important to decision making (e.g., memory, attention).

The use of processes other than arousal also might change across the life span (e.g., personality). For example, individual differences may moderate older adults' decision making in ways that are different from younger adults. Denburg et al. (2009) found that older adults who self-reported higher levels of experiencing negative emotional states also performed the most poorly on a decision task that involved learning about gains and losses, compared to older adults lower in negative emotionality. This finding contrasts with Peters and Slovic (2000) who found that younger adults high in negative emotionality learned more quickly to avoid losses in a similar decision task compared to those low in negative emotionality. Few decision studies exist examining age differences in the effects of individual-difference variables such as personality, gender, educational level, or ethnicity.

According to Hibbard and Peters (2003), making good decisions (which is what we want informed decision makers to do) requires information to be available, accurate, and timely. Information provided about Medicare Part D prescription plans, for example, meet this requirement. Decision makers also, however, must comprehend the information and comprehend the meaning of the information. The information provided about Part D plans, however, is not always understood (Hanoch et al., 2009). Beyond simple comprehension, individuals must be able to determine meaningful differences between options, weigh factors to match their needs and values, make trade-offs (e.g., between costs and benefits or pros and cons of a course of action), and ultimately choose. These steps are open to preference-construction processes. Given recent studies on the importance of cognitive and decision abilities to making good decisions about health (Peters et al., in press), these processes are important to understand.

Because older adults process information in ways that are different from younger adults, how they construct their preferences will also be different. These preference-construction processes may thus play a determining role in choices and undermine the notion of "informed choice" as aspects of the situation push individuals toward particular choices. The power of preference construction, however, can also be harnessed by understanding descriptively how decision makers make choices and normatively (or logically) what they should choose. Finally, one can examine the difference between the normative analysis and descriptive study to offer prescriptive interventions that help decision makers arrive at better choices. Applied to older adults' decisions, such an approach can recognize and describe the challenges that older people face and their successes in addressing them. It can also recognize that competence varies by individual and by decision, leading to domain-specific policies and interventions that "nudge" older adults toward better decisions (Sunstein & Thaler, 2003). Through an understanding of how older adults construct preferences in ways that differ from younger adults, researchers will begin to unlock some of the mysteries of decision making and will be able to begin to prescribe interventions that can improve decisions.

ACKNOWLEDGMENTS

Preparation of this chapter was supported by NSF Grants SES-0339204, SES-0922783, and SES-0820585. Portions of this paper are based on Peters, E., Hess, T.M., Västfjäll, D., & Auman, C. (2007). Adult age differences in dual information processes: Implications for the role of affective and deliberative processes in older adults' decision making. *Perspectives on Psychological Science, 2*(1), 1–23.

REFERENCES

Aber, M. S., & McArdle, J. J. (1991). Latent growth curve approaches to modeling the development of competence. In M. Chandler & M. Chapman (Eds.), *Criteria for competence: Controversies in conceptualization and assessment of children's abilities* (pp. 231–258). Hillsdale, NJ: Erlbaum.

Alhakami, A. S., & Slovic, P. (1994). A psychological study of the inverse relationship between perceived risk and perceived benefit. *Risk Analysis, 14*, 1085–1096.

Amieva, H., Phillips, L. H., & Della Sala, S. (2003). Behavioral dysexecutive symptoms in normal aging. *Brain and Cognition, 53*, 129–132.

Bechara, A. (2005, November). Neural basis of decision-making and implications for older adults. In National Research Council (Ed.), *Papers from the workshop on decision making by older adults*. Washington, DC: National Academy of Sciences. Retrieved June 14, 2007, from http://www7.nationalacademies.org/csbd/bechara_paper.pdf

Bennett, C. A. (2001). Evaluations and emotion: Influencing public health policy preferences via facial affect. *Dissertation Abstracts International, 62*(2-A), 375.

Blanchard-Fields, F., Chen, Y., & Norris, L. (1997). Everyday problem solving across the adult life span: Influence of domain specificity and cognitive appraisal. *Psychology and Aging, 12*, 684–693.

Blanchard-Fields, F., Jahnke, H., & Camp, C. (1995). Age differences in problem solving style: The role of emotional salience. *Psychology and Aging, 10*, 173–180.

Blanchard-Fields, F., Mienaltowski, A., & Seay, R. B. (2007). Age differences in everyday problem-solving effectiveness: Older adults select more effective strategies for interpersonal problems. *Journal of Gerontology: Psychological Sciences, 62*, P61–P64.

Brown, S. C., & Park, D. C. (2003). Theoretical models of cognitive aging and implications for translational research. *The Gerontologist, 43*, 57–67.

Bruine de Bruin, W., Parker, A. M., & Fischhoff, B. (2007). Individual differences in adult decision-making competence. *Journal of Personality and Social Psychology, 92*, 938–956.

Bruine de Bruin, W., Parker, A. M., & Fischhoff, B. (2009). Explaining adult age differences in decision-making competence. In F. Del Missier & W. Bruine de Bruin (Conveners), *Individual differences in decision making competence*. Symposium conducted at the meeting of the European Association for Decision Making, Rovereto, Italy.

Carstensen, L. L. (1993). Motivation for social contact across the life span: A theory of socioemotional selectivity. In J. E. Jacobs (Ed.), *Nebraska symposium on motivation: 1992, Developmental perspectives on motivation* (Vol. 40, pp. 209–254). Lincoln: University of Nebraska Press.

Carstensen, L. L. (2006). The influence of a sense of time on human development. *Science, 312*, 1913–1915.

Chen, Y. (2002). Unwanted beliefs: Age differences in beliefs of false information. *Aging, Neuropsychology, and Cognition, 9*, 217–228.

Chen, Y. (2004). Age differences in the correction of social judgments: Source monitoring and timing of accountability. *Aging, Neuropsychology, and Cognition, 11*, 58–67.

Chen, Y., & Blanchard-Fields, F. (2000). Unwanted thought: Age differences in the correction of social judgments. *Psychology and Aging, 15*, 475–482.

Chow, T. W., & Cummings, J. L. (2000). The amygdala and Alzheimer's disease. In J. P. Aggleton (Ed.), *The amygdala: A functional analysis* (pp. 656–680). New York: Oxford University Press.

Cohen, G. (1996). Memory and learning in normal aging. In R. T. Woods (Ed.), *Handbook of the clinical psychology of ageing* (pp. 43–58). Chichester, England: John Wiley & Sons.

Cornelius, S. W., & Caspi, A. (1987). Everyday problem solving in adulthood and old age. *Psychology, and Aging, 2*, 144–153.

Crawford, J. D., & Stankov, L. (1996). Age differences in the realism of confidence judgments: A calibration study using tests of fluid and crystallized intelligence. *Learning and Individual Differences, 8*, 83–103.

Cummings, J. R., Rice, T., & Hanoch, Y. (2009). Who thinks that part d is too complicated? Survey results on the Medicare prescription drug benefit. *Medical Care Research and Review, 66*, 97–115.

Damasio, A. R. (1994). *Descartes' error: Emotion, reason, and the human brain*. New York: Avon.

Dehaene, S. (1997). *The number sense: How the mind creates mathematics*. New York: Oxford University Press.

Denburg, N. L., Tranel, D., & Bechara, A. (2005). The ability to decide advantageously declines in some normal older persons. *Neuropsychologia, 43*, 1099–1106.

Denburg, N. L., Weller, J. A., Yamada, T. H., Shivapour, D. M., Kaup, A. R., LaLoggia, A., et al.

(2009). Poor decision making among older adults is related to elevated levels of neuroticism. *Annals of Behavioral Medicine, 37*, 164–172.

Dhar, R., & Wertenbroch, K. (2000). Consumer choice between hedonic and utilitarian goods. *Journal of Marketing Research, 27*, 60–71.

Dijksterhuis, A., Bos, M. W., Nordgren, L. F., & van Baaren, R. B. (2006). On making the right choice: The deliberation-without-attention effect. *Science, 311*, 1005–1007.

Dijksterhuis, A., & Nordgren, L. F. (2006). A theory of unconscious thought. *Perspectives on Psychological Science, 1*, 95–109.

Epstein, S. (1994). Integration of the cognitive and the psychodynamic unconscious. *American Psychologist, 49*, 709–724.

Epstein, R. M., & Peters, E. (2009). Beyond information: Exploring patients' preferences. *JAMA, 302*, 195–197.

Fein, G., McGillivray, S., & Finn, P. (2007). Older adults make less advantageous decisions than younger adults: Cognitive and psychological correlates. *Journal of the International Neuropsychological Society, 13*, 480–489.

Ferraro, F. R., King, B., Ronning, B., Pekarski, K., & Risam, J. (2003). Effects of induced emotional state on lexical processing in younger and older adults. *Journal of Psychology, 137*, 262–272.

Finucane, M. L., Slovic, P., Hibbard, J. H., Peters, E., Mertz, C. K., & MacGregor, D. G. (2002). Aging and decision-making competence: An analysis of comprehension and consistency skills in older versus younger adults considering health-plan options. *Journal of Behavioral Decision Making, 15*, 141–164.

Finucane, M. L., Alhakami, A., Slovic, P., & Johnson, S. M. (2000). The affect heuristic in judgments of risks and benefits. *Journal of Behavioral Decision Making, 13*, 1–17.

Fisk, A. D., & Rogers, W. A. (2000). Influence of training and experience on skill acquisition and maintenance in older adults. *Journal of Aging and Physical Activity, 8*, 373–378.

Fisk, J. E., & Warr, P. B. (1998). Associate learning and short-term forgetting as a function of age, perceptual speed, and central executive functioning. *Journals of Gerontology Series B: Psychological Sciences & Social Sciences, 2*, 112.

Forgas, J. P. (1995). Mood and judgment: The affect infusion model (AIM). *Psychological Bulletin, 117*, 39–66.

Fung, H. H., & Carstensen, L. L. (2003). Sending memorable messages to the old: Age differences in preferences and memory for emotionally meaningful advertisements. *Journal of Personality and Social Psychology, 85*, 163–178.

Good, C. D., Johnsrude, I. S., Ashburner, J., Henson, R. N. A., Friston, K. J., & Frackowiak, R. S. J. (2001). A voxel-based morphometric study of ageing in 465 normal adult human brains. *Neuroimage, 14*, 21–36.

Grady, C. L. (2000). Functional brain imaging and age-related changes in cognition. *Biological Psychology, 54*(1–3), 259–281.

Gregory, R., Lichtenstein, S., & Slovic, P. (1993). Valuing environmental resources: A constructive approach. *Journal of Risk and Uncertainty, 7*, 177–197.

Gross, J. J., Carstensen, L. L., Pasupathi, M., Tsai, J., Goetestam Skorpen, C., & Hsu, A. Y. C. (1997). Emotion and aging: Experience, expression, and control. *Psychology and Aging, 12*, 590–599.

Hammond, K. R. (1996). *Human judgment and social policy: Irreducible uncertainty, inevitable error, unavoidable injustice*. New York: Oxford University Press.

Hanoch, Y., Rice, T., Cummings, J., & Wood, S. (2009). How much choice is too much? The case of the Medicare prescription drug benefit. *Health Services Research, 44*, 1157–1168.

Hansson, P., Rönnlund, M., Juslin, P., & Nilsson, L. G. (2008). Adult age differences in the realism of confidence judgments: Overconfidence, format dependence, and cognitive predictors. *Psychology and Aging, 23*, 531–544.

Hasher, L., & Zacks, R. T. (1988). Working memory, comprehension, and aging: A review and a new view. In G. H. Bower (Ed.), *The psychology of learning and motivation: Advances in research and theory* (Vol. 22, pp. 193–225). San Diego: Academic Press.

Healey, M. K., & Hasher, L. (2009). Limitations to the deficit attenuation hypothesis: Aging and decision making. *Journal of Consumer Psychology, 19*, 17–22.

Hedden, T., & Park, D. (2001). Aging and interference in verbal working memory. *Psychology and Aging, 16*, 666–681.

Hershey, D. A., Walsh, D. A., Read, S. J., & Chulef, A. S. (1990). The effects of expertise on financial problem solving: Evidence for goal-directed, problem-solving scripts. *Organizational Behavior and Human Decision Processes, 46*, 77–101.

Hess, T. M. (2000). Aging-related constraints and adaptations in social information processing. In U. Von Hecker, S. Dutke, & G. Sedek (Eds.), *Generative mental processes and cognitive resources: Integrative research on adaptation and control* (pp. 129–155). Dordrecht: Kluwer.

Hess, T. M., Germain, C. M., Rosenberg, D. C., Leclerc, C. M., & Hodges, E. A. (2005). Aging-related selectivity and susceptibility to irrelevant affective information in the construction of attitudes. *Aging, Neuropsychology, and Cognition, 12*, 149–174.

Hess, T. M., McGee, K. A., Woodburn, S. M., & Bolstad, C. A. (1998). Age-related priming effects in social judgments. *Psychology and Aging, 13*, 127–137.

Hess, T. M., Pullen, S. M., & McGee, K. A. (1996). Acquisition of prototype-based information about social groups in adulthood. *Psychology and Aging, 11*, 179–190.

Hess, T. M., Waters, S. J., & Bolstad, C. A. (2000). Motivational and cognitive influences on affective priming in adulthood. *Journals of Gerontology Series B: Psychological Sciences and Social Sciences, 55*, 193–204.

Hibbard, J. H., & Peters, E. (2003). Supporting informed consumer health care decisions: Data presentation approaches that facilitate the use of information in choice. *Annual Review of Public Health, 24,* 413–433.

Hibbard, J. H., Slovic, P., Peters, E., Finucane, M. L., & Tusler, M. (2001). Is the informed-choice policy approach appropriate for Medicare beneficiaries? *Health Affairs, 20,* 199–203.

Holliday, S. G. (1988). Risky-choice behavior: A life-span analysis. *International Journal of Aging & Human Development, 27,* 25–33.

Johnson, E. J., Gächter, S., & Herrmann, A. (2006). *Exploring the nature of loss aversion* (Discussion Paper No. 2015). Retrieved from the Institute for the Study of Labor website: http://www.iza.org.

Johnson, E. J., Häubl, G., & Keinan, A. (2007). Aspects of endowment: A query theory of value construction. *Journal of Experimental Social Psychology: Learning, Memory and Cognition, 33,* 461–474.

Johnson, M. M. S. (1990). Age differences in decision making: A process methodology for examining strategic information processing. *Journals of Gerontology: Psychological Sciences, 45,* P75–P78.

Johnson, M. M. (1993). Thinking about strategies: During, before, and after making a decision. *Psychology and Aging, 8,* 231–241.

Johnson, M. M. S., & Drungle, S. C. (2000). Purchasing over-the-counter medications: The impact of age differences in information processing. *Experimental Aging Research, 26,* 245–261.

Kahneman, D. (2003). A perspective on judgment and choice: Mapping bounded rationality. *American Psychologist, 58,* 697–720.

Kahneman, D., & Tversky, A. (1979). Prospect theory: An analysis of decision under risk. *Econometrica, 47,* 263–291.

Kausler, D. H. (1990). Automaticity of encoding and episodic memory processes. In E. A. Lovelace (Ed.), *Aging and cognition: Mental processes, self-awareness, and interventions. Advances in psychology 72,* (pp. 29–67). Amsterdam: North-Holland.

Kennedy, K. M., Erickson, K. I., Rodrigue, K. M., Voss, M. W., Colcombe, S. J., Kramer, A. F., et al. (2008). Age-related differences in regional brain volumes: A comparison of optimized voxel-based morphometry to manual volumetry. *Neurobiology of aging,* doi:10.1016/j.neurobiolaging.2007.12.020.

Kensinger, E. A., Brierley, B., Medford, N., Growdon, J. H., & Corkin, S. (2002). Effects of normal aging and Alzheimer's disease on emotional memory. *Emotion, 2,* 118–134.

Kim, S., Goldstein, D., Hasher, L., & Zacks, R. T. (2005). Framing effects in younger and older adults. *Journals of Gerontology: Psychological Sciences, 60B,* 215–218.

Kim, S., & Hasher, L. (2005). The attraction effect in decision making: Superior performance by older adults. *Quarterly Journal of Experimental Psychology, 58A,* 120–133.

Kim, S., Healey, M. K., Goldstein, D., Hasher, L., & Wiprzycka, U. J. (2008). Age differences in choice satisfaction: A positivity effect in decision making. *Psychology and Aging, 23,* 33–38.

Knight, B. G., Maines, M. L., & Robinson, G. S. (2002). The effects of sad mood on memory in older adults: A test of the mood congruence effect. *Psychology and Aging, 17,* 653–661.

Knutson, B., Wimmer, G. E., Rick, S., Hollon, N. G., Prelec, D., & Loewenstein, G. (2008). Neural antecedents of the endowment effect. *Neuron, 58,* 814–822.

Kovalchik, S., Camerer, C. F., Grether, D. M., Plott, C. R., & Allman, J. M. (2005). Aging and decision making: A comparison between neurologically healthy elderly and young individuals. *Journal of Economic Behavior and Organization, 58,* 79–94.

Kruglanski, A. W., Chun, W. Y., Erb, H.-P., Pierro, A., Mannetti, L., & Spiegel, D. (2003). A parametric unimodel of human judgment: Integrating dual-process frameworks in social cognition from a single-mode perspective. In J. P. Forgas, K. D. Williams, & W. von Hippel (Eds.), *Social judgments: Implicit and explicit processes* (pp. 137–161). Cambridge, UK: Cambridge University Press.

Labouvie-Vief, G. (2003). Dynamic integration: Affect, cognition, and the self in adulthood. *Current Directions in Psychological Science, 12,* 201–206.

Labouvie-Vief, G. (2005). Self-with-other representations and the organization of the self. *Journal of Research in Personality, 39,* 185–205.

Lang, F. R., & Carstensen, L. L. (2002). Time counts: Future time perspective, goals, and social relationships. *Psychology and Aging, 17,* 125–139.

Lauriola, M., & Levin, I. P. (2001). Personality traits and risky decision-making in a controlled experimental task: An exploratory study. *Personality and Individual Differences, 31,* 215–226.

Lawton, M. P. (2001). Emotion in later life. *Current Directions in Psychological Science, 10,* 120–123.

Lee, T. M., Leung, A. W., Fox, P. T., Gao, J. H., & Chan, C. C. (2008). Age-related differences in neural activities during risk taking as revealed by functional MRI. *Social Cognitive and Affective Neuroscience, 3,* 7–15.

Lerner, J. S., Small, D. A., & Loewenstein, G. (2004). Heart strings and purse strings: Carryover effects of emotions on economic decisions. *Psychological Science, 15,* 337–341.

Levin, I. P., Schneider, S. L., & Gaeth, G. J. (1998). All frames are not created equal: A typology and critical analysis of framing effects. *Organizational Behavior & Human Decision Processes, 76,* 149–188.

Lichtenstein, S., & Slovic, P. (Eds.), (2006). *The construction of preference.* New York: Cambridge University Press.

Löckenhoff, C. E., & Carstensen, L. L. (2007). Aging, emotion, and health-related decision strategies: Motivational manipulations can reduce age differences. *Psychology and Aging, 22,* 134–146.

Löckenhoff, C. E., & Carstensen, L. L. (2008). Decision strategies in health care choices for self and others: Older but not younger adults make adjustments for the age of the decision target. *Journals of Gerontology: Psychological Sciences, 63*, P106–P109.

Loewenstein, G., Weber, E. U., Hsee, C. K., & Welch, E. S. (2001). Risk as feelings. *Psychological Bulletin, 127*, 267–286.

Lopatto, D. E., Ogier, S., Wickelgren, E. A., Gibbens, C., Smith, A., Sullivan, L., et al. (1998). Cautiousness, stereotypy, and variability in older and younger adults. *The Psychological Record, 48*, 571–589.

Luce, M. F. (2005). Decision making as coping. *Health Psychology, 24*, S23–S28.

MacPherson, S. E., Phillips, L. H., & Della Sala, S. (2002). Age, executive function, and social decision making: A dorsolateral prefrontal theory of cognitive aging. *Psychology and Aging, 17*, 598–609.

Mata, R., Schooler, L. J., & Rieskamp, J. (2007). The aging decision maker: Cognitive aging and the adaptive selection of decision strategies. *Psychology and Aging, 22*, 796–810.

Mata, R., Wilke, A., & Czienskowski, U. (2009). Cognitive aging and adaptive foraging behavior. *Journals of Gerontology: Psychological Sciences, 64*, 474–481.

Mather, M., & Johnson, M. K. (2000). Choice-supportive source monitoring: Do our decisions seem better to us as we age? *Psychology and Aging, 15*, 596–606.

Mather, M., & Knight, M. (2005). Goal-directed memory: The role of cognitive control in older adults' emotional memory. *Psychology and Aging, 20*, 554–570.

Mather, M., & Knight, M. R. (2006). Angry faces get noticed quickly: Threat detection is not impaired among older adults. *Journals of Gerontology: Psychological Sciences, 61*, P54–P57.

Mayhorn, C. B., Fisk, A. D., & Whittle, J. D. (2002). Decisions, decisions: Analysis of age, cohort, and time of testing on framing of risky decision options. *Human Factors, 44*, 515–521.

Mell, T., Heekeren, H. R., Marschner, A., Wartenburger, I., Villringer, A., & Reischies, F. M. (2005). Effect of aging on stimulus-reward association learning. *Neuropsychologia, 43*, 554–563.

Meyer, B. J. F., & Pollard, C. A. (2004). *Why do older adults make faster decisions about treatments for breast cancer?* Paper presented at the Cognitive Aging Conference, Atlanta, GA.

Meyer, B. J. F., Russo, C., & Talbot, A. (1995). Discourse comprehension and problem solving: Decisions about the treatment of breast cancer by women across the life span. *Psychology and Aging, 10*, 84–103.

Mikels, J. A., Larkin, G. R., Reuter-Lorenz, P. A., & Carstensen, L. L. (2005). Divergent trajectories in the aging mind: Changes in working memory for affective versus visual information with age. *Psychology and Aging, 20*, 542–553.

Mikels, J. A., & Reed, A. E. (2009). Monetary losses do not loom large in later life: Age differences in the framing effect. *Journals of Gerontology: Psychological Sciences, 64B*, 457–460.

Moscovitch, M., & Winocur, G. (1995). Frontal lobes, memory, and aging. *Annals of the New York Academy of Sciences, 769*, 119–150.

Murphy, S. T., & Zajonc, R. B. (1993). Affect, cognition, and awareness: Affective priming with optimal and suboptimal stimulus exposures. *Journal of Personality & Social Psychology, 64*, 723–739.

Mutter, S. A. (2000). Illusory correlation and group impression formation in young and older adults. *Journals of Gerontology: Psychological Sciences, 55*, P224–P237.

Mutter, S. A., & Goedert, K. M. (1997). Frequency discrimination vs. frequency estimation: Adult age differences and the effect of divided attention. *Journals of Gerontology Series B: Psychological Sciences & Social Sciences, 6*, 319.

Mutter, S. A., & Pliske, R. M. (1994). Aging and illusory correlation in judgments of co-occurrence. *Psychology and Aging, 9*, 53–63.

Mutter, S. A., & Pliske, R. M. (1996). Judging event covariation: Effects of age and memory demand. *Journals of Gerontology Series B: Psychological Sciences & Social Sciences, 2*, 70.

Mutter, S. A., & Williams, T. W. (2004). Aging and the detection of contingency in causal learning. *Psychology and Aging, 19*, 13–26.

Novak, D. L., & Mather, M. (2007). Aging and variety seeking. *Psychology and Aging, 22*, 728–737.

Osgood, C. E., Suci, G. J., & Tannenbaum, P. H. (1957). *The measurement of meaning*. Urbana: University of Illinois.

Pachur, T., Mata, R., & Schooler, L. J. (2009). Cognitive aging and the adaptive use of recognition in decision making. *Psychology and Aging, 24*, 901–915.

Paulos, J. A. (1988). *Innumeracy: Mathematical illiteracy and its consequences*. New York: Hill and Wang.

Payne, J. W., Bettman, J. R., & Schkade, D. A. (1999). Measuring constructed preferences: Towards a building code. *Journal of Risk and Uncertainty, 19*, 243–270.

Peters, E. (2006). The functions of affect in the construction of preferences. In S. Lichtenstein & P. Slovic (Eds.), *The construction of preference* (pp. 454–463). New York: Cambridge University Press.

Peters, E. (2008). Numeracy and the perception and communication of risk. In W. T. Tucker, S. Ferson, A. M. Finkel, & D. Slavin (Eds.), *Annals of the New York Academy of Sciences. Strategies for risk communication: Evolution, evidence, experience* (Vol. 1128, pp. 1–7). New York: The New York Academy of Sciences.

Peters, E., Baker, D., Dieckmann, N., Leon, J., & Collins, J. Explaining the education effect on health: A field study in Ghana. *Psychological Science*, in press.

Peters, E., Dieckmann, N., Västfjäll, D., Mertz, C. K., Slovic, P., & Hibbard, J. (2009). Bringing meaning to numbers: The impact of evaluative categories on decisions. *Journal of Experimental Psychology: Applied, 15*, 213–227.

Peters, E., Hibbard, J. H., Slovic, P., & Dieckmann, N. F. (2007). Numeracy skill and the communication, comprehension, and use of risk and benefit information. *Health Affairs, 26*, 741–748.

Peters, E., Lipkus, I. M., & Diefenbach, M. A. (2006).

The functions of affect in health communications and in the construction of health preferences. *Journal of Communication, 56*, S140–S162.

Peters, E., & Slovic, P. (2000). The springs of action: Affective and analytical information processing in choice. *Personality and Social Psychology Bulletin, 26*, 1465–1475.

Peters, E., & Slovic, P. (2007). Affective asynchrony and the measurement of the affective attitude component. *Cognition and Emotion, 21*, 300–329.

Peters, E., Slovic, P., & Gregory, R. (2003). The role of affect in the WTA/WTP disparity. *Journal of Behavioral Decision Making, 16*, 309–330.

Queen, T. L., & Hess, T. M. (2010). Age differences in the effects of conscious and unconscious thought in decision making. *Psychology and Aging, 25*, 251–261.

Raz, N., Lindenberger, U., Rodrigue, K. M., Kennedy, K. M., Head, D., Williamson, A., et al. (2005). Regional brain changes in aging healthy adults: General trends, individual differences and modifiers. *Cerebral Cortex, 15*, 1676–1689.

Read, D., & Read, N. L. (2004). Time discounting over the lifespan. *Organizational Behavior and Human Decision Processes, 94*, 22–32.

Reed, A. E., Mikels, J. A., & Simon, K. I. (2008). Older adults prefer less choice than young adults. *Psychology and Aging, 23*, 671–675.

Resnick, S. M., Dzung, L. P., Kraut, M. A., Zonderman, A. B., & Davatsikos, C. (2003). Longitudinal magnetic resonance imaging studies of older adults: A shrinking brain. *The Journal of Neuroscience*, 23, 3285–3301.

Reyna, V. F. (2004). How people make decisions that involve risk: A dual-processes approach. *Current Directions in Psychological Science, 13*, 60–66.

Reyna, V. F., Nelson, W., Han, P., & Dieckmann, N. F. (2009). How numeracy influences risk reduction and medical decision making. *Psychological Bulletin, 135*, 943–973.

Riggle, E. D. B., & Johnson, M. M. S. (1996). Age difference in political decision making: Strategies for evaluating political candidates. *Political Behavior, 18*, 99–118.

Rönnlund, M., Karlsson, E., Laggnäs, E., Larsson, L., & Lindström, T. (2005). Risky decision making across three arenas of choice: Are younger and older adults differently susceptible to framing effects? *The Journal of General Psychology, 132*, 81–92.

Salthouse, T. A. (1992). Why do adult age differences increase with task complexity? *Developmental Psychology, 28*, 905–918.

Salthouse, T. A. (1994). The nature of the influence of speed on adult age differences in cognition. *Developmental Psychology, 30*, 240–259.

Salthouse, T. A. (1996). The processing-speed theory of adult age differences in cognition. *Psychological Review, 103*, 403–428.

Salthouse, T. A., McGuthry, K. E., & Hambrick, D. Z. (1999). A framework for analyzing and interpreting differential aging patterns: Application to three measures of implicit learning. *Aging, Neuropsychology & Cognition, 6*, 1–18.

Schaie, K. W., & Zanjani, F. A. K. (2006). Intellectual development across adulthood. In C. Hoare (Ed.), *Handbook of adult development and learning* (pp. 99–122). New York: Oxford University Press.

Schwarz, N., & Clore, G. L. (1983). Mood, misattribution, and judgments of well-being: Information and directive functions of affective states. *Journal of Personality and Social Psychology, 45*, 513–523.

Shafir, E., Osherson, D. N., & Smith, E. E. (1993). The advantage model: A comparative theory of evaluation and choice under risk. *Organizational Behavior and Human Decision Processes, 55*, 325–378.

Shiv, B., & Fedorikhin, A. (1999). Heart and mind in conflict: Interplay of affect and cognition in consumer decision making. *Journal of Consumer Research, 26*, 278–282.

Skurnik, I., Yoon, C., Park, D. C., & Schwarz, N. (2005). How warnings about false claims become recommendations. *Journal of Consumer Research, 31*, 713–724.

Sloman, S. A. (1996). The empirical case for two systems of reasoning. *Psychological Bulletin, 119*, 3–22.

Slovic, P. (1995). The construction of preference. *American Psychologist, 50*, 364–371.

Smith, S. M., & Levin, I. (1997). Need for cognition and choice framing effects. *Journal of Behavioral Decision Making, 9*, 283–290.

Sozou, P. D., & Seymour, R. M. (2003). Augmented discounting: Interaction between aging and time-preference behavior. *Proceedings of the Royal Society of London B, 270*, 1047–1053.

Stanovich, K. E., & West, R. F. (2002). Individual differences in reasoning: Implications for the rationality debate? In T. Gilovich, D. W. Griffin, & D. Kahneman (Eds.), *Heuristics and biases: The psychology of intuitive judgment* (pp. 421–444). New York: Cambridge University Press.

Stephens, E. C., & Johnson, M. M. S. (2000). Dr. Mom and other influences on younger and older adults' OTC medication purchases. *Journal of Applied Gerontology, 19*, 441–459.

Strange, J. J., & Leung, C. C. (1999). How anecdotal accounts in news and in fiction can influence judgments of a social problem's urgency, causes, and cures. *Personality and Social Psychology Bulletin, 25*, 436–449.

Streufert, S., Pogash, R., Piasecki, M., & Post, G. M. (1990). Age and management team performance. *Psychology and Aging, 5*, 551–559.

Strough, J., Mehta, C. M., McFall, J. P., & Schuller, K. L. (2008). Are older adults less subject to the sunk-cost fallacy than younger adults? *Psychological Science, 19*, 650–652.

Sunstein, C. R., & Thaler, R. H. (2003). Libertarian paternalism is not an oxymoron. *The University of Chicago Law Review, 70*, 1159–1202.

Tanius, B. E., Wood, S., Hanoch, Y., & Rice, T. (2009). Aging and choice: Applications to Medicare Part D. *Judgment and Decision Making, 4*, 92–101.

Tentori, K., Osherson, D., Hasher, L., & May, C. (2001). Wisdom and aging: Irrational preferences in college students but not older adults. *Cognition, 81*, 87–96.

Thaler, R. H. (1980). Toward a positive theory of consumer choice. *Journal of Economic Behavior & Organization, 1*, 39–60.

Thornton, W. J. L., & Dumke, H. A. (2005). Age differences in everyday problem-solving and decision-making effectiveness: A meta-analytic review. *Psychology and Aging, 20*, 85–99.

Trostel, P. A., & Taylor, G. A. (2001). A theory of time preference. *Economic Inquiry, 39*, 379–395.

Tversky, A., & Kahneman, D. (1981). The framing of decisions and the psychology of choice. *Science, 211*, 453–458.

Weber, E. U., Shafir, S., & Blais, A.-R. (2004). Predicting risk sensitivity in humans and lower animals: Risk as variance or coefficient of variation. *Psychological Review, 111*, 430–445.

Weber, E. U., Johnson, E. J., Milch, K. F., Chang, H., Brodscholl, J. C., & Goldstein, D. G. (2007). Asymmetric discounting in intertemporal choice: A query-theory account. *Psychological Science, 18*, 516–523.

Weller, J. A., Levin, I. P., & Denburg, N. (2010). Trajectory of advantageous decision making for risky gains and losses from ages 5 to 85. *Journal of Behavioral Decision Making*, Advance online publication. Doi: 10.1002/bdm.690.

West, R. L. (1996). An application of prefrontal cortex function theory to cognitive aging. *Psychological Bulletin, 120*, 272–292.

Wilson, T. D., Dunn, D. S., Kraft, D., & Lisle, D. J. (1989). Introspection, attitude change, and attitude-behavior consistency: The disruptive effects of explaining why we feel the way we do. *Advances in Experimental Social Psychology, 22*, 287–343.

Wood, S., Busemeyer, J. R., Koling, A., Cox, C. R., & Davis, H. (2005). Older adults as adaptive decision makers: Evidence from the Iowa gambling task. *Psychology and Aging, 20*, 220–225.

Wurm, L. H., Labouvie-Vief, G., Aycock, J., Rebucal, K. A., & Koch, H. E. (2004). Performance in auditory and emotional Stroop tasks: A comparison of older and younger adults. *Psychology and Aging, 19*, 523–535.

Yoon, C., Cole, C. A., & Lee, M. P. (2009). Consumer decision making and aging: Current knowledge and future directions. *Journal of Consumer Psychology, 19*, 2–16.

Zacks, R. T., Radvansky, G., & Hasher, L. (1996). Studies of directed forgetting in older adults. *Journal of Experimental Psychology: Learning, Memory, and Cognition, 22*, 143–156.

Zamarian, L., Sinz, H., Bonatti, E., Gamboz, N., & Delazer, M. (2008). Normal aging affects decisions under ambiguity, but not decisions under risk. *Neuropsychology, 22*, 645–657.

Chapter | 10 |

Cognitive Interventions

Elizabeth A.L. Stine-Morrow, Chandramallika Basak

Beckman Institute, University of Illinois, Champaign, Illinois, USA

CHAPTER CONTENTS

Introduction and Scope of Review **153**
Varieties of Cognitive Interventions **154**
Practice and Retest Effects 154
Training Studies 155
Memory Training 155
Component-Specific Training 156
Training Core Capacities 157
Recap 159
Engagement and Lifestyle 159
Computer-Based Activities 160
Physical Exercise 160
Lifestyle Interventions 161
Recap 162
What We Know and the Hard Questions We Need to Ask **162**
What Outcomes do We Consider? 163
What is the Right Control? 163
Who Benefits from What Sort of Intervention? 163
What are the Mechanisms of (Long-Term) Effects? 164
What is the Optimal Timing in the Life Span for Cognitive Interventions of Different Sorts? 164
Conclusions **165**
References **165**

INTRODUCTION AND SCOPE OF REVIEW

As other chapters in this volume attest, there are wide individual differences in patterns of cognitive development through the adult life span. Successful cognitive aging along certain dimensions has been related to early life-span experiences, such as, education, as well as a variety of lifestyle factors from mid- and later life (Hauser, 2010; Stern, 2009; Verghese et al., 2003). Research findings in recent years from both animal models and on human learners converge clearly on the conclusion that there is plasticity in brain and behavior throughout the adult life span (Chapter 7, this volume). Faced with the pragmatic concerns for managing an aging society in which, for the first time in history, older adults will soon outnumber children (Kinsella & He, 2009) and individuals born in developed countries in the twenty-first century are as likely as not to reach their 100th birthday (Christensen et al., 2009), there is growing interest in developing a deep understanding of the principles of cognitive optimization that can be authentically applied in real social contexts. Such a research agenda serves both the practical function of informing the creation of evidence-based programs with potential to promote independence, social engagement, and continued participation in work and in civic institutions, as well as the scientific function of testing theories of cognitive aging.

Early investigations into the effects of cognitive interventions were often designed to use training as a way to test theories about the mechanisms underlying change from early to later adulthood, so that these studies directly compared the effects of training on younger and older adults. For example, the disuse hypothesis of cognitive aging, that age-related deficits are largely due to lack of practice of cognitive skills during later adulthood, would predict diminished age deficits on performance as a function of training. This test implication was rarely supported in the literature (Salthouse, 1991b), except perhaps in the case of specific age-associated production deficits (Hultsch, 1971). In fact, research examining age differences in performance as a function of extended practice

DOI: 10.1016/B978-0-12-380882-0.00010-3

(testing-the-limits) has shown that training interventions are actually likely to have a more positive effect for younger adults resulting in increased age differences (Baltes & Kliegl, 1992; Hertzog et al., 1996; Kliegl et al., 1989, 1990), a phenomenon providing strong evidence for an age-graded reduction in neural and behavioral plasticity (Baltes, 1997; Brehmer et al., 2007; Hertzog et al., 2008). In spite of this, there is every reason to believe that the plasticity that remains through adulthood in an absolute sense can be used to good advantage to increase cognitive potential. In fact, age differences in plasticity (defined as change within the testing-the-limits paradigm) vary as a function of the time available for the task and incipient pathology (Baltes et al., 1995; Kliegl et al., 1989, 1995). Older adults in good health may show relatively more capacity for change (Baltes et al., 1995). Thus, recent years have seen a plethora of research endeavors investigating the nature of interventions that are effective in enhancing cognition during the period of middle and late adulthood, and the extent to which these effects are moderated by other factors, with the ultimate goal to compress morbidity (Fries, 2006) into a period that is as short and as late in the life span as possible.

In the earlier *Handbook* chapter by Willis (2001) on behavioral interventions, she characterized this research area as in its adolescence, and anticipated the "growth spurts, mood swings, and unlimited horizons" (p. 102) consistent with this developmental phase. This prediction has been largely borne out over the ensuing decade, and a comprehensive review of the cognitive intervention literature is impossible within the current venue. We focus on behavioral interventions aimed at enhancing some facet of cognition, trying to give the reader a sense of "growth spurts" and "mood swings," but at best we can only send the reader in the general direction(s) of the "limitless horizons." We do not consider in any depth cognitive interventions involving drug or nutritional therapy (Annweiler et al., 2009; Edman & Monti, 2010). Nor do we systematically review the very large literature on interventions for late-life cognitive pathologies (Malone et al., 2007; Heyn et al., 2004). Rather, we set our sights on understanding principles of how the selection of activities and experiences in adulthood may alter the trajectory of cognitive aging. There are a number of recent sources that complement the current presentation in laying out the terrain. We refer the reader to Willis (2001) for an excellent treatment of methodological issues in the study of behavioral interventions in the elderly; to Hertzog et al. (2008) for a wide-ranging review of factors hypothesized to enrich cognitive development (see also Kramer et al., 2004); to Christiansen et al. (2008) for an excellent review of the cognitive reserve hypothesis, including the idea that education buffers against late-life declines in cognition; and to Lustig et al. (2009) for a thoughtful analysis of how behavioral and neuroimaging approaches can be integrated to develop theory-driven cognitive interventions.

Our review is organized into two parts. First, we consider different types of interventions that vary in the extent to which they involve direct exercise of target outcomes, from retest effects that are highly specific to target outcomes, to ability-specific training of different sorts, to lifestyle interventions that may only be tangentially related to measured outcomes. Second, we describe challenges for developing evidence-based principles of cognitive optimization that can be authentically translated into programs and social structures with potential to instantiate successful aging as a cultural norm.

VARIETIES OF COGNITIVE INTERVENTIONS

Practice and Retest Effects

Practice and retest effects are improvements in performance on a targeted outcome variable as a function of simply taking the test. Such a situation is devoid of instruction or adaptive feedback so that improvement depends on the development of skill or the discovery of strategies without explicit guidance or tutorial. From the standpoint of assessing the effects of training or changes in lifestyle (Salthouse, 2009) or comparative effectiveness of different interventions (Institute of Medicine, 2009), retest effects may be regarded as a nuisance factor. However, testing represents a very simple intervention with demonstrated effectiveness for near transfer to novel test items. Perhaps surprisingly older adults, even among the oldest old, show reliable improvement as a function of practice on tasks involving perceptual-motor speed, visual attention, and inductive reasoning (Yang et al., 2006, 2009). Interestingly, Yang and colleagues (2006, 2009) showed that while practice-related improvement did not depend on initial cognitive level for speed or attention tasks, the initially more able did improve more with practice on inductive reasoning problems. Fairly modest experience with testing (i.e., six hours over a three-week period) has been shown to produce retest effects that endure up to at least eight months (Yang & Krampe, 2009).

The power of retest effects is an important factor to consider in evaluating any other sort of intervention for a number of reasons. First, the effect size of the intervention needs to exceed that of the retest effect. The increasing use of growth modeling that entails multiple assessments to increase sensitivity to change (Bosworth & Hertzog, 2009; Hertzog & Nesselroade, 2003) can create a sort of catch-22: one might put in place a number of interim measurements between pre- and posttest to maximize sensitivity, but the effect of the intervention will need to be even that much more robust to compare favorably to the retest effects.

Training Studies

Gopher et al. (1989) have argued that practice may not be the best way to acquire skilled performance, since we are not necessarily "natural optimizers," and that training paradigms incorporating some guided strategies or action schemas, practice, and feedback are more likely to enhance trajectories of development. In training studies, adults are provided instruction in a particular skill, ability, or domain, as well as opportunities for practice and feedback. Such studies often have a high degree of control, enabling inferences about how training that is targeted to particular mechanisms impacts specific areas of performance. One important question here is the extent to which the targeted training generalizes to a new situation, or transfers across materials and contexts over time (Barnett & Ceci, 2002). Because age-graded declines in fluid abilities are normative, this was an early focus for cognitive training, showing clear effects of training (above and beyond retest effects) on inductive reasoning and visuospatial processing (Plemons et al., 1978; Willis & Nesselroade, 1990), with measurable improvement up to seven years post-training (Willis & Nesselroade, 1990). An important lesson from this early research was that gains were highly specific to the task without transfer to the factor level, thus mirroring effects described in the literature on expertise, a sort of "training in nature." Experts within a domain (e.g., leisure or job pursuits such as chess, bridge, or pilot performance) are ultimately able to perform well the skills they have always practiced (Ericsson & Charness, 1994; Morrow et al., 1994).

We divide our review of the training literature into three sections. We first consider training of memory, which has received much attention in part because it is the subject of frequent complaints among older adults. We then review studies that have focused on comparative training of specific cognitive skills or ability components. Finally, we examine studies that have trained what we call "core capacities," cognitive skills or resources that are hypothesized to broadly underpin specific cognitive skills.

Memory Training

A significant target outcome for cognitive training has been memory. Such training typically revolves around explicit instruction and practice with mnemonic strategies that engage organizational and elaborative processing during encoding, but can also include noncognitive interventions, such as relaxation or self-efficacy training, intended to increase the effectiveness of mnemonic training, or pre-training in a specific skill upon which the mnemonic strategy depends (e.g., practice with imagery and visualization before learning the pegword technique or method of loci). Early meta-analysis of the effects of episodic memory training on within-subject change in targeted memory performance by Verhaeghen et al. (1992) showed that older adults can benefit from memory training, with a mean effect size of 0.73, which was about twice the effect size shown by no-treatment control and placebo treatment groups. Verhaeghen et al. (1992) concluded that effects of memory training were greater for relatively younger adults, when pre-training was provided, and when training was provided in group settings relative to individual instruction, but the specific type of mnemonic used did not matter. Like early studies in ability-based training, memory training studies have generally shown effects that are tightly tied to the conditions of training (e.g., imagery-based training creates improvement in memory for concrete words but not abstract words (Stigdotter-Neely & Bäckman, 1995); older adults may find it difficult to implement trained strategies in everyday contexts (Brooks et al., 1993; see Rebok (2008) and Rebok et al. (2007) for reviews).

Recent approaches to investigating memory training emphasize the multifaceted nature of effective memory in adulthood that can depend not only on the use of skilled strategies during learning, but also attitudes and beliefs that engender persistence in learning and consistent use of these strategies. While early studies found minimal effects of explicit training in memory beliefs, such as self-efficacy (Best et al., 1992; Rebok & Balcerak, 1989), more recent studies suggest that there may be some value in augmentation of traditional memory approaches with some facet of the intervention that targets beliefs and expectations about the role of effort in learning and memory (Molden & Dweck, 2006). The Everyday Memory Clinic (EMC) program, developed by West and colleagues (Hastings & West, 2009; West et al., 2008) augments broad-based instruction in the cognitive skills underlying memory with tightly integrated training in self-efficacy. West et al. (2008) reported better performance in both name and text memory for the EMC training group relative to a wait-list control (training effects on list memory did not reach significance) after a four-week program, with gains maintained after three weeks of no contact. EMC training also improved self-efficacy at posttest and enhanced use of mnemonic strategies. Interestingly, training effects at posttest for list and text memory were larger among those with relatively higher baseline levels of self-efficacy. Because mastery experiences can contribute to a strong sense of self-efficacy (Bandura, 1989), skills in setting and monitoring progress toward goals have also been targeted for intervention (West et al., 2001, 2003, 2005, 2009; West & Thorn, 2001). Older adults may benefit more than young adults from feedback that highlights small but positive changes in improvement (West et al., 2005).

Like research on self-efficacy, approaches that target metacognitive skills also focus on the self-regulatory underpinnings of effective memory. Because older adults are sometimes found to not effectively monitor how well they have learned information (Miles & Stine-Morrow, 2004; Murphy et al., 1987) and to allocate less effort to learning than required for optimal performance (Dunlosky & Connor, 1997; Stine-Morrow et al., 2006), interventions focused on promoting monitoring of memory through self-testing have been investigated. Such metacognitive training has been found to produce training gains above and beyond strategy training under conditions in which participants can self-pace learning (even though training did not produce measureable effects in allocation of study time; Dunlosky et al., 2003; see also Murphy et al., 1987); however, these effects are not always observed, suggesting that more work is needed to isolate the factors that moderate the effectiveness of the self-testing approach (Dunlosky et al., 2007). Another angle on metacognitive training is promoting awareness of the utility of memory strategies. Cavallini et al. (in press) found that memory training in the form of imagery and generation practiced in the context of list and name learning produced transfer to a text learning task when participants were engaged in discussions about whether and how these strategies might be applied in other contexts.

Modality of memory training may also matter. Harkening back to the Verhaeghen et al. (1992) meta-analysis, some recent studies have found an advantage of memory training within a group context that can provide social support. Valentjin et al. (2006) compared the effects of group and individual training programs matched in instructional content (e.g., the nature of short- and long-term memory, normative vs. pathological age effects on memory, memory self-efficacy), and reported an advantage of group training over individual training in both objective and subjective measures of memory that was retained for at least four months. This advantage may have been due in part to the more extensive practice afforded by their group condition, however. In fact, in the Hastings and West (2009) study, in which instructional content and exercises were well-matched between training conditions, the benefits of group and individual training on memory performance were similar relative to a wait-list control group. The group training condition did show an advantage for memory self-efficacy beliefs. Hastings and West (2009) suggested that while both versions of the program provided mastery experiences without increasing anxiety, the social context of the group format offered better opportunities for vicarious success ("if she can do it, I can do it") as well as social support (e.g., verbal persuasion to continue exerting effort), and that these latter elements are important for development of self-efficacy beliefs, which may indirectly enhance memory (West et al., 2008). With the goal to enhance the capacity for dissemination, a number of studies have examined alternative venues such as a computer- or audiotape-based training. While off-the-shelf memory tapes may have limited utility, alternative venues for training have some potential (Rasmusson et al., 1999; Rebok et al., 1996, 2007).

It is important to keep in mind that there are very often individual differences in responsiveness of performance to memory training (e.g., Nyberg et al., 2003; Verhaeghen & Marcoen, 1996). Nyberg et al. (2003) used neuroimaging to show that older adults who did not benefit from method of loci training showed differential patterns of activation at encoding from those who did. Only older and younger adults who benefited from instruction showed activation of networks related to visual and spatial processing (left occipital and parietal areas). At the same time, even older adults who benefited from training did not benefit to the same extent; none of the older adults showed the increase in activation in executive control areas (left dorsal frontal areas) shown by the young. Nyberg et al. (2003) suggested that there are two sources of variability in processing that contributed to variability in performance among older adults: task-specific processing (reflected in occipitoparietal areas) and general processing capacity (more frontal). Similarly, Stine-Morrow et al. (2010) have shown that training in a conceptual integration strategy did not generally improve sentence memory, but that change in memory performance from pre- to posttest was correlated with change in the use of the strategy (as measured by increases in reading time allocation with increased conceptual load). Finally, Bagwell and West (2008) reported that individuals who actively participated in EMC sessions showed greater training gains in performance, and that participation itself was predicted by educational level and baseline levels of self-efficacy.

Collectively, research with memory training suggests that, contrary to perennial stereotypes about inevitable forgetfulness in old age, memory can be improved through intervention. Of course, even memory strategies of demonstrated effectiveness will only improve memory performance insofar as they are actually used. This research highlights the need to consider not only the need for instruction in strategic skills in memory, but also the factors that contribute to self-regulation of cognition, both in terms of motivational factors and accessibility.

Component-Specific Training

The benchmark for cognitive training research is the Advanced Cognitive Training for Independent and Vital Elderly (ACTIVE) trial (Ball et al., 2002; Jobe et al., 2001; Rebok, 2008; Willis et al., 2006). The ACTIVE trial was unique in directly comparing the effects of training on three different cognitive components thought to underlie everyday functional capacity (episodic memory, inductive reasoning, and visual speed of processing) in a multisite, randomized control trial with a large ($N = 2832$) and ethnically diverse (26% African American) sample. Intensity of training was held constant across the groups, with ten 60- to 75-min sessions devoted to strategy training and practice with laboratory exercises and everyday analogs (e.g., for reasoning, identifying serial patterns in an array of letter and patterns in a bus schedule). Booster training was offered to a randomly selected subset about one year later. Outcomes included measures of both performance (tasks of near-transfer very close to training exercises and transfer to everyday analogs) and self-reported functional capacity in each of the three domains immediately after initial training and at delays of one and two years. Importantly, effects of the interventions were evaluated using an intention-to-treat design in which posttest data are included regardless of whether the participants actually completed the intervention. Such an approach is drawn from the clinical literature in which the purpose is to draw conclusions about the effectiveness of treatment, taking into account noncompliance or inability to tolerate the treatment.

The core findings from the ACTIVE trial were clear. Training produced reliable improvement in proximal outcomes (0.26 SD for memory, 0.48 SD reasoning, and 1.46 SD for speed) that were highly specific to the domain (e.g., speed training improved visual processing speed but had no effect whatsoever on performance in reasoning or memory). Transfer to performance-based and self-reported everyday functioning was negligible up to two years post-training. For example, participants who received speed training did get faster at identifying targets in a visual field, but were no faster at looking up numbers in a phone book. Training effects faded somewhat over time but were still evident up to five years posttest (0.23 SD for memory, 0.26 SD reasoning, and 0.76 SD for speed). Those receiving booster training in reasoning and speed (but not memory) fared better in the proximal outcome measures than those who did not. Five years post-training only those who received training in reasoning reported improvement in instrumental activities of daily living (IADLs).

A thorny design problem in the study of cognitive interventions is the selection of the appropriate control group. As demonstrated in the memory training literature, motivational factors play an important role in cognition; to the extent that the control group differs from the experimental group in beliefs about their potential for improving performance, any difference in observed change might be to these expectancies, rather than or in addition to the presumed "active ingredient" in training. One of the elegant features of the ACTIVE trial was its parametric design, in which the experimental group for one intervention served as a control group for the others (Willis, 2001). The high degree of specificity of effects demonstrated given such a design suggests that generalized expectancy of doing well from training does not in itself play an important role in improving performance in the absence of component-specific training.

A number of recent follow-up reports have described effects of cognitive training in domains outside of cognition. Even though speed training did not impact IADLs, Wolinsky et al. (2006) have reported that two years post-training, it was speed training that reduced the probability of clinically significant declines in health (as measured by 0.5 SD decline on at least 4 of the 8 scales of the Health Related Quality of Life (HRQoL) scale, a self-report instrument, including assessments of frequency of physical and social activities, and perceived vitality and overall physical and mental health). Wolinsky et al. (2009) also reported that relative to the control, only speed training was protective against clinically significant increases in depression (as measured by a 0.5 SD increase threshold, the odds ratio was 0.67 for the speed group, but 0.71 and 0.87 for memory and reasoning groups, respectively).

As with memory training, other component-specific training shows variation in effectiveness among individuals. For example, more highly educated participants in the ACTIVE trial have been reported to show differential improvement on memory tasks that have a strong organizational requirement (Langbaum et al., 2009). Similarly, younger, more highly educated participants also may show stronger training effects on near-transfer measures in inductive reasoning, but also reduced transfer (McArdle & Prindle, 2008). Memory impairment at baseline may decrease training outcomes (Unverzagt et al., 2007, 2009).

Training Core Capacities

Some research has focused on developing a core skill that is hypothesized to be responsible for the wide range of cognitive deficits with aging (e.g., working memory, executive control, sensory discrimination), the key rationale is that the remediation of this core skill will have broad-based effects on the cognitive system (Buschkuehl et al., 2008; Kramer et al., 1999b; Smith et al., 2009). For example, the ability to sustain and effectively control attention is arguably a core capacity for a wide range of cognitive functions, such as memory and reasoning. Attentional control is required in the coordination and execution of complex sequences of action and thought. The more complex a task is, the larger the number of components it has, thus the greater the number of possible combinations of components it will take to behave flexibly and effectively in different contexts. Successful performance in such attentional tasks depends on the development of strategies that determine which combinations of processing components need to be selected in given situations, what aspects of performance can be emphasized, and which components can be integrated together. One might contrast three strategies for training such a complex performance. In *part-task* training, individual component processes are practiced as separate tasks and then after each is mastered, they are combined into the whole task. *Whole-task* training, by contrast, involves practicing task components in the context of the whole without initial mastery of the individual components in isolation. Whole-task training can be further distinguished into either *fixed priority* (FP) training, in which priority between the two tasks is fixed across trials (e.g., equal priority between the tasks), or *variable priority* (VP) training, in which the relative priority of components shifts unpredictably across blocks (Gopher et al., 1989). It is not the case that a complex task is simply the sum of its individual components (e.g., Damos & Wickens, 1980), but rather complex tasks involve coordination among components that can only be practiced in the context of the whole task.

Kramer et al. (1995) used an individualized adaptive approach to VP training, in which initial task difficulty was scaled to the individual, and training exercises were incremented in difficulty as skill increased. Participants were trained with a monitoring task and an alphabet arithmetic task (e.g., K−3 = ?; correct answer is H) both separately and together. Compared to those receiving FP training, both younger and older adults exposed to VP training improved more in dual-task conditions for alphabet arithmetic and in both single and dual task conditions for the monitoring task. Moreover, age differences in dual-task performance of alphabet arithmetic were reduced by VP training, but not by FP training. Both younger and older VP trainees, compared to those in the FP condition, also exhibited greater transfer to speed and accuracy in a running memory task (requiring working memory updating) and a scheduling task (requiring reasoning and attentional control) and to accuracy in a running memory task, particularly under dual task conditions. These results suggest that VP trainees learned a generalizable task coordination skill. VP trainees also showed larger long-term (six to eight weeks) retention effects (Kramer et al., 1999b). Such individualized adaptive feedback training in the dual-task paradigm has been found to reduce activation in ventral and dorsolateral prefrontal cortices that accompany improved skill acquisition (Erickson et al., 2007). It is notable that efficiency of neural networks has been related to intelligence (Neubauer & Fink, 2009).

Working memory, the capacity to store and manipulate information, has been linked to a wide range of intellectual functions such as reasoning and language comprehension (Daneman & Merikle, 1996; Kane et al., 2004), and typically shows age-related declines (Salthouse, 1991a). Thus the notion that a cognitive intervention aimed at increasing working memory capacity could broadly enhance cognitive function in late life is entirely plausible. Jaeggi et al. (2008) have demonstrated that adaptive training with an *n*-back task increases performance on a standardized measure of fluid ability (i.e., visual analogies, e.g., Raven's progressive matrices) among younger adults, and that greater training produced greater improvement in fluid ability (a dose-response effect) independent of initial ability. Buschkuehl et al. (2008) showed that even among 80 year olds, working memory could be improved through training, although transfer (to episodic memory performance) was limited.

Dahlin and colleagues (2008) showed that older adults, like younger adults, could benefit from extended practice in an updating task (i.e., from auditory sequence of letters, recall the last four letters presented). However, unlike younger adults, older adults showed no transfer to an *n*-back task (i.e., from a visual sequence of numbers report whether the current target appeared one-back, two-back, or three-back). Interestingly, patterns of brain activation at pretest (measured with fMRI) showed that among younger adults the updating task and *n*-back task produced similar patterns of activation in the left striatum (which is thought to serve a gate-keeping function for working memory) and frontoparietal regions; this pattern of overlap was also different from that produced by a Stroop control, which importantly, did not show effects of updating training. Older adults, by contrast, did not show the overlap in activation of the striatum during pretest. Dahlin et al. (2008), thus, argue that transfer of training depends on common neural systems required for target and transfer tasks, and that in this case, the lack of transfer among older adults may be due to deficiencies in striatal functioning. In other words, older adults learned to do the updating task, but did so without the activating the striatum; lack of transfer among the older group could be explained by the fact that the neural network needed for the *n*-back task was not exercised by the intervention. Another interesting facet of this study is that training effects were measured as selected increases in activation, in contrast to the Erickson et al. (2007) findings of neural efficiency described earlier. We return to this issue in our concluding comments (see also Lustig et al., 2009, for a thoughtful discussion of this issue).

An intervention developed by Mahncke and colleagues (2006; Smith et al., 2006) is predicated on the theory that age-related cognitive deficits have their roots in a reduced quality of neural information, in part, because of sensory loss (Lindenberger & Baltes, 1994). Their intervention has thus targeted sensory discrimination in which participants perform computer exercises requiring increasingly finer discriminations in auditory signal processing, requiring both speed and accuracy. As with the interventions involving VP training described earlier (Bherer et al., 2005; Erickson et al., 2007), their auditory discrimination intervention incorporates individualized adaptive training, such that exercises escalate in difficulty as competency increases. This intervention has been shown to improve both directly trained tasks and nearer transfer tasks (global auditory memory score) than active control or no contact control groups (Mahncke et al., 2006). Moreover, the training group showed long-term benefits (at a three-month follow-up) on digit span relative to the other two control groups. In a recent extension, Smith et al. (2009) showed that in a multisite randomized clinical trial, where both experimental and the active control groups received 40 hours of training, the experimental group improved more than the control group in multiple memory and attention tasks, including not just auditory but also verbal domain (e.g., backwards digit span, word list delayed recall, word list total score).

Finally, a core capacity that shows some promise for training is self-regulation, executive control, and the capacity for self-initiated processing (Berry et al., 2010; Craik & Jennings, 1992; Persson & Reuter-Lorenz, 2008; Stine-Morrow, 2007). In a memory training study, Lustig and Flegal (2008) randomly assigned older adults to learn a particular strategy for remembering (in this case, a sentence-integration strategy) or to a condition in which they were simply encouraged to use a strategy of their own choice. Transfer to a measure of executive function (Trails B) was observed only for strategy choice training. Lustig and Flegal (2008) interpreted their results as support for the idea that what adults were learning was proactive control, the self-initiation of cognitive strategies, which generalized more broadly than training any particular strategy.

Another example of training self-regulation as a core capacity can be found in the cognitive rehabilitation study from Stuss and colleagues (Craik et al., 2007; Levine et al., 2007; Stuss et al., 2007; Winocur et al., 2007), which involved multimodal training. Participants in the experimental group were provided training on three integrated modules, memory strategies (attention-related strategies that support encoding and retrieval of new information in memory), goal management (managing goal-directed behavior in everyday life), and psychosocial function (to promote well-being and confidence in using cognitive skills) for 12 weeks. Their goal of this constellation of modules was to train "'frontal lobe' strategic processes" (Stuss et al., 2007, p. 122). The training group, compared to the wait-list control, improved substantially on immediate and delayed recall of paragraph (logical stories test) as well as lists (secondary memory in Hopkins Verbal Learning Test). The training group also improved in a global measure of psychosocial well-being, as well on some measures of simulated real-life tasks such as overall goal management, goal engagement, task strategy, and monitoring behavior. The authors argue that the improvements in memory and goal management domains were primarily due to improvements in strategic processing. For example, training-related improvements in memory were observed in various organizational strategies, such as semantic clustering and subjective organization, and decreased reliance on nonoptimal strategies such as serial ordering. In goal management, they improved not only in overall score, but also on monitoring behavior and types of strategies involved in completing a task. Additionally, transfer of training to domains that were not trained, such as verbal fluency, improved. The late-training group (i.e., the wait-list control who participated in the program after the initial training group) also showed improved performance but to a lesser extent. The initial training group also showed better retention after a six-month delay. The investigators conclude that this multimodal strategic training can be effective, although expectancies associated with random assignment to a control group can impact program effectiveness.

Recap

Willis (2001) noted that the intervention literature to that point had focused on effects on proximal outcomes. Particularly with findings from the ACTIVE trial (Ball et al., 2002; Willis et al., 2006), evidence for the principle of training specificity to functionally proximal outcomes is especially strong when training is well controlled to focus on particular abilities: training in particular abilities improves performance in what is trained, and there is little evidence for transfer to functionally distal outcomes. At the same time, we also see that training has effects on temporally distant outcomes (Yang & Krampe, 2009; Willis et al., 2006). Questions about the nature of transfer and the conditions that optimize transfer are long-standing in psychology and education. Of course, transfer is possible (Barnett & Ceci, 2002; Zelinski, 2009). We return to this issue in our concluding comments.

Engagement and Lifestyle

There is now wide-ranging evidence for correlational relationships of engagement in mentally and socially stimulating activities with health, longevity, and cognitive vitality (Hultsch et al., 1999; Lennartsson & Silverstein, 2001; Scarmeas et al., 2001; Schooler & Mulatu, 2001; Shimamura et al., 1995; Stern, 2002; Stones et al., 1989; Wilson et al., 2002; but see Christiansen et al., 2001; Salthouse, 2006). The possibly broad effects of an engaged lifestyle stand in contrast to the highly specific effects observed in well-controlled training paradigms. This factor, together with suggestions from the training literature about the importance of the varying context of training, has prompted researchers to investigate the effects of lifestyle in experimental designs. The danger here is that such interventions typically entail less control in the manipulation, making it more difficult to isolate mechanisms of change. The focus of such approaches is typically to develop theory-based models of a cognitively stimulating lifestyle that are likely to be not only effective, but integrated into everyday activities. They typically capitalize on principles from more controlled studies in the design of translational models. For example, engagement exercises multiple abilities in a context in which priorities change dynamically, placing strong demands on self-regulatory skill. However, in this literature, specific mechanisms of action (e.g., ability-specific exercise, implicit VP training, interference control) are rarely, if ever, isolated. Thus, there are inevitable trade-offs between internal validity (causal mechanisms) and external validity (authenticity of life-embedded programming). The goals of such research are often to provide a framework for activities that might require a few weeks of instruction but be continued at home or in the community at a nominal cost or no cost to provide means and motivation for continued engagement by participants for years to come.

Computer-Based Activities

Engagement with videogames is one activity that uses multiple cognitive abilities, is often emotionally evocative, and is sometimes social (e.g., Wii, multiplayer videogames). A number of computer-based products purport to improve memory, attention, and processing speed (e.g., Big Brain Academy™, Brain Age™, BrainFitness™, PositScience™, and InSight™). Some of these products are marketed with broad transfer to daily life, such as reducing the risk of car accidents or improving the ability to balance a checkbook, albeit not necessarily supported by scientific data.

Although expert and novice videogame players do differ in basic attention and perceptual skills (Boot et al., 2008; Green & Bavelier, 2003, 2006), the evidence that training on videogames improves performance on untrained tasks is decidedly mixed. Training for few hours on action videogames, for as little as 10 hours (Green & Bavelier, 2003), younger adults improved perceptual and attentional skills (Frederickson & White, 1989; Green & Bavelier, 2003, 2006, 2007). Space Fortress is a videogame that is not available off-the-shelf, but rather was developed by cognitive psychologists to simulate a complex and dynamic operational environment as a research environment to study skill acquisition (Donchin, 1989). The player must simultaneously control a spaceship while both dodging enemy missiles and firing missiles to destroy a stationary enemy fortress located at the center of the screen (i.e., manual control). The player must also identify mines as those of a friend or foe by comparing its identifier with a set of three friendly letters memorized at the beginning of the game (i.e., a Sternberg memory search task). Finally, symbols are presented in a random order at a fixed location and the player must press a button when the target symbol occurs twice in succession (i.e., a one-back task with distractors). Training on Space Fortress improved performance of Israeli Air Force flight school cadets in learning flight control (Gopher, 1994), relative to a control group that practiced an off-the-shelf Apache Strike Force computer game. Yet, in a randomized intervention with novice videogamers, Boot et al. (2008) found that more than 20 hours of action video game practice in a relatively larger sample (20 adults in training group) provided no specific benefits across a wide battery of cognitive tasks even though the expert gamers outperformed the novices on many of these same tasks. The source of divergent data in the effects of videogame training on cognition is not clear, although it is possible that individual differences before training, such as brain structure (Basak et al., 2009; Erickson et al., in press), fluid intelligence, and initial gaming skills (Basak et al., 2008), could interact with skill acquisition and transfer.

Among older adults, who are typically novice game players because of generational differences, there have been but a few studies that have explored the effect of training in integrative, multimodal videogames on untrained cognitive skills. Training older adults on first-generation arcade-type video games (such as, Pac-Man, Donkey Kong, Super Tetris) improves response times, but not executive control processes (Clark et al., 1987; Dustman et al., 1992; Goldstein et al., 1997). For example, Goldstein et al. (1997) found that older adults who trained on Super Tetris for 25 hours improved in the Sternberg reaction time task, but not in Stroop Color Word Test (a measure of inhibition), more than non-gamers. However, more than 23 hours of training on a complex real-time strategy game, such as Rise of Nation, has recently been shown to improve higher level cognition (such as, task-switching, working memory, visual short-term memory, and reasoning, not perceptual or attentional skills), relative to retest controls (Basak et al., 2008). Moreover, improvements in measures of game performance predicted improvements in switching between tasks and objects in working memory, assessed by local switch cost in task-switching paradigm and focus switch cost in *n*-back task, respectively.

Physical Exercise

Epidemiological studies have shown that certain aspects of physical activity, such as peak pulmonary expiratory flow rate, walking distance, frequency, or speed (Albert et al., 1995; Weuve et al., 2004; Yaffe et al., 2001), can offset longitudinal declines in cognition in a healthy aging population. A few exercise intervention studies have been conducted to establish causation between physical activity and cognition, where participants are randomly assigned to the training or control group, with training lasting typically for a few months to a year (with occasionally longer intervals; see Rikli and Edwards (1991) for a three-year study). Blumenthal et al. (1991) conducted a randomized clinical trial over four months with an aerobic training group, a yoga training group, and a wait-list control group with multiple cognitive and psychiatric transfer tasks. Although the aerobic training group displayed improvement in peak VO_2, with the other two groups showing no improvement, they did not improve more in cognitive transfer tasks than the other two groups. On the other hand, Kramer and colleagues (Colcombe et al., 2004; Kramer et al., 1999a) found that after six months of training, the aerobic training group improved more than the toning control group in tasks of selective attention, task switching, and inhibition, all of which are functions that contribute to executive control (Miyake et al., 2000). Thus, some studies have found that aerobically trained individuals have outperformed nonaerobic control subjects on a variety of cognitive tasks (Colcombe et al., 2004; Hawkins et al., 1992; Kramer et al., 1999a; Rikli & Edwards, 1991), although others have failed to find such benefits (Blumenthal et al., 1991; Hill et al., 1993). Even though there are some discrepancies, in a meta-analysis, Colcombe and Kramer (2003) found that fitness intervention had broad and specific effects on cognition of healthy older adults; an overall moderate effect size (0.48) was obtained for fitness training with the largest benefits on executive control functions (effect size = 0.68) and the smallest on processing speed (effect size = 0.27). Also, effects were larger for programs that incorporated flexibility and strength training with aerobic activity showed greatest effects on cognition. Improved executive function has also been reported as a consequence of resistance training (Liu-Ambrose et al., 2010).

Biological changes seem to underlie this fitness-cognition relationship. Colcombe et al. (2006) found that in an exercise intervention study, the aerobic (walking) training group, compared to the toning control group, showed increased activity in the frontal and parietal regions of the brain that are thought to be involved in efficient attentional control and performance on the task used (a focused attention task), and reduced activity in the dorsal region of the anterior cingulate cortex, a region thought to be sensitive to behavioral conflict, or the need for increased cognitive control. The training group, compared to control, also showed a significant increase in gray matter volume in regions of the frontal and superior temporal lobe.

Lifestyle Interventions

Under the assumption that the optimization of cognitive vitality through adulthood will likely depend on effective functioning across a broad spectrum of psychological processes, a number of studies have attempted to intervene in lifestyle to enhance engagement. By their nature, these interventions are multimodal, involving some combination of cognitive, social, and physical activity. As noted earlier, isolating particular mechanisms of action is not typically the essential goal of this research. Rather, it serves the function of establishing models of application that exploit principles gleaned from more controlled studies. Such translational research, however, is not devoid of explanatory power. To the extent that such interventions change cognitive function in the absence of explicit ability-specific training, they may suggest "transfer" to a degree that would not be expected from laboratory training studies and perhaps challenge Gopher's view that we are not "natural optimizers." Amid a large, ever-expanding, and causally ambiguous literature showing an active lifestyle to be predictive of cognitive health and later mortality, such research also can lend somewhat stronger support to the "use it or lose it" notion, over the equally plausible explanation that "you just aren't going to use it when you are about to lose it."

There is some evidence that relatively small changes in lifestyle can have measureable effects on cognition. Small et al. (2006) have reported improvement in verbal fluency and reduced dorsolateral prefrontal activation (neural efficiency) after a 14-day lifestyle intervention involving memory training, brain-teasers, relaxation exercises, healthy diet (emphasizing fresh fruits and vegetables, low-glycemic carbohydrates, and omega-3 fats), and cardiovascular conditioning, relative to a toning and stretching control. A number of cognitive measures (e.g., verbal memory) showed no change as a function of the intervention, but even the subtle effects are interesting given the short-term nature of the intervention.

Some lifestyle interventions have involved a more serious commitment from participants. The Experience Corps project capitalizes on generativity motives in placing older adults into Baltimore elementary schools to fulfill meaningful roles in literacy development, library support, and behavior management (Fried et al., 1997, 2004; Rebok et al., 2007). Participants are primarily African American of low socioeconomic status and are paid a small stipend to first receive training and then to work in the schools for 15 hours per week. Relative to wait-list controls, Experience Corps participants report increased levels of physical activity and social contact and decreased the time spent watching television (Fried, 2004). They have also shown an increase in executive function as a result of engagement in the program (Carlson et al., 2008). The investigators attribute this enhancement in cognition to the day-to-day demands on executive processing and working memory as participants have to switch among roles in the program (e.g., filing books in the library with the Dewey decimal system one day, and working with children on reading exercises another), manage multiple perspectives in helping negotiate conflict resolution, and other problem solving in the context of an ordinary day in an elementary school.

Other programs capitalize on motives for achievement, socializing, and entertainment. Noice and Noice (2006, 2008; Noice et al., 1999, 2000) have focused on the memory skills developed among professional actors. Noice et al. (1999) reported improved word list memory among older adults participating in theatrical training using the Alexander ("active experiencing") technique involving relaxation exercises and training in concentration and sensory awareness; skills that engender effective performance. These senior actors were not explicitly trained in memory strategies, but rather worked through scenes of dialog with scripts in hand, blocking scenes with motions and gestures, and emotional expression appropriate to the larger causal structure of the narrative. Discourse memory does tend to decrease with age (Johnson, 2003), but older adults participating in this form of theatrical training learned extended passages of dialog to very high levels of accuracy. Importantly, the improvement from pre- to posttest on list memory demonstrates transfer. In a randomized experiment in which the theatrical intervention was compared to both a singing instruction intervention and a wait-list control, Noice and Noice (2008) showed that while both singing and acting increased scores on the Ryff measure of personal growth, acting (but not singing) improved performance on a wide array of cognitive measures, including immediate and delayed memory for word lists and text, verbal fluency, and problem solving. The investigators attribute the positive effects of their acting intervention on cognition in part to the embodied nature of theatrical training (Barsalou, 2008), which activates motor and emotional systems as an ordinary part of cognitive activity.

Another model of a community-based intervention is the Senior Odyssey project (Parisi et al., 2007; Stine-Morrow et al., 2007, 2008; Stine-Morrow & Parisi, to appear). Senior Odyssey is a program of team-based creative problem solving based on Odyssey of the Mind, a program that has been available to those affiliated with educational institutions for over 30 years (i.e., children through college-aged adults). Participants engage in weekly sessions of spontaneous problem solving (e.g., brain teasers and puzzles under conditions of competition that promote speeded responding) and over a period of several weeks work together in teams to develop a solution to a long-term problem, such as building a bridge out of balsa wood and glue that will hold as much weight as possible, or retelling the story of an historical event with an alternative ending, or developing a humorous performance about eccentric characters that solve a problem in the ecosystem. The long-term problem is open-ended so that solutions must be collaboratively developed, tested, and revised. While the spontaneous problems exercise component skills (e.g., reasoning, visuospatial processing, verbal fluency, divergent thinking), the completion of the long-term problem requires negotiation of long- and short-term goals and coordination of resources to achieve a product over the span of several months. The Odyssey season culminates in a tournament in which teams present their solution to a long-term problem and work together to solve a novel spontaneous problem. The tournament involves a public performance that is scored (using the same criteria as in the international program) and prizes are awarded, so that effort put into the program activities matter. Preliminary findings suggest that relative to a wait-list control, the Odyssey group shows modest improvement in a fluid ability (Stine-Morrow et al., 2008; see also Tranter and Koustall (2008) for evidence that practice with brain teasers improves working memory).

Recap

Collectively, such studies examining the effects of lifestyle interventions are promising in suggesting that engagement in ordinary activities in everyday life can promote cognitive vitality. They serve a scientific function in better establishing the causal direction of the correlation between cognitively stimulating activities and cognition (Hultsch et al., 1999; Schooler & Mulatu, 2001). They also offer an array of different models for "healthy lifestyle," so that there is potential for a "menu" of evidence-based programs to promote cognitive health. Such choice makes it more likely that individuals will find a healthy style of living to which they can adhere in the long run. Assuming that contemporary culture reduces the opportunities for intellectual engagement with aging (Riley & Riley, 2000), such lifestyle interventions also offer plausible models that may afford continued integration in enriching social institutions throughout the life span.

WHAT WE KNOW AND THE HARD QUESTIONS WE NEED TO ASK

It is abundantly clear at this point from literature in both cognitive neuroscience (Draganski et al., 2004; Maguire et al., 2000, 2003) and the behavioral data on ability training reviewed in this chapter, that mind and brain are well-suited to learn individual skills throughout the life span. The identification of principles governing how learning of particular skills with particular content in particular contexts transfers to related skills with novel content in novel situations is a long-standing problem in psychology and education. We will, of course, not be able to resolve this issue here, except to say that transfer surely exists, and that a resolution will ultimately depend on analysis of the multidimensional space of tasks, contexts, and learners (Ceci & Bennett, 2002; Mestre, 2005; Zelinski, 2009). It is an exciting time for cognitive intervention research with rich potential for transforming how we think about life span development and for yielding certain principles of transfer that feed into evidence-based educational programs that nurture cognitive vitality. At the same time, there is some distance to cover to reach these goals.

What Outcomes do We Consider?

The cognitive training literature over the last couple of decades has demonstrated quite clearly that improvement in specific tasks under certain conditions (e.g., episodic memory, certain reasoning tasks, working memory, speed) is quite possible through the life span. However, such skills in isolation are often not the ultimate goal of cognitive training. To the extent that the rationale is to compress morbidity to later points in the life span to maintain capacity above a functional floor, one might consider risk ratios for late-life pathology (e.g., Verghese et al., 2003) or IADLs (e.g., balancing a checkbook or preparing meals) that relate to independence as relevant outcomes. On the other hand, if the hypothesized intervention is geared toward slowing declines of work-related skills of different sorts, outcomes of interest may be more conventional cognitive processing (e.g., fluid ability, everyday problem solving, mental flexibility, or even work-specific skills). From the perspective of developing and maintaining human potential, relevant outcomes may also include dispositional measures such as well-being and self-efficacy, and capacities for creativity and productivity that enable satisfying work, play, and social relationships. Neuroimaging offers exciting new possibilities for measuring outcomes, such as selective growth in brain regions, and shifts in patterns of activation (e.g., Dahlin et al., 2008), that will ultimately inform issues about mechanism and principles of transfer. Entertaining questions about the appropriate outcome through which to assess the effectiveness of an intervention, one is forced to ask, "what is cognition for (at different points in the adult life span in different contexts)?" The research literature is somewhat past the point of demonstrating plasticity for the sake of plasticity. Hallmarks of adulthood include a more limited temporal horizon and more limited resources that must be selectively allocated for targeted optimization (Carstensen et al., 2008; Riediger et al., 2006). The particular functions or processes targeted by the cognitive intervention matter.

What is the Right Control?

Another perennial challenge of cognitive intervention research is the comparison against which effectiveness of the intervention is judged. Of course, individuals in the intervention group know that they are participating in cognitively enriching exercising and those in the control group (typically) know they are not. In the absence of a cognitive placebo condition (e.g., exposure to an "intelligence-stimulating light bulb"), one cannot rule out a contribution from expectancy effects. However, the high degree of specificity from training effects (e.g., ACTIVE trials) rules out an explanation in terms of some generalized belief that one is more cognitively able. Another tacky problem along these lines is the role of social context. On the one hand, social context of the treatment (e.g., trainer, other participants) might provide support for administering the cognitive intervention by providing instruction, and enhancing self-efficacy and perseverance in the cognitive exercises, without which the "dose" of cognitive training would be impossible to administer. The fear, of course, is that the operative mechanism of the cognitive training is simply the social context. The temptation is to include a social control group in which there is no obvious cognitive stimulation, but this is not a straightforward control since people are very often compelling stimuli for evoking cognitive engagement (sometimes in an emotionally satisfying way). There is no easy answer here, and the investigator needs to consider trade-offs in different designs and interpret outcomes in light of the design choices made.

Who Benefits from What Sort of Intervention?

The notion that different sorts of people benefit from different sorts of interventions (i.e., the aptitude by treatment interaction) has been in the psychological and education literature for some time, with surprisingly little empirical support to back it up (see Pashler et al. (2009) for a review). However, there is evidence that age differences in processing capacity can limit the effective use of strategies that are demanding on working memory resources (Luo et al., 2007). Recall that findings previously reviewed from the ACTIVE trial suggest that response to training may depend on initial capacities. This is a question worth pursuing. Given the different models of cognitive interventions emerging in the literature (e.g., traditional approaches, and translational approaches like home-based training, Margrett & Willis, 2006; computer-based activity, Basak et al., 2008; community-based volunteer programs, Carlson et al., 2008; Stine-Morrow et al., 2008) and the existing literature on how dispositions and interests shape cognitive engagement and the growth of crystallized abilities (Ackerman & Beier, 2006; Ackerman et al., 2001; Ackerman & Rolfhus, 1999), it is well worth exploring how individuals of particular constellations of cognitive strengths and dispositions select and benefit from different sorts of programs.

What are the Mechanisms of (Long-Term) Effects?

Ultimately, for interventions to be useful, we need to know why they work. What are the key components of the intervention that are operative and how do they affect the neural and psychological mechanisms underlying cognition? Mechanisms may be considered at different levels of analysis.

Research on mammalian brains, such as rodents, for the past four decades exploring effects of mental and physical activity in enriched environments (Nithianantharajah & Hannan, 2006) suggest biochemical and neural mechanisms underlying the effects of mental, social, and physical engagement on human cognition. Enrichment in the form of mental or physical stimulation, or both, induces brain-derived neurotrophic factor (BDNF) and nerve growth factor (Mohammed et al., 2002), vital for neural cell survival and proliferation and related to learning and memory. Mental or physical stimulation also augments synaptic plasticity (Artola et al., 2006; Vaynman et al., 2004), increases synaptogenesis (Farmer et al., 2004), and induces increase in neurogenesis in the adult and aged hippocampus (Kempermann, 2008; van Praag, 2005). BDNF also moderates the exercise effects on cognition and synaptic plasticity (Vaynman et al., 2004).

An important open question is how cognitive stimulation alters the functional architecture of the brain. Recent findings showing evidence for effects of interventions in both neural efficiency (Erickson et al., 2007) and in increased recruitment (Dahlin et al., 2008) are provocative. It is, of course, entirely plausible that efficiency in selected neural networks may enable engagement for other computations. This is an exciting area for further exploration. Neuroscience also offers a new window into transfer to suggest a "neural overlap implies functional overlap" principle (Lustig et al., 2009).

On the psychological level, we have considered a number of factors that contribute to cognitive benefits, including ability-specific exercise of different sorts, as well as exercise of more core capacities that have potential to build resources through which further ability-specific exercise is enabled. Two avenues of particular promise for promoting transfer are (a) training in multiple strategies under multiple conditions with shifting priorities (Kramer, Larish et al., 1999; Rebok et al., 2007; Swezy & Llaneras, 1997), and (b) training core capacities that depend on neural networks of broad relevance (Lustig et al., 2009). Another important question is what conditions promote self-regulatory skill in initiating and maintaining self-enhancing activity (Berry et al., 2010; Lustig & Flegal, 2008).

Finally, translational models of cognitive interventions in the context of social structures (e.g., Carlson et al., 2008) also raise questions about social and cultural mechanisms that will sustain activity in the long run. Another interesting question is how the infusion of older adults with active roles into child-centered venues shapes these institutions (Riley & Riley, 2000).

As Salthouse (2010) argues, any effects of intervention may or may not be due to the effects of remediating decline targeted by the intervention. For example, a memory intervention may improve cognition more broadly not because of the remediation of memory declines per se, but through indirect effects on the exercise of executive control or through the enhancement of self-efficacy or control beliefs that improve persistence. Salthouse (in press) recommended three strategies that can contribute to understanding mechanisms. One is, as discussed previously, comparison with appropriate controls. Another is to directly relate the effect of the intervention on cognition with change in some outcome directly related to the intervention (e.g., for a physical exercise intervention, change in VO_2 max correlated with improved cognition). A third approach is to relate effects on outcome (and mediating) variables with the dose of the intervention.

The intent-to-treat approach to analysis has the advantage of estimating effects of an intervention in the contexts in which they may be implemented (Lachin, 2000); for example, assuming that some proportion of experimental participants will not tolerate it and/or that some segment of the control group will initiate changes independently. This research model derives from a medical model in which the core concern is to develop effective treatments from a public health standpoint in which the economics of cost and benefits of treatment need to be weighed to maximize the public welfare. Such application of psychological theory to solve problems related to public health is important, as is the integration of "use-inspired science" into fabric of theory development (Stokes, 1997). It is critical that as psychologists enter in greater numbers into the arena of public health research that we do not lose sight of the need for explanatory models. Augmenting the intent-to-treat approach with analysis of dose-response relationships and mediating effects can contribute complementary information about mechanisms of effect. Of course, caution is needed in interpreting findings when there is selective subject loss across groups, but the role of program adherence in engendering change is central to understanding mechanisms of change.

What is the Optimal Timing in the Life Span for Cognitive Interventions of Different Sorts?

Neuroprotective effects of childhood and midlife education have been reported, suggesting that intellectual stimulation earlier in the life span engenders richer neural networks that can better withstand assaults later (hence, the term "cognitive reserve"; Richards & Sacker,

2003; Scarmeas & Stern, 2003; Stern, 2002, 2009). Not all facets of the cognitive reserve hypothesis enjoy equal empirical support (Christiansen et al., 2008). Theoretical development and methodological innovation are needed to define the nature of cognitive optimization at different points in the life span.

CONCLUSIONS

It is an historical and cultural oddity that we "educate" (derived from the Latin *educare* meaning to "draw out") children but provide "cognitive interventions" (implying remediation of deficits) for older adults. Our literature review suggests that a high level of mental fitness is possible longer into the life span than is often believed, but that it may depend on the coordinated enhancement of physical fitness, intellectual stimulation, and strong social networks. Educational models that are restricted to drawing out potential early in the life span do not serve us well (Riley & Riley, 2000), prompting the call for a multidisciplinary approach ("from cortex to community") to defining a life-span approach to education.

REFERENCES

Ackerman, P. L., & Beier, M. E. (2006). Determinants of domain knowledge and independent study learning in an adult sample. *Journal of Educational Psychology, 98*, 366–381.

Ackerman, P. L., Bowen, K. R., Beier, M. E., & Kanfer, R. (2001). Determinants of individual differences and gender differences in knowledge. *Journal of Educational Psychology, 93*, 797–825.

Ackerman, P. L., & Rolfhus, E. L. (1999). The locus of adult intelligence: Knowledge, abilities, and nonability traits. *Psychology and Aging, 14*, 314–330.

Albert, M. S., Jones, K., Savage, C. R., Berkman, L., Seeman, T., Blazer, D., et al. (1995). Predictors of cognitive change in older persons: MacArthur studies of successful aging. *Psychology and Aging, 10*, 578–589.

Annweiler, C., Allali, G., Allain, P., Bridenbaugh, S., Schott, A.-M., Kressig, R. W., et al. (2009). Vitamin D and cognitive performance in adults: A systematic review. *European Journal of Neurology, 16*, 1083–1089.

Artola, A., von Frijtag, J. C., Fermont, P. C. J., Gispen, W. H., Schrama, L. H., Kamal, A., et al. (2006). Long-lasting modulation of the induction of LTD and LTP in rat hippocampal CA1 by behavioural stress and environmental enrichment. *The European Journal of Neuroscience, 23*(1), 261–272.

Bagwell, D. K., & West, R. L. (2008). Assessing compliance: Active versus inactive trainees in a memory intervention. *Clinical Interventions in Aging, 3*, 371–382.

Ball, K., Berch, D. B., Helmers, K. F., Jobe, J. B., Leveck, M. D., Marsiske, M., et al. (2002). Effects of cognitive training interventions with older adults. *Journal of the American Medical Association, 288*, 2271–2281.

Baltes, P. B. (1997). On the incomplete architecture of human ontogeny: Selection, optimization, and compensation as foundation of developmental theory. *American Psychologist, 52*, 366–380.

Baltes, P. B., & Kliegl, R. (1992). Further testing of limits of cognitive plasticity: Negative age differences in a mnemonic skill are robust. *Developmental Psychology, 28*, 121–125.

Baltes, M. M., Kühl, K.-P., Gutzmann, H., & Sowarka, D. (1995). Potential of cognitive plasticity as a diagnostic instrument: A cross-validation study. *Psychology and Aging, 10*, 167–172.

Bandura, A. (1989). Human agency in social cognitive theory. *American Psychologist, 44*, 1175–1184.

Barnett, S. M., & Ceci, S. J. (2002). When and where do we apply what we learn? A taxonomy for far transfer. *Psychological Bulletin, 128*, 612–637.

Barsalou, L. W. (2008). Grounded cognition. *Annual Review of Psychology, 59*, 617–645.

Basak, C., Voss, M. W., Erickson, K. I., Boot, W. R., Kramer A. F. Regional differences in brain volume predict the acquisition of skill in a complex real-time strategy videogame, submitted.

Basak, C., Boot, W. R., Voss, M. W., & Kramer, A. F. (2008). Can training in a real-time strategy videogame attenuate cognitive decline in older adults? *Psychology and Aging, 23*, 765–777.

Basak, C., Voss, M. W., Boot, W. R., Erickson, K. I., Kramer, A. F. (July 2007). Can older adults benefit from videogame training? Relationship among cognition, game performance and brain structure. *Plenary Session 6: Training: 20th Cognitive Aging Conference–Down Under*, Adelaide, Australia.

Basak, C., Boot, W. R., Neider, M., Simons, D. J., Fabiani, M., Gratton, G., et al., (November 2009). Prioritizing subcomponents of the Space Fortress game enhances learning and engenders transfer. *Poster presented at the 2009 Annual Meeting of the Psychonomic Society*, Boston.

Berry, J. M., Hastings, E., West, R. L., Lee, C., & Cavanaugh, J. C. (2010). Memory aging: Deficits, beliefs, and interventions. In J. C. Cavanaugh & C. K. Cavanaugh (Eds.), *Aging in America* (Vol. 1. Psychological aspects, pp. 255–299). Denver, CO: Praeger.

Best, D. L., Hamlett, K. W., & Davis, S. W. (1992). Memory complaint and memory performance in the elderly: The effects of memory-skills training and expectancy change. *Applied*

Cognitive Psychology, 6, 405–416.

Bherer, L., Kramer, A. F., Peterson, J. S., Colcombe, S. J., Erickson, K., & Becic, E. (2005). Training effects on dual-task performance: Are there age-related differences in plasticity of attentional control? *Psychology and Aging, 20,* 695–709.

Blumenthal, J. A., Emery, C. F., Madden, D. J., Schniebolk, S., Walsh-Riddle, M., George, L. K., et al. (1991). Long-term effects of exercise on psychological functioning in older men and women. *Journals of Gerontology: Psychological Sciences, 46,* 352–361.

Boot, W. R., Basak, C., Erickson, K. I., Neider, M., Simons, D. J., Fabiani, M., et al. Strategy, Individual Differences, and Transfer of Training in the Acquisition of Skilled Space Fortress Performance, submitted.

Boot, W. R., Kramer, A. F., Simons, D. J., Fabiani, M., & Gratton, G. (2008). The effects of video game playing on attention, memory, and executive control. *Acta Psychologica, 129,* 387–398.

Bosworth, H. B., & Hertzog, C. (Eds.), (2009). *Aging and cognition: Research methodologies and empirical advances.* Washington, DC: American Psychological Association.

Brehmer, Y., Li, S.-C., Müller, V., von Oertzen, T., & Lindenberger, U. (2007). Memory plasticity across the life span: Uncovering children's latent potential. *Developmental Psychology, 43,* 465–478.

Brehmer, Y., Li, S.-C., Straube, B., Stoll, G., von Oertzen, T., Müller, V., et al. (2008). Comparing memory skill maintenance across the life span: Preservation in adults, increase in children. *Psychology and Aging, 23,* 227–238.

Brooks, J. O., Friedman, L., & Yesavage, J. A. (1993). A study of the problems older adults encounter when using a mnemonic technique. *International Psychogeriatrics, 5,* 57–65.

Buschkuehl, M., Jaeggi, S. M., Hutchison, S., Däpp, C., Breil, F., Perrig, W. J., et al. (2008). Impact of working memory training on memory performance in old-old adults. *Psychology and Aging, 23,* 743–753.

Carlson, M. C., Saczynski, J. S., Rebok, G. W., Seeman, T., Glass, T. A., McGill, S., et al. (2008). Exploring the effects of an "everyday" activity program on executive function and memory in older adults: Experience Corps®. *The Gerontologist, 48,* 793–801.

Carstensen, L. L., Mikels, J. A., & Mather, M. (2006). Aging and the intersection of cognition, motivation, and emotion. In J. E. Birren & K. W. Schaie (Eds.), *Handbook of the psychology of aging* (6th ed., pp. 343–362). New York: Academic Press.

Cavallini, E., Dunlosky, J., Bottiroli, S., Hertzog, C., & Vecchi, T. Promoting transfer in memory training for older adults. *Aging, Clinical, and Experimental Research,* in press.

Christensen, K., Doblhammer, G., Rau, R., & Vaupel, J. W. (2009). Ageing populations: The challenges ahead. *The Lancet, 374,* 1196–1208.

Christensen, H., Anstey, K. J., Leach, L. S., & Mackinnon, A. J. (2008). *Intelligence, education, and the brain reserve hypothesis. The handbook of aging and cognition* (3rd ed., pp. 133–188). New York: Psychology Press.

Christensen, H., Hofer, S. M., Mackinnon, A. J., Korten, A. E., Jorm, A. F., & Henderson, A. S. (2001). Age is no kinder to the better educated: Absence of an association investigated using latent growth techniques in a community sample. *Psychological Medicine, 31,* 15–28.

Clark, J. E., Lanphear, A. K., & Riddick, C. C. (1987). The effects of videogame playing on the response selection processing of elderly adults. *Journals of Gerontology, 42,* 82–85.

Colcombe, S. J., Erickson, K. I., Scalf, P. E., Kim, J. S., Prakash, R., McAuley, E., et al. (2006). Aerobic exercise training increases brain volume in aging humans. *Journals of Gerontology: Medical Sciences, 61,* 1166–1170.

Colcombe, S. J., & Kramer, A. F. (2003). Fitness effects on the cognitive function of older adults: A meta-analytic study. *Psychological Science, 14,* 125–130.

Colcombe, S. J., Kramer, A. F., Erickson, K. I., Scalf, P., McAuley, E., Cohen, N. J., et al. (2004). Cardiovascular fitness, cortical plasticity, and aging. *Proceedings of the National Academy of Science USA, 101,* 3316–3321.

Craik, F. I. M., & Jennings, J. M. (1992). Human memory. In F. I. M. Craik & T. A. Salthouse (Eds.), *The handbook of aging and cognition* (pp. 51–110). Hillsdale, NJ: Erlbaum.

Craik, F. I. M., Winocur, G., Palmer, H., Binns, M. A., Edwards, M., Bridges, K., et al. (2007). Cognitive rehabilitation in the elderly: Effects on memory. *Journal of the International Neuropsychological Society, 13,* 132–142.

Dahlin, E., Neely, A. S., Larsson, A., Bäckman, L., & Nyberg, L. (2008). Transfer of learning after updating training mediated by the striatum. *Science, 320,* 1510–1512.

Damos, D. L., & Wickens, C. D. (1980). The identification and transfer of timesharing skills. *Acta Psychologica, 46,* 15–39.

Daneman, M., & Merikle, P. M. (1996). Working memory and language comprehension: A meta-analysis. *Psychonomic Bulletin and Review, 3,* 422–433.

Donchin, E. (1989). The Learning Strategies Project. *Acta Psychologica, 71,* 1–15.

Draganski, B., Gaser, C., Busch, V., Schuierer, G., Bogdahn, U., & May, A. (2004). Changes in grey matter induced by training. *Nature, 427,* 311–312.

Dunlosky, J., Cavallini, E., Roth, H., McGuire, C. L., Vecchi, T., & Hertzog, C. (2007). Do self-monitoring interventions improve older adult learning? *Journals of Gerontology: Psychological Sciences, 62B,* 70–76.

Dunlosky, J., & Connor, L. T. (1997). Age differences in the allocation of study time account for age differences in memory performance. *Memory & Cognition, 25,* 691–700.

Dunlosky, J., Kubat-Silman, A. K., & Hertzog, C. (2003). Training monitoring skills improves older adults' self-paced associative learning. *Psychology and Aging, 18*, 340–345.

Dustman, R. E., Emmerson, R. Y., Steinhaus, L. A., Shearer, D. E., & Dustman, T. J. (1992). The effects of videogame playing on neuropsychological performance of elderly individuals. *Journals of Gerontology, 47*, 168–171.

Edman, J. S., & Monti, D. A. (2010). The use of nutritional supplements in psychiatric practice. In D. A. Monti & B. A. Beitman (Eds.), *Integrative psychiatry* (pp. 35–59). New York: Oxford University Press.

Erickson K. I, Boot W. R, Basak C, Neider, M, Prakash R. S, Voss M. W, et al. Is bigger better? Striatum volume predicts the level of video game skill acquisition. *Cerebral Cortex* (in press).

Erickson, K. I., Colcombe, S. J., Wadhwa, R., Bherer, L., Peterson, M. S., Scalf, P. E., et al. (2007). Training induced functional activation changes in dual-task processing: An fMRI study. *Cerebral Cortex, 17*, 192–204.

Ericsson, K. A., & Charness, N. (1994). Expert performance: Its structure and acquisition. *American Psychologist, 49*, 725–747.

Farmer, J., Zhao, X., van Praag, H., Wodtke, K., Gage, F. H., & Christie, B. R. (2004). Effects of voluntary exercise on synaptic plasticity and gene expression in the dentate gyrus of adult male sprague-dawley rats in vivo. *Neuroscience, 124*, 71–79.

Frederickson, J. R., & White, B. Y. (1989). An approach to training based on principled task decomposition. *Acta Psychologica, 71*, 89–146.

Fried, L. P., Carlson, M. C., Freedman, M., Frick, K. D., Glass, T. A., Hill, J., et al. (2004). A social model for health promotion for an aging population: Initial evidence on the Experience Corps model. *Journal of Urban Health: Bulletin of the New York Academy of Medicine, 81*, 64–78.

Fried, L. P., Freedman, M., Endres, T. E., & Wasik, B. (1997). Building communities that promote successful aging. *The Western Journal of Medicine, 167*, 216–219.

Fries, J. F. (2006). Compression of morbidity. In R. Schulz (Ed.), *The encyclopedia of aging* (Vol. 4, pp. 257–259). New York: Springer Publishing Company.

Goldstein, J., Cajko, L., Oosterbroek, M., Michielsen, M., Van Houten, O., & Salvedera, F. (1997). Videogames and the elderly. *Social Behavior and Personality, 25*, 345–352.

Gopher, D., Weil, M., & Bereket, Y. (1994). Transfer of skill from a computer game trainer to flight. *Human Factors, 36*(3), 387–405.

Gopher, D., Weil, M., & Siegel, D. (1989). Practice under changing priorities: An approach to the training of complex skills. *Acta Psychologica, 71*, 147–177.

Green, C. S., & Bavelier, D. (2003). Action videogame modifies visual selective attention. *Nature, 423*, 534–537.

Green, C. S., & Bavelier, D. (2006). Enumeration versus multiple object tracking: The case of action video game players. *Cognition, 101*, 217–245.

Green, C. S., & Bavelier, D. (2007). Action video game experience alters the spatial resolution of attention. *Psychological Science, 18*(1), 88–94.

Hastings, E. C., & West, R. L. (2009). The relative success of a self-help and a group-based memory training program for older adults. *Psychology and Aging, 24*, 586–594.

Hauser, R. M. (2010). Causes and consequences of cognitive functioning across the life course. *Educational Researcher, 39*, 95–109.

Hawkins, H. L., Kramer, A. F., & Capaldi, D. (1992). Aging, exercise, and attention. *Psychology and Aging, 7*, 643–653.

Hertzog, C., Cooper, B. P., & Fisk, A. D. (1996). Aging and individual differences in the development of skilled memory search performance. *Psychology and Aging, 11*, 497–520.

Hertzog, C., Kramer, A. F., Wilson, R. S., & Lindenberger, U. (2008). Enrichment effects on adult cognitive development: Can the functional capacity of older adults be preserved and enhanced? *Psychological Science in the Public Interest, 9*, 1–65.

Hertzog, C., & Nesselroade, J. R. (2003). Assessing psychological change in adulthood: An overview of methodological issues. *Psychology and Aging, 18*, 639–657.

Heyn, P., Abreu, B. C., & Ottenbacher, K. J. (2004). The effects of exercise training on elderly persons with cognitive impairment and dementia: A meta-analysis. *Archives of Physical Medicine & Rehabilitation, 85*, 1694–1704.

Hill, R. D., Storandt, M., & Malley, M. (1993). The impact of long-term exercise training on psychological function in older adults. *Journals of Gerontology, 48*, 12–17.

Hultsch, D. F. (1971). Organization and memory in adulthood. *Human Development, 14*, 16–24.

Hultsch, D. F., Hertzog, C., Small, B. J., & Dixon, R. A. (1999). Use it or lose it: Engaged lifestyle as a buffer of cognitive decline in aging? *Psychology and Aging, 14*, 245–263.

Institute of Medicine. (2009). *Initial national priorities for comparative effectiveness research*. Washington, DC: National Academies Press.

Jaeggi, S. M., Buschkuehl, M., Jonides, J., & Perrig, W. (2008). Improving fluid intelligence with training on working memory. *Proceedings of the National Academy of Sciences, 105*, 6829–6833.

Jobe, J. B., Smith, D., Ball, K., Tennstedt, S., Marsiske, M., Willis, S. L., et al. (2001). ACTIVE: A cognitive intervention trial to promote independence in older adults. *Controlled Clinical Trials, 22*, 453–479.

Johnson, R. E. (2003). Aging and the remembering of text. *Developmental Review, 23*, 261–346.

Kane, M. J., Hambrick, D. Z., Tuholksi, S. W., Wilhelm, O., Payne, T. W., & Engle, R. W. (2004). The generality of working memory capacity: A latent-variable approach to verbal and visuospatial memory span and reasoning. *Journal of Experimental Psychology: General, 133*, 189–217.

Kempermann, G. (2008). Activity dependancy and aging in regulation of adult neurogenesis. In F. H. Gage, G. Kempermann, & H. Song (Eds.), *Adult neurogenesis*. Cold Spring Harbor, NY: Cold Spring Harbor Laboratory Press.

Kinsella, K., & He, W. (2009). *International Population Reports, P95/09-1, An Aging World: 2008*. Washington, DC: U.S. Government Printing Office.

Kliegl, R., Smith, J., & Baltes, P. B. (1989). Testing-the-limits and the study of adult age differences in cognitive plasticity of a mnemonic skill. *Developmental Psychology, 25*, 247–256.

Kliegl, R., Smith, J., & Baltes, P. B. (1990). On the locus and process of magnification of age differences during mnemonic training. *Developmental Psychology, 26*, 894–904.

Kramer, A. F., Bherer, L., Colcombe, S. J., Dong, W., & Greenough, W. T. (2004). Environmental influences on cognitive and brain plasticity during aging. *Journals of Gerontology: Medical Sciences, 59A*, 940–957.

Kramer, A. F., Hahn, S., Cohen, N. J., Banich, M. T., McAuley, E., Chason, J., et al. (1999). Ageing, fitness, and neurocognitive function. *Nature, 400*, 418–419.

Kramer, A. F., Larish, J. F., & Strayer, D. L. (1995). Training for attentional control in dual task settings: A comparison of young and old adults. *Journal of Experimental Psychology: Applied, 1*, 50–76.

Kramer, A. F., Larish, J. L., Weber, T. A., & Bardell, L. (1999). Training for executive control: Task coordination strategies and aging. In D. Gopher & A. Koriat (Eds.), *Attention and Performance XVII: Cognitive regulation of performance: Interaction of theory and application* (pp. 617–652). Cambridge, MA: MIT Press.

Lachin, J. M. (2000). Statistical considerations in the intent-to-treat principle. *Controlled Clinical Trials, 21*, 167–189.

Langbaum, B. S., Rebok, G. W., Bandeen-Roche, K., & Carlson, M. C. (2009). Predicting memory training response patterns: Results from ACTIVE. *Journals of Gerontology: Psychological Sciences, 64B*, 14–23.

Langer, E. (1997). *The power of mindful learning*. Boston, MA: Addison-Wesley.

Lennartsson, C., & Silverstein, M. (2001). Does engagement with life enhance survival of elderly people in Sweden? The role of social and leisure activities. *Journals of Gerontology: Social Sciences, 56B*(6), S335–S342.

Levine, B., Stuss, D. T., Winocur, G., Binns, M. A., Fahy, L., Mandic, M., et al. (2007). Cognitive rehabilitation in the elderly: Effects on strategic behavior in relation to goal management. *Journal of the International Neuropsychological Society, 13*, 143–152.

Lindenberger, U., & Baltes, P. B. (1994). Sensory functioning and intelligence in old age: A strong connection. *Psychology and Aging, 9*, 339–355.

Liu-Ambrose, T., Nagamatsu, L. S., Graf, P., Beattie, L., Ashe, M. C., & Handy, T. C. (2010). Resistance training and executive functions. *Archives of Internal Medicine, 170*, 170–178.

Luo, L., Hendriks, T., & Craik, F. I. M. (2007). Age differences in recollection: Three patterns of enhanced encoding. *Psychology and Aging, 22*, 269–280.

Lustig, C., & Flegal, K. E. (2008). Targeting latent function: Encouraging effective encoding for successful memory training and transfer. *Psychology and Aging, 23*, 754–764.

Lustig, C., Shah, P., Seidler, R., & Reuter-Lorenz, P. A. (2009). Aging, training, and the brain: A review and future directions. *Neuropsychology Review, 18*, 504–522.

Maguire, E. A., Gadian, D. G., Johnsrude, I. S., Good, C. D., Ashburner, J., Frackowiak, R. S. J., et al. (2000). Navigation-related structural change in the hippocampi of taxi drivers. *Proceedings of the National Academy of Sciences, 97*, 4398–4403.

Maguire, E. A., Spiers, H. J., Good, C. D., Hartley, T., Frakowiak, R. S. J., & Burgess, N. (2003). Navigation expertise and the human hippocampus: A structural brain imaging analysis. *Hippocampus, 13*, 208–217.

Mahncke, H. W., Connor, B. B., Appelman, J., Ahsaduddin, O. N., Hardy, J. L., Wood, R. A., et al. (2006). Memory enhancement in healthy older adults us ing a brain plasticity-based training program: A randomized controlled study. *Proceedings of the National Academy of Sciences, 103*, 12523–12528.

Malone, M. L., Skrajner, M. J., Camp, C. J., Neundorfer, M., & Gorzelle, G. J. (2007). Research in practice II: Spaced-retrieval, a memory intervention. *Alzheimer's Care Quarterly, 8*, 65–74.

Margrett, J. A., & Willis, S. L. (2006). In-home cognitive training with older married couples: Individual versus collaborative learning. *Aging, Neuropsychology, and Cognition, 13*, 173–195.

McArdle, J. J., & Prindle, J. J. (2008). A latent change score analysis of a randomized clinical trial in reasoning training. *Psychology and Aging, 23*, 702–719.

Mestre, J. P. (Ed.), (2005). *Greenwich, CT: Information Age Publishers.*

Miles, J. R., & Stine-Morrow, E. A. L. (2004). Adult age differences in self-regulated learning in reading sentences. *Psychology and Aging, 19*, 626–636.

Miyake, A., Friedman, N. P., Emerson, M. J., Witzki, A. H., Howerter, A., & Wager, T. (2000). The unity and diversity of executive functions and their contributions to complex "frontal lobe" tasks: A latent variable analysis. *Cognitive Psychology, 41*, 49–100.

Mohammed, A. H., Zhu, S., Darmopil, S., Hjerling-Leffler, J., Ernfors, P., Winblad, B., et al. (2002). Environmental enrichment and the brain. In M. Hofman, G. Boer, & A. Hotmaat (Eds.), *Progress in brain research* (pp. 109–133). Amsterdam, The Netherlands: Elsevier.

Molden, D. C., & Dweck, C. S. (2006). Finding "meaning" in psychology: A lay thoeries approach to self-regulation, social perception, and social development. *American Psychologist, 61*, 192–203.

Morrow, D. G., Leirer, V. O., Fitzsimmons, C., & Altieri, P. A. (1994). When expertise reduces age differences in performance. *Psychology and Aging, 9*, 134–148.

Murphy, M. D., Schmitt, F. A., Caruso, M. J., & Sanders, R. E. (1987). Metamemory in older adults: The role of monitoring in serial recall. *Psychology and Aging, 2*, 331–339.

Neubauer, A. C., & Fink, A. (2009). Intelligence and neural efficiency. *Neuroscience and Biobehavioral Reviews, 33,* 1004–1023.

Nithianantharajah, J., & Hannan, A. (2006). Enriched environments, experience-dependent plasticity and disorders of the nervous system. *Nature Review Neuroscience, 7,* 697–709.

Noice, H., & Noice, T. (2006). What studies of actors and acting can tell us about memory and cognitive functioning. *Current Directions in Psychological Science, 15,* 14–18.

Noice, H., & Noice, T. (2008). An arts intervention for older adults living in subsidized retirement homes. *Aging, Neuropsychology, and Cognition, 16,* 56–79.

Noice, H., Noice, T., & Kennedy, C. (2000). Effects of enactment by professional actors at encoding and retrieval. *Memory, 8,* 353–363.

Noice, H., Noice, T., Perrig-Chiello, P., & Perrig, W. (1999). Improving memory in older adults by instructing them in professional actors' learning strategies. *Applied Cognitive Psychology, 13,* 315–328.

Nyberg, L., Sandblom, J., Jones, S., Stigsdotter Neely, A. S., Petersson, K. M., & Ingvar, M. (2003). Neural correlates of training related memory improvment in adulthood and aging. *Proceedings of the National Academy of Sciences, 100,* 13728–13733.

Parisi, J. M., Greene, J. C., Morrow, D. G., & Stine-Morrow, E. A. L. (2007). The Senior Odyssey: Participant experiences of a program of social and intellectual engagement. *Activities, Adaptation, and Aging, 31,* 31–49.

Pashler, H., McDaniel, M., Roher, D., & Bjork, R. (2009). Learning styles: Concepts and evidence. *Psychological Science in the Public Interest, 9,* 105–119.

Persson, J., & Reuter-Lorenz, P. (2008). Gaining control: Training executive function and far transfer of the ability to resolve interference. *Psychological Science, 19,* 881–888.

Plemons, J. K., Willis, S. L., & Baltes, P. B. (1978). Modifiability of fluid intelligence in aging: A short-term longitudinal training approach. *Journals of Gerontology, 22,* 224–231.

Rasmusson, D. X., Rebok, G. W., Bylsma, F. W., & Brandt, J. (1999). Effects of three types of memory training in normal elderly. *Aging, Neuropsychology, and Cognition, 6,* 56–66.

Rebok, G. W. (2008). *Cognitive training: Influence on neuropsychological and brain function in later life. State-of-Science Review: SR:E22.* UK Government Foresight Mental Capital and Mental Wellbeing Project. Government Office for Science.

Rebok, G. W., & Balcerak, L. J. (1989). Memory self-efficacy and performance differences in young and old adults: The effects of mnemonic training. *Developmental Psychology, 25,* 714–721.

Rebok, G. W., Carlson, M. C., & Langbaum, B. S. (2007). Training and maintaining memory abilities in healthy older adults: Traditional and novel approaches. Journals of Gerontology: *Psychological Sciences, 62B,* 53–61.

Rebok, G. W., Rasmusson, D. X., & Brandt, J. (1996). Prospects for computerized memory training in normal elderly: Effects of practice on explicit and implicit memory tasks. *Applied Cognitive Psychology, 10,* 211–223.

Richards, M., & Sacker, M. (2003). Lifetime antecedents of cognitive reserve. *Journal of Clinical and Experimental Neuropsychology, 25,* 614–624.

Riediger, M., Li, S.-C., & Linderberger, U. (2006). Selection, optimization, and compensation as developmental mechanisms of adaptivere resource allocation: Review and preview. In J. E. Birren & K. W. Schaie (Eds.), *Handbook of the psychology of aging* (6th ed., pp. 289–313). San Diego, CA: Elsevier.

Rikli, R., & Edwards, D. (1991). Effects of a three year exercise program on motor function and cognitive processing speed in older women. *Research Quarterly for Exercise and Sport, 62,* 61–67.

Riley, M. W., & Riley, J. W., Jr. (2000). Age integration: Conceptual and historical background. *The Gerontologist, 40,* 266–270.

Salthouse, T. A. (1991a). Mediation of adult age differences in cognition by reductions in working memory and speed of processing. *Psychological Science, 2,* 179–183.

Salthouse, T. A. (1991b). *Theoretical perspectives on cognitive aging.* Hillsdale, NJ: Erlbaum.

Salthouse, T. A. (2006). Mental exercise and mental aging: Evaluating the validity of the "use it or lose it" hypothesis. *Perspectives on Psychological Science, 1,* 68–87.

Salthouse, T. A. (2009). When does age-related cognitive decline begin? *Neurobiology of Aging, 30,* 507–514.

Salthouse, T. A. (2010). *Major issues in cognitive aging.* New York: Oxford University Press, in press.

Scarmeas, N., Levy, G., Tang, M.-X., Manly, J., & Stern, Y. (2001). Influence of leisure activity on the incidence of Alzheimer's Disease. *Neurology, 57,* 2236–2242.

Scarmeas, N., & Stern, Y. (2003). Cognitive reserve and lifestyle. *Journal of Clinical and Experimental Neuropsychology, 25,* 625–633.

Schooler, C., & Mulatu, M. S. (2001). The reciprocal effects of leisure time activities and intellectual functioning in older people: A longitudinal analysis. *Psychology and Aging, 16,* 466–482.

Small, G. W., Silverman, D. H. S., Siddarth, P., Ercoli, L. M., Miller, K. J., Lavretsky, H., et al. (2006). Effects of a 14-day healthy longevity lifestyle program on cognition and brain function. *The American Journal of Geriatric Psychiatry, 14,* 538–545.

Smith, G. E., Housen, P., Yaffe, K., Ruff, R., Kennison, R. F., Mahncke, H. W., et al. (2009). A cognitive training program based on principles of brain plasticity: Results from the Improvement in Memory with Plasticity-based Adaptive Cognitive Training (IMPACT) Study. *JAGS, 57,* 594–60.

Stern, Y. (2002). What is cognitive reserve? Theory and research application of the reserve concept. *Journal of the International Neuropsychological Society, 8,* 448–460.

Stern, Y. (2009). Cognitive reserve. *Neuropsychologia, 47,* 2015–2028.

Stigdotter-Neely, A. S., & Bäckman, L. (1995). Effects of multifactorial memory training in old age: Generalizability across tasks and individuals. *Journals of Gerontology: Psychological Sciences, 50B,* P134–P140.

Stine-Morrow, E. A. L. (2007). The Dumbledore Hypothesis of cognitive aging. *Current Directions in Psychological Science, 16,* 289–293.

Stine-Morrow, E. A. L., Noh, S. R., & Shake, M. C. (2010). Age differences in the effects of conceptual integration training on resource allocation in sentence processing. *Quarterly Journal of Experimental Psychology.*

Stine-Morrow, E. A. L., & Parisi, J. M. A practical guide to Senior Odyssey. In P. Hartman-Stein & A. LaRue (Eds.), *Enhancing cognitive fitness: A guide to the use and development of community programs.* New York: Springer, in press.

Stine-Morrow, E. A. L., Parisi, J. M., Morrow, D. G., Greene, J. C., & Park, D. C. (2007). An engagement model of cognitive optimization through adulthood. *Journals of Gerontology: Psychological Sciences, 62,* 62–69.

Stine-Morrow, E. A. L., Parisi, J. M., Morrow, D. G., & Park, D. C. (2008). The effects of an engaged lifestyle on cognitive vitality: A field experiment. *Psychology and Aging, 23,* 778–786.

Stine-Morrow, E. A. L., Shake, M. C., Miles, J. R., & Noh, S. R. (2006). Adult age differences in the effects of goals on self-regulated sentence processing. *Psychology and Aging, 21,* 790–803.

Stokes, D. E. (1997). *Pasteur's quadrant: Basic science and technological innovation.* Washington, DC: Brookings Institution Press.

Stones, M. J., Dornan, B., & Kozma, A. (1989). The prediction of mortality in elderly institution residents. *Journals of Gerontology, 44,* 72–79.

Stuss, D. T., Robertson, I. H., Craik, F. I. M., Levine, B., Alexander, M. P., Black, S., et al. (2007). Cognitive rehabilitation in the elderly: A randomized trial to evaluate a new protocol. *Journal of the International Neuropsychological Society, 13,* 120–131.

Swezy, R. W., & Llaneras, R. E. (1997). Models in training and instruction. In G. Salvendy (Ed.), *Handbook of human factor and ergonomics* (pp. 512–577). New York: Wiley.

Tranter, L. J., & Koutstall, W. (2008). Age and flexible thinking: An experimental demonstration of the beneficial effects of increased cognitively stimulating activity on fluid intelligence in healthy older adults. *Aging, Neuropsychology, and Cognition, 15,* 184–207.

Unverzagt, F., Kasten, L., Johnson, K., Rebok, G. W., Marsiske, M., Koepke, K. M., et al. (2007). Effect of memory impairment on training outcomes in ACTIVE. *Journal of the International Neuropsychological Society, 13,* 953–960.

Unverzagt, F., Smith, D., Rebok, G. W., Marsiske, M., Morris, J., Jones, R., et al. (2009). The Indiana Alzheimer Disease Center's Symposium on Mild Cognitive Impairment. Cognitive training in older adults: Lessons from the ACTIVE study. *Current Alzheimer's Disease, 6,* 375–383.

Valentijn, S. A. M., Hill, R. D., Van Hooren, S. A. H., Bosma, H., Van Boxtel, M. P. J., Jolles, J., et al. (2006). Memory self-efficacy predicts memory performance: Results from a 6-year follow-up study. *Psychology and Aging, 21,* 165–172.

van Praag, H., Shubert, T., Zhao, C., & Gage, F. H. (2005). Exercise enhances learning and hippocampal neurogenesis in aged mice. *The Journal of Neuroscience, 25,* 8680–8685.

Vaynman, S., Ying, Z., & Gomez-Pinilla, F. (2004). Hippocampal BDNF mediates the efficacy of exercise on synaptic plasticity and cognition. *European Journal of Neuroscience, 20,* 2580–2590.

Verghese, J., Lipton, R. B., Katz, M. J., Hall, C. B., Derby, C. A., Kuslansky, G., et al. (2003). Leisure activities and risk of dementia in the elderly. *New England Journal of Medicine, 348,* 2508–2516.

Verhaeghen, P., & Marcoen, A. (1996). On the mechanisms of plasticity in young and older adults after instruction in the method of loci: Evidence for an amplification model. *Psychology and Aging, 11,* 164–178.

Verhaeghen, P., Marcoen, A., & Goossens, L. (1992). Improving memory performance in the aged through mnemonic training: A meta-analytic study. *Psychology and Aging, 7,* 242–251.

West, R. L., Bagwell, D. K., & Dark-Freudeman, A. (2005). Memory and goal setting: The response of older and younger adults to positive and objective feedback. *Psychology and Aging, 20,* 195–201.

West, R. L., Bagwell, D. K., & Dark-Freudeman, A. (2008). Self-efficacy and memory ageing: The impact of a memory intervention based on self-efficacy. *Aging, Neuropsychology, and Cognition, 15,* 302–329.

West, R. L., Dark-Freudeman, A., & Bagwell, D. K. (2009). Goals-feedback conditions and episodic memory: Mechanisms for memory gains in older and younger adults. *Memory, 17,* 233–244.

West, R. L., & Thorn, R. M. (2001). Goal-setting, self-efficacy, and memory performance in older and younger adults. *Experimental Aging Research, 27,* 41–65.

West, R. L., Thorn, R. M., & Bagwell, D. K. (2003). Memory performance and beliefs as a function of goal setting and aging. *Psychology and Aging, 18,* 111–125.

West, R. L., Welch, D. W., & Thorn, R. M. (2001). Effects of goal-setting and feedback on memory performance and beliefs among older and younger adults. *Psychology and Aging, 16,* 240–250.

Weuve, J., Kang, J. H., Manson, J. E., Breteler, M. M. B., Ware, J. H., & Grodstein, F. (2004). Physical activity including walking and cognitive function in older women. *JAMA, 292,* 1454–1461.

Willis, S. L. (2001). Methodological issues in behavioral intervention research with the elderly. In J. E. Birren & K. W. Schaie (Eds.), *Handbook of the psychology of aging* (5th ed., pp. 78–108). San Diego, CA: Academic Press.

Willis, S. L., & Nesselroade, C. S. (1990). Long-term effects of fluid ability training in old-old age. *Developmental Psychology, 26,* 905–910.

Willis, S. L., Tennstedt, S. L., Marsiske, M., Ball, K., Elias, J., Koepke, K. M., et al. (2006). Long-term effects of cognitive training on everyday functional outcomes in older adults. *Journal of the American Medical Association, 296*, 2805–2814.

Wilson, R. S., Mendes de Leon, C. F., Barnes, L. L., Schneider, J. A., Bienias, J. L., Evans, D. A., et al. (2002). Participation in cognitively stimulating activities and risk of incident Alzheimer disease. *Journal of the American Medical Association, 287*, 742–748.

Winocur, G., Craik, F. I. M., Levine, B., Robertson, I. H., Binns, M. A., Alexander, M., et al. (2007). Cognitive rehabilitation in the elderly: Overview and future directions. *Journal of the International Neuropsychological Society, 13*(1), 166–171.

Wolinsky, F., Unverzagt, F., Smith, D., Jones, R., Wright, E., & Tennstedt, S. (2006). The effects of the ACTIVE cognitive training trial on clinically relevant declines in health-related quality of life. *Journals of Gerontology: Social Sciences, 61B*, S281–S287.

Wolinsky, F., Vander Weg, M., Martin, R., Unverzagt, F., Ball, K., Jones, R., et al. (2009). The effect of speed-of-processing training on depressive symptoms in ACTIVE. *Journals of Gerontology: Medical Sciences, 64A*, 468–472.

Yaffe, K., Barnes, D., Nevitt, M., Lui, L. Y., & Covinsky, K. (2001). A prospective study of physical activity and cognitive decline in elderly women. *Archives of Internal Medicine, 161*, 1703–1708.

Yang, L., & Krampe, R. T. (2009). Long-term mainenance of retest learning in young old and oldest old adults. *Journals of Gerontology: Psychological Sciences, 64B*, 608–611.

Yang, L., Krampe, R. T., & Baltes, P. B. (2006). Basic forms of cognitive plasticity extended into the oldest-old: Retest learning, age, and cognitive functioning. *Psychology and Aging, 21*, 372–378.

Yang, L., Reed, M., Russo, F. A., & Wilkinson, A. (2009). A new look at retest learning in older adults: Learning in the absence of item-specific effects. *Journals of Gerontology: Psychological Sciences, 64B*, 470–4.

Zelinski, E. M. (2009). Far transfer in cognitive training of older adults. *Restorative Neurology and Neuroscience, 27*, 455–471.

Part 3

Social and Health Factors that Impact Aging

11 The Relevance of Control Beliefs for Health and Aging *175*

12 The Speedometer of Life: Stress, Health and Aging *191*

13 Health Disparities, Social Class, and Aging *207*

14 Relationships between Adults and their Aging Parents *219*

15 Intergenerational Communication Practices *233*

16 Age Stereotypes and Aging *249*

17 Aging in the Work Context *263*

18 Wisdom, Age, and Well-Being *279*

Chapter | 11 |

The Relevance of Control Beliefs for Health and Aging

Margie E. Lachman,[1] Shevaun D. Neupert,[2] Stefan Agrigoroaei[1]

[1]Department of Psychology, Brandeis University, Waltham, Massachusetts, USA; [2]Department of Psychology, North Carolina State University, Raleigh, North Carolina, USA

CHAPTER CONTENTS

Introduction 175

Brief History and Conceptual Overview of the Construct of Control 176

Age Differences and Changes in Control Beliefs 177

Sociodemographic Variations in Control Beliefs 179

Relation of Control Beliefs to Aging-Related Domains 180

Is High Control Always Adaptive? 180

Mechanisms and Processes Linking Control Beliefs and Aging-Related Outcomes 181

Interventions to Modify Control Beliefs 184

Summary, Conclusions, and Future Directions 185

Acknowledgments 186

References 186

INTRODUCTION

Control is a pervasive concept in popular culture and in the psychological literature. On a daily basis we encounter opportunities to take control in a multitude of life domains. Advertisements promise that the best cars will give you maximum control over the road, fancy investment firms will help you to control your financial assets, and medications will allow you to control ailments and symptoms from acne, allergies, asthma, bladder problems, to high blood pressure, high blood sugar, pain, sexual dysfunction, and sleeplessness. A multitude of spiritual messages (e.g., the serenity prayer) advocate the importance of knowing what you can and cannot change. There are numerous psychological theories about control and countless treatments designed to help control behavioral problems such as gambling, excessive drinking, smoking, and overeating.

Application of the control construct to the field of aging is more recent, but the notion that one can "take control over the aging process" is now widespread. The lucrative anti-aging industry, which offers products and treatments designed to prevent, slow, reverse, or compensate for aging-related changes in the face, body, and mind, counts on the consumer to accept that there are things we can do to control aging-related changes and losses. Control over the aging process is heralded not only in the popular media and advertising industry, but also in professional journals and books such as *Successful Aging* by Rowe and Kahn (1998) and *Aging Well* by Vaillant (2002). A key message conveyed is that although aging is influenced to some degree by genetic factors, there is a large component that is determined by lifestyle choices and behavioral factors; that is, the nature of aging is to some extent under one's own control.

In stark contrast is the common notion that with aging we lose control over many aspects of life. This view is prominently embedded in stereotypes and attitudes about aging (Hess, 2006; Levy et al., 2009), with important consequences for behavior and health. These stereotypic views include images of older adults as helpless and deteriorating, and assumptions that aging-related declines are inevitable and irreversible. Such conceptions are promoted and reinforced by societal views and treatment of aging manifested in the negative views of getting older presented, for example, in birthday cards.

DOI: 10.1016/B978-0-12-380882-0.00011-5

In this chapter we focus on control beliefs, also referred to as perceived control or the sense of control. All involve expectancies about personal mastery and environmental contingencies that influence outcomes and performance. Individuals hold different views about whether and how much they can influence outcomes. Some believe there are things they can do to make a difference in the course of aging, and others see their influence as more limited. Such beliefs about control over aging may have their origins in childhood experiences and observations of parents' and grandparents' approaches and attitudes to aging, or through educational and occupational experiences with mastery or failure. The sense of control plays a pivotal role across the life span, functioning both as an antecedent and consequence of aging processes. Beliefs about control over the environment and abilities for self-regulation can serve a protective role and affect behaviors throughout life. As an outcome, a strong sense of control is an indicator of an adaptive set of beliefs about personal agency and effectiveness. Of particular interest in this chapter is to what extent control beliefs diminish or remain intact in response to aging-related changes. A sense of control also functions as a mechanism linked to performance in various domains, and may serve as a buffer for the deleterious effects of aging. Individual differences in conceptions of control are relatively stable throughout adulthood, yet they are malleable and responsive to situational influences (Hooker & McAdams, 2003), making them a viable target for interventions.

This chapter is concerned with the beliefs that individuals hold about how much they can control various outcomes in their life including the nature of their own aging. Our key focus is individual differences in multiple components of perceived control (self-efficacy, mastery, ability, or competence; and outcome expectancies, contingency, or constraints) and how such appraisals are related to behaviors and outcomes. More specifically, the goal of this chapter is to characterize the relationship between control beliefs and health, and to examine the relevance to aging. Our review of the theoretical and empirical literature suggests that attention to the sense of control can enrich the work by researchers, policy makers, clinicians, and other scientists and practitioners interested in promoting good health and well-being in adulthood and later life.

Notably, this is the first time the *Handbook of the Psychology of Aging* contains a full chapter devoted to beliefs about control. Now, more than 30 years after the first edition of this *Handbook*, there is sufficient information about the role of control beliefs in relation to aging to warrant a separate chapter. This likely reflects the enormous surge in research on this topic and the demonstrated utility of the construct with its far reaching importance across domains related to health and aging (Lachman, 2006).

In this chapter we examine four broad issues about the perceived sense of control that are relevant in the context of health and aging: (a) control is an aspect of the self that shows declines in adulthood, yet there are wide interindividual differences within age groups and variations in intra-individual change over time; (b) control shows sociodemographic variations by gender, income, education, culture, and race, which may affect the nature of health and aging; (c) control is associated with psychological well-being, cognitive functioning, and physical health, and there is emerging evidence regarding the mechanisms that link control with these outcome domains; and (d) control is an aspect of the self that can be modified, and thus is amenable to interventions that could optimize health and aging. Before addressing these topics, we begin with a summary of the theoretical and empirical origins of the control construct.

BRIEF HISTORY AND CONCEPTUAL OVERVIEW OF THE CONSTRUCT OF CONTROL

In psychology and related fields, control is studied in many different forms with many different labels and subtle variations, including self-efficacy, sense of control, personal mastery, perceived control, locus of control, learned helplessness, and primary and secondary control, just to name a few (Pearlin & Pioli, 2003; Rodin, 1990). One important distinction is between objective control and subjective perceptions of control. In this chapter we focus on the latter, with an emphasis on beliefs about control over aging and outcomes relevant to aging (e.g. health, memory). The perceptions and expectations individuals hold about their ability to control outcomes may or may not be veridical, and they may vary across domains and time. Within this framework, it is the expectancies that matter, and in many cases the actual amount of control one has is unknown. With the focus on perceived control in this chapter, what is especially of interest is that people vary in the amount of control they perceive over the same situation (independent of actual control), and these individual differences in beliefs make a difference for functioning (Lachman, 1986). We will later discuss some of the possible mechanisms involved in linking these beliefs to aging-related and health outcomes.

The control beliefs construct first emerged as the locus of control, under the rubric of social learning theory (Rotter, 1966). This work focused on the sources of control, as either internal (e.g., abilities, effort) or external (e.g., chance, fate, powerful others) to the person. Although a highly fruitful line of work, the internal-external distinction was limited especially due to a confound between the source of control and the degree of controllability. Internal sources were assumed to be within the person's control, yet some internal sources are not highly controllable (e.g., genetic influences). Other concerns raised about the early locus of control work were that (a) internal and external control was seen as opposite poles of a continuum rather than as separate dimensions that are relatively independent; and (b) control was considered a general, stable individual difference variable that applied across domains, rather than acknowledging that control beliefs also vary across time (Eizenman et al., 1997) and specific areas of life (Lachman, 1986; Lefcourt, 1984).

As the roots of the sense of control construct are in social learning theory (Rotter, 1966), control is usually considered a learned view of the self and the environment rather than a fixed personality trait, and as such it is subject to change with aging (Abeles, 1991; Hooker & McAdams, 2003; Pearlin & Pioli, 2003). Much of the locus of control work was correlational, using personality trait type items. This early work was focused on college students and children, but was not developmental. It was in the late 1970s that control was first studied in relation to aging, with the initial focus on enhancing control among institutionalized older adults (Langer & Rodin, 1976; Rodin & Langer, 1977; Schulz, 1976; Schulz & Hanusa, 1978). Studies on the control construct in relation to aging led to advancements in both theory and measurement, and have contributed to understanding the role of beliefs and expectancies for aging. This work was in large part inspired by sociologists (Brim, 1974) and social psychologists (Abeles, 1991; Rodin, 1986), and adopted by life span developmental psychologists (Heckhausen et al., 2010; Lachman, 1986, 2006; Skinner, 1996) and gerontologists (Krause & Stryker, 1984). Those interested in adult development and aging began to think about the control construct in developmental and contextual terms (Lachman, 1986). This includes work on the motivational and behavioral self-regulatory functions of control via self-efficacy and outcome expectancies (Miller & Lachman, 2000) and theories such as the life span theory of control (Heckhausen et al., 2010) and the dual process model of assimilation and accommodation (Brandtstädter & Renner, 1990).

One of the most prolific control theories focuses on self-efficacy, or the perceived ability to carry out specific goals or tasks (Bandura, 1997). Self-efficacy and control beliefs play an important role in adaptation and regulate human functioning through cognitive, motivational, affective, and selection processes (Bandura, 1990). Lowered expectancies for self-efficacy and control likely have their origin in negative stereotypes about aging and are reinforced through experiences of loss and decline (Bandura, 1997). Other related theories such as the life span developmental theory of motivation and control (Heckhausen et al., 2010), with a focus on primary (change the environment) and secondary control (change the self) and the model of assimilation (tenacious goal pursuit) and accommodation (flexible goal adjustment; Brandtstädter & Renner, 1990), focus on control strivings and strategies for exercising control, and describe approaches to goal attainment. These control strategies are best studied in time-ordered processes in which it is possible to observe responses in different circumstances (e.g., achieving a goal or after goal failure) rather than as a general predisposition. Theoretically, those with a higher sense of control should be more likely to adopt a variety of adaptive control strategies depending on the circumstances (Wrosch, Heckhausen & Lachman, 2000). Although much of the work on control has focused on stable individual differences, we now turn to consider whether and how control beliefs and strategies vary or change with age.

AGE DIFFERENCES AND CHANGES IN CONTROL BELIEFS

The general pattern of research findings suggests that with aging the sense of control declines (Lachman & Firth, 2004; Lachman & Weaver, 1998a; Mirowsky & Ross, 2007). It is perhaps not surprising that in the face of increased losses and decreased gains associated with aging (Baltes, 2006), the sense of control would wane. Indeed, many of the changes that accompany aging are not controllable. The age trends for control beliefs typically show an increase in early adulthood, with a peak in midlife, and a leveling off with a subsequent decline in later life (Lachman, 2009; Mirowsky & Ross, 2007). What is also noteworthy is the wide range of individual differences in beliefs about control over aging within age groups (Lachman, 2006) as well as the intraindividual variability in beliefs over time (Eizenman et al., 1997).

Older adults on average seem to maintain their overall sense of mastery (beliefs about one's ability or self-efficacy), perhaps because they adjust the salient domains or the standards that they use to define their competence (Bandura, 1997). With aging, we see mainly a loss of perceived control associated with an increasing acknowledgement of the constraints and limitations due to uncontrollable factors or to reduced contingency between actions and outcomes (Lachman & Firth, 2004). These age differences in control beliefs seem to occur mainly because older adults experience fewer opportunities for control and more control-limiting situations.

Although the sense of control generally shows a downward trajectory with aging, a more nuanced view shows the story is more complex, and what changes and when depends on multiple factors such as what control dimension is measured, the ages and other characteristics of the sample, the specific domains examined, and the study designs. Many of the studies about control and aging have used cross-sectional data, in which age and cohort differences are confounded, thus limiting conclusions about direct age-related changes. Longitudinal studies are helpful to move beyond the limitations of cross-sectional designs, and there is a good deal of evidence for longitudinal stability in perceived control into old age (Gatz & Karel, 1993; Grover & Hertzog, 1991; Lachman, 1985, 1986). However, findings have been mixed, as some studies report declines in perceived control late in life (Rodin & Langer, 1980).

Goal relevance may be an important contributing factor for the maintenance of control beliefs into old age. For example, Brandtstädter and Rothermund (1994) proposed a model where sense of control is maintained in later adulthood through shifts in the subjective importance of developmental goals. The degree to which perceptions of control within a particular goal domain affected an individual's general sense of control depended on the personal importance of that domain, and losses of control within a goal domain affected general perceptions of control to a lesser degree if the importance of the respective domain was downscaled within the same longitudinal interval. Within Brandtstädter's (1990) model, assimilative forms of control decline with age, whereas accommodative forms of control show increases with aging. These patterns are similar to those found by Wrosch and colleagues (2006) guided by the life span theory of control. They reported that primary control strategies remain relatively stable across adulthood, but are more likely to be replaced by secondary control strategies in later life when older adults are faced with greater obstacles to goal attainment.

Other longitudinal investigations have documented a mix of gains and losses in control beliefs. For example, Lachman et al. (2009) found evidence for changes in the sense of control over time in a national sample of adults in the United States studied over a 10-year period. The 10-year, cross-sectional differences mapped directly onto the 10-year period change data for many of the control dimensions. Average patterns of change showed both gains and losses across different dimensions and domains of control, and these patterns also varied by age cohort group. Those in midlife looked particularly strong in terms of reporting the lowest levels of perceived constraints and greatest declines in perceived constraints over time. In contrast, those in later life not only experienced increases in perceived constraints but also declines in health control. Thus, adulthood is characterized by a combination of ups and downs in the sense of control across different domains of life. Those who had a more adaptive personality profile (e.g., high in agreeableness, low in neuroticism), better quality of social relationships, better health, and higher cognitive functioning were more likely to maintain or increase control beliefs in general and in multiple domains. It is desirable to maintain a favorable balance of gains to losses in perceived control across life domains (Baltes et al., 2006). Or, as suggested by Krause (2007), what may be important is to maintain control in the domains that are most meaningful or central for the individual.

In addition to mean levels, considering and modeling intraindividual variability and within-person change has received increased attention as evidence of the processes involved in psychological adaptation (Nesselroade & Salthouse, 2004; Sliwinski et al., 2003). Based on repeated assessments within days or across days, intraindividual variability over the short term has important predictive value for aging-related outcomes (e.g., fluid intelligence, mortality; Martin & Hofer, 2004). Some studies suggest that older adults show greater intraindividual (within-person) variability in cognitive performance domains (Hultsch et al., 2002; Nesselroade & Salthouse, 2004), but less in the affective domains (Röcke et al., 2009).

Although much of the work on intraindividual variability has focused on cognitive and affective functioning, a few studies have shown that locus of control operates not just as a stable individual difference variable, but also has an important dynamic aspect (Eizenman et al., 1997; Roberts & Nesselroade, 1986). The degree of consistency of control beliefs is as important, if not more so, than the level of the beliefs (Eizenman et al., 1997), as variability in control beliefs was found to predict mortality to a greater degree than level of control. Eizenman et al. (1997) examined weekly fluctuations in general control beliefs over 25 occasions for seven months in a sample of older adults. Significant within-person fluctuations in control beliefs were found, and, importantly, these fluctuations were associated with mortality five years later.

More work is needed to examine how variability in control is linked with behavioral and physiological outcomes. One way of accomplishing this would be through the use of measurement burst designs (Nesselroade & Salthouse, 2004). These designs gather estimates of intraindividual variability within a longitudinal design by nesting daily diary measurements of control beliefs (e.g., assessing control beliefs each day for a series of consecutive days) to capture intra-individual variability within long-term longitudinal assessments of behavioral and physiological outcomes. This approach has great potential for representing the dynamics of the aging individual and addressing the relationships between fluctuations in daily control beliefs and long-term behavioral and health outcomes as people age.

Given the benefits of a high sense of control for affect and action, whether or not veridical (Thompson, 1999), a decline in perceived control with aging or fluctuations within persons may have a negative impact on health and well-being. Shupe (1985) suggested that feeling a loss of control does not cause disease, but it "alters the physiological state of the individual and leads to an increased physical and mental vulnerability" (p. 184). It is an important goal of aging research to identify those factors that enable adults to remain resilient and to maintain their sense of control in the face of aging-related declines.

SOCIODEMOGRAPHIC VARIATIONS IN CONTROL BELIEFS

In addition to variations by age, the sense of control shows systematic differences in relation to other sociodemographic variables including sex, socioeconomic status (SES; educational attainment, income), culture, and race/ethnicity. Of particular interest is whether these patterns of variation are consistent across multiple age/cohorts, or whether the course of aging differs as a function of sociodemographic characteristics. Although sex differences are not typically large, the overall pattern in surveys with representative samples shows that women have a lower general sense of control than men, although these sex differences appear to be somewhat less pronounced among the college-educated (Lachman & Weaver, 1998a), and there are some domains (e.g., social) in which women report higher control (Lachman & Weaver, 1998a). SES is also related to sense of control. Those in lower income brackets report less control over their lives, which likely reflects the constraints associated with their circumstances and environments (Adler et al., 1993; Lachman & Weaver, 1998b; Wolinsky & Stump, 1996).

A good deal of work has investigated education in relation to control beliefs during adulthood and old age, and there is consistent evidence that those with higher educational attainment have higher control beliefs on average (Lachman & Weaver, 1998a; Mirowsky & Ross, 2007). We do not know definitively if those with higher education develop a greater sense of control or whether those with greater control are more likely to seek out and achieve advanced education. Those with higher educational attainment may develop control on the basis of what they learn about solving problems, or because they have more resources (both material and psychological, e.g., coping skills) available, or greater exposure to situations in which they have the opportunity to make choices and see a contingency between their actions and outcomes. With longitudinal data and statistical controls, some have reached tentative conclusions about directionality. For example, Mirowsky and Ross (2007) found an increase in control of about 0.60 SDs with each four years of education in early adulthood. They also adjusted for the status of origin using parental education and found one's own level of education contributed additional variance to control beliefs. Although firm conclusions about directionality are not possible based on current knowledge, the results suggest that education affects control beliefs, and it is less likely that changes in control produce changes in education. In future studies, it will be interesting to consider whether providing opportunities for control of resources or stimuli (e.g., control over word presentation rate or sound volume, choice of words to recall) in experimental paradigms will help to illuminate mechanisms that can reduce educational disparities in important aging outcomes. Another important consideration for future research is whether obtaining advanced education in midlife and beyond has an effect on sense of control in later life.

There are also cultural variations in the nature and meaning of control (Ashman et al., 2006; Skaff & Gardiner, 2003). Thus, it is important to have a contextual model of control to consider variations by culture as well as by race and ethnicity. More so than citizens of any other country, Americans believe that they are in control of outcomes in their lives. A 2002 Pew Center poll of 38,000 people in 44 countries presented a typical control-belief item: "Success in life is pretty much determined by forces outside our control" (Leland, 2004). In the United States, about 65% disagreed with the statement, as did 60% in Canada. In other countries, disagreement ranged from about 10% (Bangladesh) to 50% (Japan). Variations in control beliefs across countries are likely tied to different economic conditions, values, and religious beliefs, or world views about fatalism.

Asian Americans and Asians in Asia report lower levels of perceived control than non-Asians (Sastry & Ross, 1998). When comparing Western and Eastern cultures, it is not only the level of perceived control but the salience of control that varies by individualistic (Western) and collective (Eastern) cultures (Markus & Kitayama, 1991). The importance of personal control over outcomes is more closely tied to health and well-being in Western cultures (Markus & Kitayama, 1991). Japanese men are more optimistic about their ability to control a chance event collectively, whereas American men are more optimistic about their personal ability to control such events (Yamaguchi et al., 2005). Primary control may be more central for achieving goals in Western cultures, and secondary control more common as a strategy in Eastern cultures (Schulz & Heckhausen, 1999), yet both are ways to achieve control with different emphases, as a function of variations in cultural prescriptions for independence and interdependence (Ashman et al., 2006).

There is a small body of work examining differences in control beliefs by race and ethnicity in later life (Fiorri et al., 2006; Mirowsky et al., 1996).

In general, African Americans seem to have a lower overall sense of control (Shaw & Krause, 2001), and this may be tied to level of discrimination (Bruce & Thornton, 2004), which can hinder personal efforts to reach goals. In a study of adults with type 2 diabetes, European Americans displayed significantly higher levels of global mastery than Latinos (Skaff et al., 2003). These findings have important implications for health, especially in terms of the impact of attitudes about self-regulation and control of diabetes, which has a high prevalence among Latinos.

Although there are differences in control as a function of sociodemographic factors, they are largely main effects and do not typically interact with aging effects. There is little evidence to suggest that the patterns of change in control beliefs vary by gender, education, income, culture, or race/ethnicity. Nevertheless, these group differences are relevant to aging because those who start out with lower levels of perceived control may be more vulnerable in the face of declines and less resilient. Even if patterns of decline in control are similar across sex, SES, culture, and race groups, those who start out at a disadvantage may reach a critical low point sooner than others who start out higher on control. Thus, a low sense of control may be a risk factor for those groups who already have a poor prognosis for aging outcomes, and promoting a high sense of control may be a valuable protective factor.

RELATION OF CONTROL BELIEFS TO AGING-RELATED DOMAINS

Although a majority in the United States may believe that the decrements associated with aging are preventable or modifiable (Lachman, 2006), there are many adults, especially in later life, who believe some aging-related declines are largely inevitable or irreversible. There is a great deal of evidence that such individual differences in control beliefs are associated with key aging outcomes including cognitive and physical health (Rowe & Kahn, 1998). Indeed, many studies show that a high sense of control is associated with being happy, healthy, wealthy, and wise. A high sense of control is linked to psychological and emotional well-being (Kunzmann et al., 2002; Lachman et al., 2008; Rodin, 1986). Based on cross-sectional findings from the first wave of the Midlife in the United States Study (MIDUS) national sample, those with a higher sense of control had greater life satisfaction and a more optimistic view of adulthood; they reported that things were going well and expected them to either stay that way or even to get better in the future (see Lachman & Firth, 2004). Persons with higher control were less depressed and had better self-rated health, fewer chronic conditions, and less severe functional limitations. Overall, the results suggest that a sense of control may be a key protective factor for subjective well-being in the face of declining health and other losses in later life.

Older adults are more likely than the young to believe that their memory is poor (low memory self-efficacy; MSE), and not controllable in that it has gotten worse over time and will continue to deteriorate (low memory control beliefs; Hultsch et al., 1998). Such concerns about memory emerge in middle age (Lachman & Firth, 2004; Willis & Schaie, 1999), have consequences for functioning, and may be a risk factor for accelerated decline. Control beliefs about memory and other cognitive abilities are linked to performance (Windsor & Anstey, 2008), behaviors such as strategy use (Lachman & Andreoletti, 2006) and computer use (Czaja et al., 2006), and effectiveness of cognitive training (Rebok et al., 1996). Although much of this work has been cross-sectional and correlational, there is longitudinal evidence that those who have higher control beliefs improve more on cognitive tests with practice and also are less likely to show aging-related declines in cognitive functioning over time (Caplan & Schooler, 2003).

Control beliefs are also related to health and health behaviors. Beliefs about control over aging are one key ingredient in stereotypes, which promote the view that older adults are helpless (Levy et al., 2009). Previous work has found that such stereotypes about aging affect health, including blood pressure (Levy et al., 2000), and cardiovascular events (Levy et al., 2009). Believing that one has control over outcomes is associated with better reported health, fewer and less severe symptoms, and faster recovery from illness (Lachman, 1986; Rodin et al., 1985). In the British Whitehall studies, results showed those who reported lower control in the work domain, including lower decision latitude and less autonomy, had poorer health, with higher fibrinogen levels, a risk factor for cardiovascular disease (Marmot, 2004).

Greater variability in control beliefs is associated with poorer health, poorer functional status, and more physician visits and hospital admissions, even after statistically controlling for mean perceived control level and direction of change in perceived control (Chipperfield et al., 2004). These findings suggest that health and well-being among very old individuals may be compromised by fluctuating levels of perceived control. Further research is needed to explore whether maintaining a stable sense of control is always advantageous, or whether there are circumstances when lowering or raising control expectancies may be useful.

Is High Control Always Adaptive?

Although a high sense of control is usually found to be desirable, there are some indications that a low sense of control may be protective in some circumstances, especially those in which there are limited opportunities for control (Skaff, 2007). Bisconti et al., (2006) found that recent widows with greater levels of perceived control over their social support had poorer overall adjustment across the first four months of widowhood. Further longitudinal analyses over longer periods are needed to investigate whether a high sense of control may be more beneficial for resilience and coping over the long run. Those who have a strong sense of control would be expected to be more resourceful and better at finding ways to cope with uncontrollable events or unattainable goals or outcomes by using secondary rather than primary control strategies (Wrosch et al., 2006).

In some cases, realistic assessments of control may be more beneficial than optimistic or overestimations of control, but little is known about these conditions. As Brim (1974, pp. 16–17) put it, knowing when to "shuck off responsibility over matters clearly outside one's span of control," may be a form of wisdom, and associated with increased personal well-being.

In institutional settings, relinquishing control and reducing agentic behaviors in favor of behavioral dependency may be adaptive, especially in cases of health vulnerabilities and reduced capacity (Baltes, 1995). In part, this may be because some staff inadvertently promote and reward dependency because it is easier and more efficient for them to take control of feeding, bathing, dressing, than to encourage older adults to take responsibility for these activities of daily living, and older adults may welcome this as attention and support (Baltes, 1995).

Mechanisms and Processes Linking Control Beliefs and Aging-Related Outcomes

The relationships between control beliefs and health in later life are fairly well established (Lachman, 2006). Yet, one of the most promising areas of research involves identifying the mechanisms and processes involved in linking control beliefs with aging related outcomes such as illness or memory (Carstensen & Hartel, 2006; Hess, 2006). There are wide individual differences in multiple components of perceived control (self-efficacy or competence, contingency or constraints), and such appraisals are related to behaviors and outcomes including use of adaptive compensatory memory strategies and health-promoting behaviors (Lachman, 2006). A lowered sense of control may have affective, behavioral, motivational, and physiological effects, including greater levels of stress and anxiety, lower levels of effort, and persistence and strategy use, as well as less frequent engagement in memory tasks or physical activities, which can influence aging outcomes in multiple domains. Self-efficacy and control beliefs have been postulated as a mediator of the relationship between stereotypes about aging and physiological activity and performance (Levy et al., 2000).

Miller and Lachman (1999) considered some of the possible mechanisms involved in control processes and proposed a conceptual model (see Figure 11.1) of the self-regulatory role of adaptive beliefs (e.g., control) and behaviors (e.g., strategy use, physical activity) in relation to aging-related changes. In this conceptual framework, derived from cognitive-behavioral theory (Bandura, 1997), the processes are assumed to be reciprocal and cyclical in that outcomes and experiences (e.g., memory or physical declines) can have an impact on control beliefs, which in turn can affect behavioral or physiological mediators as well as future outcomes (Bandura, 1997; Miller & Lachman, 1999). Those with a high sense of control are more likely to mobilize social support in times of need (Antonucci, 2001). However, having or giving social support can also promote a sense of control over one's life (Midlarsky & Kahana, 1994). Thus, sense of control is considered to be an antecedent and consequence of age-related losses, for example, in memory (Lachman et al., 1994; Miller & Lachman, 1999, 2000) and health (Skaff, 2007). In other words, this model depicts a multidirectional process in which control beliefs are influenced by prior performance outcomes and beliefs about control also have an influence on subsequent performance and outcomes through their impact on behavior, motivation, and affect (Lachman, 2006). For example, older adults who experience memory lapses or declines in physical strength may respond with a lowered sense of control in these domains, especially if these changes are attributed to uncontrollable factors. Such beliefs in low control can be detrimental if they are associated with distress, anxiety, inactivity, and giving up without expending the effort or using the strategies needed to support optimal outcomes (Agrigoroaei & Lachman, 2010).

In the cognitive domain, the sense of control is tied to better memory and intellectual functioning, especially among older adults (e.g., Hertzog et al., 1998; Seeman et al., 1996). Control is likely beneficial for cognitive performance by providing a necessary motivational resource for the development of effortful strategies used to compensate for cognitive limitations or losses (de Frias et al., 2003; Miller & Gagne, 2005). Control beliefs are related to effective strategy use (Hertzog et al., 1998, 2003; Lachman & Andreoletti, 2006) and goal setting (West & Yassuda, 2004). Older adults typically need to use strategies to compensate for memory losses, but past research has found that older adults are less likely to use memory strategies effectively than the young (Touron & Hertzog, 2004). Even if older adults use strategies they are less likely than the young to attribute their

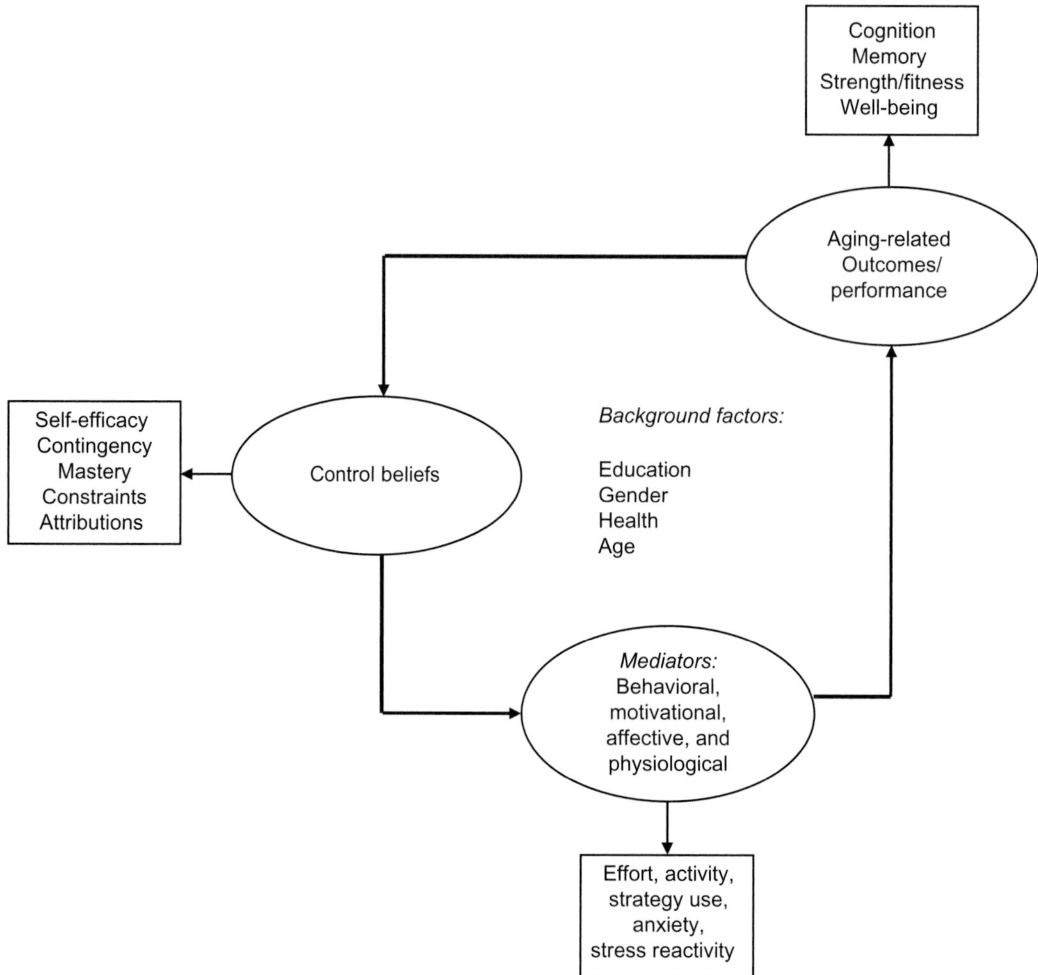

Figure 11.1 Conceptual model of the relationship between control beliefs and aging-related outcomes and performance with postulated mediators (based on Lachman, 2006; Miller & Lachman, 1999).

performance to strategies (Blatt-Eisengart & Lachman, 2004).

There are also findings regarding stress level or stress reactivity as a mediator between control beliefs and memory performance and health (Müller et al., 1998; Seeman, 1991). Experiencing personal control in a challenging situation has been shown to reduce stress-related neuroendocrine responses such as in the hypothalamic-pituitary-adrenal (HPA) axis response (Seeman & Robbins, 1994). Cognitive appraisal of challenge and threat as well as perceived controllability have an impact on response and recovery (Dickerson & Kemeny, 2004). Other results reveal that stressors can activate responses in the HPA and autonomic nervous system (e.g., slowing or increasing in heart rate), especially if the stimulus is appraised as threatening and not under personal control. Moreover, when stressors are seen as uncontrollable and the goal is important or desirable, the reactivity level is higher (Dickerson & Kemeny, 2004). Those with low control are more likely to show high levels of stress, which in turn affects memory performance among younger (Kirschbaum et al., 1996) as well as older adults (Lupien et al., 1997). The evidence suggests that acute stress affects memory performance by causing hippocampal damage (Kirschbaum et al., 1996; Lupien et al., 1997). Similarly, prolonged exposure to stress has also been associated with a loss of hippocampal neurons (McEwen & Sapolsky, 1995). Thus control may play a role in brain aging through stress mechanisms.

Self-reported anxiety is related to memory performance for older adults more so than for the young (Andreoletti et al., 2006) and may be another mediator between control and memory performance. For MSE and control beliefs, low levels may result in reduced memory performance (Berry & West, 1993); for example, by increasing the level of anxiety and arousal (Bandura, 1997), or by creating an expectation of failure (Desrichard & Köpetz, 2005) that may lead individuals to put forth less effort and be less persistent (Berry & West, 1993) in memory situations. Hultsch et al. (1998) reported a consistent small negative correlation between an individual's MSE and scores on a mnemonics usage scale, but several studies have shown that MSE is not significantly linked to the tendency to use such strategies (McDonald-Miszczak et al., 1999; Wells & Esopenko, 2008). Furthermore, in a recent study, Wells and Esopenko (2008) did not find a relationship between MSE and the amount of time participants spent on a free-recall task. MSE, however, has been shown to impact goal systems and the choice of activities (Berry & West, 1993; West et al., 2009). According to the results obtained by Bagwell and West (2008), MSE also predicts investment in memory intervention programs.

A potential mechanism linking control beliefs to better health is engagement in beneficial health-related behaviors. Those who have a higher sense of control are more likely to exercise regularly, eat a healthier diet, and therefore have better health (Lachman & Firth, 2004). According to the social-cognitive model of physical activity by Bandura (1997), self-efficacy is a primary determinant of consistent, health-promoting levels of physical activity. It is important to note, however, that the relationship between exercise self-efficacy beliefs and exercise behaviors is reciprocal. Behavior change is also determined by outcome expectations or sense of controllability; that is, whether one expects one's actions to lead to desirable outcomes. One might have high self-efficacy for exercise, but if one believes that exercise does not do anything to prevent or remediate aging-related losses, there would be little motivation to continue exercising (Lachman, 2006; Lachman et al., 1997). In a longitudinal investigation of exercise self-efficacy and control beliefs in a sample of previously sedentary older adults with at least one disability, Neupert, Lachman & Whitbourne (2009) found that exercise beliefs and exercise behavior were associated with one another and that beliefs developed during an intervention were important for maintenance of an exercise regimen. Those with higher control beliefs chose to use higher intensity and resistance levels during the intervention, and were more likely to continue exercising 9 to 12 months after the intervention program ended.

Findings about control as a moderating or buffering factor are also promising. Lachman and Weaver (1998b) found that the relationship between SES and health was moderated by a sense of control. The social gradient of health is well-documented; those with lower SES, either measured by income or educational attainment, are more likely to have poor health (Adler et al., 1993). What is less well known is under what conditions the gradient can be reduced. Findings suggest that a sense of control is one psychosocial factor that can buffer the effects of low SES. Although those in the lower SES groups, on average, have a lower sense of control, there are individual differences, and indeed overlapping distributions. Most interesting is that among middle-aged and older adults with lower SES, those who also manage to have a high sense of control have health levels comparable to their high education counterparts (Lachman & Weaver, 1998b). This is promising in that it suggests that sense of control is one modifiable factor that can help those in lower SES groups to break the cycle of poor health. One challenge is to determine how it is that some in the lower SES groups are able to develop a high sense of control in the face of the real difficulties of making ends meet. This issue is similar to the challenge of helping older adults to maintain a sense of control in the face of real changes and losses associated with aging. In future work, it would be useful to consider whether older adults with a high sense of control have health and cognitive functioning more comparable to young adults.

Rodin et al. (1985) proposed physiological explanations for the stress buffering effect of control beliefs. They argued that external control beliefs may have certain immunosuppressive tendencies that reduce the number of helper cells and lower the ability of T cells to function properly, which may lead to health problems. Bollini et al. (2004) found that locus of control moderated the relation between *control* and *cortisol* (a stress hormone); participants with more internal locus of control, who also *perceived* themselves to have *control* over the stressor, showed a reduced *cortisol* response. Higher control beliefs are also associated with physiological changes such as reduced heart rate reactivity and increased blood pressure in stressful situations (Baker & Stephenson, 2000; Sanz & Villamarín, 2001). In a study of older adults, Rodin (1983) found that those who received self-regulation/coping skills training showed a significant relationship between decreased *cortisol* level and increased *perceived control* and ratings of improved physical health. Wrosch, Miller, & Schulz (2009) found that adaptive control strategies minimized cortisol secretions associated with functional disabilities among older adults.

Whereas these summarized studies have provided insight into physiological reactions to stressors in the laboratory and individual differences in the buffering effects of control beliefs on the relationship between stressor exposure and well-being (e.g., Krause & Stryker, 1984), other recent studies have begun to examine these relationships as they unfold over time within the context of daily experiences. For example, greater personal control is related to reduced reactivity to stressors in daily life (e.g., Ong et al., 2005). When faced with stressful situations, a strong sense of control has also been linked to low levels of self-reported perceived stress and lower risk of depression (Yates Tennstedt, & Chang, 1999). Higher levels of perceived control also buffered recently bereaved wives from anxiety when they confronted daily stressors (Ong et al., 2005). Age and control beliefs played an important role in reactivity to daily interpersonal, network, and work stressors in the National Study of Daily Experiences subproject of the MIDUS survey (Neupert et al., 2007). Older age and lower perceived constraints were each related to lower emotional and physical reactivity to interpersonal stressors. High personal mastery buffered the physical effects of work stressors for younger and older adults and was important for middle-aged adults' emotional reactivity to network stressors. Those who had low perceived control, as indicated by reports of high levels of environmental constraints, had the strongest physical reactivity to network stressors for younger and older adults.

Another promising area of future research involves the examination of intraindividual variability in control beliefs as they relate to responses to stressors. Neupert, Ennis et al. (2009) examined the role of daily fluctuations in control beliefs regarding daily stressors with respect to emotional reactivity to daily stressors among older adults over eight days. Results indicated that a majority (66%) of the variance in daily control beliefs regarding stressors was due to within-person fluctuations over time, highlighting the importance of examining control beliefs with a process-oriented approach (e.g., Eizenman et al., 1997). Reactivity to stressors was heightened on days with decreased control beliefs and was buffered on days with increased control beliefs. These results suggest that fluctuations in daily control beliefs play an important role in minimizing the affective response to daily stressors in older adults, but future work examining additional responses such as physical and cognitive outcomes as well as comparisons with younger and middle-aged adults is needed.

Much of the research on physiological mechanisms linking control beliefs and health has focused on the HPA axis. Other areas showing promise for a more complete understanding of mind-body processes include immune functioning, inflammatory responses, and the autonomic nervous system (Cacioppo, 1994; Seeman, 1991).

INTERVENTIONS TO MODIFY CONTROL BELIEFS

Given the apparent benefits of high control beliefs and the likelihood of declines in sense of control in later life, it is worthwhile to consider whether and how control beliefs can be enhanced. There are a number of studies that examined whether it is possible to modify control beliefs among older adults and if this would affect outcomes in a given domain. Many adults assume they are too old to improve performance or functioning or to make up for losses in areas associated with aging, such as memory or physical ability. Given these widespread beliefs, interventions to change memory and health behaviors may be more successful if beliefs about control (abilities and contingencies) are also directly addressed in conjunction with skills training. Just focusing on performance experience does not seem to be enough to result in behavior change for older adults, perhaps because maladaptive beliefs about aging interfere (Bandura, 1997). Thus, interventions with a joint focus on modifying control beliefs (e.g., for memory or falls) and acquiring new skills and behaviors (e.g., strategy use, physical activity) may be most effective (Lachman et al., 1997). A key assumption of this multifaceted approach is that enduring behavior change is unlikely without first instilling confidence that aging-related declines can be controlled. For example, a fear of falling is relatively common among older adults and results in reduced activity. This is typically manifested as a low sense of efficacy for engaging in activities without falling and a sense that falling is uncontrollable (Tennstedt et al., 1998).

Several studies have shown that perceptions of personal control can be manipulated experimentally. They can be modified using different procedures such as presenting participants with scenarios in which they do or do not have control over the outcome (Laurin et al., 2008), asking them to recall recent events over which they did or did not have control (Kay et al., 2008), providing random feedback or feedback contingent on participants' responses (Whitson & Galinsky, 2008), or cognitive restructuring (Lachman et al., 1992). Perceived leisure control (the extent to which the individual perceives control of events and outcomes in his or her leisure experiences), but not the general sense of control, was increased in older adults by a leisure education program (Searle et al., 1995). However, over the long run (16-18 week follow-up), there also was significant improvement in the generalized measure of locus of control (Searle et al., 1998).

A classic intervention study was carried out by Langer and Rodin (1996) with nursing home residents. They were given more control over the environment (e.g., taking care of a plant, choosing activities), and this had positive long-term effects on well-being, activity, and health. Schulz (1976) found that nursing home residents who were given predictability and control over the timing of visits from student volunteers had higher well-being in the short run compared to those who did not have an influence on the visiting schedule. However, after the visiting program ended, those who had been given the most control and predictability suffered the most negative consequences, suggesting that providing control temporarily and removing it can have deleterious effects (Schulz & Hanusa, 1978).

Consistent with a cognitive behavioral framework, in which performance and beliefs interact over time, the best predictor of self-efficacy and control with respect to falling is previous fall status, and low falls self-efficacy is associated with maladaptive behavioral changes such as activity restriction, which can lead to increased risk of falling through muscle atrophy and deconditioning (Lachman et al., 1997). A multifaceted intervention, "A Matter of Balance," targeted beliefs about control over falls with older adults who reported fear of falling and were randomly assigned to an intervention or a contact comparison condition (Tennstedt et al., 1998). Cognitive-restructuring strategies were used to reframe control beliefs. This entailed analysis and challenge of maladaptive beliefs (e.g., "I can't do this," "I am too old," "It won't do any good," "I will get hurt") and information that efforts (e.g., using fall-prevention strategies; engaging in strength and balance exercises, which were also taught to participants) can make a difference for outcomes. Those who completed the treatment increased their falls self-efficacy, sense of control over falls, level of intended activity, and physical mobility functioning significantly more than the comparison group did (Tennstedt et al., 1998).

Another intervention study with older adults administered a home-based resistance training program in conjunction with cognitive restructuring of beliefs about the ability to engage in exercise and whether doing exercise would make a difference for health and well-being (Jette et al., 1999). The subjects had at least one functional limitation, and the goal was to determine if those who had already suffered some disability could break the cycle of decline. They found improvements in strength, and participation and adherence rates were higher than in previous studies, but exercise control beliefs did not increase significantly more in the treatment group. Nevertheless, those who had higher exercise control beliefs during the intervention increased their exercise intensity and resistance level significantly more than those with lower control beliefs and were more likely to be exercising three to six months after the intervention was completed (Neupert et al., 2009b).

Although there is some promise for modifying control beliefs, the effects of control interventions seem to be moderated by preexisting control beliefs (Reich & Zautra, 1990) or level of cognitive functioning. For instance, Anderson-Hanley et al. (2003) showed that following a control-enhancing intervention, those with an internal locus of control and higher levels of cognitive functioning benefitted the most in terms of perceived health efficacy. Further work is needed to develop interventions to promote a sense of control, especially among those who are most vulnerable to losing a sense of control, such as those suffering from hip fracture or memory problems or those from disadvantaged socioeconomic and minority groups.

SUMMARY, CONCLUSIONS, AND FUTURE DIRECTIONS

Adults and those in later life with a high sense of control appear better off on many indicators of health and well-being. However, those who have a lower sense of control may be at increased risk for a wide range of negative behavioral, affective, and functional outcomes, including higher levels of depression, anxiety, and stress, use of fewer health protective behaviors (e.g., exercise) and compensatory memory strategies (e.g., internal or external memory aids), and have poorer health and memory functioning. The apparent decline of the sense of control associated with aging is of concern especially given the adaptive value of maintaining beliefs in one's control over outcomes. We have presented a wealth of information about control beliefs, but there is much to explore before we understand the dynamic processes involved in changes and the linkages with outcomes. Sense of control is a promising dimension because it is amenable to change unlike more traditional stable personality traits (Hooker & McAdams, 2003). This can potentially lead us in the direction of new interventions to promote optimal aging.

Although age and education differences in health are pervasive and account for much of the variance in functioning, the sense of control has the potential to mediate or moderate some proportion of the differences. It is not just that beliefs play out as a self-fulfilling prophecy or through wishful thinking. A sense of control is a fundamental core set of self-regulatory beliefs that affects how situations are perceived and provides motivation for whether or not to exert effort or attempt new tasks (Bandura, 1997). The sense of control is a powerful psychosocial factor that influences health and well-being through behavioral and physiological means. Having a sense of control puts those from different levels of SES on a more common ground in terms of health and well-being (Lachman & Weaver, 1998b). The linkages identified between control and stress show promise for improving health and aging outcomes. Those who have a low sense of control may experience more stress with physical consequences because of the feeling that there is nothing that can be done, which goes against the basic human needs for agency and motives to be effective.

The sense of control may dwindle with age, yet it is important to note that some are able to maintain control especially in selected domains. Thus, an important direction for future research is to understand how to harness the sense of control and to widen the net of control in later life. This may lead to developing prevention-oriented interventions for young and middle-aged adults, to promote a sense of control over aging before declines and losses become salient (Lachman, 2004). Previous research has looked primarily at the consequences of control beliefs and relatively few studies have focused on their sources or directly addressed issues of causality and directionality (Lachman, 2006). Further understanding of the distal and proximal antecedents of control beliefs could reveal how to create optimal conditions for promoting a resilient sense of control.

Research on the sense of control can also teach us important lessons about the psychology of aging, more generally. Of utmost importance is that expectancies make a difference for the course of aging, and sense of control is chief among them. Despite the apparent value of perceived control, a recognition that some aspects of life are not under personal control is a key part of adaptive aging. This requires a delicate balance of knowing when to persist and when to switch gears, with the healthy realization that some aspects of aging are out of one's hands. Throughout the chapter we have made suggestions about new directions for work on control beliefs and aging. As more researchers continue to incorporate this construct in their work, it will give us the opportunities to learn more about the power and potential of control beliefs for understanding aging-related changes and for enhancing performance and functioning throughout adulthood and old age.

ACKNOWLEDGMENTS

We appreciate the multiple sources of support that facilitated preparation of this chapter, including NIA grants RO1 AG17920 and PO1 AG20166. This chapter was written while the first author was a fellow at the Center for Advanced Study in the Behavioral Sciences at Stanford University and a member of the working group sponsored by the Stanford Longevity Center.

REFERENCES

Abeles, R. (1991). Sense of control, quality of life, and frail older people. In J. E. Birren, J. E. Lubben, J. C. Rowe, & D. E. Deutschman (Eds.), *The concept and measurement of quality of life in the frail elderly* (pp. 297–314). San Diego, CA: Academic Press.

Adler, N. E., Boyce, W. T., Chesney, M. A., Folkman, S., & Syme, S. L. (1993). Socioeconomic inequalities in health: No easy solution. *Journal of the American Medical Association, 269,* 3140–3145.

Agrigoroaei, S., & Lachman, M. E. (2010). Personal control and aging: How beliefs and expectations matter: In J. C. Cavanaugh & C. K. Cavanaugh (Eds.), *Aging in America: Psychological aspects* (Vol. 1, pp. 177–201). Santa Barbara, CA: Praeger. Perspectives.

Anderson-Hanley, C., Meshberg, S. R., & Marsh, M. A. (2003). The effects of a control-enhancing intervention for nursing home residents: Cognition and locus of control as moderators. *Palliative and Supportive Care, 1,* 111–120.

Andreoletti, C., Veratti, B., & Lachman, M. E. (2006). Age differences in the relationship between anxiety and recall. *Aging & Mental Health, 10,* 265–271.

Antonucci, T. C. (2001). Social relations: An examination of social networks, social support, and sense of control. In J. E. Birren & K. W. Schaie (Eds.), *Handbook of the psychology of aging* (5th ed., pp. 427–453). San Diego, CA: Academic Press.

Ashman, O., Shiomura, K., & Levy, B. R. (2006). Influence of culture and age on control beliefs: The missing link of interdependence. *International Journal of Aging and Human Development, 62,* 143–157.

Bagwell, D. K., & West, R. L. (2008). Assessing compliance: Active versus inactive trainees in a memory intervention. *Clinical Interventions in Aging, 3,* 371–382.

Baker, S. R., & Stephenson, D. (2000). Prediction and control as determinants of behavioural uncertainty: Effects on task performance and heart rate reactivity. *Integrative Physiological and Behavioral Science, 35,* 235–250.

Baltes, M. M. (1995). Dependency in old age: Gains and losses. *Current Directions in Psychological Science, 4,* 14–19.

Baltes, M. M., Lindenberger, U., & Staudinger, U. M. (2006). Life span theory in developmental psychology. In W. Damon & R. M. Lerner (Eds.), *Handbook of child psychology: Theoretical models of human development* (Vol. 1, pp. 569–664). New York: Wiley.

Bandura, A. (1990). Perceived self-efficacy in the exercise of personal agency. *Journal of Applied Sport Psychology, 2,* 128–163.

Bandura, A. (1997). *Self-efficacy: The exercise of control.* New York: Freeman.

Berry, J. M., & West, R. L. (1993). Cognitive self-efficacy in relation to personal mastery and goal setting across the life span. *International Journal of Behavioral Development, 16,* 351–379.

Bisconti, T. L., Bergeman, C. S., & Boker, S. M. (2006). Social support as a predictor of variability: An examination of the adjustment trajectories of recent widows. *Psychology and Aging, 21,* 590–599.

Blatt-Eisengart, I., & Lachman, M. E. (2004). Attributions for memory performance in adulthood: Age differences and mediation effects. *Aging, Neuropsychology, and Cognition, 11,* 68–79.

Bollini, A. M., Walker, E. F., Hamann, S., & Kestler, L. (2004). The influence of perceived control and locus of control on the cortisol and subjective responses to stress. *Biological Psychiatry, 67*, 245–260.

Brandtstädter, J., & Renner, G. (1990). Tenacious goal pursuit and flexible goal adjustment: Explication and age-related analysis of assimilative and accommodative strategies of coping. *Psychology and Aging, 5*, 58–67.

Brandtstädter, J., & Rothermund, K. (1994). Self-percepts of control in middle and later adulthood: Buffering losses by rescaling goals. *Psychology and Aging, 9*, 265–273.

Brim, O. G. (1974). *The sense of control over one's life.* Paper presented at the American Psychological Association, New Orleans, LA.

Bruce, M. A., & Thornton, M. C. (2004). It's my world? Exploring black and white perceptions of personal control. *The Sociological Quarterly, 45*, 597–612.

Cacioppo, J. T. (1994). Social neuroscience: Autonomic, neuroendocrine, and immune response to stress. *Psychophysiology, 31*, 113–128.

Caplan, L. J., & Schooler, C. (2003). The roles of fatalism, self-confidence, and intellectual resources in the disablement process in older adults. *Psychology and Aging, 18*, 551–561.

Carstensen, L. L., & Hartel, C. R. (2006). *When I'm 64. Committee on aging frontiers in social psychology, personality, and adult developmental psychology.* National Research Council Washington DC: National Academies Press.

Chipperfield, J. G., Campbell, D. W., & Perry, R. P. (2004). Stability in perceived control: Implications for health among very old community-dwelling adults. *Journal of Aging and Health, 16*, 116–147.

Czaja, S. J., Charness, N., Fisk, A. D., Hertzog, C., Nair, S. N., Rogers, W. A. & Sharit, J. (2006). Factors predicting the use of technology: Findings from the Center for Research and Education and Aging and Technology Enhancement (CREATE). *Psychology and Aging, 21*, 333–352.

de Frias, C. M., Dixon, R. A., & Bäckman, L. (2003). Use of memory compensation strategies is related to psychosocial and health indicators. *Journals of Gerontology: Psychological Sciences, 58B*, P12–P22.

Desrichard, O., & Köpetz, C. (2005). A threat in the elder: The impact of task-instructions, self-efficacy and performance expectations on memory performance in the elderly. *European Journal of Social Psychology, 35*, 537–552.

Dickerson, S. S., & Kemeny, M. E. (2004). Acute stressors and cortisol responses: A theoretical integration and synthesis of laboratory research. *Psychological Bulletin, 130*, 355–391.

Eizenman, D. R., Nesselroade, J. R., Featherman, D. L., & Rowe, J. W. (1997). Intraindividual variability in perceived control in an older sample: The MacArthur successful aging studies. *Psychology and Aging, 12*, 489–502.

Fiorri, K. L., Brown, E. E., Cortina, K. S., & Antonucci, T. (2006). Locus of control as a mediator of the relationship between religiosity and life satisfaction: Age, race, and gender differences. *Mental Health, Religion & Culture, 9*, 239–263.

Gatz, M., & Karel, M. J. (1993). Individual change in perceived control over 20 years. *International Journal of Behavioral Development, 16*, 305–322.

Grover, D. R., & Hertzog, C. (1991). Relationships between intellectual control beliefs and psychometric intelligence in adulthood. *Journals of Gerontology: Psychological Sciences, 46B*, P109–P115.

Heckhausen, J., Wrosch, C., & Schulz, R. (2010). A motivational theory of lifespan development. *Psychological Review, 117*, 32–60.

Hertzog, C., Dunlosky, J., & Robinson, A. E. (2003). *Control beliefs influence strategic behavior in associative learning.* Paper presented at the 57th Annual Meeting of the Gerontological Society of America, San Diego, CA, November.

Hertzog, C., McGuire, C. L., & Lineweaver, T. T. (1998). Aging, attributions, perceived control, and strategy use in a free recall task. *Aging, Neuropsychology, and Cognition, 5*, 85–106.

Hess, T. M. (2006). Attitudes toward aging and their effects on behavior. In J. E. Birren & K. W. Schaie (Eds.), *Handbook of the psychology of aging* (6th ed., pp. 379–406). Boston, MA: Academic Press.

Hooker, K., & McAdams, D. P. (2003). Personality reconsidered: A new agenda for aging research. *Journals of Gerontology: Psychological Sciences, 58B*, P296–P304.

Hultsch, D. F., Hertzog, C., Dixon, R. A., & Small, B. J. (1998). *Memory change in the aged.* Cambridge, UK: Cambridge University Press.

Hultsch, D. F., MacDonald, S. W. S., & Dixon, R. A. (2002). Variability in reaction time performance of younger and older adults. *Journals of Gerontology: Psychological Sciences, 57B*, P101–P115.

Jette, A. M., Lachman, M. E., Giorgetti, M. M., Assmann, S. F., Harris, B. A., Levenson, C., Krebs, D. (1999). Exercise: It's never too late: the strong-for-life program. *American Journal of Public Health, 89*, 66–72.

Kay, A. C., Gaucher, D., Napier, J. L., Callan, M. J., & Laurin, K. (2008). God and the government: Testing a compensatory control mechanism for the support of external systems. *Journal of Personality and Social Psychology, 95*, 18–35.

Kirschbaum, C., Wolf, O. T., May, M., Wippich, W., & Hellhammer, D. H. (1996). Stress- and treatment-induced elevations of cortisol levels associated with impaired declarative memory in healthy adults. *Life Sciences, 58*, 1475–1483.

Krause, N. (2007). Age and decline in role-specific feelings of control. *Journals of Gerontology: Social Sciences, 62B*, S28–S35.

Krause, N., & Stryker, S. (1984). Stress and well-being: The buffering role of locus of control beliefs. *Social Science & Medicine, 18*, 783–790.

Kunzmann, U., Little, T., & Smith, J. (2002). Perceiving control: A double-edged sword in old age. *Journals of Gerontology: Psychological Sciences, 57B*, P484–P491.

Lachman, M. E. (1985). Personal efficacy in middle and old age: Differential and normative patterns of change. In G. H. Elder, Jr. (Ed.) *Life-course dynamics: Trajectories and transitions, 1968–1980* (pp. 188–213). Ithaca, NY: Cornell University Press.

Lachman, M. E. (1986). Locus of Control in aging research: A case for multidimensional and domain-specific assessment. *Journal of Psychology and Aging, 1,* 34–40.

Lachman, M. E. (2004). Development in midlife. *Annual Review of Psychology, 55,* 305–331.

Lachman, M. E. (2006). Perceived control over aging-related declines: Adaptive beliefs and behaviors. *Current Directions in Psychological Science, 15,* 282–286.

Lachman, M. E., & Andreoletti, C. (2006). Strategy use mediates the relationship between control beliefs and memory performance for middle-aged and older adults. *Journals of Gerontology: Psychological Sciences, 61B,* P88–P94.

Lachman, M. E., & Firth, K. M. (2004). The adaptive value of feeling in control during midlife. In O. G. Brim, C. D. Ryff, & R. Kessler (Eds.), *How healthy are we? A national study of well-being at midlife* (pp. 320–349). Chicago: University of Chicago Press.

Lachman, M. E., Jette, A., Tennstedt, S., Howland, J., Harris, B. A., & Peterson, E. (1997). A cognitive-behavioral model for promoting regular physical activity in older adults. *Psychology, Health, and Medicine, 2,* 251–261.

Lachman, M. E., Röcke, C., Rosnick, C., & Ryff, C. D. (2008). Realism and illusion in Americans' temporal views of their life satisfaction: Age differences in reconstructing the past and anticipating the future. *Psychological Science, 19,* 889–897.

Lachman, M. E., Rosnick, C. B., & Röcke, C. (2009). The rise and fall of control beliefs in adulthood: Cognitive and biopsychosocial antecedents and consequences of stability and change over nine years. In H. B. Bosworth & C. Herzog (Ed.), *Aging and Cognition: Research methodologies and empirical advances* (pp. 143–460). Washington, D.C.

Lachman, M. E., & Weaver, S. L. (1998a). Sociodemographic variations in the sense of control by domain: Findings from the MacArthur studies of midlife. *Psychology and Aging, 13,* 553–562.

Lachman, M. E., & Weaver, S. L. (1998b). The sense of control as a moderator of social class differences in health and well-being. *Journal of Personality and Social Psychology, 74,* 763–773.

Lachman, M. E., Weaver, S. L., Bandura, M., Elliott, E., & Lewkowicz, C. J. (1992). Improving memory and control beliefs through cognitive restructuring and self-generated strategies. *Journals of Gerontology: Psychological Sciences, 47B,* P293–P299.

Lachman, M. E., Ziff, M. A., & Spiro, A., III. (1994). Maintaining a sense of control in later life. In R. P. Abeles, H. C. Gift, & M. G. Ory (Eds.), *Aging and quality of life* (pp. 216–232). New York: Springer.

Langer, E., & Rodin, J. (1976). The effects of choice and enhanced personal responsibility for the aged: A field experiment in an institutional setting. *Journal of Personality and Social Psychology, 34,* 191–198.

Langer, E., & Rodin, J. (1996). Long-term effects of a control-relevant intervention with the institutionalized aged. In S. Fein & S. Spencer (Eds.), *Reading in social psychology: The art and science of research* (pp. 175–180). Boston: Houghton Mifflin.

Laurin, K., Kay, A. C., & Moscovitch, D. A. (2008). On the belief in God: Towards an understanding of the emotional substrates of compensatory control. *Journal of Experimental Social Psychology, 44,* 1559–1562.

Lefcourt, H. M. (1984). *Research with the locus of control construct: Extensions and limitations* (Vol. 3). Orlando, FL: Academic Press.

Leland, J. (2004, June 13). Faith in the future: Why America sees the silver lining. *The New York Times, Section 4,* 1.

Levy, B. R., Zonderman, A. B., Slade, M. D., & Ferrucci, L. (2009). Age stereotypes held earlier in life predict cardiovascular events in later life. *Psychological Science, 20,* 296–298.

Levy, B., Hausdorff, J. M., Hencke, R., & Wei, J. Y. (2000). Reducing cardiovascular stress with positive self-stereotypes of aging. *Journals of Gerontology: Psychological Sciences, 55B,* P205–P213.

Lupien, S. J., Gaudreau, S., Tchiteya, B. M., Maheu, F., Sharma, S., Nair, N. P. V. Meaney, M. J. (1997). Stress-induced declarative memory impairment in healthy elderly subjects: Relationship to cortisol reactivity. *Journal of Clinical Endocrinology and Metabolism, 82,* 2070–2075.

Markus, H. R., & Kitayama, S. (1991). Culture and the self: Implications for cognition, emotion, and motivation. *Psychological Review, 98,* 224–253.

Marmot, M. G. (2004). *The status syndrome. How social standing affects our health and longevity.* New York: Time Books.

Martin, M., & Hofer, S. M. (2004). Intraindividual variability, change, and aging: Conceptual and analytical issues. *Gerontology, 50,* 7–11.

McDonald-Miszczak, L., Gould, O. N., & Tychynski, D. (1999). Metamemory predictors of prospective and retrospective memory performance. *The Journal of General Psychology, 126,* 37–52.

McEwen, B. S., & Sapolsky, R. M. (1995). Stress and cognitive function. *Current Opinion in Neurobiology, 5,* 205–216.

Midlarsky, E., & Kahana, E. (1994). *Altruism in later life.* Thousand Oaks, CA: Sage Publications.

Miller, L. M. S., & Gagne, D. D. (2005). Effects of age and control beliefs on resource allocation during reading. *Aging, Neuropsychology, and cognition, 12,* 129–148.

Miller, L. M. S., & Lachman, M. E. (1999). The sense of control and cognitive aging: Toward a model of mediational processes. In T. M. Hess & F. Blanchard-Fields (Eds.), *Social Cognition and aging* (pp. 17–41). New York: Academic Press.

Miller, L. M. S., & Lachman, M. E. (2000). Cognitive performance and the role of control beliefs in midlife. *Aging, Neuropsychology, and Cognition, 7,* 69–85.

Mirowsky, J., Ross, C., & Van Willigen, M. (1996). Instrumentalism in the land of opportunity: Socioeconomic causes and emotional consequences. *Social Psychology Quarterly, 59*, 322–337.

Mirowsky, J., & Ross, C. E. (2007). Life course trajectories of perceived control and their relationship to education. *American Journal of Sociology, 112*, 1339–1382.

Müller, M. M., Günther, A., Habel, I., & Rockstroh, B. (1998). Active coping and internal Locus of Control produces prolonged cardiovascular reactivity in young men. *Journal of Psychophysiology, 12*, 29–39.

Nesselroade, J. R., & Salthouse, T. A. (2004). Methodological and theoretical implications of intraindividual variability in perceptual-motor performance. *Journals of Gerontology: Psychological Sciences, 59B*, P49–P55.

Neupert, S. D., Almeida, D. M., & Charles, S. T. (2007). Age differences in reactivity to daily stressors: The role of personal control. *Journals of Gerontology: Psychological Sciences, 62B*, P216–P225.

Neupert, S. D., Ennis, G. E., Davis, A. A., Rojas, V. A., Mroczek, D. K., & Spiro A., III. (2009). *Daily control beliefs: Implications for reactivity to daily stressors in older adults.* Paper presented at the American Psychological Association Convention, Toronto, Canada.

Neupert, S. D., Lachman, M. E., & Whitbourne, S. B. (2009). Exercise self-efficacy and control beliefs: Effects on exercise behavior after an exercise intervention for older adults. *Journal of Aging and Physical Activity, 17*, 1–16.

Ong, A. D., Bergeman, C. S., & Bisconti, T. L. (2005). Unique effects of daily perceived control on anxiety symptomatology during conjugal bereavement. *Personality and Individual Differences, 38*, 1057–1067.

Pearlin, L. I., & Pioli, M. F. (2003). Personal Control: Some conceptual turf and future directions. In S. H. Zarit, L. I. Pearlin, & K. W. Schaie (Eds.), *Personal control in social and life course contexts* (pp. 1–21). New York, NY: Springer Publishing Co.

Rebok, G. W., Rasmusson, D. X., & Brandt, J. (1996). Prospects for computerized memory training in normal elderly: Effects of practice on explicit and implicit memory tasks. *Applied Cognitive Psychology, 10*, 211–223.

Reich, J. W., & Zautra, A. J. (1990). Dispositional control beliefs and the consequences of a control-enhancing intervention. *Journals of Gerontology, 45*, P46–P51.

Roberts, M. L., & Nesselroade, J. R. (1986). Intraindividual variability in perceived locus of control in adults: P-technique factor analyses of short-term change. *Journal of Research in Personality, 20*, 529–545.

Röcke, C., Li, S.-C., & Smith, J. (2009). Intraindividual variability in positive and negative affect over 45 days: Do older adults fluctuate less than young adults? *Psychology and Aging, 24*, 863–878.

Rodin, J. (1983). Behavioral medicine: Beneficial effects of self control training in aging. *International Review of Applied Psychology, 32*, 153–181.

Rodin, J. (1986). Aging and health: Effects of the sense of control. *Science, 233*, 1271–1276.

Rodin, J. (1990). Control by any other name: Definitions, concepts, and processes. In J. Rodin, C. Schooler, & K. W. Schaie (Eds.), *Self-directedness: Cause and effects throughout the life course* (pp. 1–17). Hillsdale, NJ: Lawrence Erlbaum Associates.

Rodin, J., & Langer, E. J. (1977). Long-term effects of a control-relevant intervention with the institutionalized aged. *Journal of Personality and Social Psychology, 35*, 897–902.

Rodin, J., & Langer, E. J. (1980). Aging labels: The decline of control and the fall of self-esteem. *Journal of Social Issues, 36*, 12–29.

Rodin, J., Timko, C., & Harris, S. (1985). The construct of control: Biological and psychological correlates. *Annual Review of Gerontology and Geriatrics, 5*, 3–55.

Rotter, J. B. (1966). Generalized expectancies for internal versus external control of reinforcement. *Psychological Monographs: General and Applied, 80*, 1–28.

Rowe, J. W., & Kahn, R. L. (1998). *Successful aging*. New York: Pantheon Books.

Sanz, A., & Villamarín, F. (2001). The role of perceived control in physiological reactivity: Self-efficacy and incentive value as regulators of cardiovascular adjustment. *Biological Psychology, 56*, 219–246.

Sastry, J., & Ross, C. E. (1998). Asian ethnicity and the sense of personal control. *Social Psychology Quarterly, 61*, 101–120.

Schulz, R. (1976). Effects of control and predictability on the physical and psychological well-being of the institutionalized aged. *Journal of Personality and Social Psychology, 33*, 563–573.

Schulz, R., & Hanusa, B. H. (1978). Long-term effects of control and predictability-enhancing interventions: Findings and ethical issues. *Journal of Personality and Social Psychology, 36*, 1194–1201.

Schulz, R., & Heckhausen, J. (1999). Aging, culture and control: Setting a new research agenda. *Journals of Gerontology: Psychological Sciences, 54B*, P139–P145.

Searle, M. S., Mahon, M. J., Iso-Ahola, S. E., Sdrolias, H. A., & van Dyck, J. (1995). Enhancing a sense of independence and psychological well-being among the elderly: A field experiment. *Journal of Leisure Research, 27*, 107–124.

Searle, M. S., Mahon, M. J., Iso-Ahola, S. E., Sdrolias, H. A., & van Dyck, J. (1998). Examining the long term effects of leisure education on a sense of independence and psychological well-being among the elderly. *Journal of Leisure Research, 30*, 331–340.

Seeman, T. E. (1991). Personal control and coronary artery disease: How generalized expectancies about control may influence disease risk. *Journal of Psychosomatic Medicine, 35*, 661–669.

Seeman, T. E., McAvay, G., Merrill, S., Albert, M., & Rodin, J. (1996). Self-efficacy beliefs and change in cognitive performance: MacArthur studies of successful aging. *Psychology and Aging, 11*, 538–551.

Seeman, T. E., & Robbins, R. J. (1994). Aging and hypothalamic-pituitary-adrenal response to challenge in humans. *Endocrine Reviews, 15*, 233–260.

Shaw, B. A., & Krause, N. (2001). Exploring race variations in aging and personal control. *Journals of Gerontology: Social Sciences, 56B*, S119–S124.

Shupe, D. R. (1985). Perceived control, helplessness, and choice: Their relationship to health and aging. In J. E. Birren & J. Livingston (Eds.), *Cognition, stress, and aging* (pp. 174–197). Englewood Cliffs, NJ: Prentice Hall.

Skaff, M. M. (2007). Sense of control and health: A dynamic duo in the aging process. In C. M. Aldwin, C. L. Park, & A. Spiro, III. (Eds.), *Handbook of health psychology and aging* (pp. 186–209). New York: Guilford Press.

Skaff, M. M., & Gardiner, P. (2003). Cultural variations in meaning of control. In S. H. Zarit, L. I. Pearlin, & K. W. Schaie (Eds.), *Personal control in social and life course contexts* (pp. 83–105). New York: Springer Publishing Co.

Skaff, M. M., Mullan, J. T., Fisher, L., & Chesla, C. A. (2003). A contextual model of control beliefs, behavior, and health: Latino and European Americans with type 2 diabetes. *Psychology and Health, 18*, 295–312.

Skinner, E. A. (1996). A guide to constructs of control. *Journal of Personality and Social Psychology, 71*, 549–570.

Sliwinski, M. J., Hofer, S. M., & Hall, C. (2003). Correlated and coupled cognitive change in older adults with and without preclinical dementia. *Psychology and Aging, 18*, 672–683.

Tennstedt, S., Howland, J., Lachman, M. E., Peterson, E. W., Kasten, L., & Jette, A. (1998). A randomized, controlled trial of a group intervention to reduce fear of falling and associated activity restriction in older adults. *Journals of Gerontology: Psychological Sciences, 53B*, P384–P392.

Thompson, S. C. (1999). Illusions of control: How we overestimate our personal influence. *Current Directions in Psychological Science, 8*, 187–190.

Touron, D. R., & Hertzog, C. (2004). Distinguishing age differences in knowledge, strategy use, and confidence during strategic skill acquisition. *Psychology and Aging, 19*, 452–466.

Vaillant, G. E. (2002). *Aging Well: Surprising guideposts to a happier life from the landmark Harvard study of adult development.* Little, Brown and Company.

Wells, G. D., & Esopenko, C. (2008). Memory self-efficacy, aging, and memory performance: The roles of effort and persistence. *Educational Gerontology, 34*, 520–530.

West, R. L., Dark-Freudeman, A., & Bagwell, D. K. (2009). Goals-feedback conditions and episodic memory: Mechanisms for memory gains in older and younger adults. *Memory, 17*, 233–244.

West, R. L., & Yassuda, M. S. (2004). Aging and memory control beliefs: Performance in relation to goal setting and memory self-evaluation. *Journals of Gerontology: Psychological Sciences, 59B*, P56–P65.

Whitson, J. A., & Galinsky, A. D. (2008). Lacking control increases illusory pattern perception. *Science, 322*, 115–117.

Willis, S. L., & Schaie, K. W. (1999). Intellectual functioning in midlife. In S. L. Willis & J. D. Reid (Eds.), *Life in the middle: Psychological and social development in middle age* (pp. 233–247). San Diego, CA: Academic Press.

Windsor, T. D., & Anstey, K. J. (2008). A longitudinal investigation of perceived control and cognitive performance in young, midlife and older adults. *Aging, Neuropsychology, and Cognition, 15*, 744–763.

Wolinsky, F. D., & Stump, T. E. (1996). Age and sense of control among older adults. *Journals of Gerontology: Social Sciences, 51B*, S217–S220.

Wrosch, C., Heckhausen, J., & Lachman, M. E. (2000). Primary and secondary control strategies for managing health and financial stress across adulthood. *Psychology and Aging, 15*, 387–399.

Wrosch, C., Heckhausen, J., & Lachman, M. E. (2006). Goal management across adulthood and old age: The adaptive value of primary and secondary control. In D. K. Mroczek & T. D. Little (Eds.), *Handbook of personality development* (pp. 399–421). Mahwah, NJ: Lawrence Erlbaum Associates.

Wrosch, C., Miller, G. E., & Schulz, R. (2009). Cortisol secretion and functional disabilities in old age: The importance of using adaptive control strategies. *Psychosomatic Medicine, 71*, 996–1003.

Yamaguchi, S., Gelfand, M., Ohashi, M. M., & Zemba, Y. (2005). The cultural psychology of control: Illusions of personal versus collective control in the United States and Japan. *Journal of Cross-Cultural Psychology, 36*, 750–761.

Yates, M. E., Tennstedt, S., & Chang, B. H. (1999). Contributors to and mediators of psychological well-being for informal caregivers. *Journals of Gerontology: Psychological Sciences, 54B*, P12–P22.

Chapter | 12 |

The Speedometer of Life: Stress, Health and Aging

David M. Almeida, Jennifer R. Piazza, Robert S. Stawski, Laura C. Klein

Department of Human Development and Family Studies, The Pennsylvania State University, University Park, Pennsylvania, USA

CHAPTER CONTENTS

Introduction **191**

Concepts and Measurement of Stress Processes **192**

Stressor Pathways to Health and Well-Being **192**

Changes in Stress Processes Across Middle and Later Adulthood **193**

The Theory of Strength and Vulnerability Integration 194

Individual Differences in Stress Processes **194**

Physiology of the Stress Response and Age-Related Changes **196**

The SAM Axis 196

Age, Exposure to Stressors, and the SAM Axis 196

The HPA Axis 196

Age, Exposure to Stressors, and the HPA Axis 197

Gender Difference in Responses to Stress: Tend and Befriend **197**

Stress Age and Cognitive Health **198**

Summary and conclusions **199**

Acknowledgments **200**

References **200**

INTRODUCTION

The study of stress has long played an important role in the understanding of adult development and health. Over 50 years ago, Hans Selye wrote in the final pages of *The Stress of Life*: "Stress is the sum of all of the wear and tear caused by any kind of vital reaction throughout the body at any one time. That is why it can act as a common denominator of all of the biologic changes which go on in the body; it is a kind of 'speedometer of life'" (1956, p. 274). Indeed, since the pioneering work of Cannon (1932) and Selye (1956), research has focused on the biological and physiological effects of stressor exposure. Biological responses elicited by physical and psychological stressors include the release of catecholamines (e.g., norepinephrine, epinephrine release from the adrenal medulla), sympathetic arousal (e.g., increased blood pressure, elevated heart rate), and hypothalamic-pituitary-adrenal (HPA) axis activation (e.g., cortisol secretion from the adrenal cortex; see Klein & Corwin, 2007; Stratakis & Chrousos, 1995; Taylor et al., 2000 for reviews). Chronic exposure to these stress hormones leads to accumulated wear and tear on the body, referred to as "allostatic load" (McEwen & Stellar, 1993), which, in turn, contributes to an increased risk of illness and mortality (Kiecolt-Glaser et al., 2002). As such, the study of stress and aging are closely aligned. The purpose of this chapter is to describe the links between stress, health, and aging; to identify stress processes that lead to changes in key psychological and physiological indicators; and to examine the associations between biological indicators, health, and well-being.

Our view is grounded in a life-span developmental theory of stress and health that highlights variations and differences within and between individuals as they develop in multidimensional sociohistorical contexts (Baltes et al., 1999; Spiro, 2001). This theory posits that life experiences accumulate throughout the life course, with each stage of life reflecting both the consequences of prior experiences, as well

DOI: 10.1016/B978-0-12-380882-0.00012-7

as the antecedents for subsequent life experiences. In this chapter we provide a broad framework for incorporating the role of stress into the study of health and aging by describing: (1) concepts and measurement of stress processes, (2) life-span and life course perspectives on stressors and their consequences, (3) biomarkers that provide a link between stressors and health, and (4) emerging research documenting the effects of stress on cognitive health.

CONCEPTS AND MEASUREMENT OF STRESS PROCESSES

There are two prominent ways to think about the links between stress, health, and aging. One approach focuses on the molar impact of major life changes, and is referred to as the life event tradition (e.g., Dohrenwend, 2006; Holmes & Rahe, 1967). This approach examines the discrete, observable, and objectively reportable life changes that are relatively rare (e.g., divorce or job loss) and require significant adjustment on the part of the individual (Wheaton, 1997). The other approach takes a microscopic dynamic approach to stress processes, with a focus on the accumulation of daily stressors (Bolger et al., 2003; Pearlin, 1999). A growing body of research suggests that it is the myriad of these everyday events, or quotidian stressors (Almeida, 2005; Pearlin & Skaff, 1996), rather than the major, but less frequent, life events that most severely impact individual well-being (Lazarus & Folkman, 1984; Pearlin, 1982).

Quotidian stressors are divided into two classes: chronic stressors and daily hassles. Chronic stressors are the persistent or recurrent difficulties of life. One source of chronic stressors is the strains associated with the enactment of certain social roles (Pearlin, 1982, 1999; Pearlin et al., 1981; Wheaton, 1996), such as caregiving for a sick spouse. Another source of chronic stressors may arise from conflicting social roles experienced by individuals, such as being a working parent (Pearlin, 1999). Irrespective of the origin, there is agreement that it is the ongoing and open-ended nature of the stressor that qualifies it as chronic. Furthermore, it is often difficult to identify when the chronic stressor began and when — or even if — it will end (Wheaton, 1996, 1999).

In contrast to chronic stressors, daily hassles are defined as relatively minor events arising from day-to-day living, such as spousal conflict, specific caregiving activities, and work deadlines (Almeida, 2005). An emerging literature has shown that day-to-day stressors play an important part in health and emotional adjustment (Zautra, 2003). Daily stressors represent tangible, albeit minor interruptions that tend to have a more proximal effect on well-being than do major life events. In terms of their physiological and psychological effects, reports of life events may be associated with prolonged arousal, whereas reports of daily stressors may be associated with spikes in arousal or psychological distress during a particular day (Almeida, 2005). Minor daily stressors exert their influence through separate and immediate direct effects on emotional and physical functioning, and by piling up over a series of days to create persistent irritations, frustrations, and overloads that increase the risk of serious stress reactions, such as anxiety and depression (Lazarus, 1999; Pearlin et al., 1981; Zautra, 2003).

Many studies have established an association between health and life events (Dohrenwend, 2006; Brown & Harris, 1978), chronic stressors (Bolger et al., 1996; Eckenrode, 1984; Pillow et al., 1996), and daily hassles (Almeida, 2005; Bolger et al., 1989; Folkman et al., 1987). More recent work has extended this research by examining the linkages between these multiple dimensions of stress and their combined effect on psychological and physical health. Research that includes multiple types of stressors, such as those combining both life events, chronic stressors, and daily hassles, suggests that it is the interaction of stressors and the accumulation over time that leads to poor health outcomes, rather than the immediate and unique effects of a single stressor or type of stressor (Almeida & Wong, 2009; Chiriboga, 1997; Pearlin et al., 1981; Serido et al., 2004; Turner et al., 2000). Prior to being able to make the linkages between stress and health, however, it is necessary to understand developmental processes in stressor exposure and reactivity.

STRESSOR PATHWAYS TO HEALTH AND WELL-BEING

There are two primary pathways through which stressors impact well-being: stressor exposure and stressor reactivity. Stressor exposure is the likelihood that an individual will experience a stressor based on combinations of resilience and vulnerability factors. Experiencing stressors is not simply a matter of chance or bad luck; rather differences in stressor exposure more often emerge from individual sociodemographic, psychosocial, and situational factors (Pearlin, 1993a, 1999; Wheaton, 1997, 1999). There is substantial evidence that stable sociodemographic, psychosocial, and situational factors, such as age (Aldwin, 1990, 1991; Almeida & Horn, 2004; Hamarat et al., 2001), personality (Bouchard, 2003; Penley & Tomaka, 2002), and social support (Brewin et al., 1989; Felsten, 1991) play a significant role in differences in stressor frequency, content, and appraisal. The stressor exposure path contends that stressors and appraisals emerge from a combination of factors that in turn lead to changes in both self-reports and physiological markers of well-being.

Reactivity is the likelihood that an individual will show emotional or physical reactions to the stressors he or she encounters (Almeida, 2005; Bolger & Zuckerman, 1995; Cacioppo, 1998). In this sense, stressor reactivity is not defined as well-being (i.e., negative affect or physical symptoms), but is operationally defined as the within-person relationship between stressors and well-being. Reactivity, therefore, is a dynamic process that links stressors and well-being over time. Previous research shows that people who are more reactive to daily stressors are more susceptible to physical disease than are people who are less reactive (Cacioppo et al., 1998). Because resources of individuals and their environments (e.g., education, income, chronic stressors) limit or enhance possibilities and choices for coping (Lazarus, 1999), reactivity to stressors is likely to differ across people and across situations. The stressor reactivity path therefore contends that sociodemographic, psychosocial, and other situational factors modify reactivity to daily stressors. To this end, researchers can examine whether the same stressors produce different responses in various people, whether the same person responds differently to disparate stressors, and whether these responses vary according to self-report and physiological measures. A primary purpose of this chapter is to consider how these stress processes inform and are informed by research on aging. The next section articulates how stressor exposure and reactivity changes throughout adulthood, followed by a section on how stress plays an important role in biological and cognitive aging.

CHANGES IN STRESS PROCESSES ACROSS MIDDLE AND LATER ADULTHOOD

One vital component of our life-span perspective is to track intra-individual changes in exposure and reactivity to stressors. Several theoretical perspectives predict *decreases in stressor exposure and reactivity* across adulthood. One set of theories posits that with age, adults exercise more control over their social interactions and avoid situations that are stressful. According to Socioemotional Selectivity Theory (SST; Carstensen, 1987; Carstensen et al., 1999), for example, goals shift across adulthood, from a focus on knowledge-based goals during youth to a focus on emotion-based goals in later adulthood. As a consequence of these shifting goals, the composition of social networks changes, such that young adults broaden the size of their networks, whereas older adults strive to maintain their existing, close networks. These shifting social networks have implications for stressor exposure and reactivity. For example, daily experiences for younger adults may involve meeting new people and putting oneself in novel situations. As people age, however, their daily interactions become more predictable. These differences are reflected in the types of stressors people encounter. Compared to younger adults, older adults report fewer stressors overall and fewer overload stressors (i.e., meeting many demands). They do, however, experience more network stressors (i.e., events occurring to a network of friends and relatives that are experienced vicariously by the individual; Almeida & Horn, 2004). From this perspective, age-related changes in the stress process may emanate from differences in the frequency and type of daily stressors experienced across adulthood.

In a related vein, some theorists argue that adults become less reactive to stressors with age because of the knowledge, resources, and understanding they have accumulated from prior experiences (Whitbourne, 1985, 1986). This adaptation perspective suggests that it is the individual's evaluation of life experience rather than the experience itself that changes across adulthood. Simply stated, when exposed to daily stressors, older adults may interpret their experiences differently based on previous life experiences. Diehl et al. (1996), for example, found that older adults display greater impulse control than do younger adults when dealing with stressors, suggesting that as people age they may cope better with stress and perhaps become less reactive to stressors. These findings are consistent with a growing body of literature suggesting that people regulate emotions more effectively with age. Lawton (1996) suggested that repetition of negative affect states over many years may decrease the likelihood of triggering such states in the future. Such increases in the threshold for experiencing negative affect due to repeated activation are known as "dampening" effects. Certain life-span theories of emotion regulation are also consistent with the idea of lessened emotional reactivity to stress with age (Labouvie-Vief & DeVoe, 1991; Lang et al., 1998). In sum, the association between stress and well-being may shift throughout the life span as a result of reduced stressor exposure with age, reduced stressor reactivity, or a combination of both.

An alternative perspective suggests that the same process (i.e., repeated exposure to stressful events) may actually *increase stressor reactivity with age* in certain people (Mroczek & Almeida, 2004; Sliwinski et al., 2009). In this view, repeated activation may lead to sensitization as opposed to habituation or dampening. Several theoretical perspectives give rise to this idea. Changes in the aging brain alter the way people experience emotion, especially negative affect. The structures that mediate negative affect, the amygdala and limbic system, become more sensitive as we age (Adamec, 1990; Panksepp & Miller, 1996) as does the HPA axis (Seeman et al., 2001). Such heightened sensitivity may lead to an easier activation of the neural substrates that underlie the experience of negative affect when a stressor is encountered. These neurophysiologic changes make it conceivable that negative affect is more likely to become activated as a consequence of frequent activation. Thus, due to a lifetime of repeated activations of the neural systems that mediate negative affect, reactivity to stressors may increase as people age.

These heightened sensitivities are akin to kindling effects, a process in which repeated exposure to some stimulus causes sensitization (Kendler et al., 2001; van der Kolk, 1997; Woolf & Costigan, 1999). It is believed that kindling effects are a result of neuroplasticity, which refers to the ability of neurons to change and realign themselves in response to repeated exposure. The neural network that governs some processes (e.g., the sensation of pain, an epileptic seizure, and feelings of depression or negative affect) can itself become molded by the stimulus, causing these networks to become even more sensitive to the stimulus (van der Kolk, 1997; Woolf & Costigan, 1999). We suggest that a similar process might be occurring in the affective response to stressful events, especially among individuals who view stressors in a negative light. Indeed, some of our prior work has shown that older adults high in neuroticism display the greatest reactivity to stressors (Mroczek & Almeida, 2004; Mroczek et al., 2006, Sliwinski et al., 2009).

The Theory of Strength and Vulnerability Integration

The theory of Strength and Vulnerability Integration (SAVI) attempts to explain why some research shows increased reactivity to stressors with age and other research shows age-related decreases (Chapter 19, this volume; Charles & Piazza, 2009). According to SAVI, later adulthood is comprised of both strengths and vulnerabilities that affect emotion regulation. Strengths include the motivation to maintain affective well-being due to a shift in time perspective (as described in SST) and the cognitive-behavioral skills to do so, which are acquired over a lifetime of dealing with difficult experiences. These strengths, however, are coupled with age-related physiological vulnerabilities that make it difficult to recover once a stressor has been experienced. Thus, although age may bring with it an improved ability to avoid stressors and/or reappraise them as being innocuous, it also brings with it the vulnerabilities that occur as a result of a less flexible physiological system. For this reason, SAVI posits that age-related changes in emotion regulation are least likely to occur during exposure to a stressor that creates high levels of physiological arousal. At times such as these, physiological cues will largely override emotion regulation strategies. As time from the stressor passes, however, and physiology normalizes, age differences in emotional experience will increase because people's assessments of their emotional states will be less influenced by their physiological experience and more influenced by their appraisals of an event. Although this is hypothesized to be the normative pattern of age-related strengths and vulnerabilities, some life experiences make it difficult to avoid stressors or to modify one's appraisals of an event. Such experiences include loss of social belonging; exposure to chronic, uncontrollable stressors; and neurological dysregulation. Under these circumstances, age-related gains in affective well-being are unlikely to occur, regardless of the time that has passed since the emotion-eliciting event. Thus, although the motivation to maintain affective well-being exists, certain circumstances may impinge upon older adults' ability to do so (Chapter 19, this volume; Charles & Piazza, 2009).

INDIVIDUAL DIFFERENCES IN STRESS PROCESSES

While it is important to document general age trends in daily stress processes, life-span developmental theory asserts that aging does not represent a monolithic predictable trajectory (e.g., Baltes & Baltes, 1990; Rowe & Kahn, 1987, 1997). Thus, researchers should assess group and individual differences in patterns of change in stress processes as a function of resilience and vulnerability factors. Although there is emerging research documenting how factors such as SES, personality, perceived control, and genetic endowment predict exposure and reactivity to daily stressors concurrently, future research should extend this line of inquiry by assessing how stable and changing characteristics of individuals predict changes in stress processes.

Several researchers have asserted that *personal dispositions* interact with stressful situations in determining stressful experiences (Ben-Porath & Tellegen, 1990; Costa et al., 1996; Watson, 1990). For example, people who report high levels of neuroticism also report greater overall psychological distress. However, neuroticism is also associated with elevated distress and negative affect in the context of specific stressful situations (e.g., an argument with a spouse or boss). This tendency is referred to as hyperreactivity (Bolger & Schilling, 1991; Suls, 2001), and is perhaps the central theoretical concept in understanding individual differences in mood regulation. When people high in neuroticism encounter stressful events, they tend to experience them as more aversive and react with much higher levels of negative affect than do those low in this trait (Bolger & Schilling, 1991; Bolger & Zuckerman, 1995; David & Suls, 1999; Gunthert et al., 1999).

The repercussions of hyperreactivity, which refers to an inability (or lessened ability) to regulate back to a more optimal emotional state, are best understood in a developmental framework. In hyperreactivity, the state of distress remains continually activated, which is detrimental if it occurs too frequently, as it does among people high in neuroticism. Kendler et al. (2001) and Wilson et al. (2003, 2004) have hypothesized that neuroticism, and the constant elevated levels of distress that accompany this trait over periods of many years or decades, leads to a negative emotion "hair-trigger" in older adulthood. They suggest that as people high in neuroticism age, they become more, not less, susceptible to elevated distress. In theoretical terms, earlier experiences influence later experiences, accumulating in a manner suggested by Spiro (2001). This developmental accumulation may potentially result in greater hyperreactivity among certain older adults, namely those who have remained high in neuroticism over time. A study examining the long-term effect of neuroticism on physical health supports the hyperreactivity hypothesis (Charles et al., 2008). In this study, neuroticism was assessed among twin pairs who ranged in age from 15 to 47 in 1973. These individuals were contacted again 25 years later and asked about their physical health conditions. Results indicated that even when controlling for familial influences, those individuals who had a history of neuroticism had a higher likelihood of reporting a physical condition during the follow-up interview. Neuroticism, therefore, appears to have long-lasting physiological consequences.

Socioeconomic factors are also hypothesized to shape patterns of change in stress processes. Individuals with lower levels of socioeconomic status (SES) are at increased risk for major stressful events and chronic difficulties (e.g., violence, discrimination) and are thus more likely to suffer distress (Dohrenwend, 1970, 1973; Ettner, 2000; Marmot et al., 1997; Myers et al., 1972). One mechanism for this association is that lower SES individuals are more emotionally vulnerable to major stressors (Brown & Harris, 1978; Kessler & Cleary, 1980). Our work has shown that this is true for day-to-day stressors as well (Almeida et al., 2005; Grzywacz et al., 2004). On days individuals reported stressors (e.g., arguments, work demands), those with lower levels of education experienced greater psychological distress than did their better educated counterparts. Our cross-sectional analysis found no age differences (from 25 to 74 years) in this effect, but longitudinal analysis would permit testing longer-term effects of this differential reactivity. Over time, for example, people with lower SES may exhibit less optimal affective and physical functioning compared to people with higher SES, a premise consistent with findings of greater morbidity and mortality associated with each incremental decrease in SES (Marmot et al., 1997). In addition, not all people with low SES display poor affective and physical functioning, nor do all people with high SES do well. Using longitudinal data, researchers could examine the wide variability in the profiles of physical and mental health, focusing on people with high levels of functioning despite their lack of access to education, income, and other advantages that accompany higher SES.

Race/ethnicity also plays an important role in stress processes. For example, African Americans are at greater risk for morbidity and mortality compared to European Americans. Although SES and access to health care certainly play a role in these differences (Wagner, 1998), they do not explain why African Americans of the same SES as European Americans tend to be less healthy. Researchers suggest that several factors play a role, including a higher prevalence of risky health behaviors, environmental stressors, and genetic vulnerabilities. In addition, societal factors such as racial discrimination may also result in different health trajectories for African Americans. African American men, for example, are at higher risk for hypertension and experience more rapid progression of end-organ damage from hypertension than European American men (Wagner, 1998), which may be indicative of cardiovascular hyperactivity (Anderson, 1989). In one study, for example, African Americans who attributed mistreatment to discrimination exhibited higher than average diastolic blood pressure reactivity, an effect that was not evident among European Americans. African Americans also exhibited larger increases in mean arterial blood pressure in threat conditions compared to European Americans. Moreover, after exposure to racist stimuli, diastolic blood pressure levels remained elevated, suggesting that even indirect exposure to discrimination elicits significant and long-lasting reactivity (Fang & Myers, 2001). Racial discrimination may thus be a chronic stressor that negatively impacts the cardiovascular health of African Americans through pathogenic processes associated with physiological reactivity (Guyll et al., 2001). Future stress research should investigate linkages between daily psychosocial stressors (e.g., perceived discrimination, perceived inequalities) and biological health (e.g., allostatic load).

Life transition also contributes to stress processes. Changes in stress processes may also be reflected in the timing and transitions into and out of social roles, including role changes in the family and work domains (Almeida & Wong, 2009). These role changes may be precipitated by grown children leaving home (Lowenthal et al., 1975), career transitions (Moen, 2003), and the renegotiation of family relationships (Blatter & Jacobsen, 1993; Kim & Moen, 2002). Role transitions often entail transformations in multiple domains of responsibilities, such as combining work responsibilities and caretaking for one's aging parents and/or children. Such roles expose adults not only to specific types of major life events, but also to unique daily stressors. For example, in some of our work we examine how timing of retirement shapes daily experiences (Wong & Almeida, 2005, 2006). Although the average retirement age in the United States is rising and there are older workers in the labor force (Bureau of Labor Statistic, 2008), the question of whether delayed retirement is beneficial to the psychological and physical well-being of older workers requires further examination (Moen, 2003). Our analyses indicate that older workers (age 65 and older) report higher levels of daily negative affect as well as greater stressor severity compared to younger workers, and younger and older retirees (Wong & Almeida, 2006). Older workers' reports of higher levels of daily negative mood and greater stressor severity were not attributed to a greater number of total stressors experienced. Rather, older workers appraised stressors as more disruptive and unpleasant than did younger workers and retirees. The area where older workers appraised stressors as having the greatest impact was in the way other people felt about them. These findings suggest that older workers may face issues of discrimination not simply in the work force but in other areas of their lives. It is important to note that these findings were based on a cross-section of workers, and it is necessary to examine social roles longitudinally to assess whether and for whom changes in role status coincide with changes in stress processes.

PHYSIOLOGY OF THE STRESS RESPONSE AND AGE-RELATED CHANGES

Our review thus far has focused on how stressors may influence physical health and how these processes change throughout adulthood. Next, we briefly review two physiological systems that are involved in the stress response: the sympathetic-adrenal-medullary (SAM) axis and the HPA axis. We also discuss normative age-related changes in these two systems and how exposure to psychological stressors may accelerate these changes.

The SAM Axis

Physiological adaptation to stressors is essential for survival. The stress response mobilizes the body's resources to ward off or run from a potential threat, assists in wound repair during times of injury, and motivates an organism during times of challenge (Segerstrom & Miller, 2004). After a stressor is perceived, it is the immediate action of the sympathetic (SNS) branch of the autonomic nervous system that enables an organism to fight or flee. The SNS stimulates the adrenal medulla and the sympathetic neurons to secrete the catecholamines epinephrine and norepinephrine into the blood stream; the process where by the SNS enervates the adrenal medulla to release epinephrine and norepinephrine is known as the SAM axis. Epinephrine and norepinephrine prepare the body against threat by increasing heart rate, blood pressure and perspiration, dilating the pupils and bronchioles, and inhibiting gastrointestinal activity. Although SAM-axis arousal is necessary in the context of acutely stressful situations, continual activation of this system may ultimately arise in damage to the organism. For this reason, cessation of the stress response is imperative to physical health (McEwen & Stellar, 1993).

Age, Exposure to Stressors, and the SAM Axis

There are a number of age-related changes in SAM-axis activity (for a review, see Crimmins et al., 2008), which are oftentimes magnified when an individual is exposed to stressors. After the age of 60, for example, systolic blood pressure tends to increase, whereas diastolic blood pressure tends to decrease (Franklin et al., 2001). Older age is associated with even greater increases in systolic blood pressure in the context of acute psychosocial stressors (Uchino et al., 1999). Age may also be associated with higher levels of norepinephrine (e.g., Barnes et al., 1983) and lower levels of epinephrine (e.g., Esler et al., 1995), both of which may increase in magnitude when older adults are exposed to stressors (Barnes et al., 1983; Ester et al., 1995), though not all studies show these trends (e.g., Lindheim et al., 1992). The associations between age, stress, and SAM-axis activation is further illustrated in a study examining reactivity to a laboratory stressor among spousal caregivers (Aschbacher et al., 2008). In this study, older adult caregivers had higher levels of plasma norepinephrine than did non-caregivers. Moreover, among caregivers, higher perceived role overload was related to higher levels of plasma norepinephrine during recovery from the stressor. Illnesses appear to compound these age differences. For example, resting heart rate is heightened among older adults with cardiovascular disease (Gillum et al., 1991). The associations between age, SAM-axis activity, and stressor exposure may therefore be most pronounced among people with preexisting physical conditions.

The HPA Axis

Stressor-induced SNS activation also stimulates the HPA axis, which begins with the release of corticotrophin-releasing hormone (CRH) from the paraventricular nucleus of the hypothalamus. CRH stimulates adrenocorticotropin hormone (ACTH) release from the anterior pituitary, and arginine vasopressin (AVP) from the posterior pituitary gland. AVP acts centrally to support the "fight-or-flight" response, whereas ACTH circulates to the adrenal cortex to simulate glucocorticoid release, including corticosteroids such as cortisol (Chrousos & Gold, 1992; for a review see Dickerson & Kemeny, 2004). Corticosteroids regulate HPA-axis function through a negative feedback loop by dampening further release of CRH and ACTH and, consequently, corticosteroids. This negative feedback loop is necessary; although adaptive in the short-term, prolonged and repeated activation of the HPA axis can lead to adverse health outcomes, including the development and progression of chronic disease, dampened immune response, and destruction of hippocampal neurons (McEwen, 1998; Sapolsky, 1996, 2000a,b, 2001).

Age, Exposure to Stressors, and the HPA Axis

There are several changes in the HPA axis that occur with age, both in terms of an altered diurnal pattern and a disruption of the negative feedback loop that essentially stems the tide of cortisol overproduction (for a review, see Epel et al., 2009). With age, for example, the diurnal pattern of cortisol remains relatively flat, with an attenuated awakening response (Almeida et al., 2009b) and a higher evening nadir (Van Cauter et al., 1996). Age is also associated with a greater HPA-axis response to stressors (e.g., Otte et al., 2005; Peskind et al., 1995). As with the SAM axis, psychological stress appears to accelerate the effects of aging on the HPA axis. For example, in a study examining distress and urinary cortisol levels among people of different ages, age was not associated with urinary cortisol levels among people reporting milder distress. Among people experiencing more severe distress, however, urinary cortisol levels increased with age (Jacobs et al., 1984). As with the SAM axis, the associations between age, stressor exposure, and the HPA axis may be strongest among people in poor health (McEwen, 1998).

GENDER DIFFERENCE IN RESPONSES TO STRESS: TEND AND BEFRIEND

Men and women also may differ in their responses to stress as they age. For example, both sexes have similar cortisol levels at rest, yet between puberty and menopause, the HPA-axis response during stress tends to be lower (as indexed by cortisol) in women compared to men (Kajantie & Phillips, 2006). It is hypothesized that this is the time when estrogen levels are higher for women, which may exert a protective effect on some aspects of health functioning (i.e., cardiovascular system), but could increase vulnerability to autoimmune illness. Interestingly, these sex differences may be dependent upon the nature of the stressor. For example, men respond more (increased cortisol) to achievement-oriented challenges whereas women respond more intensely to social rejection (Stroud et al., 2002).

A relatively new theory may help explain the underlying sex difference in reactivity to social stressors. Taylor and colleagues (2000) suggest that although both males and females display the traditional fight-or-flight response to some stressors, a behavioral pattern of "tend-and-befriend" might be a more adaptive response to some stressors for women. Designed to increase the likelihood of survival when faced with a threat, "tending-and-befriending" promotes safety and diminishes distress through creating and maintaining social networks (i.e., befriending), along with nurturing activities that protect the female and her offspring (i.e., tending). The underlying neurobiological system of the tend-and-befriend response differs from the fight-or-flight response in that it appears to be modulated by the posterior pituitary hormone oxytocin (Taylor et al., 2000), which may mediate many of the biobehavioral health effects of stress (e.g., Carter & Altemus, 1997; McCarthy, 1995; McCarthy & Altemus, 1997; Uvnas-Moberg, 1997), including reduced blood pressure (Light et al., 2000), perceived stress levels (Mezzacappa & Katlin, 2002), anxiety (Turner et al., 1999), aggression (Lubin et al., 2003), depression (Anderberg & Uvnas-Moberg, 2000), and, perhaps, improved attention and social memory (e.g., Brett & Baxendale, 2001; Ferguson et al., 2002).

With regard to aging, it is important to note that the effects of oxytocin are enhanced in the presence of estrogen (McCarthy, 1995). Thus, age-related declines in estrogen in women may result in a loss of the stress-buffering benefits of oxytocin and, perhaps, the tend-and-befriend response. In a study of post-menopausal women, Taylor et al. (2006) suggested that higher plasma oxytocin levels signal relationship stress and are associated with elevated cortisol levels. Klein and colleagues (Klein & Corwin, 2002; Klein et al., 2006) suggested that sex differences in stressor reactivity may make women particularly vulnerable to social stressors such as family, work, and social relationships. More specifically, women may be particularly vulnerable to the health consequences (e.g., depression) of social stressors ranging from social isolation and interpersonal conflict to romantic and marital relationships (e.g., Hammen, 2003a,b). Indeed, women are more vulnerable to developing classic signs of depression in response to stressful life events than are men (e.g., Maciejewski et al., 2001; Sherrill et al., 1997; Weich et al., 2001). Unfortunately, how these sex differences in sensitivity to interpersonal stressors change across the life span is unknown. Our review of the literature suggests that age-related sex differences in tend-and-befriend responses to stress have not been studied and that this is a promising area of research.

STRESS AGE AND COGNITIVE HEALTH

Research has provided considerable evidence of a link between the experience of stressors including major trauma and negative life events, as well as daily hassles and a number of adverse health outcomes (Baum & Posluszny, 1999). An emerging area of inquiry complementing the study of stressors and their links to health and well-being is that of understanding how stressful experiences, as well as self-reported and biological indicators of stress, are linked to cognitive health, including cognitive performance and the structural and functional integrity of the brain. Furthermore, stress has been identified as particularly relevant for understanding cognitive health during old age because of age-related increases in vulnerability to stress (Smith, 2003).

In terms of linking stressful experiences to cognitive health, previous research has shown associations between different types of stressful experiences including major trauma, negative life events, chronic stressors, and daily hassles with compromised cognitive function. Major traumatic experiences including combat and childhood abuse have been associated with both impaired cognitive function and smaller hippocampal volume (Bremner, 1999; Sapolsky, 1996). Similarly, the chronic effects of these major traumatic events, specifically post-traumatic stress disorder (PTSD), has also been linked to impaired memory and attention function in combat veterans (Vasterling et al., 2002). Negative life events have also been adversely associated with cognitive function. Klein and her colleagues (Baradell & Klein, 1993; Klein & Barnes, 1994) showed that younger adults reporting greater numbers of negative life events exhibited poorer decision making, problem solving (Klein & Barnes, 1994), and working memory performance (Klein & Boals, 2001). Similar findings have been observed among older adults. Rosnick et al. (2007) found that older adults reporting greater numbers of stressful life events exhibited poorer memory performance, while Stawski et al. (2006) found that cognitive interference associated with the most stressful life event older adults self-identified was associated with poorer episodic memory, working memory, and processing speed performance. Chronic stressors, such as caregiving, have been shown to be associated with poorer processing speed (Caswell et al., 2003), as well as lower overall general cognitive function (Lee et al., 2004), among older adults. Finally, the experience of daily hassles has been linked to poorer working memory performance among both younger and older adults (Sliwinski et al., 2006), as well as self-reported memory failures in older adults (Neupert et al., 2006). Together, the results of these studies provide evidence that a wide variety of stressful experiences are associated with cognitive health.

The study of biological indicators of stress, as they relate to cognition, has primarily focused on cortisol, which is thought to impair cognitive function by binding to receptors in the hippocampus and frontal lobes and interfering with effective neural function and transmission. Cortisol is thought to have proximal effects on brain function and cognition by interfering with neural function and subsequent behavioral performance (Lupien & Lapage, 2001; Wolf, 2003; however also see Roozendaal, 2002), and more durable and distal effects by causing neuronal death from repeated and prolonged exposure to high levels of cortisol (Sapolsky, 1992; Sapolsky et al., 1986). Consistent with this biological perspective, research has shown that, in old age, higher basal cortisol levels and longitudinal increases in basal cortisol levels are associated with poorer episodic memory performance (Lupien et al., 1994, 1996; Seeman et al., 1997) and smaller hippocampal volume (Lupien et al., 1998). Similarly, McEwen's seminal work on the wear-and-tear hypothesis and the construct of allostatic load (McEwen, 1998) has also been important in motivating the understanding of the biological consequences of stress and their relation to cognitive and brain function. Allostatic load is a multiple-indicator (including cortisol) biological index of the cumulative effects of stressful experiences, permitting the consideration of how multidimensional, multisystemic biological indicators of stress can be used to understand cognitive health. Seeman et al. (2001) showed that higher levels of allostatic load were associated with the most precipitous seven-year declines in global cognitive function among older adults. Together, the results of these studies indicate that biological indicators of stress are predictive of cognitive and brain health.

Psychological indicators of stress, including psychological distress, proneness to distress, and stress-related cognitive interference have all been linked to cognitive performance. The role of these psychological indicators of stress and their link to cognitive function emerged from social psychological perspectives on the stress-cognition link, which suggests that stress competes for limited resources that can otherwise be devoted to information processing (Kahneman, 1973; Mandler, 1979; Wegner, 1988), and also serves to prolong physiological activation in response to stress (Brosschot et al., 2006). Work from Wilson and colleagues has shown that individual differences in distress and proneness to distress are associated with lower levels of and more precipitous declines in cognitive function, particularly episodic memory performance in both healthy older adults (Wilson et al., 2006) and lower levels of episodic memory among older adults diagnosed with Alzheimer's disease (Wilson et al., 2004). In addition to links between distress and cognitive function, Wilson and colleagues have shown psychological distress and proneness to distress to be associated with an increased likelihood of being diagnosed with Alzheimer's disease, suggesting that proneness to distress may compromise the structural and functional integrity of the brain, rendering older adults more susceptible to age-related pathologies linked to dementia (Wilson et al., 2006, 2007).

Complementing the use of distress as a psychological indicator of stress, cognitive interference, defined as intrusive off-task thoughts and images, and the intentional suppression of such intrusions, has been employed as a useful predictor of cognitive function. Klein and Boals (2001) showed that stress-related cognitive interference, as measured by the Impact of Events Scale (Horowitz et al., 1979), was associated with poorer working memory performance among younger adults. Also using the Impact of Events Scale, Stawski et al. (2006) found that higher levels of stress-related cognitive interference were associated with poorer processing speed, working memory, and episodic memory.

Together, the small portion of the stress-cognition literature reviewed here presents a promising emerging field of research for understanding aging. There is fairly consistent evidence that the experience of discrete and specific stressful events is negatively associated with cognitive health, as are biological and psychological indicators of stress. There are, however, a number of challenges and opportunities that require attention. The existing research linking stressful experiences to cognitive function has not always included and identified relevant mechanisms for explaining the effect of stressor exposure on cognitive health. Similarly, biological and psychological indicators are proxies for exposure to stressors, without demonstrating that stressful experiences are antecedent factors. Finally, stress is a process, as is how stressful experiences are associated with cognitive function. Research linking stressful experiences to level and change in cognitive function, as well as the mechanisms responsible for these links, needs to be thoughtful regarding issues of the appropriateness of study design and the sampling of time for studying these phenomena (Neupert et al., 2008). For instance, the mechanisms linking daily stressors to daily fluctuations in cognitive function may not be the same as linking the chronic stressor of caregiving to longitudinal changes in cognitive function. The field of stress-cognitive health research is growing and is ripe for empirical inquiry. While many challenges for understanding stress-cognition linkages are on the horizon, these challenges present exciting opportunities for melding stress, health, and aging research with research on cognitive aging.

SUMMARY AND CONCLUSIONS

The overarching goal of this chapter was to provide a broad overview on how stress processes play a role in heath and aging. There are multiple dimensions of stressors ranging from major life events to chronic stressors to daily hassles. Adult developmental researchers have examined how stressors affect health by assessing intra-individual change in exposure and reactivity to these types of stressors. Research has also begun to document individual and group differences in changes in these stress processes. Much of the psychological literature on stress and aging has assessed affective reactivity, but emerging work has begun to incorporate biological as well as cognitive outcomes of stress processes. These are all important advances in understanding how stress may speed not only biological aging but also cognitive aging.

Of course the next step in this enterprise is to begin to develop interventions that target stress processes. For example, one intervention designed to reduce stress and its negative effects on health and well-being is the mindfulness-based stress reduction (MBSR) program (Kabat-Zinn, 1990). This program focuses on the cultivation of mindfulness (a form of meditation) and associated practices. Participation has been associated with decreases in medical symptoms (Carmody et al., 2008) and positive changes in brain and immune function in adults (Davidson et al., 2003). In addition, patients recently diagnosed with early stage breast cancer who took part in the MBSR program displayed improved coping, quality of life, and immune function, as well as lower cortisol levels, than those in a control group (Witek-Janusek et al., 2008). Future work could adapt to this approach to other chronic illnesses as well as cognitive outcomes.

Future research on stress and aging will need to consider how multiple dimensions of stressors and their putative outcomes are embedded in one other. Research on the relationship between stressor processes and physical, mental, and cognitive health is rapidly evolving toward perspectives that emphasize the accumulation, associations, and interactions of stressors over time rather than the impact of a single stressor or category of stressors (Almeida et al., 2009a; Chiriboga, 1997; Turner et al., 2000). Stressors often co-occur across multiple levels (Pearlin et al., 1981). The presence of chronic stressors (persistent or recurrent difficulties of life) may increase exposure to daily hassles, such as troubled relationships giving rise to more frequent arguments. Chronic stressors may also exacerbate emotional and physical reactions to daily stressors, either by increasing negative appraisal (Lazarus, 1999) or by depleting resources such as time or finances needed for successful coping (Serido et al., 2004). Chronic stress or prolonged stressor exposure has profound negative effects on physiological systems including the pathological overproduction of corticosteroids (e.g., cortisol). Similarly, chronic stress exposure can impair immune function, leading to increased susceptibility to infectious disease (e.g., influenza, common cold) and overactivation of the immune response (e.g., allergic and autoimmune responses; Segerstrom & Miller, 2004). Daily stressor exposure also appears to increase risk factors for the development of cardiovascular disease (e.g., Hallman et al., 2001; Twisk et al., 1999). Chronic stressors and daily stressors often share a common etiology rising out of enduring social roles (i.e., worker, parent, or caregiver) that structure demands and create exposure to crises in real life (Eckenrode, 1984; Pearlin et al., 1981; Serido et al., 2004). Future research should track how role transitions, chronic stressors, and daily stressors coalesce to create patterns of vulnerability that impact mental and physical health.

One way to capture multiple levels of stressful experiences is to embed intensive repeated measurements in traditional longitudinal designs (Almeida et al., 2009b). Using data collected over a long period would permit an examination of how major life events and chronic stressors are linked to daily stress processes. Repeated measurement of various domains on the same individuals over the life course allows important questions to be addressed. How do early life experiences shape adult stressor exposure and reactivity? In particular, how does chronic stress such as poverty in childhood, or residing in a high-crime neighborhood affect stressor reactivity and biomarkers in life, net of current SES? What are mechanisms through which such effects might occur, such as a trajectory of low education, poor job, and resulting financial stressors? Importantly, what aspects of one's life circumstances may modify these relationships? Do many severe stressors early in life have additive or multiplicative effects on reactivity? How are such effects dependent upon the characteristics of the life events themselves in terms of content, severity, persistence, and timing? What aspects of life experience (e.g., quality of interpersonal relationships, educational attainment, SES, and health) can reduce stressor exposure and reactivity? And how does stressor exposure and reactivity influence achievement in the future, including SES and educational attainment?

Data obtained over many waves can be used to tease apart the pathways through which economic, social, and psychological factors affect the daily experience of stressor exposure and reactivity. Using the full life course allows further specificity of life cycle variation in these relationships, as well as an exploration of economic and social factors that contribute to alterations in these pathways (Almeida & Wong, 2009). Moreover, going forward in time, the effects of multiple sources of stressor exposure and reactivity on future experiences can also be examined to elucidate how and under what conditions stress processes may speed aging processes.

ACKNOWLEDGMENTS

This paper was supported by grants from the National Institute on Aging (P01 AG020166 and R01AG019239).

REFERENCES

Adamec, R. E. (1990). Does kindling model anything clinically relevant? *Biological Psychiatry, 27*, 249–279.

Aldwin, C. M. (1990). The elders life stress inventory: Egocentric and nonegocentric stress. In M. A. P. Stephens, J. H. Crowther, S. E. Hobfoll, & D. L. Tennenbaum (Eds.), *Stress and coping in later-life families* (pp. 49–69). Washington, DC: Hemisphere.

Aldwin, C. M. (1991). Does age affect the stress and coping process? Implications of age differences in perceived control. *Journals of Gerontology, 46*, 174–180.

Almeida, D. M. (2005). Resilience and vulnerability to daily stressors assessed via diary methods. *Current Directions in Psychological Science, 14*, 64–68.

Almeida, D. M., & Horn, M. C. (2004). Is daily life more stressful during middle adulthood? In C. D. Ryff & R. C. Kessler (Eds.), *How healthy are we? A portrait of midlife in the United States* (pp. 425–451). Chicago: The University of Chicago Press.

Almeida, D. M., McGonagle, K., & King, H. (2009a). Assessing daily stress processes in social surveys by combining stressor exposure and salivary cortisol. *Biodemography and Social Biology, 55*, 220–238.

Almeida, D. M., Piazza, J. R., & Stawski, R. S. (2009b). Inter-individual differences and intra-individual variability in the cortisol awakening response: An examination of age and gender. *Psychology and Aging, 24*, 819–827.

Almeida, D. M., & Wong, J. D. (2009). Life transition and stress: A life course perspective on daily stress processes. In G. H. Elder & J. Z. Giele (Eds.), *The craft of life course research* (pp. 141–162). New York: Guilford Press.

Anderberg, U. M., & Uvnas-Moberg, K. (2000). Plasma oxytocin levels in female fibromyalgia syndrome patients. *Zeitschrift fur Rheumatologie, 59*, 373–379.

Anderson, N. B. (1989). Racial differences in stress-induced cardiovascular reactivity and hypertension: Current status and substantive issues. *Psychological Bulletin, 105*, 89–105.

Aschbacher, K., Mills, P. J., von Känel, R., Hong, S., Mausbach, B. T., Roepke, S. K., et al. (2008). Effects of depressive and anxious symptoms on norepinephrine and platelet P-selectin responses to acute psychological stress among elderly caregivers. *Brain, Behavior, and Immunity, 22*, 493–502.

Baltes, P. B., & Baltes, M. M. (1990). Psychological perspectives on successful aging: The model of selective optimization with compensation. In P. B. Baltes & M. M. Baltes (Eds.), *Successful aging: Perspectives from the behavioral sciences* (pp. 1–34). Cambridge: Cambridge University.

Baltes, P. B., Staudinger, U. M., & Lindenberger, U. (1999). Lifespan psychology: Theory and application to intellectual functioning. *Annual Review of Psychology, 50*, 71–507.

Baradell, J. G., & Klein, K. (1993). Relationship of life stress and body consciousness to hypervigilant decision making. *Journal of Personality and Social Psychology, 64*, 267–273.

Barnes, R. F., Raskind, M., Gumbrecht, G., & Halter, J. B. (1982). The effects of age on the plasma-catecholamine response to mental stress in man. *Journal of Clinical Endocrinology and Metabolism, 54*, 64–69.

Baum, A., & Posluszny, D. M. (1999). Health psychology: Mapping biobehavioral health contributions to health and illness. *Annual Review of Psychology, 50*, 137–163.

Ben-Porath, Y. S., & Tellegen, A. (1990). A place for traits in stress research. *Psychological Inquiry, 1*, 14–17.

Blatter, C. W., & Jacobsen, J. J. (1993). Older women coping with divorce: Peer support groups. *Women & Therapy, 14*, 141–155.

Bolger, N., Davis, A., & Rafaeli, E. (2003). Diary methods: Capturing life as it is lived. *Annual Review of Psychology, 54*, 579–616.

Bolger, N., DeLongis, A., Kessler, R. C., & Schilling, E. A. (1989). Effects of daily stress on negative mood. *Journal of Personality and Social Psychology, 57*, 808–818.

Bolger, N., Foster, M., Vinokur, A. D., & Ng, R. (1996). Close relationships and adjustments to a life crisis: The case of breast cancer. *Journal of Personality and Social Psychology, 70*, 283–294.

Bolger, N., & Schilling, E. A. (1991). Personality and the problems of everyday life: The role of neuroticism in exposure and reactivity to daily stressors. *Journal of Personality. Special Issue: Personality and Daily Experience, 59*, 355–386.

Bolger, N., & Zuckerman, A. (1995). A framework for studying personality in the stress process. *Journal of Personality and Social Psychology, 69*, 890–902.

Bouchard, G. (2003). Cognitive appraisals, neuroticism, and openness as correlates of coping strategies: An integrative model of adaptation to marital difficulties. *Canadian Journal of Behavioural Science, 35*, 1–12.

Bremner, J. D. (1999). Does stress damage the brain? *Biological Psychiatry, 45*, 797–805.

Brett, M., & Baxendale, S. (2001). Motherhood and memory: A review. *Psychoneuroendocrinology, 26*, 339–362.

Brewin, C. R., MacCarthy, B., & Furnham, A. (1989). Social support in the face of adversity: The role of cognitive appraisal. *Journal of Research in Personality, 23*, 354–372.

Brosschot, J. F., Gerin, W., & Thayer, J. F. (2006). The perseverative cognition hypothesis: A review of worry, prolonged stress-related physiological activation, and health. *Journal of Psychosomatic Research, 60*, 113–124.

Brown, G. W., & Harris, T. O. (1978). *Social origins of depression: A study of psychiatric disorder in women*. London: Tavistock.

Bureau of Labor Statistic (2008). American time use survey summary. USDL 08-0859. *Bureau of Labor Statistics*. US Department of Labor, Washington DC.

Cacioppo, J. T. (1998). Somatic responses to psychological stress: The reactivity hypothesis. In M. Sabourin, F. Craik, & M. Robert (Eds.), *Advances in psychological science* (Vol. 2, pp. 87–112). East Sussex, UK: Psychology Press.

Cannon, W. B. (1932). *The Wisdom of the Body*. New York: Norton.

Carmody, J., Reed, G., Kristeller, J., & Merriam, P. (2008). Mindfulness, spirituality, and health-related symptoms. *Journal of Psychosomatic Research, 64*, 393–403.

Carstensen, L. L. (1987). Age-related changes in social activity. In L. L. Carstensen & B. A. Edelstein (Eds.), *Handbook of clinical gerontology: Vol. 146. Pergamon general psychology series* (pp. 222–237). New York: Pergamon Press.

Carstensen, L. L., Isaacowitz, D. M., & Charles, S. T. (1999). Taking time seriously: A theory of socioemotional selectivity. *American Psychologist, 54*, 165–181.

Carter, C. S., & Altemus, M. (1997). Integrative functions of lactational hormones in social behavior and stress management. *Ann NY Acad Sci, 807*, 164–174.

Caswell, L. W., Vitiliano, P. P., Croyle, K. L., Scanlan, J. M., Zhang, J., & Daruwala, A. (2003). Negative associations of chronic stress and cognitive performance in older adults spouse caregivers. *Experimental Aging Research, 29*, 303–318.

Charles, S. T., Gatz, M., Kato, K., & Pedersen, N. L. (2008). Physical health 25 years later: The predictive ability of neuroticism. *Health Psychology, 27*, 369–378.

Charles, S. T., & Piazza, J. R. (2009). Age differences in affective well-being: Context matters. *Social and Personality Psychology Compass, 3*, 711–734.

Chiriboga, D. A. (1997). Crisis, challenge, & stability in the middle years. In M. E. Lachman & J. B. James (Eds.), *Multiple paths of midlife development* (pp. 293–322). Chicago: The University of Chicago Press.

Chrousos, G. P., & Gold, P. W. (1992). The concepts of stress and stress system disorders: Overview of physical and behavioral homeostasis. *JAMA Journal of the American Medical Association, 267,* 1244–1252.

Costa, P. T., Jr., Somerfield, M. R., & McCrae, R. R. (1996). Personality and coping: A reconceptualization. In M. Zeidner & N. S. Endler (Eds.), *Handbook of coping: Theory, research, applications* (pp. 44–61). New York: Wiley.

Crimmins, E., Vasunilashorn, S., Kim, J. K., & Alley, D. (2008). Biomarkers related to aging in human population. *Advances in Clinical Chemistry, 46,* 161–216.

David, J. P., & Suls, J. (1999). Coping efforts in daily life: Role of Big Five traits and problem appraisals. *Journal of Personality, 67,* 265–294.

Davidson, R. J., Kabat-Zinn, J., Schumacher, J., Rosenkranz, M., Muller, D., & Santorelli, S. F. (2003). Alterations in brain and immune function produced by mindfulness meditation. *Psychosomatic Medicine, 65,* 564–570.

Dickerson, S. S., & Kemeny, M. E. (2004). Acute stressors and cortisol responses: A theoretical integration and synthesis of laboratory research. *Psychological Bulletin, 130,* 355–391.

Diehl, M., Coyle, N., & Labouvie-Vief, G. (1996). Age and sex differences in strategies of coping and defense across the life span. *Psychology and Aging, 11,* 127–139.

Dohrenwend, B. S. (1970). An experimental study of directive interviewing. *Public Opinion Quarterly, 34,* 117–125.

Dohrenwend, B. S. (1973). Social status and stressful life events. In E. H. Hare & J. K. Wing (Eds.), *Psychiatric epidemiology* (pp. 313–319). London: Oxford University.

Dohrenwend, B. P. (2006). Inventorying stressful life events as risk factors for psychopathology: Toward resolution of the problem of intracategory variability. *Psychological Bulletin, 132,* 477–495.

Eckenrode, J. (1984). The impact of chronic and acute stressors on daily reports of mood. *Journal of Personality and Social Psychology, 46,* 907–919.

Epel, E. S., Burke, H. M., & Wolkowitz, O. M. (2009). The psychoneuroendocrinology of aging: Anabolic and catabolic hormones. In C. M. Aldwin, C. L. Park, & A. Spiro (Eds.), *Handbook of health psychology and aging* (pp. 119–141). New York, NY: Guilford Press.

Esler, M., Kaye, D., Thompson, J., Jennings, G., Cox, H., Turner, A., et al. (1995). Effects of aging on epinephrine secretion and regional release of epinephrine from the human heart. *Journal of Clinical Endocrinology & Metabolism, 80,* 435–442.

Ettner, S. (2000). The relationship between labor market outcomes and mental and physical health: Exogenous human capital or endogenous health production? In D. S. Sakevaer & A. Sorkin (Eds.), *The economics of disability.* Stamford, CT: JAI Press.

Fang, C. Y., & Myers, H. F. (2001). The effects of racial stressors and hostility on cardiovascular reactivity in African American and Caucasian men. *Health Psychology, 20,* 64–70.

Felsten, G. (1991). Influences of situation-specific mastery beliefs and satisfaction with social support on appraisal of stress. *Psychological Reports, 69,* 483–495.

Ferguson, J. N., Young, L. J., & Insel, T. R (2002). The neuroendocrine basis of social recognition. *Frontiers in Neuroendocrinology, 23,* 200–224.

Folkman, S., Lazarus, R. S., Pimley, S., & Novacek, J. (1987). Age differences in stress and coping processes. *Psychology and Aging, 2,* 171–184.

Franklin, S. S., Larson, M. D., Kahn, S. A., Wong, N. D., Leip, E. P., Kannel, W. B., et al. (2001). Does the relation of blood pressure to coronary heart disease risk change with aging? The Framingham heart study. *Circulation, 103,* 1245–1249.

Gillum, R. F., Makuc, D. M., & Feldman, J. J. (1991). Pulse rate, coronary heart disease, and death: The NHANES-I epidemiologic follow-up study. *American Heart Journal, 121,* 172–177.

Grzywacz, J. G., Almeida, D. M., Neupert, S. D., & Ettner, S. L. (2004). Socioeconomic status and health: A microlevel analysis of exposure and vulnerability to daily stressors. *Journal of Health and Social Behavior, 45,* 1–16.

Gunthert, K. C., Cohen, L. H., & Armeli, S. (1999). The role of neuroticism in daily stress and coping. *Journal of Personality and Social Psychology, 77,* 1087–1100.

Guyll, M., Matthews, K. A., & Bromberger, J. T. (2001). Discrimination and unfair treatment: Relationship to cardiovascular reactivity among African American and European American women. *Health Psychology, 20,* 315–325.

Hallman, T., Burell, G., Setterlind, S., Oden, A., & Lisspers, J. (2001). Psychosocial risk factors for coronary heart disease, their importance compared with other risk factors and gender differences in sensitivity. *Journal of Cardiovascular Risk, 8,* 39–49.

Hamarat, E., Thompson, D., Zabrucky, K. M., Steele, D., Matheny, K. B., & Aysan, F. (2001). Perceived stress and coping resource availability as predictors of life satisfaction in young, middle-aged, and older adults. *Experimental Aging Research, 27,* 181–196.

Hammen, C. (2003a). Interpersonal stress and depression in women. *Journal of Affective Disorders, 74,* 49–57.

Hammen, C. (2003b). Social stress and women's risk for recurrent depression. *Archives of Women's Mental Health, 6,* 9–13.

Holmes, T. H., & Rahe, R. H. (1967). Holmes-Rahe life changes scale. *Journal of Psychosomatic Research, 11,* 213–218.

Horowitz, M., Wilner, N. J., & Alvarez, W. (1979). Impact of Event Scale: A measure of subjective stress. *Psychosomatic Medicine, 41,* 209–218.

Jacobs, S., Mason, J., Kosten, T., Brown, S., & Ostfeld, A. (1984). Urinary-free cortisol excretion in relation to age in acutely stressed persons with depressive symptoms. *Psychosomatic Medicine, 46,* 213–221.

Kahneman, D. (1973). *Attention and effort.* Englewood Cliffs, NJ: Prentice-Hall.

Kajantie, E., & Phillips, D. I. W. (2006). The effects of sex and hormonal status on the physiological response to acute psychosocial stress. *Psychoneuroendocrinology, 31*, 151–178.

Kendler, K. S., Thornton, L. M., & Gardner, C. O. (2001). Genetic risk, number of previous depressive episodes, and stressful life events in predicting onset of major depression. *The American Journal of Psychiatry, 158*, 582–586.

Kessler, R. C., & Cleary, P. D. (1980). Social class and psychological distress. *American Sociological Review, 47*, 752–764.

Kiecolt-Glaser, J. K., McGuire, L., Robles, T. F., & Glaser, R. (2002). Emotions, morbidity, and mortality: New perspectives from psychoneuroimmunology. *Annual Review of Psychology, 53*, 83–107.

Kim, J. E., & Moen, P. (2002). Retirement transitions, gender, and psychological well-being: A life-course, ecological model. *Journals of Gerontology: Psychological Sciences and Social Sciences, 57*, 212–222.

Klein, K., & Barnes, D. (1994). The relationship of life stress to problem solving: Task complexity and individual differences. *Social Cognition, 12*, 187–204.

Klein, K., & Boals, A. (2001). The relationship of life events stress and working memory capacity. *Applied Cognitive Psychology, 15*, 565–579.

Klein, L. C., & Corwin, E. J. (2002). Seeing the unexpected: how sex differences in stress responses may provide a new perspective on the manifestation of psychiatric disorders. *Current Psychiatry Reports, 4*, 441–448.

Klein, L. C., & Corwin, E. J. (2007). Homeostasis and the stress response. In E. J. Corwin (Ed.), *Handbook of pathophysiology* (3rd ed., pp. 159–172). Philadelphia, PA: Lippincott Williams & Wilkins.

Klein, L. C., Corwin, E. J., & Ceballos, R. M. (2006). The social costs of stress: How sex differences in stress responses can lead to social stress vulnerability and depression in women. In C. L. M. Keyes & S. H. Goodman (Eds.), *Women and Depression: A handbook for the social, behavioral, and biomedical sciences* (pp. 199–218). New York: Cambridge University Press.

Labouvie-Vief, G., & Devoe, M. (1991). Emotional regulation in adulthood and later life: A developmental review. In K. W. Schaie (Ed.), *Annual review of gerontology and geriatrics* (pp. 172–194). New York: Springer.

Lang, F. R., Staudinger, U. M., & Carstensen, L. L. (1998). Perspectives on socioemotional selectivity in late life: How personality and social context do (and do not) make a difference. *Journals of Gerontology: Psychological Sciences and Social Sciences, 53*, 21–30.

Lawton, M. P. (1996). Quality of life and affect in later life. In C. Magai & S. McFadden (Eds.), *Handbook of emotion, adult development and aging* (pp. 327–348). Orlando, FL: Academic Press.

Lazarus, R. S. (1999). *Stress and emotion: A new synthesis*. New York: Springer.

Lazarus, R. S., & Folkman, S. (1984). *Stress, appraisal, and coping*. New York: Springer.

Lee, S., Kawachi, I., & Grodstein, F. (2004). Does caregiving stress affect cognitive function in older women? *Journal of Nervous and Mental Diseases, 192*, 51–57.

Light, K. C., Smith, T. E., Johns, J. M., Brownley, K. A., Hofheimer, J. A., & Amico, J. A. (2000). Oxytocin responsivity in mothers of infants: A preliminary study of relationships with blood pressure during laboratory stress and normal ambulatory activity. *Health Psychology, 19*, 560–567.

Lindheim, S. R., Legro, R. S., Bernstein, L., Stanczyk, F. Z., Vijod, M. A., Pressor, S. C., et al. (1992). Behavioral stress responses in premenopausal and post menopausal women and the effects of estrogen. *American Journal of Obstetrics and Gynecology, 167*, 1831–1836.

Lowenthal, M. F., Thurner, M., & Chiriboga, D. A. (1975). *Four stages of life: A comparative study of men and women facing transitions.* San Francisco: Jossey-Bass.

Lubin, D. A., Elliott, J. C., Black, M. C., & Johns, J. M. (2003). An oxytocin antagonist infused into the central nucleus of the amygdala increases maternal aggressive behavior. *Behavioral Neuroscience, 117*, 195–201.

Lupien, S. J., de Leon, M., de Santi, S., Convit, A., Tarshish, C., Nair, N. P. V., et al. (1998). Cortisol levels during human aging predict hippocampal atrophy and memory deficits. *Nature Neuroscience, 1*, 69–73.

Lupien, S. J., & Lapage, M. (2001). Stress, memory, and the hippocampus: Can't live with it, can't live without it. *Behavioural Brain Research, 127*, 137–158.

Lupien, S., Lecours, A. R., Lussier, I., Schwartz, G., Nair, N. P. V., & Meaney, M. J. (1994). Basal cortisol levels and cognitive deficits in human aging. *Journal of Neuroscience, 14*, 2893–2903.

Lupien, S. J., Lecours, A. R., Schwartz, G., Sharma, S., Hauger, R. L., Meaney, M. J., et al. (1996). Longitudinal study of basal cortisol levels in health elderly subjects: Evidence for subgroups. *Neurobiology of Aging, 17*, 95–105.

Maciejewski, P. K., Prigerson, H. G., & Mazure, C. M. (2001). Sex differences in event-related risk for major depression. *Psychological Medicine, 31*(4), 593–604.

Mandler, G. (1979). Thought processes, consciousness and stress. In V. Hamilton & D. W. Warburton (Eds.), *Human stress and cognition: An information processing approach*. New York: Wiley.

Marmot, M., Ryff, C. D., Bumpass, L. L., Shipley, M., & Marks, N. F. (1997). Social inequalities in health: Converging evidence and next questions. *Social Science and Medicine, 44*, 901–910.

McCarthy, M. M. (1995). Estrogen modulation of oxytocin and its relation to behavior. In R. Ivell & J. Russell (Eds.), *Oxytocin: Cellular and molecular approaches in medicine and research* (pp. 235–242). New York: Plenum Press.

McCarthy, M. M., & Altemus, M. (1997). Central nervous system actions of oxytocin and modulation of behavior in humans. *Molecular Medicine Today, 3*, 269–275.

McEwen, B. S. (1998). Protective and damaging effects of stress mediators. *The New England Journal of Medicine, 338*, 171–180.

McEwen, B. S., & Stellar, E. (1993). Stress and the individual: Mechanisms leading to disease.

Archives of Internal Medicine, 153, 2093–2101.

Mezzacappa, E. S., & Katlin, E. S. (2002). Breast-feeding is associated with reduced perceived stress and negative mood in mothers. *Health Psychology, 21*, 187–193.

Moen, P. (2003). Midcourse: Navigating retirement and a new life stage. In J. Mortimer & M. J. Shanahan (Eds.), *Handbook of the life course* (pp. 269–291). New York: Kluwer Academic.

Mroczek, D. K., & Almeida, D. M. (2004). The effect of daily stress, personality, and age on daily negative affect. *Journal of Personality, 72*, 355–378.

Mroczek, D. K., Spiro, A., III, Griffin, P. W., & Neupert, S. D. (2006). Social influences on adult personality, self-regulation, and health. In K. W. Schaie & L. L. Carstensen (Eds.), *Social structures, aging, and self-regulation in the elderly* (pp. 70–122). New York: Springer.

Myers, J. K., Lindenthal, J. J., Pepper, M. P., & Ostrander, D. R. (1972). Life events and mental status: A longitudinal study. *Journal of Health and Social Behavior, 13*, 398–406.

Neupert, S. D., Almeida, D. M., Mroczek, D. K., & Spiro, A., III. (2006). Daily stressors and memory failures in a naturalistic setting. *Psychology and Aging, 21*, 242–249.

Neupert, S. D., Stawski, R. S., & Almeida, D. M. (2008). Considerations for sampling time in aging research. In S. M. Hofer & D. F. Alwin (Eds.), *The handbook of cognitive aging: Interdisciplinary perspectives* (pp. 492–505). Thousand Oaks, CA: Sage Publications.

Otte, C., Hart, S., Neylan, T. C., Marmar, C. R., Yaffe, K., & Mohr, D. C. (2005). A mete-analysis of cortisol response to challenge in human aging: Importance of gender. *Psychoneuroendocrinology, 30*, 80–91.

Panksepp, J., & Miller, A. (1996). Emotions and the aging brain: Regrets and remedies. In C. Magai & S. H. McFadden (Eds.), *Handbook of emotions, adult development, and aging* (pp. 3–26). San Diego, CA: Academic Press.

Pearlin, L. I. (1993). The sociological study of stress. *Journal of Health and Social Behavior, 30*, 241–256.

Pearlin, L. I. (1993). The social contexts of stress. In L. Goldberger & S. Goldberger (Eds.), *Handbook of stress: Theoretical and clinical aspects* (2nd ed., pp. 303–315). New York: Free Press.

Pearlin, L. I. (1982). Discontinuities in the study of aging. In T. K. Hareven (Ed.), *Aging and the life course* (pp. 55–74). NY: Guilford.

Pearlin, L. I. (1999). The stress process revisited: Reflections on concepts and their interrelationships. In C. S. Aneshensel & J. C. Phelan (Eds.), *Handbook of the sociobiology of mental health* (pp. 395–415). New York: Kluwer Academic.

Pearlin, L. I., Menaghan, E. G., Lieberman, M. A., & Mullan, J. T. (1981). The stress process. *Journal of Health and Social Behavior, 22*, 337–356.

Pearlin, L. I., & Skaff, M. M. (1996). Stress and the life course: A paradigmatic alliance. *The Gerontologist, 36*, 239–247.

Penley, J. A., & Tomaka, J. (2002). Associations among the Big Five, emotional responses and coping with acute stress. *Personality and Individual Differences, 32*, 1215–1228.

Peskind, E. R., Raskind, M. A., Wingerson, D., Pascualy, M., Thal, L. J., Dobie, D. J., et al. (1995). Enhanced hypothalamic-pituitary-adrenocortical axis responses to physostigmine in normal aging. *Journals of Gerontology: Biological Sciences and Medical Sciences, 50*, M114–M120.

Pillow, D. R., Zautra, A. J., & Sandler, I. (1996). Major life events and minor stressors: Identifying meditational links in the stress process. *Journal of Personality and Social Psychology, 70*, 381–394.

Roozendaal, B. (2002). Stress and memory: Opposing effects of glucocorticoids on memory consolidation and retrieval. *Neurobiology of Learning and Memory, 78*, 578–595.

Rosnick, C. B., Small, B. J., McEvoy, C. L., Borenstein, A. R., & Mortimer, J. A. (2007). Negative life events and cognitive performance in a population of older adults. *Journal of Aging and Health, 19*(4), 612–629.

Rowe, J. W., & Kahn, R. L. (1987). Human aging: Usual and successful. *Science, 237*, 143–149.

Rowe, J. W., & Kahn, R. L. (1997). Successful aging. *The Gerontologist, 37*, 433–440.

Sapolsky, R. M. (1992). *Stress, the aging brain, and the mechanisms of neuron death*. Cambridge, MA: MIT Press.

Sapolsky, R. M. (1996). Why stress is bad for your brain. *Science, 273*, 749–750.

Sapolsky, R. M. (2000a). Glucocorticoids and hippocampal atrophy in neuropsychiatric disorders. *Archives of General Psychiatry, 57*, 925–935.

Sapolsky, R. M. (2000b). The possibility of neurotoxicity in the hippocampus in major depression: A primer on neuron death. *Biological Psychiatry, 48*, 755–765.

Sapolsky, R. M. (2001). Atrophy of the hippocampus in posttraumatic stress disorder: How and when? *Hippocampus, 11*, 90–91.

Sapolsky, R. M., Krey, L. C., & McEwen, B. S. (1986). The neuroendocrinology of stress and aging: The glucocorticoid cascade hypothesis. *Endocrine Reviews, 7*, 284–301.

Seeman, T. E., McEwen, B. S., Rowe, J. W., & Singer, B. H. (2001). Allostatic load as a marker of cumulative biological risk: MacArthur studies on successful aging. *Proceedings of the National Academy of Sciences, 98*, 4770–4775.

Seeman, T. E., McEwen, B. S., Singer, B. H., Albert, M. S., & Rowe, J. W. (1997). Increase in urinary cortisol excretion and memory declines: MacArthur studies on successful aging. *Journal of Clinical Endocrinology and Metabolism, 82*, 2458–2465.

Segerstrom, S. C., & Miller, G. E. (2004). Psychological stress and the human immune system: A meta-analytic study of 30 years of inquiry. *Psychological Bulletin, 130*, 601–630.

Selye, H. (1956). *The stress of life*. New York: McGraw-Hill.

Serido, J., Almeida, D. M., & Wethington, E. (2004).

Chronic stressors and daily hassles: Unique and interactive relationships with psychological distress. *Journal of Health and Social Behavior, 45*, 17–33.

Sherrill, J. T., Anderson, B., Frank, E., Reynolds, C. F., III, Tu, X. M., Patterson, D., et al. (1997). Is life stress more likely to provoke depressive episodes in women than in men? *Depression and Anxiety, 6*, 95–105.

Sliwinski, M. J., Almeida, D. M., Smyth, J. M., & Stawski, R. S. (2009). Intra-individual change and variability in daily stress processes: Findings from two diary burst studies. *Psychology and Aging, 24*, 828–840.

Sliwinski, M. J., Smyth, J. M., Hofer, S. M., & Stawski, R. S. (2006). Intra-individual coupling of daily stress and cognition. *Psychology and Aging, 21*, 545–557.

Smith, J. (2003). Stress and aging: Theoretical and empirical challenges for interdisciplinary research. *Neurobiology of Aging, 24*, S77–S80.

Spiro, A. (2001). Health in midlife: Toward a life-span view. In M. E. Lachman (Ed.), *Handbook of Midlife Development* (pp. 156–185). New York: Wiley.

Stawski, R. S., Sliwinski, M. J., & Smyth, J. M. (2006). Stress-related cognitive interference predicts cognitive function in old age. *Psychology and Aging, 21*, 535–544.

Stratakis, C. A., & Chrousos, G. P. (1995). Neuroendocrinology and pathophysiology of the stress system. In G. P. Chrousos, R. McCarty, K. Pacák, G. Cizza, E. Sternberg, P. W. Gold, & R. Kvet anský (Eds.), *Stress: Basic mechanisms and clinical implications* (Vol. 771, pp. 1–18). New York: The New York Academy of Sciences.

Stroud, L. R., Salovey, P., & Epel, E. S. (2002). Sex differences in stress responses: Social rejection versus achievement stress. *Biological Psychiatry, 52*, 318–327.

Suls, J. (2001). Affect, stress, and personality. In J. P. Forgas (Ed.), *Handbook of affect and social cognition* (pp. 392–409). Mahwah, NJ: Lawrence Erlbaum.

Taylor, S. E., Gonzaga, G. C., Klein, L. C., Hu, P., Greendale, G. A., & Seeman, T. E. (2006). Relation of oxytocin to psychological stress responses and hypothalamic-pituitary-adrenocortical axis activity in older women. *Psychosomatic Medicine, 68*, 238–245.

Taylor, S. E., Klein, L. C., Lewis, B. P., Gruenewald, T. L., Gurung, R. A. R., & Updegraff, J. A. (2000). Female responses to stress: Tend-and-befriend, not fight-or-flight. *Psychological Review, 107*, 411–429.

Turner, R. A., Altemus, M., Enos, T., Cooper, B., & McGuinness, T. (1999). Preliminary research on plasma oxytocin in healthy, normal cycling women investigating emotion and interpersonal distress. *Psychiatry, 62*, 97–113.

Turner, R. J., Sorenson, A. M., & Turner, J. B. (2000). Social contingencies in mental health: A seven-year follow-up study of teenage mothers. *Journal of Marriage and the Family, 62*, 777–791.

Twisk, J. W. R., Snel, J., Kemper, H. C. G., & van Mechelen, W. (1999). Changes in daily hassles and life events and the relationship with coronary heart disease risk factors: A 2-year longitudinal study in 27–29 year-old males and females. *Journal of Psychosomatic Research, 46*, 229–240.

Uchino, B. N., Uno, D., Holt-Lunstad, J., & Flinders, J. B. (1999). Age-related differences in cardiovascular reactivity during acute psychological stress in men and women. *Journals of Gerontology Series B-Psychological Sciences and Social Sciences, 54*, 339–346.

Uvnas-Moberg, K. (1997). Oxytocin linked antistress effects — the relaxation and growth response. *Acta Psychologica Scandinavica, 640*, 38–42.

Van Cauter, E., Leproult, R., & Kupfer, D. J. (1996). Effects of gender and age on the levels and circadian rhythmicity of plasma cortisol. *Journal of Clinical Endocrinology and Metabolism, 81*, 2468–2473.

van der Kolk, B. A. (1997). Traumatic memories. In P. S. Appelbaum, L. A. Uyehara, & M. R. Elin (Eds.), *Trauma and memory: Clinical and legal controversies* (pp. 243–260). New York: Oxford University Press.

Vasterling, J. J., Duke, L. M., Brailey, K., Constans, J. I., Allain, A. N., Jr., & Sutker, P. B. (2002). Attention, learning, and memory performances and intellectual resources in Vietnam veterans: PTSD and no disorder comparisons. *Neuropsychology, 16*, 5–14.

Wagner, L. (1998). Hypertension in African-American males. *Clinical Excellence for Nurse Practitioners: The International Journal of NPACE, 2*, 225–231.

Watson, D. (1990). On the dispositional nature of stress measure: Stable and nonspecific influences on self-reported hassles. *Psychological Inquiry, 1*, 34–37.

Wegner, D. M. (1988). Stress and mental control. In S. Fisher & J. Reason (Eds.), *Handbook of life stress, cognition and health* (pp. 683–697). London: John Wiley & Sons Ltd.

Weich, S., Sloggett, A., & Lewis, G. (2001). Social roles and the gender difference in rates of the common mental disorders in Britain: a 7-year, population-based cohort study. *Psychological Medicine, 31*, 1055–1064.

Wheaton, B. (1996). The domains and boundaries of stress concepts. In H. B. Kaplan (Ed.), *Psychosocial stress* (pp. 29–70). San Diego, CA: Academic Press.

Wheaton, B. (1997). The nature of chronic stress. In B. H. Gottlieb (Ed.), *Coping with chronic stress. The Plenum series on stress and coping* (pp. 43–73). New York: Plenum Press.

Wheaton, B. (1999). The nature of stressors. In A. V. Horowitz & T. L. Scheid (Eds.), *A handbooks for the study of mental health: Social contexts, theories, and systems* (pp. 176–197). New York: Cambridge University Press.

Whitbourne, S. K. (1985). The psychological construction of the life span. In J. E. Birren & K. W. Schaie (Eds.), *Handbook of the psychology of aging* (2nd ed., pp. 594–618). New York: Van Nostrand Reinhold.

Whitbourne, S. K. (1986). Openness to experience, identity flexibility, and life change in adults. *Journal of Personality and Social Psychology, 50*, 163–168.

Wilson, R. S., Arnold, S. E., Schneider, J. A., Kelly, J. F., Tang, Y., & Bennett, D. A. (2006).

Chronic psychological distress and risk of Alzheimer's disease in old age. *Neuroepidemiology, 27*, 143–153.

Wilson, R. S., Arnold, S. E., Schneider, J. S., Li, Y., & Bennett, D. A. (2007). Chronic distress, age-related neuropathology, and late-life dementia. *Psychosomatic Medicine, 69*, 47–53.

Wilson, R. S., Bienias, J. L., Mendes de Leon, C. F., Evans, D. A., & Bennett, D. A. (2003). Negative affect and mortality in older persons. *American Journal of Epidemiology, 158*, 27–35.

Wilson, R. S., Mendes de Leon, C. F., & Bienias, J. L. (2004). Personality and mortality in old age. *Journals of Gerontology: Psychological Sciences and Social Sciences, 59B*, 110–116.

Witek-Janusek, L., Albuquerque, K., Chroniak, K. R., Chroniak, C., Durazo-Arvizu, R., & Mathews, H. L. (2008). Effect of mindfulness based stress reduction on immune function, quality of life and coping in women newly diagnosed with early stage breast cancer. *Brain, Behavior & Immunity, 22*, 969–981.

Wong, J. D., & Almeida, D. M. (2005, November). *Is daily life stressful after retirement?* Poster presented for the meeting of the Gerontological Society of America, Orlando, FL.

Wong, J. D., & Almeida, D. M. (2006, August). *Does retirement status affect how older adults spend their time?* Poster presented at the 114th Annual Scientific Meeting of the American Psychological Association, New Orleans, LA.

Woolf, C. J., & Costigan, M. (1999). Transcriptional and posttranslational plasticity and the generation of inflammatory pain. *Proceedings of the National Academy of Sciences, 96*, 7723–7730.

Zautra, A. (2003). *Emotions, stress, and health*. New York: Oxford University Press.

Chapter | 13 |

Health Disparities, Social Class, and Aging

Keith E. Whitfield[1], Roland Thorpe[2], Sarah Szanton[2]

[1]Department of Psychology and Neuroscience, Duke University, Durham, North Carolina, USA [2]School of Public Health, Johns Hopkins University, Baltimore, Maryland, USA

CHAPTER CONTENTS

Introduction	**207**
SES and Health	**208**
Education	208
Income	209
The Relationship Between Income and Education	209
Wealth	210
Race and SES	210
Distribution of Chronic Conditions, Acute Conditions, and Disability	**211**
Chronic Conditions	211
Disability	211
By Ethnicity	211
Biobehavioral Explanations of Health Disparities	**212**
Weathering	212
Allostatic Load	212
The Role of Genetics in Health Disparities Research	**213**
New Challenges	**214**
References	**214**

INTRODUCTION

The composition of the United States is quickly becoming more demographically diverse, particularly in the proportion of people of color (Macera et al., 2000). The significant increase in diversity has made policy makers and social science and medical researchers recognize the enormous disparities that exist in health across racial and ethnic populations. In 1998, President Clinton committed the United States to the elimination of health disparities in racial and ethnic minority populations by the year 2010 and the National Institutes of Health (NIH) has responded by creating the Office for Research on Minority Health. The mission of that office is to identify and support research opportunities to close the gap in health status of underserved populations, promote the inclusion of minorities in clinical trials, enhance the capacity of the minority community to address health problems, increase collaborative research and research training between minority and majority institutions, and improve the competitiveness and increase the numbers of well-trained minority scientists applying for NIH funding. This "call to arms" requires a better understanding of the current status as well as the sources of variability in health among minorities. Investigations of the origins of health disparities across ethnic groups have traditionally emphasized hypotheses that concentrate on social and economic inequities related to differential health outcomes.

Health disparities are described as differences in the incidence, prevalence, mortality, burden of diseases, and other adverse health conditions or outcomes between minority and majority population groups. Health disparities have been observed in gender, age, ethnicity, socioeconomic status (SES), geography, sexual orientation, disability, and special health care needs. Disparities occur among groups who have persistently experienced historical trauma, social disadvantage, or discrimination, and systematically experience worse health or greater health risks than more advantaged social groups.

There is a growing literature on health disparities among members of racial and ethnic groups in the United States (Collins et al., 1999). While differences do not exist for every group on every health index, health disparities are represented by the general

DOI: 10.1016/B978-0-12-380882-0.00013-9

pattern of poorer health (e.g., life expectancy, self-reported health status, incidence of disease) among members of racial or ethnic minority groups when compared to the majority group(s). Disparities in health care are thought to arise from many sources including but not limited to disparities in the access to care and quality of care that is received (Smedley et al., 2002). Disparities in health reflect not only the lack of health insurance but the combined effects of poverty and lack of health insurance (Isaacs & Schroeder, 2004). While some research on disparities in care due to health insurance have focused on individuals insured through either the Medicare or Medicaid programs or private insurance, there is also evidence of racial/ethnic disparities in quality of care within SES /Medicaid recipients (Ali & Osberg, 1997; Bradley et al., 2001; Lillie-Blanton et al., 2001; Lozano et al., 1995; Moore & Hepworth, 1994). "Disparity," in the context of public health and social science, has also begun to include the implications of injustice. A health disparity specifically should be viewed as a chain of events signified by a difference in (1) environment; (2) access to, utilization of, and quality of care; (3) health status; or (4) a particular health outcome that deserves scrutiny (National Association of Chronic Disease Directors, 2009).

The goal of this chapter is to discuss previous research on the interrelationships between health disparities, social class, and aging as they relate to psychological dimensions of the human condition. To understand the psychology of aging for ethnic and social minority groups, we will draw from disciplines that include medical, biomedical, sociology, public health, and the humanities. To accomplish this goal, we operate under several assumptions: (1) we will provide information about each component (social class and health disparities) and provide insights about the interactions between these main effects, and (2) we will not be exhaustive in every example of these interrelationships, instead we will provide useful examples for understanding how each of these main effects contribute to the psychology of aging for ethnic minority groups.

SES AND HEALTH

SES is one of the most critical variables in understanding health (Smedley et al., 2002). It is defined as an individual's position in a system of social stratification that differentially allocates the major resources enabling people to achieve health and other desired goals (House & Williams, 2000). These resources centrally include education, occupation, income, assets, or wealth (House & Williams, 2000). Although SES disparities in health and functional outcomes are well established, our understanding of this persistent relationship remains incomplete. This is in large part because of insufficient assessment of key dimensions of SES and evaluation of interrelationships among SES parameters. Research has repeatedly shown a residual effect even after controlling for several variables known to be related to SES and the outcome of interest (Braveman et al., 2005; Williams & Collins, 1995). This highlights the importance of a more complete understanding of SES and how it affects health and function by examining measures of SES beyond income and education (Braveman et al., 2005; LaVeist, 2005a; Thorpe et al., 2008a). This is particularly true for older adults whose income is potentially reduced due to retirement and their educational attainment level is not likely to change. Additional SES factors such as financial strain (Szanton et al., 2010) and educational quality have been shown to be associated with health and cognitive functioning (Allaire & Whitfield, 2004). Moreover to complicate the relationship even more, SES operates at different levels throughout the life course, and each SES measure may have a different pathway to the health outcome of interest (Herd et al., 2007; Zimmer & House, 2003). Furthermore SES factors also have been shown to interact with other social factors such as race and gender to produce different health outcomes (Williams & Collins, 1995). Interestingly, while SES is multidimensional and complex, most research in the United States focuses on the three primary measures of SES — education, income, and wealth.

Education

Education is one of the most widely obtained measures of SES because it is largely determined early in the life course and remains relatively stable across adulthood. There are several pathways that educational attainments are associated with such as improved health and extended life expectancy. For example, an individual's reading, writing, and problem-solving skills are enhanced with the number of years of education achieved and this in turn potentially provides more opportunities such as better employment in society (Liu & Hummer, 2008; Mirowsky & Ross, 2003). High educational attainment is also associated with individuals engaging in favorable health behaviors such as increased physical activity, abstinence from tobacco use, and maintenance of healthy and ideal body weight (Link & Phelan, 1995; Mirowsky & Ross, 2003). Additionally, higher levels of education provide improved access to new health information and technologies that may ameliorate some health problems and not only promote longevity but quality of life as well (Link & Phelan, 1995). With regard to race differences in education, the Black/White gap in education (measured by high school graduates and college completion) has narrowed over the last two decades, but blacks are still disadvantaged with lower rates of life expectancy (Buchmann & DiPrete, 2006; Lin et al., 2003; U.S. Bureau of the Census, 2005). Lin et al. (2003) stratified by education, income, and employment status and still found that Blacks still had higher rates of mortality.

Education is a very important indicator of SES that is easily obtained in research studies. However, when studying SES disparities, particularly across the life course and among older adults, it is imperative to account for educational quality because for many groups, particularly African Americans, there have been significant changes in education during their lifetime. For example, Allaire & Whitfield (2004) examined whether there were differences in the structure of specific cognitive abilities and their association with age and education in a sample of African American elders with two different early educational experiences; one group that had attended desegregated schools and the other that had not. The results indicated that the pattern of age differences in cognition differed between the two groups. The desegregated sample exhibited significant negative age differences for some cognitive abilities while the segregated group did not, suggesting that it is important to consider the nature of the educational experience when examining dimensions of aging in African American older adults. Yet, studies examining the association between educational histories and health indicators are limited, but have the potential to provide important and fine distinctions in understanding SES disparities in health outcomes.

Income

SES is often implicitly associated with income. Yet income is regarded as confidential information and is not measured or poorly captured in many studies. Unlike education, income is a resource that increases from early adulthood to middle age, after which it tends to stabilize and even decline (Duncan, 1988). There is a consistent inverse association between income and health. People with low incomes consistently exhibit higher rates of morbidity, physical impairments, functional limitations, disability, mortality, and lower rates of self-rated health compared to their more affluent counterparts (House et al., 1994; Kington & Smith, 1997; McDonough et al., 1997; Mirowsky & Ross, 2003; Mulatu & Schooler, 2002). Although there are several pathways for how income influences morbidity and mortality, we will elaborate on material deprivation, psychosocial, and behavioral factors. Material deprivation including not being able to afford basic amenities like housing, food, and clothing has been shown to explain a considerable part of the association between low income and health. This finding suggests that income policies could and need to be developed to ensure that the basic needs of low income people are met (Stronks et al., 1998).

The second pathway that links income to health is through psychosocial factors (House & Williams, 2000). For instance, low-income people typically live in stressful and despondent environments, endure discrimination and racism, and have fewer opportunities afforded to them thereby altering biological processes that lead to disease manifestation (Adler et al., 1994; Byrne & Whyte, 1980; Cohen et al., 1993; Hayward et al., 1997). Low-income individuals tend to be more socially isolated, depressed, and feel they have less control over their lives, all of which are known to be associated with poor health (House & Williams, 2000; Rowe & Kahn, 1987; Turner & Marino, 1994).

The third pathway linking income to health is behavioral risk factors. People with low income tend to engage in negative health behaviors such as smoking, physical inactivity, and consuming too much food or alcohol. These negative health behaviors have been shown to be associated with higher rates of morbidity and mortality (Hayward et al., 2000). However, any single set of these factors (e.g., health behaviors, stress, social relationships and support, or psychological disparities) can account for just 10 to 20% of the association between SES and health (Lantz et al., 1998, 2005; Marmot, 2004). The relationship between income and health requires further examination, especially other possible pathways that may link income to health and if these pathways vary by gender and race.

One potential problem with measuring income is that it is subject to reverse causation (also referred to as downward drift; LaVeist, 2005b); that is, typically low income is thought to produce poor health. However, the reverse is also true; poor health leads to low income. For example, individuals with poor health and functioning often achieve lower education, occupation, and income relative to persons without those conditions. In contrast, persons who experience serious illness and limitations in physical functioning face unemployment and downward mobility. Although health status can influence income, there is more evidence that income strongly affects health and function (Adler & Newman, 2002; Fiscella & Williams, 2004; LaVeist, 2005a; Lynch et al.,1997; Ross & Wu, 1995).

The Relationship Between Income and Education

Often researchers hesitate to include both income and education in one statistical model because of the possibility of collinearity (Braveman et al., 2005). While several studies have shown that education and income are correlated, these correlations are not strong enough to justify using education as a proxy for income (or vice versa; Abramson et al., 1982; Braveman et al., 2001; Gazmararian et al., 1996; Winkleby et al., 1992). While high educational attainment might provide specific kinds of health-promoting knowledge, this information is of little use without the material resources to act on it. For example, those with higher incomes can better afford to live in clean and safe neighborhoods, buy healthier foods, and engage in leisure-time physical activity. Higher incomes may reduce exposure to psychosocial hazards such as stress and enhance coping mechanisms ranging from social relationships to psychological dispositions such as control (e.g., House & Williams, 2005). Furthermore, Blacks and women earn less than Whites and men at similar educational levels (Hamil-Luker, 2005; LaVeist, 2005a; Liu & Hummer, 2008). Both income and education can influence the etiology of many health outcomes, in part through common pathways involving material resources. However the pathway linking income and education to health may also be different (Zimmer & House, 2003). Thus, income and education are correlated but represent two different measures of SES and should be treated as such.

Wealth

Wealth is a measure of SES that has not received much attention among public health researchers compared to other SES indicators in the United States. This is largely because wealth, similar to income, can be considered confidential for the interviewee and methods and measurement needed to calculate wealth are time-consuming. Wealth refers to the accumulated assets that an individual has, and it is the possession of these assets that can provide additional resources beyond income including investment real estate, land, car, and home ownership, and investments (e.g., savings, stocks, mutual funds). However, the major source of wealth for most Americans is equity from home ownership. Because wealth can modify the effects of restricted income due to job loss or retirement, it may be more important than income with respect to health and particularly true for older adults.

Net worth is another measure of wealth and is defined as one's assets minus one's liabilities (LaVeist, 2005b). It is rarely collected in health-related studies, in part, because it requires several additional questions to the questionnaire, which may not always be feasible. Alternatively, one could collect only assets and use it as a proxy for wealth as has been done in several studies (LaVeist et al., 2007; Rooks et al., 2002; Thorpe et al., 2008a). While racial differences in income and education have declined over the past four decades (LaVeist, 2005b; Orzechowski & Sepielli, 2003; U.S. Bureau of the Census, 2005), there are still disparities in wealth.

Past research that has collected data on wealth shows that race differences in wealth are much larger than those in income (Williams & Collins, 2001) due to the large differences in the inheritance and intergenerational transfers of wealth across race. Eller reported that the median net worth of White households in the United States was $44,408 compared to $4,604 for blacks and $5,345 for Hispanics (Eller, 1994). At every income level the net worth of Black and Hispanic households was dramatically lower than their White counterparts. Thus, measures of assets are important to capture a broad picture of the economic status of households (LaVeist, 2005a; Thorpe et al., 2008a; Williams & Collins, 1995).

It has been argued that wealth is a more appropriate SES indicator than income particularly among older adults because their income is often fixed (Robert & House, 1996), and thus can provide a more accurate picture of the overall SES in older ages (Crystal & Shea, 1990; Hurd, 1989).

Race and SES

A key objective of the public health agenda is to reduce, if not eliminate, health disparities (U.S. Department of Health and Human Services, 2000; U.S. Department of Health and Human Services, 2001). However, over the past two decades little progress has been achieved as African Americans continue to exhibit poorer health and physical and cognitive functioning relative to Whites (Bell et al., 2010; Hayward et al., 2000; Mehta et al., 2004). Many investigators believe race differences are a manifestation of SES differences, yet our understanding of SES disparities is limited because race and SES are inextricably linked in the United States with African Americans having markedly fewer socioeconomic resources than Whites (House & Williams, 2000; Rooks et al., 2002; Sudano & Baker, 2006; Thorpe et al., 2008a). Moreover, the overlap between race and SES complicates efforts to determine whether it is, "race *and* class" or "race *or* class" that produces disparities in health status (Braveman et al., 2005; LaVeist et al., 2007; Navarro, 1990).

Typically this problem is addressed by using multivariate modeling in national samples to simultaneously specify the effects of race and measures of SES (such as income or education) on a dependent variable. However, this approach is inadequate (LaVeist et al., 2007; Thorpe et al., 2008a) because even after adjusting for income and education, unmeasured differences remain in SES between race groups, and there remains unmeasured heterogeneity associated with extreme differences in the historical and social contexts of various race groups in the United States (e.g., historical discrimination and intergenerational transfers of wealth). Even multivariate modeling may not be sufficient to overcome this source of heterogeneity (Braveman et al., 2005; LaVeist, 2005a). Moreover, even in a large national survey, multivariate modeling may lead to biased results because of small cell sizes in some race/SES groupings. For example, small numbers of low income Whites or high income Blacks (LaVeist et al., 2007).

Some investigators have developed or employed approaches to overcome the confounding of race and SES. One approach is to conduct within-group investigations, which provides the opportunity to examine how social variables contribute to heterogeneity within that particular group (e.g., Whitfield et al., 2008); that is, if one is interested in understanding how SES and race affects health, then stratifying by race and examining the SES effects on health within each race group is a logical strategy. This will provide additional information that could not be gleaned from merely examining a parameter estimate for race (Kaufman et al., 1997; LaVeist, 2005a; Williams, 1997). Another approach that is gaining attention is to control for the cofounding of race and SES in the study design. Currently we are aware of two studies that have employed this approach (LaVeist et al., 2008; Kuczmarski et al., 2010). Investigators who seek to understand the relationship between SES and health in older populations should carefully consider one of the above approaches, particularly when trying to understand how social variables contribute to this relationship.

DISTRIBUTION OF CHRONIC CONDITIONS, ACUTE CONDITIONS, AND DISABILITY

The prevalence of disability and chronic and acute conditions increases as adults age. As mentioned previously, SES is consistently related to health status, which includes but is not limited to chronic conditions, acute conditions, and disability. These relationships also vary by ethnicity. Each of these components are discussed in this section.

Chronic Conditions

Those of lower SES are more likely to develop chronic conditions earlier in life and with greater severity at any age. For example, low income people are more likely to develop diabetes; the average age at onset is younger than their higher income counterparts, and their glucose level is more likely to be dangerously high than the glucose levels of their higher income counterparts (Bachmann et al., 2003). These disparities are due to a complex web of factors including decreased access to active physical settings (Gordon-Larsen et al., 2006; Lovasi et al., 2009) decreased leisure time, decreased access to supermarkets that sell healthy foods (Moore & Diez Roux, 2006), increased life stress (Braveman, 2009), and decreased access to preventive health care (Hoffman & Schwartz, 2008) among other important factors.

Partly due to the increased burden of chronic disease, with accompanying underlying inflammation and immune status, people of lower SES are more likely to develop acute conditions such as pneumonia (Flory et al., 2009).

Disability

With the exception of birth-related disabilities, most older adults with disabilities developed them from sequelae of chronic diseases (i.e., uncontrolled hypertension leading to stroke causing hemiplegia) or work-related accidents/conditions (i.e., asbestosis from coal mining). Since chronic diseases can lead to disabilities, and dangerous, repetitive work conditions are more likely to be experienced by those of low SES, it follows that older adults of low SES bare much higher rates of disability (Schoeni et al., 2005) than do their higher SES counterparts. These disabilities include essential tasks such as bathing, getting dressed, and toileting (i.e., activities of daily living; ADLs) as well as mobility disability and functional limitations (Thorpe et al., 2008b). There is considerable but not complete overlap between those with disabilities and those who are considered frail. Those of lower SES have greater odds of being frail (Szanton et al., 2010). Another reason those of low SES suffer increased rates of disabilities is that intrinsic in the definition of disability is the gap between what one can do and the environment one is in (Verbrugge & Jette, 1994). Low income people are less likely to have access to services and adaptations that allow them to bathe, cook, and be mobile for themselves such as shower chairs, adjustable countertops, and electric scooters. Thus, they are more likely to have severe physical limitations *and* less likely to have access to successful adaptations for the physical limitations.

By Ethnicity

African Americans have higher rates of diseases that can have disabling effects such as diabetes, cardiovascular disease, and hypertension (Bowen, 2009) as well as less access to high quality health care (Committee on Understanding and Eliminating Racial and Ethnic Disparities in Health Care, 2003). For example, in the nationally representative Health and Retirement Study sample of more than 14,000 people over age 50, Bowen found that 59% of African Americans had hypertension compared to 40% of Caucasians. Similarly, African Americans had twice the prevalence of diabetes as Caucasians (22% compared to 11%) and 53% of African American had arthritis while 46% of Caucasians had arthritis. Despite great strides toward equality over the past century, older African American adults have significantly greater rates of disability (Thorpe et al., 2008b), disease, and mortality than their White counterparts (Hummer et al., 2004). Among women 60 to 64 years old, African Americans have 173% greater rate of disability than Caucasians (Hummer et al., 2004).

BIOBEHAVIORAL EXPLANATIONS OF HEALTH DISPARITIES

The well-documented disparities in life expectancy and morbidity across socioeconomic and racial groups (Adler & Newman, 2002) have led scientists to move beyond documentation to seeking explanations for these inequalities. Life course research on disparities has mainly focused on differential exposure to specific social and environmental risks, or biobehavioral explanations. A life course perspective provides the opportunity to assess the impact of long-term negative (or positive) experiences including the timing of earlier life experiences (George, 2005). Both the weathering hypothesis (Geronimus & Hillemeier, 1992; Geronimus et al., 2006) and cumulative disadvantage theory (Dannefer, 1987) contend that long-term exposure to social and environmental inequalities leads to increases in disparities in middle and later life both within and across groups. Some health disparities may be the result of cumulative exposure to lifetime stressors that are more frequent, worse, and less remitting than those that higher SES or non-minority older adults face. Two prominent frameworks to describe stressors' impact on aging are "weathering" and "allostatic load."

Weathering

The weathering hypothesis asserts that African Americans experience earlier morbidity and mortality as a consequence of the cumulative effect of social and economic adversity. Originally proposed in the context of adolescent childbearing (Geronimus, 2001), it has been used to examine health disparities in cumulative biological risk (Geronimus et al., 2006), hypertension (Geronimus et al., 2007), and mortality (Astone et al., 2002) in adults. Weathering helps explain the interaction between age and race/ethnicity such that African Americans acquire conditions normally associated with aging at younger ages than Whites (Geronimus et al., 2006). The weathering hypothesis suggests that the consequences of social inequality on health in certain populations may compound with age, leading to a widening gap in health status for individuals within and across racial/ethnic groups. Thus, observed health disparities in the onset of age-related diseases by racial/ethnic groups reflect accelerated aging in African Americans.

The theoretical concept of weathering may be seen in other research that focuses on unique stressors and "high coping strategies" in explaining morbidity among middle class African Americans. This health deterioration leads to methodological problems in that African Americans may not survive to be sampled in research on older adults, which leaves relatively healthy African Americans to be compared with their healthy and unhealthy White counterparts. Furthermore, a high prevalence of comorbidity experienced earlier in the life course has long-term, adverse effects for chronic conditions later in life (Blackwell et al., 2001). In a variety of health indicators, such as reproductive health (Hudson, 2004; LaClere et al., 1998; Rauh et al., 2008), mortality (Lantz et al., 2001; Wildsmith, 2002), allostatic load (Geronimus et al., 2006), and functional status (Geronimus, 2001), age patterns by race consistent with the weathering hypothesis have been found to underlie the disparities observed across ethnic groups. Behavioral studies of health and the complex interrelationship between disadvantage across the life course, health, and ethnicity would benefit from integrating this hypothesis into their design.

Allostatic Load

The allostatic load framework is sometimes referred to as the mechanism for weathering. Allostatic load is a construct theorized to quantify stress-induced biological risk that the weathering hypothesis predicts. Differences in allostatic load may reflect the accumulation of physiological changes induced by differences in exposure to psychological stressors and thus provide a mechanistic link to understanding and studying biobehavioral interfaces that create health disparities.

The multisystem approach to the construct of allostatic load is a descendant of the work of Hans Selye, who proposed stress-reacting "agents" had "a general effect on large portions of the body" (Selye, 1946). While there is no scientific consensus on the definition of stress, this chapter defines "stress" as "physical or perceived threat to homeostasis" (Pacak & Palkovits, 2001). More modern stress researchers such as Sterling and Eyer (1981) developed the concept of allostasis and allostatic load. Allostasis comes from the word *allo*, which means *change* and *stasis*, which means *stability*. Further refined by McEwen and Stellar (1993), allostasis refers to the body's adaptation to stressors. Healthy functioning requires ongoing physiologic adjustment that responds to stressors such as isolation, hunger, danger, and infection (McEwen, 1998). These systems are the sympathetic nervous system, and the neuroendocrine system, in particular the hypothalamic-pituitary-adrenal (HPA) axis and the immune system. Together, they constitute the physiologic stress response. The stress response temporarily subjugates internal needs in response to external ones (Porges, 1995), which are essential for survival. In his refinement of the concept into a framework that can be used in a research context, McEwen theorized that a person with multiple acute or chronic stressors or stress exposure would suffer physiologic consequences from this continued subjugation (McEwen & Stellar, 1993). Thus, multiple recurring stressors leave the body with a physiologic stamp (Seplaki et al., 2004) reflected in biomarkers, and in derangement of the body systems they affect. This physiologic stamp is the allostatic load, which then impairs one's ability to adapt to future stressors.

Allostatic load has been shown to be a preclinical marker of pathophysiologic processes hypothesized to precede the onset of disease or disability (Karlamangla et al., 2002). Importantly for health disparities, allostatic load has been found to vary by sociodemographic factors such as race and SES (Geronimus et al., 2006) as well to predict cardiovascular disease, cognitive decline, and mortality (Seeman et al., 2001, 2004) and been associated with frailty (Szanton et al., 2010). While this construct has great utility across many domains critical to understanding aging, more longitudinal studies using this framework are warranted with diverse populations of midlife and older adults.

There is an apparent paradox in disparities observed for physical and mental health by ethnicity. In contrast to higher rates of all cause mortality among Blacks and other racial and ethnic minority groups, there is evidence from epidemiological and clinical studies that in comparison to non-Hispanic whites, African Americans have either the same or lower rates of mental disorders (Jackson, 2002). Jackson has argued that many African Americans faced with stressful conditions engage in behaviors that alleviate the pressing stressful reactions to these exposures (Jackson, 2006; Jackson et al., 2009). Those exposures are thought to be the same ones that increase morbidity and mortality. Engaging in some poor health behaviors may interfere or mask the stress response exhibited by responses through the HPA axis, which could lead to mental disorders (Barden, 2004).

THE ROLE OF GENETICS IN HEALTH DISPARITIES RESEARCH

The role of genetics in the origin of racial health disparities is receiving growing attention but has been susceptible to considerable misinterpretation (Whitfield, 2004, 2005; Whitfield & McClearn, 2005). The misinterpretation of genetically informative samples should not deter this line of inquiry. Instead, scientifically sound studies examining biobehavioral relationships, such as studying the health of minority families with older family members, will provide an excellent avenue for advancing the science of aging, particularly as it relates to health disparities.

The frequent misuse of genetic research to justify racist viewpoints is one likely reason for the avoidance of explanations about health disparities using genetic approaches as a means for understanding health disparities. It is a correct assumption that investigations of health differentials across ethnic groups solely on the basis of genetic differences will not yield accurate identification of the mechanisms responsible for health disparities (Whitfield, 2005). Preconceived notions about genetically based racial inferiority have hindered advances in understanding and reducing health disparities. Attempting to explain the differential health burden ethnic minorities experience by genetic differences goes against probability given there are only small genetic differences across racial groups and more variability within each group. The role of genetic influences, however, cannot be completely dismissed. Recent discussions about the complexity of how genes work within networks of genetic and environmental effects to produce phenotypes has provided salient points to be mindful of in considering the potential of genetic approach for understanding health disparities (Whitfield & McClearn, 2005). First, while the amount of the genome that is related to disease risk is currently unknown, what risks are related to genetic influences are likely of a multi-genetic fashion rather than a single gene manner (Hamer, 2002). Additionally, genes do not operate without significant input from the environment (Whitfield, 2004). Examples of environmental factors include such things as diet, education, health care, and sources of stress and coping like family, neighborhood, and friends.

The manner in which genes have the potential for playing a role in creating health differentials requires even greater explanation. These explanations require attention to not only the phenotype under consideration but to the distinctions of race compared to ethnicity. It is not genes defining individuals from different ethnic groups that is key to the elucidation of health differentials per se. Instead, describing health differentials as arising from insults to a complex system represented by the interaction between genes and environments, which creates excess burden of chronic illness and disease within some groups is a more accurate perspective.

In contrast to simply focusing on genetic explanations, there is ample information that differences in environmental factors between ethnic groups account for disparities in health status. Recent research on the multifactorial nature of risks for disease processes and understanding behaviors is perhaps our best indicator that science must avoid a reductionistic view (Whitfield & McClearn, 2005). Genetic reductionism assumes knowing and manipulating the genome will cure all our ills. Rather, we must understand how genetic and environmental influences work in concert to account for health conditions and the psychosocial variables that impact health. Much of previous research has focused on the behaviors and social structures that produce differences in health and disease across ethnic groups. One of the future and formidable challenges to using the information ascertained from adding genetic information to examinations of health differentials is to understand the underlying effect genes have on health and aging within complex environments or contexts. We may find that the polymorphisms that occur in genotypes are destructive or protective factors related to disease and health that are created, modified, or triggered by cultural and contextual factors (see Hernandez & Blazer, 2006). An additional layer of complexity to thinking about these possibilities is that they may change over the life course. For example, in a recent study stressed mice were found to produce hormones that influenced the way vasopressin genes reacted, which in turn affected their behavior throughout their life span (Murgatroyd et al., 2009). This complex cascade of interconnecting effects between genes and environment need much more examination.

Recent advances in molecular genetics have significantly increased our ability to understand the contribution of genes to health disparities. The National Human Genome Research Institute (NHGRI) of the NIH announced in June of 2000 that they had developed a working draft of the human genome. This historic event places science on the doorstep of limitless possibilities including new insights about diseases and how to treat and prevent them. The trepidation by some scientists about using genetic approaches in the study of health differentials may arise from previous research that used poorly or inappropriately defined phenotypic characteristics to make generalizations about group differences. Knowing the sequence of the genome, however, is only the beginning. Equally important will be knowing what phenotype is truly of interest and our knowledge of how the environment influences health, disease, and complex behaviors associated with health differentials.

NEW CHALLENGES

The development and testing of explanatory hypotheses about the underlying mechanisms that produce health differentials between ethnic groups will be crucial in identifying solutions for reducing the current disparities. These solutions will not only be seen in the reform of health care practices, health worker training, and health care access, but will also include improved transfer of information about health conditions and reform of some social practices. It is clearly evident that behavioral and social influences like racial discrimination contributes in a myriad of ways to health disparities. What is not clear are the ways we can create environments that are rich in protective psychosocial factors. For example, the intersection of age curves of mortality at the older ages commonly called a "cross-over effect" has been observed that arises from lower Caucasian mortality rates at younger ages and lower rates for African Americans at the oldest ages. It has been argued as to whether the cross-over effect really occurs (Whitfield et al., 2002). If it is true, the question is why and how does this occur. The answer may lie in understanding sources of individual variability in health outcomes that can be described in the balance between the contributions of environmental as well as genetic factors. New models of the contribution of genetic and environmental factors that account for social inequities are being posed (Whitfield, 2005). These models suggest there are complex pathways that account for the mortality and morbidity observed among individuals and groups to produce health differentials. Furthermore, the interplay and interrelationship among the psychosocial factors represent risk as well as protective factors in the variability observed in pathways that lead to or away from health disparities.

The ability to include genetic information with assessments of environmental factors will greatly aid in the search for the underpinnings of health disparities. Harnessing the current technology while avoiding past pitfalls of genetic determinism and inappropriate interpretations of the meaning of genetic contributions will advance the science of health disparities research (Whitfield & McClearn, 2005). Advancing this science of health disparities would also benefit from longitudinal studies that include family data, sufficient numbers of minorities, and more in-depth examination of social, biological, and behavioral factors that impact health and disparities across racial/ethnic as well as economic status groups.

REFERENCES

Abramson, J. H., Gofin, R., Habib, J., Pridan, H., & Gofin, J. (1982). Indicators of social class: A comparative appraisal of measures for use in epidemiological studies. *Social Science & Medicine, 16*(20), 1739–1746.

Adler, N., Boyce, T., Chesney, M., Folkman, S., & Syme, S. L. (1994). SES and health. *American Psychologist, 49*(1), 15–24.

Adler, N. E., & Newman, K. (2002). Socioeconomic disparities in health: Pathways and policies. *Health Affairs, 21*, 60–76.

Ali, S., & Osberg, J. S. (1997). Differences in follow-up visits between African-American and white Medicaid children hospitalized for asthma. *Journal of Health Care for the Poor and Underserved, 8*(1), 83–98.

Allaire, J. C., & Whitfield, K. E. (2004). Relationships among education, age, and cognitive functioning in older African Americans: The impact of desegregation. *Aging, Neuropsychology, and Cognition S2 — Aging & Cognition, 11*(4), 443–449. doi:10.1080/13825580490521511.

Astone, N. M., Ensminger, M., & Juon, H. S. (2002). Early adult characteristics and mortality among inner-city African American women. *American Journal of Public Health, 92*(4), 640–645.

Bachmann, M. O., Eachus, J., Hopper, C. D., Davey Smith, G., Propper, C., Pearson, N. J., et al. (2003). Socio-economic inequalities in diabetes complications, control, attitudes and health service use: A cross-sectional study. *Diabetic Medicine: A Journal of the British Diabetic Association, 20*(11), 921–929.

Barden, N. (2004). Implications of the hypothalamic-pituitary-adrenal axis in the physiopathology of depression. *Journal of Psychiatry Neuroscience, 29*(3), 185–193.

Bell, C. B., Thorpe, R. J. Jr., & LaVeist, T. A. (2010). Race/ethnicity and hypertension: The role of social support. *American Journal of Hypertension* 23(5), 534–540.

Blackwell, D. L., Hayward, M. D., & Crimmins, E. M. (2001). Does childhood health affect chronic morbidity in later life? *Social Science & Medicine (1982), 52*(8), 1269–1284.

Bowen, M. E. (2009). Childhood socioeconomic status and racial differences in disability: Evidence from the health and retirement study (1998–2006). *Social Science & Medicine (1982), 69*(3), 433–441.

Bradley, C. J., Given, C. W., & Roberts, C. (2001). Disparities in cancer diagnosis and survival. *Cancer, 91*(1), 178–188.

Braveman, P. (2009). A health disparities perspective on obesity research. *Preventing Chronic Disease, 6*(3), A91.

Braveman, P., Cubbin, C., Marchi, K., Egerter, S., & Chavez, G. (2001). Measuring socioeconomic status/position in studies of racial/ethnic disparities: Maternal and infant health. *Public Health Reports, 116*(5), 449–463.

Braveman, P. A., Cubbin, C., Egerter, S., Chideya, S., Marchi, K. S., Metzler, M., et al. (2005). Socioeconomic status in health research: One size does not fit all. *Journal of the American Medical Association, 294*(22), 2879–2888.

Buchmann, C., & DiPrete, T. (2006). The growing female advantage in college completion: The role of family background and academic achievement. *American Sociological Review, 71*(4), 515–541.

Byrne, D. G., & Whyte, H. M. (1980). Life events and myocardial infarction revisited: The role of measures of individual impact. *Psychosomatic Medicine, 42*(1), 1–10.

Cohen, S., Tyrell, D. A., & Smith, A. P. (1993). Negative life events, perceived stress, and susceptibility to the common cold. *Journal of Personality and Social Psychology, 64*(1), 131–140.

Collins, K. S., Hall, A., & Neuhaus, C. (1999). *U.S. minority health: A chartbook*. New York: The Commonwealth Fund.

Committee on Understanding and Eliminating Racial and Ethnic Disparities in Health Care. (2003). In B. Smedley, A. Stith, & A. Nelson (Eds.), *Unequal treatment: Confronting racial and ethnic disparities in healthcare*. Washington DC: National Academies Press.

Crystal, S., & Shea, D. (1990). Cumulative advantage, cumulative disadvantage, and inequality among elderly people. *The Gerontologist, 30*(4), 437–443.

Dannefer, D. (1987). Aging as intracohort differentiation: Accentuation, the Matthew effect, and the life course. *Sociological Forum, 2*, 211–236.

Duncan, G. (1988). The volatility of family income over the life course. In P. Bates, D. Featherman, & R. Lerner (Eds.), *Life span development and behavior* (pp. 31–58). Hillsdale, NJ: Lawrence Erlbaum Associates.

Eller, T. J. (1994). *Household wealth and asset ownership: 1991: Current population reports* No. P70-34). Washington, DC: U.S. Government Printing Office.

Fiscella, K., & Williams, D. R. (2004). Health disparities based on socioeconomic inequities: Implications for urban health care. *Academic Medicine, 79*(12), 1139–1147.

Flory, J. H., Joffe, M., Fishman, N. O., Edelstein, P. H., & Metlay, J. P. (2009). Socioeconomic risk factors for bacteraemic pneumococcal pneumonia in adults. *Epidemiology and Infection, 137*(5), 717–726.

Gazmararian, J. A., Adams, M. M., & Pamuk, E. R. (1996). Associations between measures of socioeconomic status and maternal health behavior. *American Journal of Preventive Medicine, 12*(2), 108–115.

George, L. K. (2005). Socioeconomic status and health across the life course: Progress and prospects. *Journals of Gerontology: Psychological Sciences and Social Sciences, 60, Spec No 2*, 135–139.

Geronimus, A. T. (2001). Understanding and eliminating racial inequalities in women's health in the united states: The role of the weathering conceptual framework. *Journal of the American Medical Women's Association, 56*(4), 133–150.

Geronimus, A. T., Bound, J., Keene, D., & Hicken, M. (2007). Black-White differences in age trajectories of hypertension prevalence among adult women and men, 1992–2002. *Ethnicity and Disease, 17*, 40–48.

Geronimus, A. T., Hicken, M., Keene, D., & Bound, J. (2006). "Weathering" and age patterns of allostatic load scores among blacks and whites in the united states. *American Journal of Public Health, 96*(5), 826–833.

Geronimus, A. T., & Hillemeier, M. M. (1992). Patterns of blood lead levels in US black and white women of childbearing age. *Ethnicity & Disease, 2*(3), 222–231.

Gordon-Larsen, P., Nelson, M. C., Page, P., & Popkin, B. M. (2006). Inequality in the built environment underlies key health disparities in physical activity and obesity. *Pediatrics, 117*(2), 417–424.

Hamer, D. (2002). Rethinking behavior genetics. *Science, 298*, 71–72.

Hamil-Luker, J. (2005). Women's wages: Cohort differences in returns to education and training over time. *Social Science Quarterly, 86*(5), 1261–1278.

Hayward, M., Pienta, A., & McLaughlin, D. (1997). Inequality in men's mortality: The socioeconomic status gradient and geographic context. *Journal of Health and Social Behavior, 38*(4), 313–330.

Hayward, M. D., Miles, T. P., Crimmins, E. M., & Yang, Y. (2000). The significance of socioeconomic status in explaining the racial gap in chronic health conditions. *American Sociological Review, 65*(6), 910–930.

Health aging in neighborhoods of diversity across the life span (HANDLS): Study design. Retrieved 03/24, 2010, from http://handls.nih.gov/HANDLS-2design.php.

Herd, P., Goesling, B., & House, J. S. (2007). Socioeconomic position and health: The differential effects of education versus income on the onset versus progression of health problems. *Journal of Health and Social Behavior, 48*(3), 223–238.

Hernandez, L. M., & Blazer, D. G. (2006). *Genes, behavior, and the social environment: Moving beyond the nature nurture debate.* Washington, DC: National Academies Press.

Hoffman, C., & Schwartz, K. (2008). Eroding access among nonelderly U.S. adults with chronic conditions: Ten years of change. *Health Affairs (Project Hope), 27*(5), w340–w348.

House, J. S., Lepkowski, J. M., Kinney, A. M., Mero, R. P., Kessler, R. C., & Herzog, A. R. (1994). The social stratification of aging and health. *Journal of Health and Social Behavior, 35*(3), 213–234.

House, J. S., & Williams, D. (2000). Understanding and reducing socioeconomic and racial/ethnic disparities in health. In B. D. Smedly & S. L. Syme (Eds.), *Promoting health: Intervention strategies from social and behavioral* (pp. 82–124). Washington, DC: National Academies Press.

Hudson, P. (2004). Positive aspects and challenges associated with caring for a dying relative at home. *International Journal of Palliative Nursing, 10*(2), 58–65.

Hummer, R., Benjamins, M., & Rogers, R. (2004). Racial and ethnic disparities in health and mortality among the U.S. elderly population. In N. Anderson, R. Bulatao, & B. Cohen (Eds.), *Critical perspectives on racial and ethnic differences in health in late life* (pp. 69–110). Washington, DC: National Academies Press.

Hurd, M. D. (1989). The economic status of the elderly. *Science, 244*(4905), 659–664.

Isaacs, S. L., & Schroeder, S. A. (2004). Class — the ignored determinant of the nation's health. *New England Journal of Medicine, 351*(11), 1137–1142.

Jackson, J. S. (2002). Health and mental health disparities among Black Americans. In M. Hager (Ed.), *Modern psychiatry: Challenges in educating health professionals to meet new needs* (pp. 246–254). New York: Josiah Macy Jr. Foundation.

Jackson, J. S., & Knight, K. M. (2006). Race and self-regulatory health behaviors: The role of stress and the HPA axis in physical and mental health disparities. In K. W. Schaie & L. L. Carstensen (Eds.), *Social structures aging, and self regulation in the elderly* (pp. 189–208). New York: Springer Publishing Co.

Jackson, J. S., Knight, K. M., & Rafferty, J. A. (2009). Race and unhealthy behaviors: Chronic stress, the HPA Axis, and physical and mental health disparities over the life course. *American Journal of Public Health, 99*(12), 1–7.

Karlamangla, A. S., Singer, B. H., McEwen, B. S., Rowe, J. W., & Seeman, T. E. (2002). Allostatic load as a predictor of functional decline. MacArthur studies of successful aging. *Journal of Clinical Epidemiology, 55*(7), 696–710.

Kaufman, J. S., Cooper, R. S., & McGee, D. L. (1997). Socioeconomic status and health in blacks and whites: The problem of residual confounding and the resiliency of race. *Epidemiology, 8*(6), 621–628.

Kington, R. S., & Smith, J. P. (1997). Socioeconomic status and racial and ethnic differences in functional status associated with chronic diseases. *American Journal of Public Health, 87*(5), 805–810.

Kuczmarski, M. F., Sees, A. C., Hotchkiss, L., Contugna, N., Evans, M. K., & Zuderman, A. B. (2010). Higher Healthy Eating Index-2005 Scores Associated with Reduced Symptoms of Depression in an Urban Population: Findings from the Healthy Aging in Neighborhoods of Diversity Across the Life Span (HANDLS) Study. *Journal of the American Dietetic Association,* doi:10.1016/j.jada.2009.11.025.

LaClere, F., Rogers, R., & Peters, K. (1998). Neighborhood social context and racial differences in women's heart disease mortality. *Journal of Health and Social Behavior, 39,* 91–107.

Lantz, P. M., House, J. S., Lepkowski, J. M., Williams, D. R., Mero, R. P., & Chen, J. (1998). Socioeconomic factors, health behaviors, and mortality: Results from a nationally representative prospective study of US adults. *Journal of the American Medical Association, 279*(21), 1703–1708.

Lantz, P. M., House, J. S., Mero, R. P., & Williams, D. R. (2005). Stress, life events, and socioeconomic disparities in health: Results from the Americans' Changing Lives study. *Journal of Health and Social Behavior, 40*(3), 274–288.

Lantz, P. M., Lynch, J. W., House, J. S., Lepkowski, J. M., Mero, R. P., Musick, M. A., et al. (2001). Socioeconomic disparities in health change in a longitudinal study of US adults: The role of health-risk behaviors. *Social Science & Medicine (1982), 53*(1), 29–40.

LaVeist, T., Thorpe, R., Jr., Bowen-Reid, T., Jackson, J., Gary, T., Gaskin, D., et al. (2008). Exploring health disparities in integrated communities: Overview of the EHDIC study. *Journal of Urban Health, 85*(1), 11–21.

LaVeist, T. A. (2005a). Disentangling race and socioeconomic status: A key to understanding health inequalities. *Journal of Urban Health: Bulletin of the New York Academy of Medicine, 82*(2 Suppl. 3), iii26–iii34. doi:10.1093/jurban/jti061.

LaVeist, T. A. (2005b). *Minority populations and health: An introduction to health disparities in the United States* (1st ed.). San Francisco, CA: Jossey-Bass.

LaVeist, T. A., Thorpe, R. J., Jr., Mance, G. A., & Jackson, J. (2007). Overcoming confounding of race with socio-economic status and segregation to explore race disparities in smoking. *Addiction (Abingdon, England), 102*(Suppl. 2), 65–70. doi:10.1111/j.1360-0443.2007.01956.x.

Lillie-Blanton, M., Martinez, R. M., & Salganicoff, A. (2001). Site of medical care: Do racial and ethnic differences persist? *Yale Journal of Health Policy, Law, and Ethics, 1*, 15–32.

Lin, C. C., Rogot, E., Johnson, N. J., Sorlie, P. D., & Arias, E. (2003). A further study of life expectancy by socioeconomic factors in the national longitudinal mortality study. *Ethnicity and Disease, 13*(2), 240–247.

Link, B. G., & Phelan, J. (1995). Social conditions and fundamental causes of disease. *Journal of Health and Social Behavior, Spec. No.*, 80–94.

Liu, H., & Hummer, R. A. (2008). Are educational differences in U.S. self-rated health increasing?: An examination by gender and race. *Social Science & Medicine, 67*(11), 1898–1906.

Lovasi, G. S., Hutson, M. A., Guerra, M., & Neckerman, K. M. (2009). Built environments and obesity in disadvantaged populations. *Epidemiologic Reviews* 31, 7–20. doi:10.1093/epirev/mxp005.

Lozano, P., Connell, F. A., & Koepsell, T. D. (1995). Use of health services by African-American children with asthma on Medicaid. *Journal of the American Medical Association, 274*(6), 469–473.

Lynch, J. W., Kaplan, G. A., & Shema, S. J. (1997). Cumulative impact of sustained economic hardship on physical, cognitive, psychological, and social functioning. *The New England Journal of Medicine, 337*(26), 1889–1895.

Macera, C., Armstead, C., & Anderson, N. (2000). Sociocultural influences on minority health. In A. S. Baum, T. A. Revenson, & J. E. Singer (Eds.), *Handbook of health psychology*. Mahwah, NJ: Lawrence Erlbaum Associates.

Marmot, M. (2004). *Status syndrome*. London. UK: Bloomsbury Publishing.

McDonough, P., Duncan, G. J., Williams, D., & House, J. (1997). Income dynamics and adult mortality in the United States, 1972 through 1989. *American Journal of Public Health, 87*(9), 1476–1483.

McEwen, B. S. (1998). Stress, adaptation, and disease. Allostasis and allostatic load. *Annals of the New York Academy of Sciences, 840*, 33–44.

McEwen, B. S., & Stellar, E. (1993). Stress and the individual. mechanisms leading to disease. *Archives of Internal Medicine, 153*(18), 2093–2101.

Mehta, K. M., Simonsick, E. M., Rooks, R., Newman, A. B., Pope, S. K., Rubin, S. M., et al. (2004). Black and white differences in cognitive function test scores: What explains the difference? *Journal of the American Geriatrics Society, 52*(12), 2120–2127.

Mirowsky, J., & Ross, C. E. (2003). *Education, social class, and health*. New York: Aldine de Gruyter.

Moore, L. V., & Diez Roux, A. V. (2006). Associations of neighborhood characteristics with the location and type of food stores. *American Journal of Public Health, 96*(2), 325–331.

Moore, P., & Hepworth, J. T. (1994). Use of perinatal and infant health services by Mexican-American Medicaid enrollees. *Journal of the American Medical Association, 272*(4), 297–304.

Mulatu, M. S., & Schooler, C. (2002). Causal connections between socioeconomic status and health: Reciprocal effects and mediating mechanisms. *Journal of Health and Social Behavior, 43*(2), 22–41.

Murgatroyd, C., Patchev, A. V., Wu, Y., Micale, V., Bockmühl, Y., Fischer, D., et al. (2009). Dynamic DNA methylation programs persistent adverse effects of early-life stress. *Nature Neuroscience, 12*, 1559–1566.

National Association of Chronic Disease Directors. (2009). http://www.chronicdisease.org/i4a/pages/index.cfm?pageid=3447

Navarro, V. (1990). Race or class versus race and class: Mortality differentials in the United States. *Lancet, 336*(8725), 1238–1240.

Orzechowski, S., & Sepielli, P. (2003). *Net worth and asset ownership of households: 1998 and 2000* (No. P70-88) U.S. Census Bureau.

Pacak, K., & Palkovits, M. (2001). Stressor specificity of central neuroendocrine responses: Implications for stress-related disorders. *Endocrine Reviews, 22*(4), 502–548.

Porges, S. W. (1995). Cardiac vagal tone: A physiological index of stress. *Neuroscience and Biobehavioral Reviews, 19*(2), 225–233.

Rauh, V. A., Landrigan, P. J., & Claudio, L. (2008). Housing and health: Intersection of poverty and environmental exposures. *Annals of the New York Academy of Sciences, 1136*, 276–288.

Robert, S., & House, J. S. (1996). SES differentials in health by age and alternative indicators of SES. *Journal of Aging Health, 8*(3), 359–388.

Rooks, R. N., Simonsick, E. M., Miles, T., Newman, A., Kritchevsky, S. B., Schulz, R., et al. (2002). The association of race and socioeconomic status with cardiovascular disease indicators among older adults in the health, aging, and body composition study. *Journals of Gerontology: Social Sciences, 57B*(4), S247–S256.

Ross, C. W., & Wu, C. (1995). The links between education and health. *American Sociological Review, 60*(5), 719–749.

Rowe, J. W., & Kahn, R. L. (1987). Human aging: Usual and successful. *Science, 237*(4811), 143–149.

Schoeni, R. F., Martin, L. G., Andreski, P. M., & Freedman, V. A. (2005). Persistent and growing socioeconomic disparities in disability among the elderly: 1982–2002. *American Journal of Public Health, 95*(11), 2065–2070.

Seeman, T. E., Crimmins, E., Huang, M. H., Singer, B., Bucur, A., Gruenewald, T., et al. (2004).

Cumulative biological risk and socio-economic differences in mortality: MacArthur studies of successful aging. *Social Science & Medicine (1982)*, *58*(10), 1985–1997.

Seeman, T. E., McEwen, B. S., Rowe, J. W., & Singer, B. H. (2001). Allostatic load as a marker of cumulative biological risk: MacArthur studies of successful aging. *Proceedings of the National Academy of Sciences of the United States of America*, *98*(8), 4770–4775.

Selye, H. (1946). The general adaptation syndrome and the diseases of adaptation. *The Journal of Clinical Endocrinology*, *6*(2), 117–230.

Seplaki, C. L., Goldman, N., Weinstein, M., & Lin, Y. H. (2004). How are biomarkers related to physical and mental well-being? *Journals of Gerontology Series A: Biological Sciences. Medical. Sciences*, *59*(3), 201–217.

Smedley, B. D., Stith, A. Y., & Nelson, A. R. (Eds.), (2002). *Unequal treatment: Confronting racial and ethnic disparities in health care*. Washington, DC: National Academies Press.

Sterling, P., & Eyer, J. (1981). Biological basis of stress-related mortality. *Social Science & Medicine. Part E, Medical Psychology*, *15*(1), 3–42.

Stronks, K., van der Mheen, H. D., & Mackenbach, J. P. (1998). A higher prevalence of health problems in low income groups: Does it reflect relative deprivation? *Journal of Epidemiology and Community Health*, *52*(9), 548–557.

Sudano, J. J., & Baker, D. W. (2006). Explaining US racial/ethnic disparities in health declines and mortality in late middle age: The roles of socioeconomic status, health behaviors, and health insurance. *Social Science & Medicine*, *62*(4), 909–922.

Szanton, S. L., Seplaki, C. L., Thorpe, R. J., Jr., Allen, J. K., & Fried, L. P. (2010). Socioeconomic status is associated with frailty: The women's health and aging studies. *Journal of Epidemiology and Community Health*, *64*(1), 63–67.

Thorpe, R. J., Jr., Brandon, D. T., & LaVeist, T. A. (2008a). Social context as an explanation for race disparities in hypertension: Findings from the exploring health disparities in integrated communities (EHDIC) study. *Social Science & Medicine (1982)*, *67*(10), 1604–1611. doi:10.1016/j.socscimed.2008.07.002.

Thorpe, R. J., Jr., Kasper, J. D., Szanton, S. L., Frick, K. D., Fried, L. P., & Simonsick, E. M. (2008b). Relationship of race and poverty to lower extremity function and decline: Findings from the women's health and aging study. *Social Science & Medicine (1982)*, *66*(4), 811–821.

Turner, R. J., & Marino, F. (1994). Social support and social structure: A descriptive social epidemiology. *Journal of Health and Social Behavior*, *35*(3), 193–212.

U.S. Bureau of the Census. (2005). *Statistical abstract of the United States: 2004–2005*. Washington, DC: U.S. Government Printing Office.

U.S. Department of Health and Human Services. (2000). *Tracking healthy people 2010*. Washington, DC: U.S. Department of Health and Human Services.

U.S. Department of Health and Human Services. (2001). *Healthy people 2010*. Washington, DC: U.S. Department of Health and Human Services.

Verbrugge, L. M., & Jette, A. M. (1994). The disablement process. *Social Science & Medicine*, *38*(1), 1–14.

Whitfield, K. E., Weidner, G., Clark, R., & Anderson, N. B. (2002). Sociodemographic diversity and behavioral medicine. *Journal of Consulting and Clinical Psychology*, *70*(3), 463–481.

Whitfield, K. E. (2004). Behavioral genetic studies of health. In N. B. Anderson, & M. Kemeny, (Eds.), *Encyclopedia of health and behavior: Vol. 1* (pp. 85–89). Thousand Oaks, CA: Sage Publications.

Whitfield, K. E. (2005). Studying biobehavioral aspects of health among older adult minorities. *Journal of Urban Health*, *82*(2 Suppl. 3), iii103–iii110.

Whitfield, K. E., & McClearn, G. (2005). Genes, environment, race, and health. *American Psychologist*, *60*(1), 104–114.

Wildsmith, E. M. (2002). Testing the weathering hypothesis among Mexican-origin women. *Ethnicity & Disease*, *12*(4), 470–479.

Williams, D. R. (1997). Race and health: Basic questions, emerging directions. *Annals of Epidemiology*, *7*(5), 322–333.

Williams, D. R., & Collins, C. (1995). US socioeconomic and racial differences in health: Patterns and explanations. *Annual Review of Sociology*, *21*, 349.

Williams, D. R., & Collins, C. (2001). Racial residential segregation: A fundamental cause of racial disparities in health. *Public Health Reports (Washington, DC: 1974)*, *116*(5), 404–416.

Winkleby, M. A., Jatulis, D. E., Frank, E., & Fortmann, S. P. (1992). Socioeconomic status and health: How education, income, and occupation contribute to risk factors for cardiovascular disease. *American Journal of Public Health*, *82*(6), 816–820.

Zimmer, Z., & House, J. S. (2003). Education, income, and functional limitation transitions among American adults: Contrasting onset and progression. *International Journal of Epidemiology*, *32*(6), 1089–1097.

Chapter | 14 |

Relationships between Adults and their Aging Parents

Karen L. Fingerman,[1] Kira S. Birditt[2]

[1]Child Development and Family Studies, Purdue University, West Lafayette, IN, USA; [2]Institute for Social Research, University of Michigan, Ann Arbor, MI, USA

CHAPTER CONTENTS

Introduction 219

Variability in Relationships between Adults and Parents 220

Exchanges of Support between Adults and their Parents 221

Support of Grown Children and The Generational Flow of Support 221

Caregiving Relationships 223

Emotional Qualities of Ties between Adults and Parents 223

Solidarity and the Developmental Stake 224

Conflict Perspective 224

Intergenerational Ambivalence Theory 225

Gender and Race Differences in Emotional Qualities of the Relationship 226

Well-Being and Qualities of the Parent-Offspring Tie 226

Lessons in Understanding the Psychology of Aging and Future Directions for Research 227

References 229

INTRODUCTION

One of the most profound changes of the past century pertains to the duration of relationships between parents and children. Throughout human history, adults rarely had the opportunity to have relationships with aging parents. In 1900, one in four children in the United States lost a parent prior to the age of 15. Today, parents and children often share five or six decades of life; the majority of adults aged 50 to 59 in industrialized nations have at least one aging parent (Hagestad & Uhlenberg, 2007). Indeed, the parties spend more years together as adults than they do as parents raising children. This relatively new phenomenon in human experience warrants research attention.

Relationships between adults and their parents are distinct from other types of social ties due to their long shared history and the evolving nature of the relationship from infancy through adulthood. The tie begins at birth and typically endures until one party dies (usually the parent). With the exception of twins, no other relationship lasts as long. Dramatic discontinuity is evident from the childhood years into adulthood, however, both in structural and emotional qualities. The childhood years are marked by high dependency on parents, coordination of schedules, and shared environments. In adulthood, the vast majority of parents and children in the United States reside in separate households, attain their own livelihoods, and retain distinct social networks. Research examining parent-child ties longitudinally reveals only modest associations between qualities of parent-child relationships from early childhood into adulthood (Aquilino, 2006).

Nonetheless, for most adults, ties with parents and children are highly salient and involve frequent interaction and support. With the exception of divorced or absent fathers (Amato, 2000), parents and children rarely sever contact. Adults typically rate relationships with their parents or grown children as among their most important ties, second only to romantic partners (Fingerman et al., 2004). In late life, when parents are widowed, grown children may become their primary social tie (Ha, 2008). In the United States, when aging parents incur health declines, grown children often step in to provide care (Wolff & Kasper, 2006).

DOI: 10.1016/B978-0-12-380882-0.00014-0

Even in the absence of such crises, grown children and aging parents engage in exchanges of daily support, companionship, and conversation (Fingerman, 2000; Silverstein et al., 2006).

The resource rich nature of these relationships is intriguing. Laws obligate parents to provide a minimum threshold of care for children under age 18 in the United States. But in Western countries, few laws require people to provide support or companionship to their aging parents or grown children. Likewise, social sanctions do not provide collective oversight of these ties. Co-workers might inquire about weekend activities with a romantic partner or dependent children, but rarely ask about calls to an elderly mother or father.

Historically, ties to parents provided a means of livelihood via vocation, land, and inheritance (Hareven, 1995). Industrialization and educational opportunities have disbanded strict economic imperatives for most adults and parents in Western societies, however. Some exceptions are evident, as in situations where individuals expect to inherit a business, farm, or wealth from parents, but most American adults find a nonparental income source. Similar changes are evident in values observed in other cultures. East Asian societies espouse traditional Confucian ideals of obligation, but strict implementation of these formal values has eroded in recent years (Sung, 2000). Thus, for most adults and their parents, relationships are predicated on obligations and emotions. In other words, people retain connections to grown children and parents because they care about them or they believe they should.

Indeed, researchers have been interested in *why* adults retain ties with aging parents. Theory regarding adults and aging parents during the World War II era predicted the disenfranchisement of the elderly adult. Parsons (1943) hailed the rise of the nuclear family as America shifted from an agrarian to a manufacturing economy, arguing that elderly parents were increasingly irrelevant to their offspring's families of procreation. Family solidarity theory arose to refute this premise by articulating mechanisms underlying strong bonds or solidarity including: structures (e.g., proximity), affection, norms, and exchanges of support (Homans, 1950). Family solidarity theory took hold as an explanatory model for close intergenerational ties and dominated research on adults and their parents into the 1990s (e.g., Atkinson et al., 1986; Rossi & Rossi, 1990; Silverstein & Bengtson, 1997). Throughout the 1980s and 1990s, a parallel literature also described the role of offspring as caregivers for the frail elderly at the end of life (Aneshensel et al., 1995; Zarit et al., 1980). Thus, research at the end of the twentieth century portrayed relationships between adults and their parents as generally close, positive, and a source of support (even at sacrifice for offspring as caregivers).

During the past decade, scholars have moved beyond explanations for why these ties endure to examine complexities in these relationships. This shift in focus reflects theoretical and methodological advances, as well as increased recognition of the role of social relationships for health and well-being (Cohen & Janicki-Deverts, 2009). Recent research also documents the effects of ties to parents and offspring on well-being (Fingerman et al., 2008; Lowenstein, 2007; Pudrovska, 2009; Ward, 2008). Relationships exert influence on individual well-being via several mechanisms, but two that receive particular attention in the literature regarding adults and parents include emotional reactions (with accompanying downstream mental health and physiological implications) and social support.

In this chapter, we address three important questions regarding adults and aging parents: (a) What do people gain from relationships with grown children or parents, and who provides what for whom?; (b) What are the emotional qualities of these ties?; and (c) How do these ties affect individual well-being? In the remainder of this chapter, we describe recent research relevant to each of these issues. First, however, we address variability in these ties.

VARIABILITY IN RELATIONSHIPS BETWEEN ADULTS AND PARENTS

Although this chapter addresses commonalities in relationship patterns between adults and parents, it would be irresponsible to ignore diversity in these patterns. Much of what is known about variability involves social structural variables such as gender, marital status, geographic distance, and ethnicity.

Research on family life necessarily entails consideration of gender. Women typically report greater investment in their social relationships than men, and provide cohesion between generations by planning family events, offering support, and maintaining connections (Troll, 1987). Similarly, daughters are more emotionally involved in their relationships with parents than are sons (Fingerman, 2003; Willson et al., 2003). When mothers select favorites both in terms of emotional connection and support, they disproportionately select daughters (Suitor et al., 2006, 2007a).

Studies of recent cohorts suggest these gender differences may be attenuating, however. Due to changing gender roles and men's greater involvement with family, sons' reports of contact and assistance to parents has increased and studies report fewer gender differences in offspring's ties to parents (Fingerman et al., 2007; Logan & Spitze, 1996). Studies also find fewer gender differences between mothers and fathers than previously documented (Fingerman et al., 2008). These mixed findings suggest well-established gender roles placing mothers and daughters at the center of family life may be shifting. Nonetheless, treating parents and offspring as gender-neutral would be premature.

Gender is a relatively stable characteristic with enduring effects on this tie. Across the life course, status transitions also may generate increased or decreased contact and closeness in this tie. Marital status is a case in point. Married parents, particularly fathers, are more involved with their grown children than divorced fathers (Amato, 2000). By contrast, widowhood may induce increased contact and reliance on offspring (Ha, 2008). Offspring marriage may generate detachment from parents, as young adults become consumed with their romantic ties (Sarkisian & Gerstel, 2008). Similar patterns can be observed for student status; young adults who are students receive more support than young adults who have completed education (Aquilino, 2006; Fingerman et al., 2009). A unifying theme underlying these patterns reflects the available social and material resources and competition for resources that parents and offspring experience. In situations where they have few social partners, time, or material resources, parents and offspring find succor in one another.

Likewise, family size may play a central role in the nature of any given offspring's tie with his or her aging parents (Davey et al., 2005). Family size is a determinant of resources and competition for resources. Researchers interested in adults' relationships with aging parents rarely mention family size, despite the fact that today's aging cohorts are the parents of the Baby Boomers. These parents have a greater number of progeny than future cohorts of older adults will have, and a great array of potential caregivers. By contrast, each offspring may receive less parental support and closeness in a large sibship (Fingerman et al., 2010; Grundy & Henretta, 2006), and future cohorts of older adults may have fewer offspring to step in when their health declines.

Ethnic and racial variation in relationships between adults and parents also has been observed (Becker et al., 2003; Sarkisian & Gerstel, 2004), but researchers in the field of aging often are not attentive to race and ethnic variability in parent-offspring ties. This dearth of attention may reflect difficulties in pinpointing implications of such variability. For example, Black and Hispanic families have high rates of intergenerational coresidence (Chatters et al., 2002; Kamo, 2000). But these presumed cultural preferences may be motivated by structural factors such as larger family size, lower income, housing discrimination, and lack of access to mortgages.

Current conceptions of variability in patterns of relationships between adults and parents tend to be sociological in orientation. As such, we know more about structural variables than intrapsychic ones. Nonetheless, appraisals and personality may generate systematic differences as well. For example, a study of elderly mothers found that they placed higher importance on ties with a given child when they had fewer children. Moreover, the psychological importance of the tie played a greater role in relationship qualities than family size (Fingerman, 2003). Likewise, another study including parents and offspring of both genders found adult offspring who scored high on indicators of neuroticism generated conflicted feelings for their parents (controlling for parental neuroticism; Fingerman et al., 2006).

In sum, future research may elaborate when and why relationship pattern varies by considering these individual factors as well as the social structural positions individuals occupy. We turn next to consider patterns of support and emotional qualities of these ties.

EXCHANGES OF SUPPORT BETWEEN ADULTS AND THEIR PARENTS

Relationships between adults and their parents are resource rich; that is, both parties depend on the other for support in everyday life and when crises arise. Scholarly work on older adults' interpersonal ties has often portrayed relationships as a repository from which needed help is withdrawn. Such an economic metaphor for aging parents' relationships with children may be particularly relevant in the United States where significant gaps in public programs for the elderly render families the mainstay of support in late life. Moreover, parents provide many forms of support to their grown children, up to the final years of life (when the flow of support may reverse; Fingerman et al., 2010; Zarit & Eggebeen, 2002).

SUPPORT OF GROWN CHILDREN AND THE GENERATIONAL FLOW OF SUPPORT

Most generational support flows downstream, from parents to offspring. Parents provide financial gifts and loans (McGarry, 1999) and practical support (Suitor et al., 2006) to grown children in the United States and in Europe (Kohli, 2005; Lowenstein & Daatland, 2006). Research also documents an array of nontangible support including advice, emotional support, companionship, and simply lending an ear to listen to them talk about their day (Fingerman, 2000; Fingerman et al., 2009).

Parents do not offer all grown offspring the same level of assistance, however. We have proposed a model of intergenerational support that accounts for rewards parents may experience in assisting offspring as well as responses to offspring's needs (Fingerman et al., 2009). When choosing among offspring, parents typically engage in support that is personally rewarding in the present (i.e., helping a child they love), that fulfills a child's everyday needs or for the future (i.e., helping a grown child who will support the parents' needs later), or in response to a grown child's problems (Fingerman et al., 2009; Suitor et al., 2006).

These behaviors may reflect nurturing behaviors established earlier in life that persist after the children are grown. A recent study in Israel found young-old Jewish parents sought to extend their role as parents by helping their grown children (Levitzki, 2009). After decades of investment in the parental role, parents may view their grown children as a reflection on their own accomplishments as parents. Indeed, parents may still experience their grown children as a narcissistic extension of themselves. Research on different ethnic groups in the United States also finds parents assist grown children they deem most successful (Fingerman et al., 2009; Lee & Aytec, 1998) or with whom they have particularly close ties (Suitor et al., 2006).

Parental support also reflects a desire to alleviate children's needs. Parents today may view offspring as requiring more support than in the past. Data regarding parental support of different cohorts are not available, but some findings support this assertion. For example, analysis of parents and a randomly selected child in the 1988 National Survey of Family and Households (NSFH) found that fewer than half (46%) of parents had provided advice in the past month, and only a third had provided practical assistance (Eggebeen, 1992). More recent data revealed that 75% of offspring received parental advice, and nearly 50% received practical assistance on a monthly basis (Fingerman et al., 2009).

Current parental support may reflect the nature of opportunities and social structures of young adulthood. Middle-class young adults obtain parental support during extended schooling and "explorations"; they may work in a series of trial jobs or careers, and revolve through a succession of relationships or living arrangements. By contrast, young working class adults need support from parents to offset uncertain and poorly paid jobs that provide few benefits or involve irregular shifts (Aquilino, 2006; Furstenberg, 2010). Thus, the nature of parental support varies by socioeconomic circumstances, but young adults receive parental support across contexts.

Although few studies have traced the flow of generational support longitudinally, cross-sectional data suggest a temporal sequence in support from parents to offspring. A life course perspective suggests a trajectory in intergenerational support shifting across adulthood. A typical pattern might change from parental investment in offspring during young adulthood, to mutual respect and reciprocal exchanges in midlife, to a short period when parents require intensive care from offspring at the end of life. Evidence supports this premise. Younger adult offspring receive more support than older offspring, even controlling for differences in parental health or age (Aquilino, 2006; Fingerman et al., 2009). Studies in both Europe and the United States also find greater parental support associated with statuses that are pervasive in early adulthood including being a student (Attias-Donfut & Wolff, 2000; Schoeni & Ross, 2005), unmarried (Eggebeen, 1992; Fingerman et al., 2010), coresiding with parents (Schoeni & Ross, 2005), or having labor-intensive young children of one's own (Casper & Bianchi, 2002).

Theorists have proposed a period of filial maturity beginning in the child's 30s, when offspring no longer receive this onslaught of support from parents, and relationships are predicated on mutual exchanges and respect (Birditt et al., 2008). Evidence for this transition is scant, however. It is not clear whether individual differences are pervasive when grown children are in their 30s or whether researchers simply have not adequately assessed filial maturity. Given the heterogeneity of pathways into adulthood, some offspring may remain dependent, whereas other offspring are independent by their 30s.

An apparent temporal sequence of generational support over the course of the relationship is consistent with our model suggesting crises may transcend personally rewarding support patterns. Parents typically provide greater support to offspring rather than the reverse, but when parents incur crises and ongoing health problems, the generational flow of support alters (Fingerman et al., 2010). In most families, as parental health declines, parents proffer less support to offspring and offspring increase the range of tasks they complete for parents (Fingerman et al., 2007). Variability in these patterns is evident when offspring suffer developmental delays (Ha et al., 2008) or grandchildren are dependent on the older generation (Hughes et al., 2007), but the typical flow of support shifts upstream to parents in late old age.

Middle-aged offspring who must support aging parents typically also have adult children of their own. The premise of a sandwich generation, with a middle-generation caring for young children and elderly parents, is relatively rare in the United States. Yet, a "pivot" generation, altering their attention between demands from above (from aging parents) and below (from grown children), is fairly common (Fingerman et al., 2009; Grundy & Henretta, 2006). In these situations, a central question is whether resources are reallocated from the younger generation to the older generation when parents incur health declines. Studies in the United States and Britain suggest middle-aged adults expand time and energy they exert to family support when parents' needs increase, rather than taking resources from the younger generation (Fingerman et al. 2010; Grundy & Henretta, 2006). Nonetheless, the middle generation may reach a point where support cannot be expanded, and decisions are made to give less to grown offspring or to place the elderly parent in an institution.

CAREGIVING RELATIONSHIPS

Although everyday support of offspring is the normative pattern, popular lore often situates caregiving for an elderly parent at the center of this relationship. The emphasis on caregiving reflects the importance of this care in the U.S. public health system. Due to a dearth of formal support programs in the United States, many grown children assume a wide range of activities that are time-consuming, physically challenging, unpleasant, and emotionally draining.

Nonetheless, the period of elder care is typically brief in the life cycle of the parent-offspring tie, particularly in comparison to decades when both parties are likely to be in good health. At any given time in the United States or Britain, only one-fifth of middle-aged adults are engaged in caregiving for an elderly parent (Fingerman et al., 2010; Grundy & Henretta, 2006). A recent national study documented that the majority of elder care now involves a grown child as care provider for a parent. This pattern is a shift from a decade ago when the most common care provider was a spouse (Wolff & Kasper, 2006). Offspring may fill in because parents are less likely to be partnered or married in old age (Swarz, 2009).

The literature pertaining to caregiving is vast, and justice in covering this topic is beyond the scope of this chapter (for reviews see: Schulz & Martire, 2004; Zarit & Zarit, in press). There has been little attention to longitudinal patterns of intergenerational support; some studies examine everyday intergenerational exchanges and other studies examine parental caregiving. Yet, this division obscures the aging process. Few older adults incur precipitous declines (with notable exceptions such as stroke). Rather, disability accrues via a cumulative downhill process over the course of chronic illness, perhaps culminating in a distinct crisis shifting the relationship into one defined as caregiving. As such, aging parents transition from independence to increasing dependence on grown children over many years (Fingerman et al., 2007). Much caregiving in the United States involves dementia care, but many chronic illnesses generate frailty or disabilities requiring hands-on care from offspring (Pinquart & Sorensen, 2007). Throughout this period, parents may continue to help their offspring (Lowenstein & Daatland, 2006) before caregiving becomes intensive at the end of life.

Caregiving patterns in the United States may not generalize to other cultures, however. In other Western nations, government agencies provide a range of services for the elderly. For example, the Swedish welfare system offers older adults help with shopping, administering medication, transportation, and cleaning (Sundstrom et al., 2006). Moreover, there is considerable variability in patterns of support in the United States, with some parents or offspring involved in more support exchanges than others.

Explanations for variability in support have drawn on models of reciprocity. For example, studies find that adults who received support from their parents in young adulthood are more likely to provide care to their aging parents in the future (Silverstein et al., 2002). Nonetheless, a strict economic interpretation of "payback" is overly simplistic. Although relationships between adults often are predicated on norms of reciprocity (Antonucci, 2001), the idea of directly repaying debts to parents is unlikely.

Associations in intergenerational support from one point in time to another point in time may reflect third factors, such as characteristics of the offspring or the relationship, rather than efforts to retain a reciprocal balance. For example, middle-aged parents provide considerable help to offspring they deem successful, via investment in education or other forms of practical support (Fingerman et al., 2009). Parents also are likely to turn to such successful offspring for their own care needs in old age (Suitor et al., 2007a). Likewise, women receive more support from parents in early adulthood and are more likely to provide care in later life.

Furthermore, parental support patterns vary by race, culture, and family structure. For example, Hispanic and Black Americans endorse greater norms of filial obligation to support aging parents than White Americans do (Swartz, 2009). A qualitative study of elderly parents in four ethnic groups (i.e., African American, Cambodian, Filipino, and Latino) revealed considerable complexities in beliefs and preferences for support (Becker et al., 2003). African American older adults were likely to offer their children housing and to seek a degree of independence for themselves. By contrast, the Cambodian elders moved in with their children and considered this pattern normative. Norms of support also vary by family structure. Adults espouse less obligation to care for a stepparent than a biological parent (Ganong & Coleman, 1999). Finally, in societies that offer formal support structures for older adults, offspring may offer parents companionship, but not be involved in meeting their physical needs (Sundstrom et al., 2006). In sum, norms for providing care of the elderly are multidetermined and reflect earlier patterns in the relationships, cultural beliefs, and available resources.

EMOTIONAL QUALITIES OF TIES BETWEEN ADULTS AND PARENTS

The parent-child tie not only involves a great deal of contact and support exchange but also is emotionally complex involving intense closeness and positivity as well as negativity, tension, and conflict. Three dominant theoretical perspectives exist in the parent-child literature regarding the emotional qualities of the relationship including solidarity theory, the conflict perspective, and ambivalence theory.

Solidarity and the Developmental Stake

According to solidarity theory, emotional aspects of the parent-child relationship are characterized by affective solidarity and the developmental stake. Affective solidarity refers to positive sentiments between family members, including emotional closeness, trust, and respect (Bengtson et al., 2002). The developmental stake hypothesis suggests that parents are more emotionally invested in the relationship than are their children due to their investment in their offspring as their future. Specifically, parents view their children as extensions of themselves and are concerned with passing on their values and with feeling emotional closeness (Giarrusso et al., 2005). Research has found that parents often report feeling closer and more positive regarding the relationship than do their children and these generational differences persist over time (Giarrusso et al., 2005; Shapiro, 2004). In contrast, because children desire independence and are invested in developing their own families, they tend to underreport closeness and positive relationship quality with parents.

The majority of parents and children report feeling close to one another and have frequent contact often involving positive interactions. For example, Fingerman (2000) described enjoyable visits between dyads of young adult daughters and their mothers, and dyads of middle-aged daughters and their mothers. Regardless of age, mothers and daughters talked on the phone or visited in person frequently. The content of their visits, however, varied by age. Younger daughter-mother dyads focused more attention on the young adult and her emergence into adulthood, whereas older mothers and midlife daughters focused on the broader family. In addition, cross-sectional research suggests that these feelings of closeness and positive relationship quality increase as parents and children grow older together (Rossi & Rossi, 1990).

Conflict Perspective

Research on parent-child conflict began in late 1990s. The conflict perspective attempts to describe the areas of tension in this relationship and the strategies parents and children use to cope with those tensions. The majority of parents and children report having at least some tensions with one another (Fingerman, 2003; Fingerman et al., 2004).

Longitudinal research indicates that parental reports of negative relationship quality with their children decreases over time but studies have yet to examine change over time in children's reports of negative relationship qualitys (Birditt et al., 2009a).

To understand tensions and conflict in the parent-child tie, Fingerman (2003) developed the developmental schism hypothesis, which postulates that parents and children experience conflict because they have competing developmental needs. Two predominate schisms in the parent and adult child tie include independence (also referred to as care of self) and the importance placed on the relationship (Birditt et al., 2009b). These schisms may lead to different topics of tension and variations in perceptions of tensions between family members.

Specific tensions arising from these schisms typically reflect either the parameters of the relationship (relationship tensions) or the behaviors of one of the individuals in the relationship (individual tensions; Fingerman, 2003). Relationship tensions refer to how the dyad interacts and encompasses issues of emotional closeness and cohesion or lack thereof. Individual tensions pertain to the behaviors of one member of the dyad and often have to do with independence or self-care. Relationship tensions include unsolicited advice, contact frequency, personality differences, childrearing, and past relationship problems. Individual tensions include job or education, finances, housekeeping, lifestyle, and health.

Parents and offspring often view the tensions in their relationship differently (Fingerman, 2003). Birditt et al. (2009b) found that mothers and fathers reported more intense individual tensions than did adult children. This generation difference may be due to the parent's need for their children to be well-established adults, validating their own success in raising them. Thus parents become tense about children's lack of progress (e.g., financial trouble). Both types of tensions predicted lower quality relationships, but relationship tensions were more highly associated with poor relationship quality than individual tensions. Relationship tensions may represent more fundamental problems between the two parties, whereas they may be able to view individual problems as something outside the purview of their relationship.

Researchers have also examined how parents and children cope with the tensions that they experience and have found generation differences in strategies. Fingerman (2003) found that mothers and daughters were least likely to use destructive strategies, but that daughters were more open about discussing problems than were mothers, who preferred avoidance. Birditt et al. (2009c) found that mothers, fathers, and their adult children were most likely to report using constructive conflict strategies (e.g., discussing the problem) followed by avoidant and destructive/aggressive strategies least frequently. Constructive strategies predicted better relationship quality, whereas avoidant and destructive e strategies predicted lower quality relationships.

Tensions and coping strategies vary with age. Older adult children report less strain with parents than younger adult children (Umberson, 1992). Surprisingly however, Birditt and colleagues (2009b) found that families with middle-aged offspring reported experiencing more intense relationship tensions than did families with younger adult children. They suggested that this finding may be due to age-related disparities in feelings of closeness. Middle-aged children become more invested in their own families and have less time to spend with parents, whereas parents may have more time and increased investment in the relationship.

Intergenerational Ambivalence Theory

Ambivalence theory provides a useful framework for understanding the complexity of the positive and negative aspects of the parent-child relationship. In the literature addressing adults and aging parents, intergenerational ambivalence is defined both sociologically and psychologically. Sociological ambivalence involves conflicting feelings or cognitions that arise when social structures do not provide clear guidelines for interpersonal behaviors or relationships (Connidis & McMullin, 2002). This sociological or structural ambivalence occurs when roles include incompatible norms or expectations that cause contradictory emotions or beliefs. According to this approach, people with fewer social and economic resources are more likely to experience ambivalence. For example, the competing need to work at an hourly wage job to support a family but to provide care for elderly parents generates ambivalence. Gender and generation are important structural determinants of ambivalence in the parent and adult child relationship. Women are more likely to occupy roles that generate conflicting norms.

Psychological ambivalence refers to the simultaneous experience of positive and negative sentiments about the same relationship (Luescher & Pillemer, 1998). For example, a person may experience intense love and irritation regarding a son or daughter. Ambivalence is distinct from feelings of confusion or indifference involving low levels of positive and negative feelings.

Ambivalence is most likely to occur when conflicting needs for independence and closeness in relationships arise. For example, parents are more likely to report ambivalence when their adult children have not achieved expected adult statuses (e.g., career, children), when they have financial problems, or when they do not visit their parents often enough (Peters et al., 2006). Success of grown children also is important with regard to ambivalence. Parents experience less ambivalence when their grown children report success and investment in work, spouse, and children (Birditt et al., 2010; Fingerman et al., 2006), and more ambivalence when their grown children have problems (Pillemer & Suitor, 2002). Adult children, on the other hand, tend to feel ambivalent when they experienced parental rejection earlier in life or when they anticipate having to provide support for elderly or sick parents (Fingerman et al., 2007; Willson et al., 2003).

Parents and children who report having more intense tensions, or who report using more destructive and avoidant strategies also report more ambivalence (Birditt et al., 2009c). Overall, adult children tend to report greater ambivalence than do their parents across situations (Fingerman et al., 2006; Willson et al., 2003).

As with positive and negative emotional qualities of the tie, ambivalence also varies by age and personality. Ambivalence seems to be higher in adolescence and early adulthood but seems to dissipate when adults are in their 30s and increase again in later adulthood when parental health declines (Pillemer & Suitor, 2002; Tighe et al., 2009). Research has shown that offspring's worries about their parents are associated with feelings of ambivalence (Hay et al., 2007). Watching parents decline with age also may generate fears in offspring for the own future declines, contributing to the ambivalence they feel.

Overall, ambivalence has negative implications for well-being. Researchers have found that ambivalence in the parent-child tie predicts depression, lower quality of life, lower self-rated health, and lower relationship satisfaction (Fingerman et al., 2008; Lowenstein, 2007). Indeed studies of ambivalent ties in general reveal that ambivalent relationships are associated with lower self-reported well-being than solely negative relationships (Uchino et al., 2004). Uchino and his colleagues have provided two possible explanations for these findings: (1) ambivalent relationships are more unpredictable than solely negative or positive relationships, which may lead to increased distress; or (2) ambivalent ties may not provide support when it is needed most.

Other research has suggested that ambivalence may reflect negativity more so than positivity in the relationship. Negative relationship quality measures tend to have more variance whereas measures of positive qualities of relationship may be biased by ceiling effects. Thus, much of the variance in the indirect assessments of ambivalence is due to negative relationship quality rather than positive relationship quality. Rather than referring to both high positive and negative quality, ambivalence may actually refer to relationships that have high levels of positive quality coupled with moderate negative quality. In addition, studies that examine the separate components of ambivalence often find parallel predictors of negative relationship quality and ambivalence suggesting that negative quality represents the majority of the "action" in ambivalence (Ha & Ingersoll-Dayton, 2008).

Gender and Race Differences in Emotional Qualities of the Relationship

Emotional qualities of the parent-child tie may vary by gender and race. Women often report feeling closer to, and more positive about their children than do men (Fingerman, 2003; Rossi & Rossi, 1990). Mothers also tend to express more intimacy and negativity with young children and adolescents than do fathers (Collins & Russell, 1991). Birditt et al. (2009b) found that families with daughters reported relationship and individual tensions were more intense than families with sons. Some studies have found that women report greater ambivalence (Willson et al., 2003), but other studies have found no gender difference (Fingerman et al., 2006).

Because of structural (economic) and cultural variations, African Americans are highly reliant on family support (Neighbors, 1997) and may be more reliant on the parent-child tie for support than European Americans (Umberson, 1992). Thus, the parent-child tie may be a source of support as well as strain and ambivalence for African Americans (Chatters et al., 1989; Umberson, 1992). Research regarding race differences in the emotional qualities of the parent-child tie has been inconclusive. Birditt et al. (2009c) found no difference in affective solidarity between African American and European American families, but found that African Americans reported greater ambivalence than did European Americans. In contrast, Umberson (1992) found Black respondents reported more positive relations with mothers than did White respondents. Pillemer et al. (2007) found that race differences in ambivalence dissipated once sociostructural control variables were added to models.

WELL-BEING AND QUALITIES OF THE PARENT-OFFSPRING TIE

Research has clearly established the influence of social relationships on physical and psychology well-being (see Cohen & Janicki-Deverts, 2009). Mechanisms explaining these associations include emotional pathways (e.g., stresses and positive emotions in the context of relationships exert health implications), and supportive behaviors (e.g., social partners enhance well-being directly or buffer against stress during crises). Given the high support and emotional intensity of ties between adults and their parents, their relationships appear to affect well-being.

It is important to ask whether ties with parents or grown children have distinct effects on well-being or whether they are simply prototypes of relationships that affect well-being. Loneliness is a risk factor for adverse psychological and physical outcomes throughout adulthood (Cacioppo & Hawkley, 2003). A relationship with a parent or grown child may mitigate such effects by fulfilling needs for affiliation. Likewise, the supportive aspects of ties to parents or offspring could be fulfilled by a different relationship partner. In these respects, benefits of the tie are interchangeable with other types of relationships (e.g., spouse, friend).

Evidence suggests, however, that specific features of ties to parents or offspring exert effects on well-being. Indeed, the implications of the relationship appear to differ for the parent and the offspring. Several recent studies have linked relationships with grown children to aging parents' well-being (Fingerman et al., 2008; Lowenstein, 2007; Milkie et al., 2008; Pudrovska, 2009; Ward, 2008). From a theoretical perspective, parental investment may explain why grown children influence parental well-being. Throughout the twentieth century, middle-class parenting was reshaped as an investment in the child, and children became emotionally rewarding for the self rather than economically rewarding (Hulbert, 2003). In the twenty-first century, after two decades of childrearing, parents may view their grown children as a reflection of their own success or failure as parents (Fingerman et al., 2006). Both offspring's achievements and problems may affect parents' well-being.

Evidence supporting this premise is found in recent studies. Parents report poorer well-being when offspring have not achieved normative markers of adulthood or when they suffer difficulties. For example, in cultures where adult coresidence with parents is not normative, offspring who coreside with parents have a deleterious impact on those parents (Pudrovska, 2009). Parents may empathize with their children, and suffer when their children feel distress (Birditt et al., 2009b) or grown children suffering problems may treat their parents badly (Milkie et al., 2008). As such, parents report poorer well-being when offspring incur problems (e.g., financial crisis, health problem, victim of a crime), particularly when those problems are associated with the offspring's own behaviors (e.g., alcoholism; Pillemer & Suitor, 2002). Parents report better adjustment when their offspring make them feel important and acknowledge their support (Byers et al., 2008).

There is some inconsistency in the literature with regard to gender differences in the effects of offspring on the well-being of mothers and fathers. Negative events in offspring's lives may affect mothers more than fathers (Milkie et al., 2008). Research also finds poor quality relationships with offspring have a greater effect on mothers than on fathers (Wickrama et al., 2001). By contrast, a recent study examined parents' ties to each of their grown children and found no parental gender differences in well-being; even one poor quality tie with a grown child had deleterious effects on well-being for mothers and fathers (Ward, 2008). Lest we overstate the case for offspring effects on parents, Lowenstein (2007) examined positive and negative qualities of ties to grown children in five countries (Norway, Israel, Germany, Spain, and England) and found that positive qualities of ties to offspring showed only a small association with well-being, whereas parents' own education and income had much stronger effects.

In sum, the quality of the relationship that mothers and fathers have with their grown children may affect their well-being. Likewise, the grown children's achievement or statuses have implications for parental well-being above and beyond the quality of the relationship.

The effects of relationships with parents on grown children's well-being are less clear. Historically, psychoanalytic theory placed qualities of early ties to parents at the center of adults' mental health (e.g., Erikson, 1950; Freud, 1938). Although research on adults and their parents has not validated psychodynamic theories, recent studies have found deleterious effects on adult well-being stemming from trauma with parents in childhood such as abuse or parental loss through death or divorce (Irving & Ferraro, 2006), although many individuals appear to be resilient following experiences of early stress with parents (Pitzer & Fingerman, in press).

In addition to early experience, current ties to parents in adulthood have been linked to adults' psychological well-being. Nearly twenty years ago, Umberson (1992) found negative qualities of ties to parents had a greater effect on grown children's well-being than positive qualities of these ties. This finding is consistent with a broader literature on social ties suggesting negative qualities of relationships are more salient than positive aspects (Rook, 2001).

Studies reveal that caregiving for parents can have detrimental effects on children's well-being, but these effects appear to vary depending on personal and contextual factors (for meta-analyses see Pinquart & Sorensen, 2007). Provision of care appears to be more deleterious for spouses than for offspring. Indeed, benefits of providing care to an ailing parent also have been detected. For women, caring for a non-coresident parent has been associated with increased sense of purpose in life (Marks et al., 2002). Moreover, a high quality marriage appears to mitigate adverse mental health implications of caregiving for middle-aged adults (Choi & Marks, 2006), suggesting it is not simply the tie to the parent that affects well-being. Rather, middle-aged adults typically have ties to a wide array of family members and other social roles, and may benefit from their involvement in more central roles when also providing care to aging parents (Martire et al., 2000).

Overall, the parent-child tie is a long-term close relationship that usually involves a great deal of contact, support exchange, closeness, tension, and ambivalence. Indeed, because of the emotional intensity of this tie, it often has profound effects on the well-being of both parents and their children. Although the literature on the parent-child tie is growing rapidly, there are many unanswered questions and areas in need of future research.

LESSONS IN UNDERSTANDING THE PSYCHOLOGY OF AGING AND FUTURE DIRECTIONS FOR RESEARCH

The literature regarding relationships between adults and their aging parents may help provide an understanding of late-life development more generally. Many aging processes enacted in this tie apply to studies of aging in general. Addressing gaps in the study of adults and their parents also might contribute to the field of gerontology more broadly.

Perhaps the most important issue that haunts gerontological research involves potential biases due to sample selection reflecting factors such as health, mortality, and refusals to participate. For example, older adults who are healthier, more cognitively fit, and socially integrated are more likely to participate and continue participation in studies. With regard to adults and parents, the finding that most adults have fairly positive ties with their parents and offspring (e.g., Fingerman et al., 2006; Silverstein & Bengtson, 1997; Umberson, 1992) may partially reflect the fact that people with conflictual relationships refuse to participate in studies. Moreover, selective mortality determines who is available to participate. For example, poorer ties to offspring have been linked to higher incidence of mortality following widowhood (Silverstein & Bengtson, 1991). Although the samples in many studies of adults and parents are generally representative of the population with regard to economic dispersion, researchers cannot claim representation of people who will not participate in studies. Instead, more research should attempt to include adults who have poor relationships or lack contact with aging parents, and researchers should interpret findings in light of potential biases.

Relationships between adults and parents also are subject to other biases common to late life. The premise that old age is a return to childhood is pervasive in popular writing and cartoons and often referred to as a "role reversal" in old age between parents and offspring. Empirical research has demonstrated that offspring often do expand their own role when parents experience the transition to old age by taking on increasing tasks and emotional concerns for parents, but the roles do not reverse (Fingerman et al., 2007). The experience of parenting a child who is maturing is orthogonal to the experience of caring for an elderly adult who faces chronic decline after a lifetime of experience. Gerontologists might seek to understand the factors that lead members of the public to perpetuate perceptions that are unfounded in research literature.

Moreover, the implications of holding such beliefs warrant consideration. Beliefs that older adults are losing competence can undermine older adults' functioning and well-being (Baltes, 1995; Levy et al., in press). Thus, an offspring's belief that they have reversed roles could undermine the parent's esteem and autonomy. Likewise, adult children may fear losing their independence, and feel anger and sadness over the loss of a parent who supported them. By contrast, these beliefs may translate into offspring's compassionate care for the parent. Indeed, negative attributions about older adults' behaviors have been linked to more positive treatment of older adults in several contexts (Fingerman & Charles, 2010). As such, researchers might consider when and how negative beliefs about aging can result in adaptive behaviors rather than simply disproving such negative beliefs.

A second area of consideration regarding adults and parents pertains to new technologies and the aging process. In the twenty-first century, personal electronics, cell phones, and software-enhancing social networking sites (i.e., Facebook) are ubiquitous. Of course, throughout history, technologies have determined the nature of family ties. Beginning with the Pony Express, people were able to connect with social partners residing at a distance (Adams & Stevenson, 2004). Nonetheless, technologies reshaped family life dramatically in the twenty-first century, as inexpensive travel and communication allowed individuals to traverse greater distances at increasing speed with lower costs. Such technologies permit adults and parents to retain frequent contact regardless of whether they live nearby.

The role of technologies in parent-child ties also pertains to the broader field of gerontology. A generational gap in use of technologies may reflect timing in the introduction of such technologies. Current cohorts of older adults are less technically savvy than their children because such equipment or software became widely accessible after they had established careers. Such trends may not persist in future cohorts. For example, currently, only 26% of adults over the age of 70 use the Internet, but 57% of adults aged 65 to 69 are online (Pew Internet Survey, 2009), and they are unlikely to quit after they turn 70. Thus, a focus on generational disparities in use of technologies should consider these complexities; a focus on how technologies contribute to relationships between adults and parents and the aging process more broadly remains relevant.

Finally, several areas of investigation have not yet been brought to bear on understanding aging parents. Scholars who study intergenerational ties have been surprisingly reserved when it comes to borrowing theoretical perspectives to apply to this tie. Literature regarding social learning theory, family systems theory, and behavioral genetics might inform our understanding of the parent-offspring tie in late life. We need more comprehensive models of the parent-child tie that include the characteristics of the relationship (e.g., support, relationship quality), the predictors of those relationship characteristics, and their implications.

Another area of research that has not been considered in the parent-child relationship is the incorporation of biological systems to understand the predictors and implications of the parent-child relationship for health and well-being. For example, researchers have found that genetic and hormonal factors predict variations in the parental and child behavior among nonhuman mammals and humans (Bakermans-Kranenburg & Ijzendoorn, 2008; Broad et al., 2006). For example, human mothers with particular variants of the serotonergic (5-HTT ss) and oxytonergic (AA/AG) genes were less sensitive to their toddlers during observed interactions (Bakermans-Kranenburg & Ijzendoorn). Further, activation of the endogenous opioid system predicts variation in maternal bonding among humans and nonhuman primates and maternal behaviors predict variations in the development of infants (Broad et al., 2006). This research should be expanded to research on the adult parent-child tie to examine the implications of genetics and hormonal factors in the prediction of relationship quality, transmission of behaviors across generations, and other factors.

Further, the parent-child relationship has important implications for health, well-being, and mortality (Fingerman et al., 2008; Lowenstein, 2007). We need to start examining the possible mechanisms that account for those linkages. For example, on the one hand, the strain of having problematic children may cause chronic stress reactions and lead to later health problems. On the other hand, having successful and supportive children may lead to the reduction of stress reactivity and better health outcomes.

Overall, we hope that this chapter serves to highlight the great complexity of the parent-child tie in adulthood. To understand this relationship it is important to take a life span and life course perspective and to consider the multitude of conflicting emotions and cognitions that exist within dyads and families. Although research in this area is growing, there are many unanswered questions and areas ripe for future research. We need more complex models of the parent-child tie that include the context and the multitude of relationship characteristics and their implications. In addition, we need to incorporate biopsychosocial models to understand the biological and social underpinnings and the implications of this important and long-lasting tie. The parent-child relationship is an exceedingly complicated close relationship that has profound implications for parents and children across the life span.

REFERENCES

Adams, R. G., & Stevenson, M. L. (2004). A lifetime of relationships mediated by technology. In F. R. Lang & K. L. Fingerman (Eds.), *Growing together: Personal relationships across the lifespan* (pp. 368–394). New York: Cambridge University Press.

Amato, P. R. (2000). The consequences of divorce for adults and children. *Journal of Marriage and Family, 62*, 1269–1287.

Aneshensel, C., Pearlin, L. I., Mullan, J. T., Zarit, S. H., & Whitlatch, C. J. (1995). *Profiles in caregiving: The unexpected career*. New York: Academic Press.

Antonucci, T. C. (2001). Social relations: An examination of social networks, social support, and sense of control. In J. E. Birren (Ed.), *Handbook of aging and psychology* 5th edition (pp. 427–453). San Diego, CA.: Academic Press.

Aquilino, W. (2006). Family relationships and support systems in emerging adulthood. In J. J. Arnett & J. L. Tanner (Eds.), *Emerging adults in the America: Coming of age in the 21st century* (pp. 193–217). Washington, DC: American Psychological Association.

Atkinson, M. P., Kivett, V. R., & Campbell, R. T. (1986). Intergenerational solidarity: An examination of a theoretical model. *Journals of Gerontology, 41*, 408–416.

Attias-Donfut, C., & Wolff, F. C. (2000). The redistributive effects of generational transfers. In S. Arbur & C. Attias-Donfut (Eds.), *The myth of generational conflict: The family and state in ageing societies* (pp. 22–46). New York: Routledge.

Bakermans-Kranenburg, M. J., & van Ijzendoorn, M. H. (2008). Oxytocin receptor (OXTR) and serotonin transporter (5-HTT) genes associated with observed parenting. *Social Cognitive and Affective Neuroscience*, 1–7.

Baltes, M. M. (1995). Dependency in old age: Gains and losses. *Current Directions in Psychological Science, 4*, 14–19.

Becker, G., Beyene, Y., Newsom, E., & Mayen, N. (2003). Creating continuity through mutual assistance: Intergenerational reciprocity in four ethnic groups. *Journals of Gerontology: Social Sciences, 58*, S151–S159.

Bengtson, V., Giarrusso, R., Mabry, J. B., & Silverstein, M. (2002). Solidarity, conflict, and ambivalence: Complementary or competing perspectives on intergenerational relationships? *Journal of Marriage and the Family, 64*, 568–576.

Birditt, K. S., Fingerman, K. L., Lefkowitz, E. S., & Kamp Dush, C. M. (2008). Parents perceived as peers: Filial maturity in adulthood. *Journal of Adult Development, 15*, 1-12.

Birditt, K. S., Fingerman, K. L., & Zarit, S. (2010). Adult children's problems and successes: Implications for intergenerational ambivalence. *Journals of Gerontology: Psychological Sciences, 65B, 145–153.*

Birditt, K. S., Jackey, L. M. H., & Antonucci, T. C. (2009a). Longitudinal patterns of negative relationship quality across adulthood. *Journals of Gerontology: Psychological Sciences, 64B*, 55–64.

Birditt, K. S., Miller, L. M., Fingerman, K. L., & Lefkowitz, E. S. (2009b). Tensions in the parent and adult child relationship: Links to solidarity and ambivalence. *Psychology and Aging, 24*, 287–295.

Birditt, K. S., Rott, L., & Fingerman, K. L. (2009c). 'If you can't say something nice, don't say anything at all': Coping with interpersonal tensions in the parent-child relationship during adulthood. *Journal of Family Psychology, 23*, 769–778.

Broad, K. D., Curley, J. P., & Keverne, E. B. (2006). Mother-infant bonding and the evolution of mammalian social relationships. *Philosophical Transactions of the Royal Society B, 361*, 2199–2214.

Byers, A. L., Levy, B. R., Allore, H. G., Bruce, M. L., & Kasl, S. V. (2008). When parents matter to their adult children: Filial reliance associated with parents' depressive symptoms. *Journals of Gerontology: Psychological Sciences, 63*, P33–P40.

Cacioppo, J. T., & Hawkley, L. C. (2003). Social isolation and health, with an emphasis on underlying mechanisms. *Perspectives in Biology and Medicine, 46*, S39–S52.

Casper, L. M., & Bianchi, S. M. (2002). *Continuity and change in the American family*. Thousand Oaks, CA: Sage Publications.

Chatters, L. M., Taylor, R. J., & Neighbors, H. W. (1989). Size of the informal health network mobilized in response to serious personal problems. *Journal of Marriage and the Family, 51*, 667–676.

Chatters, L. M., Taylor, R. T., Lincoln, K. D., & Schroepfer, T. (2002). Patterns of informal support from family and church members among African Americans. *Journal of Black Studies, 33*, 66–85.

Choi, H., & Marks, N. F. (2006). Transition to caregiving, marital disagreement, and psychological well-being: A prospective US national study. *Journal of Family Issues, 27*, 1701–1722.

Cohen, S., & Janicki-Deverts, D. (2009). Can we improve our physical health by altering our social networks? *Perspectives on Psychological Science, 4*, 375–378.

Collins, A., & Russell, S. (1991). Mother-child and father-child relationships in middle childhood and adolescence: A developmental analysis. *Developmental Review, 11*, 99–136.

Connidis, I. A., & McMullin, J. A. (2002). Sociological ambivalence and family ties: A critical perspective. *Journal of Marriage and Family, 64*, 558–567.

Davey, A., Janke, M., & Savla, J. (2005). Antecedents of intergenerational support: Families in contact and families as context. In M. Silversten (Ed.), *Intergenerational relations across time and place*. New York: Springer Publishers.

Eggebeen, D. J. (1992). Family structure and intergenerational exchanges. *Research on Aging, 14*, 427–447.

Erikson, E. K. (Ed.), (1950). Eight ages of man. *Childhood and society* (pp. 247–273). New York: W.W. Norton.

Fingerman, K. L. (2000). "We had a nice little chat": Age and generational differences in mothers' and daughters' descriptions of enjoyable visits. *Journals of Gerontology: Psychological Sciences, 55*, P95–P106.

Fingerman, K. L. (2003). *Mothers and their adult daughters: Mixed emotions, enduring bonds.* Amherst, NY: Prometheus Books.

Fingerman, K. L., & Charles, S. T. (2010). It takes two to tango: Why older people have the best relationships. *Current Directions in Psychological Science,* 19, 172–176.

Fingerman, K. L., Chen, P. C., Hay, E. L., Cichy, K. E., & Lefkowitz, E. S. (2006). Ambivalent reactions in the parent and offspring relationship. *Journals of Gerontology: Psychological Sciences, 61B*, 152–160.

Fingerman, K. L., Hay, E. L., & Birditt, K. S. (2004). The best of ties, the worst of ties: Close, problematic, and ambivalent relationships across the lifespan. *Journal of Marriage and Family, 66*, 792–808.

Fingerman, K. L., Hay, E. L., Kamp Dush, C. M., Cichy, K. E., & Hosterman, S. (2007). Parents' and offspring's perceptions of change and continuity when parents experience the transition to old age. *Advances in Life Course Research, 12*, 275–306.

Fingerman, K. L., Miller, L. M., Birditt, K. S., & Zarit, S. (2009). Giving to the good and the needy: Parental support of grown children. *Journal of Marriage and Family, 71*, 1220–1233.

Fingerman, K. L., Pitzer, L., Lefkowitz, E. S., Birditt, K. S., & Mroczek, D. (2008). Ambivalent relationship qualities between adults and their parents: Implications for both parties' well-being. *Journals of Gerontology: Psychological Sciences, 63B*, P362–P371.

Fingerman, K. L., Chan, W., Pitzer, L. M., Birditt, K. S., Franks, M. M., & Zarit, S. (2010). Who gets what and why: Help middle-aged adults provide to parents and grown children. *Journals of Gerontology: Social Sciences*, doi:10.1093/geronb/gb9009.

Freud, S. (1938). *The basic writings of Sigmund Freud.* (A. A. Brill, Translator). New York: The Modern Library.

Furstenberg, F. (2010). On a new schedule: Transitions to adulthood and family change. *Future of the Child, 20*, 67–87.

Ganong, L. H., & Coleman, M. (1999). *Changing families, changing responsibilities: Family obligations following divorce and remarriage.* Mahwah, NJ: Lawrence Erlbaum Publishers.

Giarrusso, R., Feng, D., & Bengtson, V. L. (2005). The intergenerational stake over 20 years. In M. Silverstein (Ed.), *Annual review of gerontology and geriatrics* (pp. 55–76). New York: Springer.

Grundy, E., & Henretta, J. C. (2006). Between elderly parents and adult children: A new look at the "sandwich generation." *Aging & Society, 26*, 707–722.

Ha, J. H. (2008). Changes in support from confidants, children, and friends following widowhood. *Journal of Marriage and Family, 70*, 306–318.

Ha, J. H., Hong, J., Seltzer, M. M., & Greenberg, J. S. (2008). Age and gender differences in the well-being of midlife and aging parents with children with mental health or developmental problems: Report of a national study. *Journal of Health and Social Behavior, 49*, 301–316.

Ha, J. H., & Ingersoll-Dayton, B. (2008). The effect of widowhood on intergenerational ambivalence. *Journals of Gerontology: Social Sciences, 63B*, S49–S58.

Hagestad, G. O., & Uhlenberg, P. (2007). The impact of demographic changes on relations between age groups and generations: A comparative perspective. In K. W. Schaie & P. Uhlenberg (Eds.), *Social structures: Demographic changes and the well-being of older persons* (pp. 239–261). New York: Springer.

Hareven, T. K. (1995). Historical perspectives on the family and aging. In R. Blieszner & V. H. Bedford (Eds.), *Handbook of aging and the family* (pp. 13–31). Westport, CT: Greenwood Press.

Hay, E. L., Fingerman, K. L., & Lefkowitz, E. S. (2007). The experience of worry in parent-adult child relationships. *Personal Relationships, 14*, 605–622.

Homans, G. F. (1950). *The human group.* New York: Harcourt, Brace, & World.

Hughes, M. E., Waite, L. J., LaPierre, T. A., & Luo, Y. (2007). All in the family: The impact of caring for grandchildren on grandparents' health. *Journals of Gerontology: Social Sciences, 62*, S108–S199.

Hulbert, A. (2003). *Raising America: Experts, parents, and a century of advice about children.* New York: Alfred A. Knopf.

Irving, S., & Ferraro, K. (2006). Reports of abusive experiences during childhood and adult health ratings: Personal control as a pathway. *Journal of Aging and Health, 18*, 458–485.

Kamo, Y. (2000). Racial and ethnic differences in extended family households. *Sociological Perspectives, 43*, 211–229.

Kohli, M. (2005). Intergenerational transfers and inheritance: A comparative view. In M. Silverstein & K. W. Schaie (Eds.), *Intergenerational relations across time and place: Annual review of gerontology and geriatrics* (pp. 266–289). New York: Springer.

Lee, Y. J., & Aytac, I. A. (1998). Intergenerational financial support among Whites, African Americans, and Latinos. *Journal of Marriage and Family, 60*, 426–441.

Levitzki, N. (2009). Parents are always parents: Parenting of adult children in an Israeli sample. *Journal of Family Psychology, 23*, 226–235.

Levy, B. R., Chung, P., & Caravan, M. (in press). Impact of explanatory style and age stereotypes on health across the lifespan. To appear in Fingeman, K. L., Berg, C., Smith, J., & Antonucci, T. C. (Eds.), (in press). *Handbook of lifespan psychology.* New York: Springer Publishers.

Logan, J. R., & Spitze, G. D. (1996). *Family ties: Enduring relations between parents and their grown children.* Philadelphia: Temple University Press.

Lowenstein, A. (2007). Solidarity-conflict and ambivalence: Testing two conceptual frameworks and their impact on quality of life for older family members. *Journals of*

Gerontology: Social Sciences, 62B, S100–S107.

Lowenstein, A., & Daatland, S. O. (2006). Filial norms and family support in a comparative cross-national context: Evidence from the OASIS study. *Ageing & Society, 26*, 203–223.

Luescher, K., & Pillemer, K. (1998). Intergenerational ambivalence: A new approach to the study of parent-child relations in later life. *Journal of Marriage and Family, 60*, 413–425.

Marks, N. F., Lambert, J. D., & Choi, H. (2002). Transitions to caregiving, gender, and psychological well-being: A prospective U.S. national study. *Journal of Marriage and Family, 64*, 657–667.

Martire, L. M., Stephens, M. A. P., & Townsend, A. L. (2000). Centrality of women's multiple roles: Beneficial and detrimental consequences for psychological well-being. *Psychology and Aging, 15*, 148–156.

McGarry, K. (1999). Inter-vivos transfers and intended bequests. *Journal of Public Economics, 73*, 321–351.

Milkie, M. A., Bierman, A., & Schieman, S. (2008). How adult children influence older parents' mental health: Integrating stress-process and life course perspectives. *Social Psychology Quarterly, 71*, 86–105.

Neighbors, H. W. (1997). Husbands, wives, family, and friends: Sources of stress, sources of support. In R. J. Taylor, J. S. Jackson, & L. M. Chatters (Eds.), *Family life in Black America* (pp. 277–292). Thousand Oaks, CA: Sage Publications.

Parsons, T. (1943). The kinship system of the contemporary United States. *American Anthropologist, 45*, 22–28.

Peters, C. L., Hooker, K., & Zvonkovic, A. M. (2006). Older parents' perceptions of ambivalence in relationships with their children. *Family Relations, 55*, 539–551.

Pew Internet Survey. (2009, September). Generations online. *Pew Internet & American Life Project*. Retrieved September 1, 2009 from http://www.pewinternet.org/Reports/2006/Generations-Online.aspx?r=1.

Pillemer, K., Suitor, J. J., Mock, S. E., Sabir, M., Pardo, T. B., & Sechrist, J. (2007). Capturing the complexity of intergenerational relations: Exploring ambivalence within later-life families. *Journal of Social Issues, 63*, 775–791.

Pillemer, K., & Suitor, J. J. (2002). Explaining mothers' ambivalence toward their adult children. *Journal of Marriage and Family, 64*, 602–613.

Pinquart, M., & Sorensen, S. (2007). Correlates of physical health of informal caregivers: A meta-analysis. *Journals of Gerontology: Psychological Science, 62*, P126–P137.

Pitzer, L. M., & Fingerman, K. L. Psychosocial resources and associations between childhood physical abuse and adult well being. *Journals of Gerontology: Psychological Sciences*, in press.

Pudrovska, T. (2009). Parenthood, stress, and mental health in late midlife and early old age. *International Journal of Aging and Human Development, 68*, 127–147.

Rook, K. S. (2001). Emotional health and positive versus negative social exchanges: A daily diary analysis. *Applied Developmental Science, 5*, 86–97.

Rossi, A. S., & Rossi, P. H. (1990). *Of human bonding: Parent-child relations across the life course*. New York: Aldine de Gruyter.

Sarkisian, N., & Gerstel, N. (2004). Kin support among Blacks and Whites: Race and family organization. *American Sociological Review, 69*, 812–837.

Sarkisian, N., & Gerstel, N. (2008). Till marriage do us part: Adult children's relationship with their parents. *Journal of Marriage and Family, 70*, 360–376.

Schoeni, R. F., & Ross, K. E. (2005). Material assistance from families during the transition to adulthood. In R. A. Settersten, F. F. Furstenberg, & R. G. Rumbaut (Eds.), *On the frontier of adulthood: Theory, research, and public policy* (pp. 396–417).

Schulz, R., & Martire, L. M. (2004). Family caregiving of persons with dementia: Prevalence, health effects, and support strategies. *American Journal of Geriatric Psychiatry, 12*, 240–249.

Shapiro, A. (2004). Revisiting the generation gap: Exploring the relationships of parent/adult-child dyads. *International Journal of Aging and Human Development, 58*, 127–146.

Silverstein, M., & Bengtson, V. L. (1991). Do close parent-child relations reduce the mortality risk of older parents? *Journal of Health and Social Behavior, 32*, 382–395.

Silverstein, M., & Bengtson, V. L. (1997). Intergenerational solidarity and the structure of adult child-parent relationships in American families. *American Journal of Sociology, 103*, 429–460.

Silverstein, M., Conroy, S., Wang, H., Gairrusso, R., & Bengtson, V. L. (2002). Reciprocity in parent-child relations over the adult life course. *Journals of Gerontology: Social Sciences, 57*, S3–S13.

Silverstein, M., Gans, D., & Yang, F. M. (2006). Intergenerational support to aging parents: The role of norms and needs. *Journal of Family Issues, 27*, 1068–1084.

Suitor, J. J., Pillemer, K., & Sechrist, J. (2006). Within-family differences in mothers' support to adult children. *Journals of Gerontology, 61B*, S10–S17.

Suitor, J. J., Sechrist, J., & Pillemer, K. (2007a). When mothers have favorites: Conditions under which mothers differentiate among their adult children. *Canadian Journal on Aging, 26*, 85–100.

Suitor, J. J., Sechrist, J., & Pillemer, K. (2007b). Within-family differences in mothers' support to adult children in Black and White families. *Research on Aging, 29*, 410–435.

Sundstrom, G., Malmberg, B., & Johansson, L. (2006). Balancing family and state care: Neither, either, or both? The case of Sweden. *Ageing & Society, 26*, 767–782.

Sung, K. T. (2000). Respect for elders: Myths and realities in East Asia. *Journal of Aging and Identity, 5*, 197–205.

Swartz, T. T. (2009). Intergenerational family relations in adulthood: Patterns, variations, and implications in the contemporary United States. *Annual Review of Sociology, 25*, 191–212.

Tighe, L., Birditt, K. S., & Antonucci, T. (2009, April). It's a love/hate relationship: Adolescents' ambivalence towards their parents. Poster presented at the annual meeting of the Society for Research on Child Development, Denver, CO.

Troll, L. E. (1987). Mother-daughter relations across the lifespan. *Applied Social Psychology Annual, 7*, 284–305.

Uchino, B. N., Holt-Lunstad, J., Smith, T. W., & Bloor, L. (2004). Heterogeneity in social networks: A comparison of different models linking relationships to psychological outcomes. *Journal of Social and Clinical Psychology, 23*, 123–139.

Umberson, D. (1992). Relationships between adult children and their parents: Psychological consequences for both generations. *Journal of Marriage and the Family, 544*, 664–674.

Ward, R. A. (2008). Multiple parent-adult child relations and well-being in middle and later life. *Journals of Gerontology: Social Sciences, 63B*, S239–S248.

Wickrama, K. A. S., Lorenze, F. O., Wallace, L. E., Peiris, L., Conger, R. D., & Elder, G. H. (2001). Family influence on physical health during the middle years: The case of onset of hypertension. *Journal of Marriage and the Family, 63*, 527–539.

Willson, A. E., Shuey, K. M., & Elder, G. H. (2003). Ambivalence in the relationship of adult children to aging parents and in-laws. *Journal of Marriage and Family, 65*, 1055–1072.

Wolff, J. L., & Kasper, J. D. (2006). Caregivers of frail elders: Updating a national profile. *The Gerontologist, 46*, 344–356.

Zarit, S. H., & Eggebeen, D. J. (2002). Parent-child relationships in adulthood and later years. In M. H. Bornstein (Ed.), *Handbook of parenting: Children and parenting* (2nd ed.) (pp. 135–161). Mahwah, NJ: Lawrence Erlbaum.

Zarit, S. H., Reever, K. E., & Bach-Peterson, J. (1980). Relatives of the impaired elderly: Correlates of feelings of burden. *The Gerontologist, 20*, 649–655.

Zarit, S. H., & Zarit, J. M. (2008). Flexibility and change: The fundamentals for families coping with dementia. In M. Downs & B. Bowers (Eds.), *Excellence in dementia care.* (pp. 85–102) Berkshire, UK: Open University Press.

Chapter | 15 |

Intergenerational Communication Practices

Howard Giles, Jessica Gasiorek

Department of Communication, University of California Santa Barbara, Santa Barbara, California, USA

CHAPTER CONTENTS

Introduction **232**
Overaccommodation **234**
Forms and Functions 234
Social and Cultural Evaluations 236
Management and Prevention 237
Theoretical Models 238
Problematic Elder-To-Young Communications **240**
Communicative Constructions of Aging **241**
Epilogue **242**
Acknowledgments **243**
References **243**

INTRODUCTION

Research on communication and aging has increased considerably in the last two to three decades (Coupland & Nussbaum, 2004; Harwood, 2007), fueled by the expansion of the Communication discipline and demographic shifts in the world's population, particularly as they have impacted the number of older people living longer. In many ways, communicative practices and processes define and mediate individuals' understanding of what it means to be a certain age, and this necessarily connects with a range of issues integral to the psychology of aging (Hummert, 2010). As individuals age, they must increasingly contend with ageist remarks, humor, and deeds (Williams & Giles, 1998). Although it is often likened to other "isms" such as racism or sexism, ageism is unique in a number of communicative ways.

First, while one's race or sex generally does not change across a lifetime, everyone ages. As such, ageism is a form of prejudice that nearly everybody – including those who have manifested, expressed, and likely internalized ageist sentiments themselves – come to experience. Second, unlike sexism and racism, ageism has not really been the subject of any major activist movement. Although there are laws in the United States prohibiting age-related discrimination in the workplace (see McCann & Giles, 2002), many expressions of ageism are so thoroughly integrated into Western social norms and communicative practices that they are taken for granted and go unremarked upon. Such biased messages are frequently expressed by both young and old (Coupland, 2004) and are compounded by the ageist diet of mainstream media (e.g., Robinson et al., 2004; Vasil & Wass, 1993). These manifestations are not taboo in the way that sexist and racist expressions are and, hence, the result is the reinforcement and perpetuation of ageist sentiments and values that, in turn, contribute to the problematic nature of much intergenerational communication.

Across contexts, intergenerational communication is often characterized as dissatisfying or otherwise problematic (e.g., Coupland et al., 1988a; Ryan et al., 1986). Younger speakers often report feeling unsure about how to respond to their elderly conversational partners, accommodating to them reluctantly, and feeling discomfort during such interactions (e.g., Barker, 2007; Williams & Giles, 1996). Age stereotypes, and both parties' beliefs and attitudes about the others' communicative styles, play significant roles in mediating this process (Ryan et al., 1992). The lesser the extent to which young adults stereotype older adults as benevolent and personally vital, for example, the more they report avoiding communication with them and that, in turn, predicts intergenerational dissatisfaction (e.g., Giles et al., 2007; McCann et al., 2005).

A significant area of inquiry within communication and aging has been exploring the antecedents and

DOI: 10.1016/B978-0-12-380882-0.00015-2

outcomes attending young people's use of diverse forms of overaccommodation with older adults (Caporael, 1981); for a discussion of this kind of communication and its kindred forms in other intergroup contexts, see DePaulo and Coleman (1986) and Hummert and Ryan (2001). This chapter explores important parameters of intergenerational communication, with a focus on older people being targets of overaccommodation, also known variously across studies as patronizing talk, elderspeak, or infantilizing talk (e.g., Whitbourne et al., 1995). The latter are considered by us as (interchangeable) forms in that they can be subsumed under or treated as exemplars of the more superordinate category of overaccommodative moves. We first consider the different forms overaccommodation can take, its social effects, the variable ways it can be managed by recipients, and the theoretical mechanisms proposed to underlie this process. Other forms problematic intergenerational communication may take will then be considered, including elderly-to-young overaccommodation, painful self-disclosures, and off-target verbosity. Finally and consequentially, this chapter concludes with a discussion of how *communicative* practices are endemic in the social construction of successful and unsuccessful aging.

OVERACCOMMODATION

Forms and Functions

Overaccommodation is a construct derived from communication accommodation theory (CAT; see Gallois et al., 2005 for an historical overview) that has been operationalized in terms of a speaker perceiving to exceed or overshoot the level of implementation of communicative behaviors necessary for a smooth and successful interaction (Coupland et al., 1988a). In intergenerational encounters, this sort of talk typically consists of a younger speaker adjusting their communication to compensate for perceived physical or psychological deficits of an older adult (for example, hearing loss or dementia). As there are genuine changes in communicative capabilities and characteristics as individuals age (e.g., Kemper & Kliegl, 1999), some of these adjustments can be beneficial to older communicators (see Gould & Dixon, 1997; Kemper et al., 1995). For example, certain linguistic modifications — specifically, semantic elaborations, focal stress on key words, and a reduction in the use of subordinate and embedded clauses — can improve older adults' comprehension and recall (Cohen & Faulkner, 1986; Kemper & Harden, 1999). Such adjustments may be appropriate when they are in response to genuine changes or deficits in others' communicative abilities.

However, perceived deficits of older adults are often derived from age-based stereotypes, rather than the actual communicative characteristics of the target. In this case, the adjustments made are often in excess of what is appropriate (Hummert et al., 2004). Indeed, it has been shown that older adults perceived as fitting negative age stereotypes are more likely to be the recipients of overaccommodation (Hummert et al., 1998). Examples of common young-to-elderly overaccommodation include simplified vocabulary and syntax; limited topic selection; and exaggerated intonation, pitch, and volume (e.g., Edwards & Noller, 1993; Hummert & Ryan, 2001). As Table 15.1 (from Ryan et al., 1995, p. 159) indicates, features of overaccommodation (therein termed patronizing talk) may be verbal or nonverbal, and many potential combinations thereof. As such, overaccommodation may take a wide range of forms across different contexts and can vary in the degree of patronization expressed (see Giles et al., 2004). Overaccommodation can also manifest as so-called "third-party talk" in which speakers direct questions not to elders themselves but, instead, to those people accompanying or caring for them (e.g., Coupland & Coupland, 1999).

Overaccommodation is most likely to occur — albeit far from always — in intergenerational encounters with unfamiliar elders, as such circumstances often dictate a reliance on first impressions and physical cues. Health and related institutional or caregiving contexts (such as nursing homes) are also settings wherein overaccommodation is particularly prevalent (LaTourette & Meeks, 2001; Ryan et al., 1995). In Salari's (2006) ethnographic study of five "model" Northeast adult day centers, all sites exhibited either verbal or environmental "infantilizations" (such as baby talk, nicknames, reprimands, child-oriented décor, use of confinement, and the invasion of privacy), with two of the five exhibiting these examples severely (see Kemper, 1994). It is worth highlighting that in these situations, such infantalizations are not only present in talk, but also manifest in older adults' physical locales and, as such, these messages permeate elders' verbal and visual experiences. Interviews indicated that older adults at these centers resented this kind of treatment, with other consequences including apparent negative impact on elders' well-being and their relationships with staff and peers.

However, overaccommodation does not only occur in institutional situations, and is clearly an issue older adults are aware of and consider both pervasive and problematic. It can occur in public settings like grocery stores or banks, as well as in ongoing relationships, with many older adults reporting overaccommodation from their own (adult) children (Hummert & Mazloff, 2001) and grandchildren reporting nonaccommodative experiences with their grandparents (Soliz & Harwood, 2006). When asked, a majority (58%) of older adults surveyed believed overaccommodation (in this study, patronizing talk) was something older adults in general experienced and just over

Table 15.1 A taxonomy of patronizing talk features in communication with older adults.

VERBAL	NONVERBAL
A. Vocabulary	A. Voice
Simple	High pitch
Few multisyllabic words	Exaggerated intonation
Childish terms	Loud
Minimizing words (e.g., *just, tittle, short*)	Slow
Pronoun modifications (e.g., over inclusive *we*, exclusive *we*, avoidance of me/you in favor of name substitutions)	Exaggerated pronunciation
Grammar	B. Gaze
B. Simple clauses and sentences	Low eye contact
Repetitions	Staring
Tag questions	Roll eyes
Imperatives	Wink
Fillers	C. Proxemics
Fragments	Stand too close
Forms of address	Stand over a person seated or in bed
C. First names and nicknames	Stand too far off
Terms of endearment (e.g., *sweetie, dearie, honey*)	D. Facial expression
Childlike terms (e.g., *good girl, naughty boy, cute little man*)	Frown
Third-person reference	Exaggerated smile
D. Topic management	Raised eyebrows
Limited topic selection and topic reinforcement (e.g., focus on past, shallow, task oriented, or overly personal/intimate)	E. Gestures
Interruptions	Shake head
Dismissive of other-generated topics	Shrug shoulders
Exaggerated praise for minor accomplishments	Hands on hips
	Cross arms
	Abrupt movements
	F. Touch
	Pat on head
	Pat on hand, arm, shoulder

From Ryan et al. (1995, p. 154).

a third believed it occurred often. However, perhaps self-protectively and in line with the process of "social downgrading" (Heckhausen & Brim, 1997), only 36% reported that they themselves had actually been "victims" of this kind of communication – and of those, 13% often. In any case, responses to overaccommodation were clearly unfavorable; of those: 58% reported feeling patronized, while only a small minority (less than 8%) felt "cared for" following such communications (Giles et al., 1993).

In addition to negative affect and lowered self-esteem associated with being patronized, this kind of talk can have a number of harmful consequences. Studies of its effects have suggested that its recipients may internalize the negative evaluation this kind of talk implies (see communication predicament of aging model; CPAM in the section Theoretical Models), resulting in perceptions of less competent independent behaviors, and even learned helplessness (Coupland et al., 1988a; Ryan et al., 1986). In a recent study of patients in an Alzheimer's care facility, it was found that residents were significantly more likely to engage in resistive or disruptive behavior (such as shouting, pushing staff away, or refusing requests) after being addressed in a patronizing manner, as compared to those being addressed more "neutrally" (Williams et al., 2009).

Investigations into overaccommodation and its effects most often take the form of vignette studies (e.g., Edwards & Noller, 1993; Giles et al., 1993; Ryan et al., 1994a). These typically consist of transcripts and audio- or video-recordings of interactions between two or more individuals, elements of which are manipulated for different (independent variable) dimensions. Because they are scripted, vignettes allow for the highly specific manipulation of interactional content and features that would be largely impossible with other methods. Study participants are asked to consider the version of the vignette they are presented with, and then respond to it along a number of judgmental dimensions. Interestingly, participants report "hearing" and "seeing" nonverbal features of overaccommodation (e.g., loud, shrill, and exaggerated pronunciations) when reading these vignettes (Ryan et al., 1991).

Social and Cultural Evaluations

In comparison with so-called neutral speakers, overaccommodative speakers are generally evaluated as more dominant, less respectful, less nurturant, and less warm. Such encounters are also inferred to be less satisfying than accommodative ones (Ryan et al., 1994a). Recipients of overaccommodation are, in turn, viewed as more frustrated with the interaction (Ryan et al., 1991) and less competent (Ryan et al., 1994b). In an exploratory study, Cunningham and Williams (2007) reported that recipiency of overaccommodation among elderly patients with dementia was associated with such observable, resistive behaviors as turning and pulling away, crying, screaming, and threatening.

As previously stated, evaluations of overaccommodation are not uniformly negative in all situations; the picture is somewhat more complex. Indeed, a number of behaviors associated with intergenerational overaccommodation are inherently ambiguous; for example, the nicknames like "dearie" or exaggerated praise have both supportive *and* patronizing connotations (Ryan et al., 1995). In this vein, Hummert and Ryan (1996) conceptualized motives for this kind of communication along two dimensions (high-low for each) of caring and control, thereby providing four quadrants of combinations (e.g., low control and high caring). How older adults would construe and define these two dimensions is, however, for future research to uncover. All else being equal, individuals tend to infer overaccommodative speakers' intentions as more controlling and domineering in nature rather than reflections of genuine supportiveness (Harwood & Giles, 1996). Although overaccommodation is often discussed in terms of its communicative ingredients, it is important to note that it is ultimately the recipient's perception of a behavior — not objective qualities of the behavior itself — that determines whether or not it is considered overaccommodative. Thus, labels such as "overaccommodation" are ultimately *social attributions* (Ytsma & Giles, 1997) rather than communicative behaviors per se. That said, as Table 15.1 illustrates, there are a number of behaviors that are routinely associated with this kind of communication such that they may be considered "features" of this sort of talk.

As Jones et al. (1994) observed, experiences and social roles of observers and interactants affect perceptions of accommodation. What one individual perceives as overaccommodative may not be considered overaccommodative by another (including the other individual in the interaction). Edwards and Noller (1993), for example, found that overaccommodative interactions between an older adult and a caretaker were evaluated more favorably; that is, as less patronizing, by elderly participants than by nursing students or a neutral third party (psychology students). Sachweh (1998) reported similar findings in her study of communication with German nursing home residents. Indeed, communication that would likely be considered overaccommodative by third parties has been rated positively (as supportive and caring) by those who are extremely frail (Ryan & Cole, 1990), perhaps because of its (potentially) caring connotations. All this notwithstanding, there are data to suggest that older community-dwelling elders tend to be even more sensitive to overaccommodation than younger adults, and attribute age-peer recipients of it as much lower in competence (Giles et al., 1993). In other words, overaccommodation can make its "victims" feel stigmatized, an emotion that can be exacerbated if other elders or family members are in potential earshot of it.

As these findings suggest, there appear to be certain circumstances in which negative evaluations of overaccommodation are attenuated. In addition to the tendency for (institutionalized) older adults to evaluate overaccommodation less negatively than other groups, there are indications that this type of communication is evaluated as more acceptable in institutional settings (such as hospitals; Hummert et al., 1994). Overaccommodation has also been judged more acceptable when directed toward "cognitively confused" older adults (relative to those cognitively alert) as well as to institutionalized older adults (as opposed to community residents; e.g., LaTourette & Meeks, 2001; Ryan & Cole, 1990). There is also evidence that reactions to overaccommodation are more positive when there are cues present suggesting that a speaker's motives are caring (Harwood & Giles, 1996). These findings underscore the importance of attributed motives in both characterizing overaccommodation and determining individuals' affective as well as behavioral reactions to it. Interestingly, in a vignette study where a police officer was depicted as patronizing an older woman who had lost a child, raters viewed the officer less and the elder more competent, the more the officer patronized her (Giles et al., 2003).

While the majority of research into overaccommodation, and problematic communication more broadly, has been conducted in Anglophone Western contexts, recent years have seen an increasing interest in a more global exploration of these issues. A number of consistent findings have emerged across cultures with rather profound longer term consequences. In particular, older adults' perceptions of recurrent non-accommodative talk over time from younger acquaintances and family (as well as elder peers) can be associated with self-reported lowered self-esteem and life satisfaction, as well as increased depressive symptomatology (e.g., Cai et al., 1998; Giles et al., 2008; Noels et al., 2001). However, and with respect to overaccommodation specifically, it is clear that such messages are not evaluated uniformly across cultures. In other words, what might be considered overaccommodation (in terms of a given set of psycholinguistic features; see Table 15.1) in one culture is not necessarily considered overaccommodative in another, with consequent differences in associated attributions about the individuals involved.

For example, talk considered overaccommodative by Anglo American students was not rated as overaccommodative when translated into Chinese and rated by Hong Kong students, suggesting that it is conceptualized differently in (written) Chinese than English (Giles et al., 1998). Similarly, young Chinese respondents did not downgrade a "patronizing" overaccommodative) speaker (i.e., rate them lower on status and nurturance traits) as did students from California, nor did they perceive a recipient of supposed patronizing talk as less satisfied with the interaction. In sum, overaccommodation, at least in the prototypical forms portrayed above, "incurs nowhere near the attributional costs it invokes for patronizing [overaccommodating] in the West —at least in terms of the (arguably Western-biased) inferential traits adopted" (p. 173). Further research (and with older raters) is needed to discover why Chinese respondents reacted differently from their American counterparts. Indeed, what might be considered overaccommodative in China (or elsewhere in Asia) but not in the United States is an intriguing issue yet to be explored.

Although problematic communication involving older adults is generally discussed in relation to intergenerational communication, overaccommodation can occur in peer interactions between older adults, too. In both Western and Eastern contexts, and intriguingly so, older adults have rated their peers as even more non-accommodating than younger adults (e.g., Cai et al., 1998; Giles et al., 2008; Ota et al., 2007). As in intergenerational communication, non-accommodation from elderly peers was associated with avoidance of them (Giles et al., 2008) as well as decreased subjective well-being (Ota et al., 2007).

Management and Prevention

Overaccommodation generally occurs as an ingredient of an ongoing interaction and, as such, evaluations of it and its participants may be shaped by how individuals respond to it. A number of studies have examined how different response styles (that are assertive, cooperative, passive, or humorous) affect evaluations of overaccommodative encounters, and thus their relative effectiveness in managing overaccommodation. Generally, assertive reactions to overaccommodation result in the respondent being considered more competent, but evaluated less favorably along other dimensions, such as warmth (Harwood & Giles, 1996). Harwood et al. (1993) found that assertive respondents were seen as of a higher status, but also more controlling, less nurturing, and less satisfied, than more passive respondents. Overaccommodative speakers receiving an assertive response were, in turn, seen as less in control, and less satisfied. Similarly, in the study of Harwood et al. (1997) involving a car-accident scenario, assertive respondents were evaluated as more competent but less respectful and less benevolent than non-assertive respondents. Recipients of overaccommodation were also judged more likely to have caused the accident in question for age-related reasons, indicating that overaccommodation may invoke age-related stereotypes of elderly incompetence.

Such results appear to leave recipients of overaccommodation in a bind: while an assertive response makes them appear more competent, it is also associated with a range of other more negative evaluations, such as threatening to a control-inclined patronizer. Nonetheless and again, the cultural parameters in which overaccommodation are embedded can, of course, be crucial. Giles et al. (1998) showed how young adults from Hong Kong were not favorably disposed toward an older person who adopted assertive tactics when being overaccommodated. The authors explained this reaction in terms of a Chinese value for avoiding overt retaliation or interactive aggression.

There are, however, modest data to suggest that a third potential response — humor — may be an effective response that acts as a foil to overaccommodation. Comparing passive, assertive, and humorous responses to overaccommodation directed toward older adults in an institutional setting, Ryan et al. (2000) found that assertive responses led to the least favorable ratings of the recipient for manner, appropriateness, *and* competence. It is worth observing that these results contrast with those of other studies, which found higher competence ratings for assertive responses. However, this difference may be due to the nursing home context of the study compared to the community context of other studies in that it is possible a dependency-oriented context makes assertive response seem less appropriate. Humorous responses, however, were rated positively on all three factors of manner, appropriateness, and competence. In this study, rather than answering an overly accommodative request to engage in some crafts work in a passive manner, the humorous response was, instead, "I think I'll just pass today. I've made more crafts in my lifetime than an overachieving Girl Guide group at Christmas." As humor has been shown to be an effective tool in coping with stressful situations (e.g., Thorson et al., 1997) and generally prevents a negative end to encounters in a socially acceptable manner, it may be considered a "best-of-both-worlds" reaction: Humorous responses permit a speaker to express opposition to overaccommodation, while maintaining a creative, lively competence, benevolence, and politeness on the part of the respondent. Effectively striking the "right" humorous note, however, appears to be something of a fine art as the benefits of humorous responses may not apply to those perceived as sarcastic (Ryan et al., 2000).

Another obvious way of mitigating the negative effects of overaccommodation on older adults is to diminish its use. In institutional contexts, communication training programs for nurses and staff are one possible means of recourse and, to date, some intervention programs have shown promising results. Williams et al. (2003) designed a course of three, one-hour educational sessions targeting nursing home staff about their use of overaccommodative talk and its consequences. Following the training program, they saw a significant reduction in use of diminutives (e.g., "honey" or "dear"), collectives (i.e., "we should get up now" versus "you should…"), and controlling emotional tone (all characteristics of this kind of overaccommodation) by nursing staff. The authors also claimed that "...anecdotal reports suggest that residents were aware of a change in staff talk and participated more in dialogue after training" (p. 247; see also, Williams, 2006). This suggests that communication training programs aimed at raising awareness of overaccommodation, at least in institutional settings, may be effective in reducing both its prevalence and related negative outcomes.

Theoretical Models

Given the range of negative consequences associated with overaccommodation, an understanding of its origins and mechanisms is clearly important. To this end, a number of models addressing the cognitive processes mediating intergenerational communication have been proposed. Both the CPAM (Hummert et al., 2004; Ryan et al., 1986) and the age stereotypes in interactions model (ASIM; Hummert, 1994; Hummert et al., 2004) seek to describe the potential role and impact of age stereotypes on communication in an encounter with an older adult. The CPAM primarily addresses the consequences of negative stereotypes for interaction, while the ASIM incorporates both positive and negative stereotypes (and consequent action) in its framework.

The CPAM contends that individuals' particular stereotypes of older adults can trigger a negative feedback cycle that results in overaccommodative talk and, ultimately, a reinforcement of age stereotypes. According to this framework, in an encounter with an older adult, individuals recognize age cues (e.g., gray hair or voice quality) that prime or evoke negative age stereotypes. These stereotypes often include conceptions of communicative characteristics (or deficiencies) associated with aging, such as poor hearing or difficulty following complex trajectories of information. Drawing on CAT (see the section Forms and Functions), the model suggests that speakers will adapt their language to accommodate the older adult's perceived communicative needs (i.e., by talking louder or simplifying explanations). When stereotyped expectations do not match the older adult's actual abilities, however, overaccommodation is the result. This overaccommodation reinforces age stereotypes for both parties in the interaction which may, in turn, limit older adults' opportunities for communication. Older adults may also internalize the negative stereotypes (and evaluations) implicit in such an interaction, leading to a loss of self-esteem as well as physical and cognitive declines (as stereotypes essentially become a self-fulfilling prophecy). A revision of the model (see Figure 15.1) incorporated cooperative and assertive response types, proposing how each can affect subsequent interaction as well as physical and psychological well-being (Harwood et al., 1993).

Hummert's (1994) ASIM extends and elaborates on the CPAM by including both positive and negative stereotypes in its framework and identifying specific contextual and communicator factors that contribute to age stereotyping in interaction. The model suggests that three characteristics of individuals — age, cognitive complexity, and quality of past contact with older adults — will affect the nature and valence of individuals' age stereotypes. The physical and communicative characteristics of the older adult target and the context of the interaction (which may make age stereotypes salient and/or highlight a particular stereotype) will also influence the stereotyping process. The degree of these components' impacts is seen as moderated by accessible cognitive schemas available to the individual speaker in question. If unfavorable stereotypes are triggered, the negative feedback cycle of the CPAM is played out. If positive stereotypes result, then communication beliefs related to what Hummert refers to as "normal adult speech" are invoked, and appropriate accommodative talk should occur (with an accompanying positive feedback cycle for the older adult target in terms of self-esteem, competence, etc.). Finally, the ASIM suggests that the older adult's communicative behavior (in response to the individual-speaker's talk) may either reinforce or disrupt the individual-speaker's perceptions. An unexpected (non-stereotypical) response; for example, an assertive one as previously mentioned, potentially results in an interruption of either the CPAM's negative feedback cycle or the positive stereotype's positive feedback cycle. To provide a foil, Ryan et al. (1995) proposed the "communicative enhancement model of aging." Here, those interacting with older adults make sure that they do not succumb to social stereotyping but, rather, accommodate the idiosyncratic characteristics of elder *persons* (see also, Barker et al., 2004).

As, perhaps, a complement to these models, Harwood (1998) has proposed the existence of what he terms intergenerational communication schemas (ICSs); thus far and restrictively, these have only been studied from young people's perspectives. Defined as cognitive structures that delineate how an intergenerational communication episode is expected to play

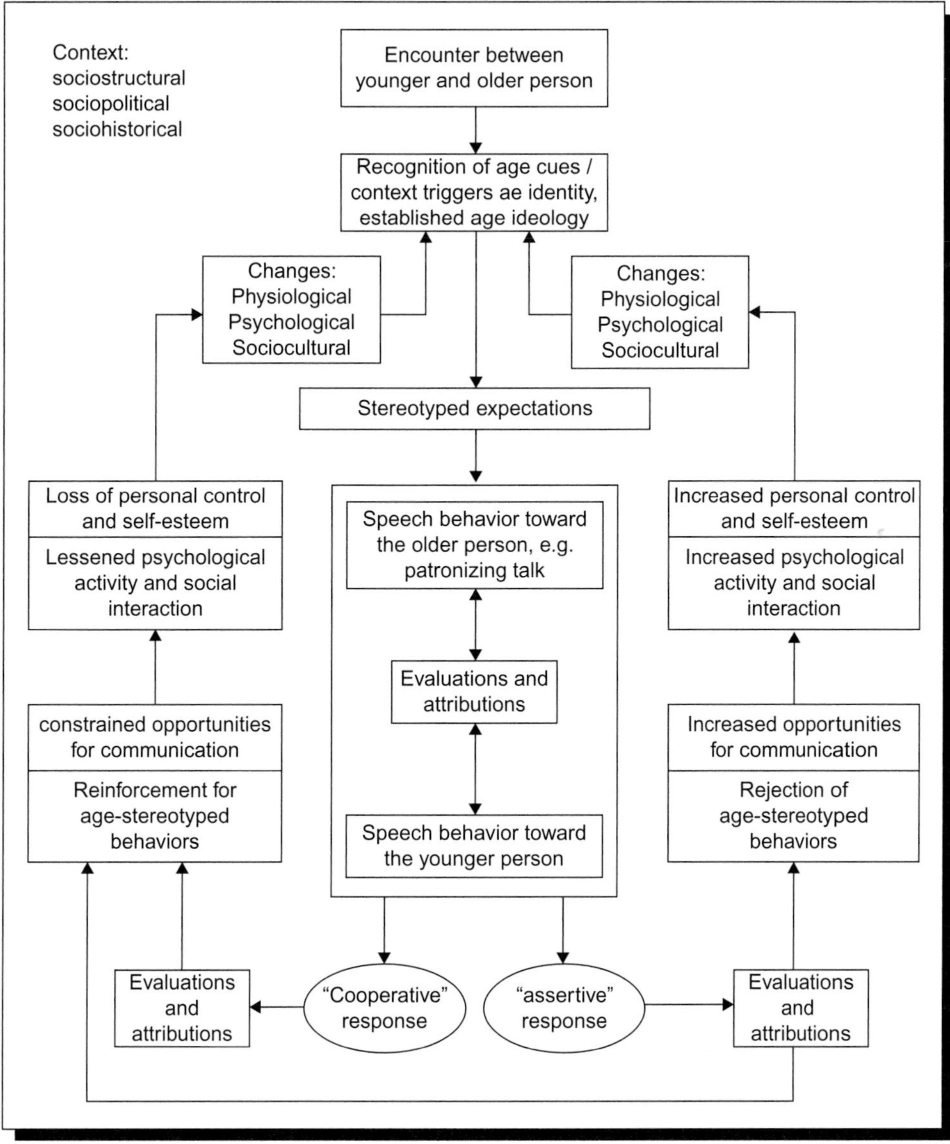

Figure 15.1 The revised communication of aging predicament model (after Harwood et al., 1993, p. 213).

out, ICSs are conceived as a constellation of expectations for the process of a conversation (Harwood et al., 2000). Elements include topics of discussion, emotional responses, what interactants are saying, who is talking (when), interactants' attitudes toward each other, the tone of the discussion and interaction, and expected outcomes of the interaction. Communication schemas include trait-based information about a conversational partner and expected sequences of conversational events (scripts), but will also include additional information about the interaction (Harwood et al., 2000). Multidimensional scaling and cluster analyses of schemas derived from a content analysis of descriptions of intergenerational encounters resulted in several categories of young-to-elder ICSs varying across a number of dimensions, including valence (positive/negative/neutral), respect, helpfulness, and level of connection. These schemas appear to differ between cultures (see Lin et al., 2008).

While not detailed explicitly in Harwood and colleagues' (2000) analyses, it would be expected that different ICSs would contain different expectations and prescriptions for the type of talk the younger speaker should engage in. Overaccommodation might result from helping-oriented schemas (where, in an effort to be as helpful as possible to an older adult, a younger adult might easily overcompensate for any perceived or imagined interactional issues) or negative schemas (where a younger adult is more likely to perceive an older adult as somehow deficient). Explicitly investigating such links to overaccommodation and its variants should be an area for future research, as Harwood (1998) has suggested.

PROBLEMATIC ELDER-TO-YOUNG COMMUNICATIONS

Thus far, problematic intergenerational communication has primarily been considered in terms of how younger speakers patronize older recipients. However, overaccommodation does not just occur in young-to-elderly communication; younger people may be the targets of such talk from older adults as well. In the exploration of this issue by Giles and Williams (1994), younger adults reported that they were frequently patronized (overaccommodated) by older adults. Following a multidimensional scaling analysis of characteristics of young adults' accounts of such encounters, three clusters of elderly-to-young overaccommodation were identified; namely *non-listening* (e.g., "Older people never listen to your opinion"), *disapproving/disrespecting youth* (e.g., "You're just beer-drinking dopeheads that don't know any better"), and *overprotective/parental* (e.g., "When you get older you will see this was best"). Vignettes were then devised to assess any attributions associated with each type. Parental talk was found to be the least offensive (although it was still considered less appropriate than non-overaccommodative talk), while non-listening was associated with the most negative affective reactions. Disapproving patronization, in turn, evoked the most negative attributions of speaker intent. Whether these same types of language and associated attributions also characterize young-to-elderly overaccommodation remains an empirical question, although at least some overlap seems likely.

Not surprisingly, negative outcomes are associated with elderly-to-young overaccommodation. Like older adult recipients of overaccommodation, young adults reported being bothered by this kind of talk, and generally judged overaccommodative speech as less polite and appropriate than neutral talk (Giles & Williams, 1994). Negative encounters of this sort with older adults may also reinforce negative age stereotypes (e.g., that communication with older adults is awkward or unpleasant), with attendant negative consequences for young-to-elderly communication as outlined in the CPAM. Disapproving elderly-to-young communication can also result in expressed conflict; when young adult participants were asked to recall a conflict in a relationship with an older adult age 60+, old-to-young criticism was the most common source in both Chinese (Zhang, 2004) and American (Zhang & Lin, 2009) contexts.

As discussed above, overaccommodation is conceptualized as a speaker transcending or overshooting the communicative behaviors a participant judges necessary for appropriate talk (Coupland et al., 1988a). However, contrasting situations arise when, from a participant's perspective, a speaker does not do enough to implement the communicative behaviors judged necessary for appropriate talk. Examples include not listening, failing to adjust language or topic choice for another interactant, or interrupting a fellow speaker. According to the communication accommodation framework, this is labeled *underaccommodation* (Coupland et al., 1988a), and is another type of potentially problematic intergenerational communication. Painful self-disclosures and off-target verbosity are two forms this type of communication may take.

Painful self-disclosures (PSDs; Coupland et al., 1988a) are defined as the disclosure of relatively intimate, negative information. This phenomenon frequently follows on from older peoples' disclosure of their own ages, itself taking various forms, such as "I remember Goleta in the old days," "We senior citizens these days...," etc. (Coupland et al., 1989). In the context of intergenerational communication, PSDs frequently take the form of older adults talking about ill health, ongoing medical problems, hospital stays and operations, sensory decrements, accidents, bereavement, immobility, and loneliness, among other debilitating topics. Because of the nature of their content, such disclosures often feel inappropriate, and can leave the other interactant unsure of how to respond and/or unable to engage in the conversation, as the topic does not represent a domain of shared experience for the other interactant. In many respects and because of their explosive management consequences, PSDs can be metaphorically considered "communicative grenades." Both younger and older individuals tend to rate those who engage in PSDs less favorably, although this tendency appears amplified in younger respondents. There is also evidence that younger adults experience elder PSDs as more painful and less appropriate than do older adults (Bonneson & Hummert, 2002), and that discomfort relating to PSDs is a more significant differentiator of positive and negative aspects of grandparent-grandchild relationships than neutral self-disclosure (Fowler & Soliz, 2010). As such, PSDs are arguably more of a communicative issue in intergenerational encounters than in same-age adult interactions (see, however, Collins and Gould, 1994). As with overaccommodative talk, attributed motives also appear to at least partially mediate reactions to PSDs. For instance, Barker (2007) found that young adult grandchildren were less likely to report discomfort in response to grandparent PSD when they perceived grandparents' motives for communicating to be related to identity expression or positive affect, as opposed to control.

PSDs from older adults are generally viewed negatively by younger people and, clearly, further research needs to address elder peers' reactions to it, too. As noted above, they often result in discomfort on the part of others in the interaction, as well as less favorable evaluations of the discloser. Coupland et al. (1988a) identified a number of potential causes of elder PSDs. The first of these have been identified and include self-stereotyping (Turner et al., 1987), in which older adults view themselves as "elderly" and thus discuss topics and enact behaviors they view as typical of "elderly" people (see Levy, 2003). Second, PSDs may also be a means of coping with life circumstances, that is, of seeking social support when faced with difficulties associated with aging. Third, PSDs may be used as a form of self-handicapping and/or self-protection: the content of these disclosures may be used as a face-saving device or disclaimer, providing an excuse should the speaker not communicatively "perform" in a manner considered up to par in whatever interaction may follow (Coupland et al.,1988b).

Yet there is also some evidence of potential benefits and, hence perhaps, other causal agents, for such disclosures. Particularly with more isolated older adults, PSDs provide speakers with an opportunity to engage in conversation with "newsworthy" information to share which is, arguably, beneficial for the discloser's positive face (Coupland et al., 1988b). There also may be a cathartic benefit to discussing one's problems for the speaker, particularly if they evoke a sympathetic or otherwise supportive response. As such, PSDs should not necessarily be seen as simple evidence of natural decline (both mental and physical) in old age but, rather, as a function of more complex, *socially* constituted phenomena. Future research may allow us to determine which factor (or combination of them) enables one form of PSD over others. Such a realization, through educational interventions yet to be actually devised to foster, for example, empathy, might lead to more sensitive ways of managing the recipiency of PSDs. Furthermore, underaccommodating language is not only a feature of older-to-younger talk, but has also been documented with regard to young people's inattentiveness in intergenerational conversations, sometimes even admitting to not "having their hearts in it" (Lin et al., 2004). The converse can also emerge, and with seemingly harmful emotional consequences, when younger caregivers verbally deflect and minimize the legitimacy of elderly people's physical and heart-felt, dire complaints (see Grainger, 1993).

Off-target verbosity, that is, prolific speech judged to be irrelevant, tangential, and away-from-the-prevailing-topic (Pushkar et al., 1994) at least by younger people, is another form of underaccommodation often associated with other adults, as is repeating the same content time after time (Brenes, 2010; termed *lao dao* in Chinese, see Zhang and Hummert, 2001). Similar to PSDs, off-target verbosity generally represents a failure to make appropriate adjustments to the topic and/or content of a conversation from the perspective of at least one interactant. What constitutes "off-target," however, is, again, a subjective judgment in which the age of the perceiver appears to play an important role. There is evidence, for example, that older evaluators rated (particularly female) older speakers to be less off-target than do younger evaluators (Odato & Keller-Cohen, 2009).

Younger and older adults have also shown differences in communicative goals (objective versus expressive) for a given type of topic, with younger adults favoring objective goals and older adults favoring a combination of objective (comprehensible and logical) and expressive (entertaining and educational) goals. These goals predict ratings of off-topic speech by listeners, with older adults rated as less clear, less focused, and more talkative (Trunk & Abrams, 2009). Thus, it appears that at least some of perceived age-related differences in off-topic speech may in fact reflect differences in speakers' goal-related communicative strategies, rather than, for example, simple (attributions of) age-related cognitive decline, as age stereotypes might suggest. Exploring the range of factors that contribute to this process and its outcome is a potentially fruitful area for future research.

COMMUNICATIVE CONSTRUCTIONS OF AGING

While age and age boundaries are chronologically determined numbers, they are also states of mind that can be *expressed* (see, for example, Giles et al., 2005). As individuals age, they must repeatedly redefine themselves; most encounter ageism, challenging their age-based views of themselves, arguably far earlier than perhaps they would have anticipated (see the next section). We each have senses of what it means to be a certain age; for example, what a fifty-year-old *is* and *does*, which are, in large part, determined by the social models, expectations, and stereotypes that have been communicated to us across our lifetimes (see Brenes, 2010; Pecchioni et al., 2005). How we see others treat and communicate with individuals of different ages, and how we are treated and spoken to as we pass through different life stages, contribute to these understandings which we, in turn, enact in our interactions with others. As such, communication plays a central role in social constructions of age and aging and in ways that, arguably, the rich array of conceptual definitions of both objective and subjective successful aging have neglected (see, e.g., Depp & Jeste, 2006; Montrose et al., 2006). A life span perspective on communication and aging emphasizes how the accumulation of experiences with ageism and ageist communication across the decades influence both attitudes toward aging and age-related behaviors.

However, negative outcomes are not of course inevitable (see Baltes & Baltes, 1990). In the same way that negative stereotypes and ageism can contribute to unsuccessful aging, conscious attention to age-positive attitudes and behavior can help foster healthy aging. A number of empirically based suggestions and recommendations for successfully negotiating the aging process and communicatively combating ageism can be proffered. These "anti-ageist" tactics may take a range of forms, from explicit interventions in institutional settings to shifts in individual outlooks on what it means to age. Indeed, there should be greater emphasis on a life span perspective that values individuals at *all* stages of the aging process. In other words, successful adaptation to elderliness is, arguably for most people, engaged and anticipated in much earlier decades. This is the foundation of Giles and Dorjee's (2004) proposed framework for successful aging in later life, which builds on ideological and cognitive kinds of adjustments (e.g., not to *think or feel* "old"), but behaviorally focuses on communicative practices necessary for productive aging. Six of these are highlighted next.

The first acknowledges that *colluding* in negative age categorizing with others (e.g., by sending them ageist birthdays and even humorously expressing and anticipating their supposed age decrements) can be problematic and harmful. The second encourages wariness about imposing readily accessible *self*-age attributions age excuses (in middle-age and beyond) can also be detrimental to long-term well-being (Ryan et al., 2002). The third factor advocates, instead, accommodating to, and caring for when appropriate, the personal idiosyncratic characteristics of older adults (Ryan et al., 1995). It also views this from the other side of the coin and recommends older people personalizing younger people and their (actually, somewhat alien and ever-changing) cultures and doing so in ways that avoid being perceived as overaccommodating and, thereby, potentially sounding false (Brenes, 2010). The fourth encourages effectively managing (by selective assertiveness and adroit humor) being the inevitable recipient of interactional ageisms (Ryan et al., 2006). The fifth recommends promoting media literacy among older adults to combat depictions of ageism on TV and elsewhere (see Donlon & Levy, 2005). The final prescription would be, even in light of recent cognitive data showing well-being can be associated with negative expectations for one's future self (Cheng et al., 2009), to consistently communicate for others, in parallel, positive emotions and optimism about the aging process (see Danner et al., 2001). In sum, this perspective underscores the need for individuals to construct, sustain, and redefine communicative climates and social networks (see Nussbaum & Fisher, 2009, in press) as they age and develop. This way, each life phase, as well as the crucial transitions between them (see Giles & Reid, 2005), becomes absorbing and a fascinating challenge.

EPILOGUE

In a celebratory editorial announcing the 65th anniversary of the *Journals of Gerontology: Psychological Sciences*, Blieszner and Sanford (2010) took stock of the topics of articles submitted between 2000 and 2008. The top seven topics were identified, and communication did not figure at all in this list. In the Social Sciences section to this same journal issue, however, communication was mentioned — though only to the extent of acknowledging that new communication technologies might now foster closer academic exchanges between scholars (Silverstein, 2010). In other words, matters of communication have not emerged as a focal theme in this mainstream forum of the psychology of aging. This chapter has tried to make the case that *communicative* phenomena and processes are integral to the social construction of aging and we hope that, as such, our contribution might be a modest impetus for encouraging more work on this vital topic. More specifically, this chapter has argued that problematic and avoidant intergenerational communication climates can be a function of younger people overaccommodating their elders by adopting various forms of overaccommodation, while the latter (and perhaps, sometimes, simultaneously) underaccommodating the former by their use of PSDs and off-target verbosity. In other words and as the model in Figure 15.2 depicts, younger and older people can often be communicatively "missing each other." Even when mutual accommodation is evident, it, too, can be expressed, rather reluctantly, on the part of younger people (Williams & Giles, 1996) and demeaned as false when conveyed by elders (Brenes, 2010). Oftentimes, the motives for these communicative practices are pro-social, benevolent, and nurturant, yet they can all too quickly lead to inferences that are mutually negative and miscommunicative; that is, they are attributed to young people's pernicious desires for control and subordination on the one hand, and invoked as evidence of elders' decline and incompetence on the other. Such a sequence, as was previously alluded to, is complicated and reciprocated by older adults sometimes overaccommodating (e.g., over-parenting) younger people and younger people underaccommodating their elders (e.g., by dismissing their legitimate concerns). Clearly, communication practices are shaped by age schemas which, in turn,

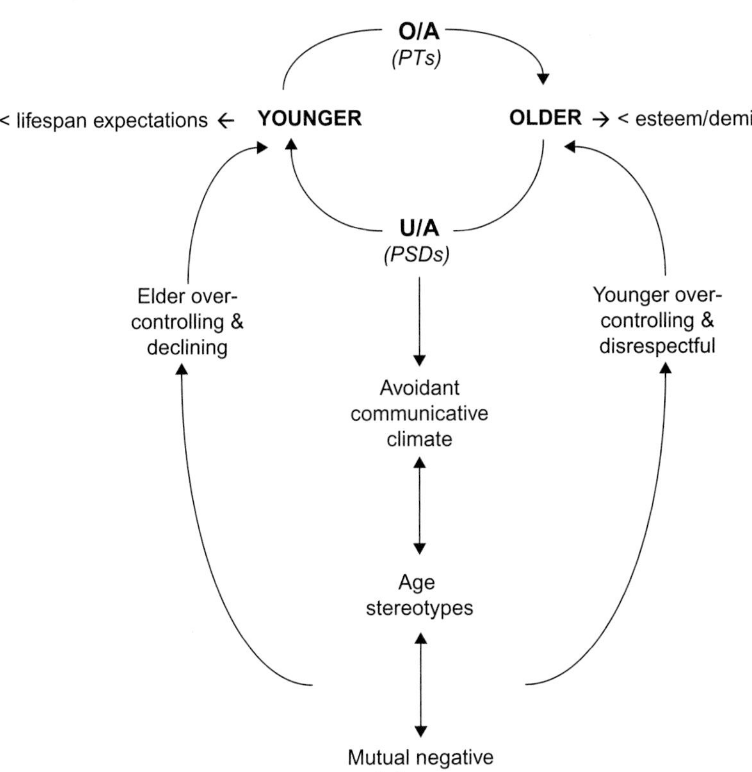

Figure 15.2 Model of the non-accommodative parameters of intergenerational communication.

are molded transactively by these linguistic devices. The emergent communication climates have been shown to be associated with lowered self-esteem, life satisfaction, and demise from the elderly's perspective and can lead to negative outcomes for younger people, too, in personally reinforcing diminished life span expectations for them.

In closing, this model is ripe for empirical scrutiny and might benefit from the recognition of moderating variables, such as cognitive complexity and intergenerational contact, found in other models previously outlined. Moreover, while we have veered in the direction of parsimony in Figure 15.2, future refinements and elaborations might be enriched by adding cultural variables such as filial piety, acknowledging communication dynamics operating beyond the dichotomous "younger-versus-older" to include other social categories such as adolescents and middle-aged people (Brenes, 2010), and considering the communication climates operating within peer-elderly encounters (see Barker et al., 2004). Finally, we advocate that educational interventionists who wish to promote intergenerational harmony empower their applications with due attention to the communication intricacies that can foster successful aging across the life span as well as recognize the different expressive cultures (e.g., Millennialism) that each generation can foster.

ACKNOWLEDGMENTS

We would like to express our gratitude to K. Warner Schaie and an anonymous reviewer for their cogent feedback on an earlier draft of this chapter.

REFERENCES

Baltes, P. B., & Baltes, M. M. (1990). Psychological perspectives on successful aging: The model of selective optimization with compensation. In P. B. Baltes & M. M. Baltes (Eds.), *Successful aging: Perspectives from the behavioral sciences* (pp. 1–34). New York: Cambridge University Press.

Barker, V. (2007). Young adults' reactions to grandparent painful self-disclosure: The influence of grandparent sex and overall motivations for communication. *International Journal of Aging and Human Development*, *64*, 195–215.

Barker, V., Giles, H., & Harwood, J. (2004). Intra- and intergroup perspectives on intergenerational communication. In J. F. Nussbaum & J. Coupland (Eds.), *Handbook of communication and aging research* (2nd ed.) (pp. 139–165). Mahwah, NJ: Erlbaum.

Blieszner, R., & Sanford, N. (2010). Editorial: Looking back and looking ahead as *Journals of Gerontology: Psychological Sciences* turns 65. *Journals of Gerontology: Psychological Sciences, 65B*, 3–4.

Bonneson, J. L., & Hummert, M. L. (2002). Painful self-disclosures of older adults in relation to age stereotypes and perceived motivations. *Journal of Language and Social Psychology, 21*, 275–301.

Brenes, M. (2010). *Intergenerational communication in Costa Rica*. San José: Psychological Research Institute, University of Costa Rica.

Cai, D., Giles, H., & Noels, K. (1998). Elderly perceptions of communication with older and younger adults in China: Implications for mental health. *Journal of Applied Communication Research, 26*, 32–51.

Caporael, L. R. (1981). The paralanguage of caregiving: Baby talk to the institutionalized aged. *Journal of Personality and Social Psychology, 40*, 876–884.

Cheng, S-T., Fung, H. H., & Chan, A. C. M. (2009). Self-perception and psychological well-being: The benefits of foreseeing a worse future. *Psychology and Aging, 24*, 623–633.

Cohen, G., & Faulkner, D. (1986). Does "elderspeak" work? The effect of intonation and stress on comprehension and recall of spoken discourse in old age. *Language and Communication, 6*, 91–98.

Collins, C. L., & Gould, O. N. (1994). Getting to know you: How own age and other's own age relate to self-disclosure. *International Journal of Aging and Human Development, 39*, 55–66.

Coupland, J., & Nussbaum, J. F. (Eds.), (2004). *Handbook of communication and aging research*. Mahwah, NJ: Erlbaum.

Coupland, N. (2004). Age in social and sociolinguistic theory. In J. Coupland & J. F. Nussbaum (Eds.), *Handbook of communication and aging research* (pp. 61–90). Mahwah, NJ: Erlbaum.

Coupland, N., & Coupland, J. (1999). Ageing, ageism, and anti-ageism: Moral stance in geriatric medical discourse. In H. Hamilton (Ed.), *Language and communication in old age: Multidisciplinary perspectives* (pp. 177–208). New York: Garland.

Coupland, N., Coupland, J., & Giles, H. (1989). Telling age in later life: Identity and face implications. *Text, 9*, 129–151.

Coupland, N., Coupland, J., Giles, H., & Henwood, K. (1988a). Accommodating the elderly: Invoking and extending a theory. *Language in Society, 17*, 1–41.

Coupland, N., Coupland, J., Giles, H., Henwood, K., & Wiemann, J. (1988b). Elderly self disclosure: Interactional and intergroup issues. *Language and Communication, 8*, 109–133.

Cunningham, J., & Williams, K. N. (2007). A case study of resistiveness to care and elderspeak. *Research and Theory for Nursing Practice, 21*, 45–56.

Danner, D., Snowdon, D., & Friesen, W. (2001). Positive emotions in early life and longevity: Findings from the Nun Study. *Journal of Personality and Social Psychology, 80*, 804–813.

DePaulo, B. M., & Coleman, L. M. (1986). Verbal and nonverbal communication of warmth to children, foreigners, and retarded adults. *Journal of Nonverbal Behavior, 11*, 75–88.

Depp, C. A., & Jeste, D. V. (2006). Definitions and predictors of successful aging: A comprehensive review of larger quantitative studies. *American Journal of Geriatric Psychiatry, 14*, 5–20.

Donlon, M. M., & Levy, B. R. (2005). Re-vision of older television characters: A stereotype-awareness intervention. *Journal of Social Issues, 61*, 307–319.

Edwards, H., & Giles, H. (1998). Prologue on two dimensions: The risk and management of intergenerational miscommunication. *Journal of Applied Communication Research, 26*, 1–12.

Edwards, H., & Noller, P. (1993). Perceptions of overaccommodation used by nurses in communication with the elderly. *Journal of Language and Social Psychology, 12*, 207–223.

Fowler, F., & Soliz, J. (2010). Responses of young adult grandchildren to grandparents' painful self-disclosures. *Journal of Language and Social Psychology, 29*, 75–100.

Gallois, C., Ogay, T., & Giles, H. (2005). Communication accomodation theory: A look back and a look ahead. In W. B. Gudykunst (Ed.), *Theorizing about inter-cultural communication* (pp. 121–148). Thousand Oaks, CA: Sage.

Giles, H., Dailey, R. M., Sarkar, J. M., & Makoni, S. (2007). Intergenerational communication beliefs across the lifespan: Comparative data from India. *Communication Reports, 20*, 75–89.

Giles, H., & Dorjee, T. (2004). Communicative climates and prospects in cross-cultural gerontology. *Journal of Cross-Cultural Gerontology, 19*, 261–274.

Giles, H., Fox., S., & Smith, E. (1993). Patronizing the elderly. *Research on Language and Social Interaction, 26*, 129–149.

Giles, H., Harwood, J., Pierson, H., Clément, R., & Fox., S. (1998). Stereotypes of the elderly and evaluations of patronizing speech: A cross-cultural foray. In R. K. Agnihotri, A. L. Khanna, & I. Sachdev (Eds.), *Social psychological perspectives on second language learning* (pp. 151–186). New Dehli: Sage.

Giles, H., Makoni, S., & Dailey, R. M. (2005). Intergenerational communication beliefs across the lifespan: Comparative data from West and South Africa. *Journal of Cross-Cultural Gerontology, 20*, 191–211.

Giles, H., & Reid., S. A. (2005). Ageism across the lifespan: Towards a self-categorization model of ageing. *Journal of Social Issues, 61*, 389–404.

Giles, H., Ryan, E. B., & Anas, A. P. (2008). Perceptions of intergenerational communication by young, middle-aged, and older Canadians. *Canadian Journal of Behavioural Science, 40*, 21–30.

Giles, H., & Williams, A. (1994). Patronizing the young: Forms and evaluations. *International Journal of Aging and Human Development, 39*, 33–53.

Giles, H., Zwang-Weissman, Y., & Hajek, C. (2004). Patronizing and policing elderly people. *Psychological Reports, 95*, 754–756.

Gould, O. N., & Dixon, A. (1997). Recall of medication instructions by young and adult women: Is overaccommodative speech helpful? *Journal of Language and Social Psychology, 16*, 50–69.

Grainger, K. (1993). "That's a lovely bath, dear": Reality construction in the discourse of elderly care. *Journal of Aging Studies, 7*, 247–262.

Harwood, J. (1998). Young adults' cognitive representations of intergenerational conversations. *Journal of Applied Communication Research, 26*, 13–31.

Harwood, J. (2007). *Understanding communication and aging*. Mahwah, NJ: Erlbaum.

Harwood, J., & Giles, H. (1996). Reactions to older people being patronized: The roles of response strategies and attributed thoughts. *Journal of Language and Social Psychology, 15*, 395–421.

Harwood, J., Giles, H., Fox, S., Ryan, E. B., & Williams, A. (1993). Patronizing young and elderly adults: Response strategies in a community setting. *Journal of Applied Communication Research, 21*, 211–226.

Harwood, J., McKee, J., & Lin, M. (2000). Younger and older adults' schematic representations of intergenerational communication. *Communication Monographs, 67*, 20–41.

Harwood, J., Ryan, E. B., Giles, H., & Tysoski, S. (1997). Evaluations of patronizing speech and three response styles in a non-service-providing context. *Journal of Applied Communication Research, 25*, 170–195.

Heckhausen, J., & Brim, O. (1997). Perceived problems for self and others: Self-protection by social downgrading throughout adulthood. *Psychology and Aging, 12*, 610–619.

Hummert, M. L. (1994). Stereotypes of the elderly and patronizing speech style. In M. L. Hummert, J. M. Wiemann, & J. F. Nussbaum (Eds.), *Interpersonal communication in older adulthood: Interdisciplinary theory and research* (pp. 162–185). Newbury Park: Sage.

Hummert, M. L. (2010). Age group identity, age stereotypes, and communication in a life span context. In H. Giles, S. A. Reid, & J. Harwood (Eds.), *The dynamics of intergroup communication* (pp. 41–52). New York: Peter Lang.

Hummert, M. L., Garstka, T. A., Ryan, E. B., & Bonneson, J. L. (2004). The role of age stereotypes in interpersonal communication. In J. Coupland & J. F. Nussbaum (Eds.), *Handbook of communication and aging research* (pp. 91–114). Mahweh, NJ: Erlbaum.

Hummert, M. L., Garstka, T. A., Shaner, J. L., & Strahm, S. (1994). Stereotypes of the elderly held by young, middle-aged, and elderly adults. *Journal of Gerontology: Psychological Sciences, 49*, P240–P249.

Hummert, M. L., & Mazloff, D. (2001). Older adults' responses to patronizing advice: Balancing politeness and identity in context. *Journal of Language and Social Psychology, 1–2*, 168–196.

Hummert, M. L., & Ryan, E. B. (1996). Toward understanding variations in patronizing talk addressed to older adults: Psycholinguistic features of care and control. *International Journal of Psycholinguistics, 12*, 149–169.

Hummert, M. L., & Ryan, E. B. (2001). Patronizing. In W. P. Robinson & H. Giles (Eds.), *The new handbook of language and social psychology* (pp. 253–269). Chichester: John Wiley & Sons.

Hummert, M. L., Shaner, J. L., Garstka, T. A., & Henry, C. (1998). Communication with older adults: The influence of age stereotypes, context, and communicator age. *Human Communication Research, 25*, 124–151.

Jones, E., Gallois, C., Barker, M., & Callon, V. J. (1994). Evaluations of interactions between students and academic staff: Influence of communication accommodation, ethnic group, and status. *Journal of Language and Social Psychology, 13*, 158–191.

Kemper, S. (1994). "Elderspeak": Speech accommodation to older adults. *Aging and Cognition, 1*, 17–28.

Kemper, S., & Harden, T. (1999). Experimentally disentangling what's beneficial about elderspeak from what's not. *Psychology and Aging, 14*, 656–670.

Kemper, S., & Kliegl, R. (Eds.), (1999). *Constraints on language: Aging, memory, and grammar.* New York: Kluwer Academic.

Kemper, S., Vandeputte, D., Rice, K., Cheung, H., & Gubarchuk, J. (1995). Speech adjustments to aging during a referential communication task. *Journal of Language and Social Psychology, 14*, 40–59.

LaTourette, T., & Meeks, S. (2001). Perceptions of patronizing speech by older women in nursing homes and in the community: Impact of cognitive ability and place of residence. *Journal of Language and Social Psychology, 19*, 66–82.

Levy, B. R. (2003). Mind matters: Cognitive and physical effects of aging self-stereotypes. *Journals of Gerontology: Psychological Sciences, 58B*, 203–211.

Lin, M-C., Harwood, J., & Hummert, M. L. (2008). Young adults' intergenerational communication schemas in the U.S. and Taiwan: Association between schematic components. *Journal of Language and Social Psychology, 27*, 28–50.

Lin, M-C., Zhang, Y. B., & Harwood, J. (2004). Taiwanese young adults' intergenerational communication schemas. *Journal of Cross-Cultural Gerontology, 19*, 321–342.

McCann, R., Dailey, R. M., Giles, H., & Ota, H. (2005). Beliefs about intergenerational communication across the lifespan: Middle age and the roles of age stereotyping and respect norms. *Communication Studies, 56*, 293–311.

McCann, R., & Giles, H. (2002). Ageism in the workplace: A communication perspective. In T. D. Nelson (Ed.), *Ageism: Stereotyping and prejudice against older persons* (pp. 163–200). Cambridge, MA: MIT Press.

Montrose, L. P., Depp, C., Daly, J., Reichstadt, J., Golshan, S., Moore, D., et al. (2006). Correlates of self-rated successful aging among community-dwelling older adults. *American Journal of Geriatric Psychiatry, 14*, 43–51.

Noels, K., Giles, H., Gallois, C., & Ng, S. H. (2001). Intergenerational communication and health across the Pacific Rim. In M. L. Hummert & J. F. Nussbaum (Eds.), *Communication, aging, and health: Multidisciplinary perspectives* (pp. 249–278). Mahwah, NJ: Erlbaum.

Nussbaum, J. F., & Fisher, C. (2009). A communication model for the competent delivery of geriatric medicine. *Journal of Language and Social Psychology, 28*, 190–208.

Nussbaum, J.F., & Fisher, C.L. Communication wellness in older adults: Lessons from two decades of research within the United States. In Y. Matsumoto (Ed.), *Faces of aging:* The lived experiences of the elderly in Japan Palo Alto, CA: Stanford University Press, in press.

Odato, C. V., & Keller-Cohen, D. (2009). Evaluating the speech of younger and older adults: Age, gender, and speech situation in press. *Journal of Language and Social Psychology, 28*, 457–475.

Ota, H., Giles, H., & Somera, L. P. (2007). Beliefs about intra- and intergenerational communication in Japan, the Philippines, and the United States: Implication for older adults' subjective well-being. *Communication Studies, 58*, 173–188.

Pecchioni, L. L., Wright, K. B., & Nussbaum, J. F. (2005). *Life-span communication.* Mahwah, NJ: Erlbaum.

Pushkar, D. P., Arbuckle, T. Y., & Andres, D. (1994). Verbosity in older adults. In M. L. Hummert, J. M. Wiemann, & J. F. Nussbaum (Eds.), *Interpersonal communication in older adulthood* (pp. 107–129). Thousand Oaks, CA: Sage.

Robinson, J. D., Skill, T., & Turner, J. T. (2004). Media usage patterns and portrayals of seniors. In J. Coupland & J. F. Nussbaum (Eds.), *Handbook of communication and aging research* (pp. 423–446). Mahweh, NJ: Lawrence Erlbaum Associates.

Ryan, E. B., Anas, A., & Gruneir, A. J. S. (2006). Evaluations of over-helping and under-helping communication: Do old age and physical disabilities matter? *Journal of Language and Social Psychology, 25*, 97–107.

Ryan, E. B., Bieman-Copland, S., Kwong See, S. T., Ellis, C. H., & Anas, A. P. (2002). Age excuses: Conversational management of memory failures in older adults. *Journals of Gerontology: Psychological Sciences, 57B*, P256–P267.

Ryan, E. B., Bourhis, R. Y., & Knops, U. (1991). Evaluative perceptions of patronizing speech addressed to elders. *Psychology and Aging, 6*, 442–450.

Ryan, E. B., & Cole, R. (1990). Evaluative perceptions of interpersonal communication with elders. In H. Giles, N. Coupland, & J. Wiemann (Eds.), *Communication, health, and the elderly* (pp. 172–190). Manchester, England: Manchester University Press.

Ryan, E. B., Giles, H., Bartolucci, G., & Henwood, K. (1986). Psycholinguistic and social psychological components of communication by and with the elderly. *Language and Communication, 6*, 1–24.

Ryan, E. B., Hummert, M. L., & Boich, L. H. (1995). Communication predicaments of aging: Patronizing behavior toward older adults. *Journal of Language and Social Psychology, 14*, 144–166.

Ryan, E. B., Kennaley, D. E., Pratt, M. W., & Shumovich, M. A. (2000). Evaluations by staff, residents, and community seniors of patronizing speech in the nursing home: Impact of passive, assertive, or humorous responses. *Psychology and Aging, 15*, 272–285.

Ryan, E. B., Kwong See, S., Meneer, W. B., & Trovato, D. (1992). Age-based perceptions of Language performance among young and older adults. *Communication Research, 19*, 423–444.

Ryan, E. B., Maclean, M., & Orange, J. B. (1994a). Inappropriate accommodation in communication to elders: Inferences about nonverbal correlates. *International Journal of Aging and Human Development, 39*, 273–291.

Ryan, E. B., Meredith, S. D., & Shantz, G. D. (1994b). Evaluative perceptions of patronizing speech addressed to institutionalized elders in contrasting conversational contexts. *Canadian Journal of Aging, 13*, 216–248.

Sachweh, S. (1998). Granny darling's nappies: Secondary babytalk in German nursing homes for the aged. *Journal of Applied Communication Research, 26*, 52–65.

Salari, S. M. (2006). Infantilization as elder mistreatment: Evidence from five adult day centers. *Journal of Elder Abuse and Neglect, 17*, 53–91.

Silverstein, M. (2010). It is not getting old: The rejuvenation of social gerontology. *Journals of Gerontology: Social Sciences, 65B*, 67–68.

Soliz, J., & Harwood, J. (2006). Shared family identity, age salience, and intergroup contact: Investigation of the grandparent-grandchild relationship. *Communication Monographs, 73*, 87–107.

Thorson, J. A., Powell, F. C., Sarmany-Schuller, I., & Hampes, W. P. (1997). Psychological health and sense of humor. *Journal of Clinical Psychology, 53*, 605–619.

Trunk, D. L., & Abrams, L. (2009). Do younger and older adults' communicative goal influence off-topic speech in autobiographical narratives? *Psychology and Aging, 24*, 324–337.

Turner, J. C., Hogg, M. A., Oakes, P. J., Reicher, S. D., & Wetherell, M. S. (1987). *Rediscovering the social group: A self-categorization theory.* Oxford: Basil Blackwell.

Vasil, L., & Wass, H. (1993). Portrayal of the elderly in the media: A literature review and implications for educational gerontologists. *Educational Gerontology, 19*, 71–85.

Whitbourne, S. K., Culgin, S., & Cassidy, E. (1995). Evaluation of infantilizing intonation and content of speech directed at the aged. *International Journal of Aging and Human Development, 41*, 109–116.

Williams, A., & Giles, H. (1996). Intergenerational conversations: Young adults' retrospective accounts. *Human Communication Research, 23,* 220–250.

Williams, A., & Giles, H. (1998). Communication of ageism. In M. L. Hecht (Ed.), *Communicating prejudice* (pp. 136–160). Thousand Oaks, CA: Sage.

Williams, K. N. (2006). Improving outcomes of nursing home interactions. *Research in Nursing and Health, 29,* 121–133.

Williams, K. N., Herman, R., Gajewski, B., & Wilson, K. (2009). Elderspeak communication: Impact on dementia care. *American Journal of Alzheimer's Disease and Other Dementias, 24,* 11–20.

Williams, K. N., Kemper, S., & Hummert, M. L. (2003). Improving nursing home communication: An intervention to reduce elderspeak. *The Gerontologist, 43,* 242–247.

Ytsma, J., & Giles, H. (1997). Reactions to patronizing talk: Some Dutch data. *Journal of Sociolinguistics, 1,* 259–268.

Zhang, Y. B. (2004). Initiating factors of Chinese intergenerational conflict: Young adults' written accounts. *Journal of Cross-Cultural Gerontology, 19,* 299–319.

Zhang, Y. B., & Hummert, M. L. (2001). Harmonies and tensions in Chinese intergenerational communication: Younger and older adults' accounts. *Journal of Asian Pacific Communication, 11,* 203–230.

Zhang, Y. B., & Lin, M. (2009). Conflict initiating factors in intergenerational relationships in press. *Journal of Language and Social Psychology, 28,* 343–363.

Chapter | 16 |

Age Stereotypes and Aging

Mary Lee Hummert

Vice Provost for Faculty Development, University of Kansas, Lawrence, Kansas, USA

CHAPTER CONTENTS

Introduction 249

Nature of Age Stereotypes 250

Culture as an Influence on the Structure and Content of Age Stereotypes 251

The Stereotype Content Model and the Valence of Age Stereotypes 251

Multiple Stereotypes and the Stereotype Content Model 252

The Age Stereotyping Process 252

Activating Age Stereotypes: Stereotype Salience, Attitudes, and Behaviors 253

Implicit Processes in Age Stereotyping 254

Self-Stereotyping and Its Effects 256

Self-Stereotyping and Stereotype Threat 256

Self-Stereotyping and Health 257

Conclusions 258

References 259

INTRODUCTION

In October of 1984, the two candidates for president of the United States, incumbents President Ronald Reagan and former Vice President Walter Mondale, participated in two debates prior to the general election. Mondale was a forceful speaker and well in command of the facts during the first debate, while the consensus was that Reagan "appeared tired and somewhat confused" (All Politics, 1996). This raised concerns about whether Reagan's age (73) was hurting his performance. Reagan tackled this concern directly in the second debate. Responding to a question about his competence from reporter Henry Trewhitt of the *Baltimore Sun*, Reagan stated: "I want you to know that also I will not make age an issue of this campaign. I am not going to exploit, for political purposes, my opponent's youth and inexperience" (All Politics, 1996).

Fast forward 24 years to the 2008 presidential campaign, in which the age of the candidates, Senator John McCain (71 years) and Senator Barack Obama (47 years), again entered into political discourse. In March, *Fox News* commentator Brit Hume characterized McCain's misstatements about Iran and Al-Quaeda as a sign of his age and a "senior moment" (Goodman, 2008). A second incident occurred in May. When Senator Obama said on CNN that his opponent was "losing his bearings," a McCain adviser accused Obama of intentionally "raising John McCain's age as an issue" (Walsh, 2008). Discussing these events in the *New York Times*, Adam Nagourney (2008) argued that age had become "the New Race and Gender"(2008), and *Boston Globe* columnist Ellen Goodman (2008) summarized the question behind voters' concerns about the ages of the two candidates as how to "balance the incline of wisdom against the decline of, say, memory."

Clearly two quite different aspects of age stereotypes were brought into both the 1984 and 2008 campaigns: declines in competence and vitality versus gains in wisdom and experience. Notably, those stereotypes appear to have changed little over the intervening years. Recognition of the power of age stereotypes to affect social evaluations not only in the political arena, but also in the private arena, has contributed to social psychologists' interest in understanding their nature and operation.

For over 30 years, the cognitive perspective has dominated the study of stereotypes, including the study of age stereotypes (Ashmore & Del Boca, 1981; Hummert, 1999; Operario & Fiske, 2004). Accordingly, social psychologists have examined age stereotypes as cognitive schemas that represent widely shared beliefs

DOI: 10.1016/B978-0-12-380882-0.00016-4

about the defining characteristics of older individuals, and which function as resources in the process of person perception. Adopting the cognitive perspective has enabled social psychologists to explore and reconcile the sometimes contradictory components of age stereotypes noted above, as well as to investigate age stereotyping as a process that influences individual perceptions and behaviors (Leyens et al., 1994). As a result, this research has yielded key insights into quite diverse effects of age stereotypes, including the psychological factors underlying ageism and discrimination against older people (see Nelson, 2002) at one extreme and, at the other extreme, illuminating the link between positive self-stereotyping, longevity, and health status of older adults (Levy et al., 2002b).

This chapter will build on previous reviews of the research on age stereotypes and age attitudes (Crockett & Hummert, 1987; Hess, 2006; Hummert, 1999; Kite & Johnson, 1988; Kite et al., 2005; Kite & Wagner, 2002), but will emphasize recent research that provides insights into the complexity of age stereotypes and their influence on perceptions and behaviors, particularly those of older individuals. This chapter is organized into three sections: the nature of age stereotypes, the age stereotyping process, and self-stereotyping and its effects. Cultural influences on age stereotypes are considered within each section. The chapter concludes with a discussion of the implications of this research for understanding the psychology of aging and an outline of directions for future research.

NATURE OF AGE STEREOTYPES

In the 1980s and 1990s, age stereotype research focused on identifying the content and structure of age stereotypes (Hummert, 1999). For example, Schmidt and Boland (1986) invited one group of young adult participants to list all of the traits they associated with older adults, and then asked a second group to sort the resulting traits into groups defining different types of older people. Results revealed three major trait clusters: one general consisting of eight traits signaling chronological age (e.g., gray haired, retired, wrinkled skin), one negative containing 59 traits (e.g., sick, senile, sad, complaining, poor), and one positive with 32 traits (e.g., wise, capable, healthy, wealthy, patriotic). Within the negative and positive trait clusters, twelve subcategories or stereotypes were evident, eight negative (e.g., Severely Impaired, Shrew/Curmudgeon, Despondent) and four positive (e.g., Perfect Grandmother, John Wayne Conservative).

Hummert et al. (1994) replicated the Schmidt and Boland (1986) procedures, but involved middle-aged and older participants as well as younger ones. Analysis showed that inclusion of the two older age groups added new traits to the Schmidt and Boland trait list, and that the number of age stereotype subcategories — both positive and negative — increased from the young to the middle-aged to the older age group. The greater number of older participants' stereotypes in comparison to those of young participants was consistent with research demonstrating that individuals have more complex views of their ingroup than of an outgroup (Linville, 1982). However, the number of stereotype subcategories held by middle-aged participants fell between those of the young and older groups, consistent with developmental processes reflecting the unique nature of age as a social category; that is, as individuals move from youth, to middle-age, to old age across the life span, they integrate their own experiences of aging into their stereotype schemas, resulting in increased refinement and elaboration of those stereotypes with advancing age (Heckhausen et al.,1989).

While the study revealed age differences in the complexity of age stereotypes, it also identified four negative and three positive stereotypes that were shared across the three age groups. These stereotypes and representative traits are presented in Table 16.1.

Table 16.1 Age stereotypes shared by young, middle-aged, and older participants as reported in Hummert et al., 1994.

NEGATIVE STEREOTYPES & REPRESENTATIVE TRAITS	POSITIVE STEREOTYPES & REPRESENTATIVE TRAITS
Severely Impaired[a]: Slow-thinking, incompetent, feeble, incoherent, inarticulate, senile	**Golden Ager**[b]: Alert, active, sociable, independent, well-informed, productive, capable, happy, healthy, sexual
Despondent[a]: Depressed, sad, hopeless, afraid, neglected, lonely	**Perfect Grandparent**[a]: Interesting, kind, loving, family-oriented, generous, supportive, trustworthy, intelligent, wise
Shrew/Curmudgeon[a]: Complaining, ill-tempered, prejudiced, demanding, inflexible, selfish, jealous, stubborn, nosy	**John Wayne Conservative**[a]: Patriotic, religious, nostalgic, reminiscent, retired, conservative, determined, proud
Recluse[a]: Quiet, timid, naïve	

[a]Stereotype label reflects subtype first reported by Schmidt & Boland (1986).
[b]Stereotype label reflects subtype first reported by Hummert et al. (1994).

Six of these stereotypes echoed those reported earlier by Schmidt and Boland (1986).

These two studies and research by Brewer and colleagues (1981; Brewer & Lui, 1984) supported four conclusions about the content and structure of age stereotypes: (1) the social category of *older person* constitutes a superordinate category that encompasses multiple stereotypes of older individuals, just as *bird* defines a superordinate category that subsumes robins, sparrows, eagles, and so on (Rosch, 1978); (2) some age stereotypes reflect negative beliefs about older individuals and others reflect positive beliefs, but the number of negative stereotypes exceeds that of positive stereotypes; (3) age stereotype content includes beliefs about physical characteristics (e.g., sick, gray haired), personality traits (e.g., wise, inflexible), social status (e.g., retired, wealthy), and behavioral tendencies (e.g., complaining, active); (4) although age stereotypes have a basis in shared beliefs, they exist only as cognitive representations within individuals; therefore their structure and content will vary across individuals as a function of experience, life span development, and so on.

Culture as an Influence on the Structure and Content of Age Stereotypes

The majority of the work on the nature of age stereotypes has been conducted in the United States and other Western cultures, and therefore may be indicative of a cultural bias favoring younger people over older ones not present in other cultures. As Liu et al. (2003) stated, "What we know about stereotypes of older persons is based primarily on what Caucasians think of other Caucasians" (p. 149). In Asian cultures, allegiance to *Xiao* or filial piety confers high status on older people, requiring that they be treated with respect by those younger (Ho, 1994). In turn, filial piety may mean that stereotypes of older people are more positive in Asian than in Western cultures (Levy & Langer, 1994; Liu et al., 2003; Zhang et al., 2002).

Some results support this view. Levy and Langer (1994) asked older adults from the People's Republic of China (PRC) and the United States to list five traits descriptive of older people. They found that the Chinese participants offered more positive traits than those from the United States. Zhang et al. (2002) found additional support for this view in the responses of young, middle-aged, and older participants from the PRC on the trait generation task used by Schmidt and Boland (1986) and Hummert et al. (1994). In contrast to the U. S. participants in the earlier studies, the Chinese participants in all three age groups listed more positive than negative age traits.

On the other hand, some results indicate that stereotypes about aging are more negative in Asia than in Western cultures. Harwood and colleagues (2001; Harwood et al., 1996) have reported that young people in Asian Pacific Rim cultures (China, Philippines, Hong Kong, Japan, Taiwan, South Korea) rate older persons as less vital (e.g., attractive, healthy, strong) and benevolent (e.g., warm, generous, wise) than do young people in Western Pacific Rim cultures (United States, Australia, New Zealand, Canada). Similarly, Yun and Lachman (2006) found that in comparison to U. S. participants in the same age groups, South Korean young, middle-aged, and older participants reported greater fears about psychological aging, physical aging, and old people.

The majority of the research, however, has revealed broad cross-cultural agreement on the general nature of age stereotypes that subsumes culturally specific beliefs about individual components of those stereotypes. For example, Korean and Chinese participants associate increased cognitive, physical, and socioemotional decline with advancing age just as do those in Western cultures (Boduroglu et al., 2006; Jin et al., 2001; Yun & Lachman, 2006). Likewise, over two-thirds of the age traits provided by Chinese participants in Zhang et al. (2002) corresponded to age traits named by the U.S. participants in Hummert et al. (1994); and Liu et al. (2003) found that young and middle-aged ethnic Chinese and ethnic European New Zealanders held several age stereotypes for older people (e.g., Nurturant, Curmudgeon, Elder Statesperson, Golden Ager, Impaired) that were similar not only across the ethnic groups, but also to those reported in Hummert et al. (1994) and Schmidt and Boland (1986).

This cross-cultural agreement on the general nature of age stereotypes coexists with cultural specificity, however. The participants in the Zhang et al. (2002) study described older adults in some terms that were uniquely Chinese, such as *Laodao* (endless repeating) and male-favoritism, and in other terms (e.g., experienced, superstitious, principled) that were related to, but distinct from, those reported by Hummert et al. (1994; e.g., wise, religious, trustworthy). Boduroglu et al. (2006) and Liu et al. (2003) found evidence that culture may influence the relative emphasis on content domains, with mental and physical traits more prominent in the age stereotypes of those from Western cultures, and social or emotional traits more central to the stereotypes of those from East Asian cultures. These results are consistent with the cognitive perspective on age stereotypes, showing that culture, like life experience and age, can influence the content and structure of individuals' age stereotypes.

The Stereotype Content Model and the Valence of Age Stereotypes

The stereotype content model (Fiske et al., 2002) provides an alternative to the multiple stereotype perspective on the dual valence of age stereotypes. This model is built on the premise that warmth and competence are the fundamental dimensions underlying group stereotypes, just as they are in person perception (Cuddy et al., 2008; Fiske et al., 2007). Fiske et al. (2002) posited that perceptions of the competition or threat posed by a group would predict the warmth dimension of its stereotype, while the group's status would predict the competence dimension. They expected that competition and warmth would be inversely related, so that groups viewed as less competitive would be seen as warmer than more competitive groups, whereas status and competence would be positively related, with high status groups seen as more competent than low status groups. Accordingly, within the stereotype content model, groups can be viewed as high in both warmth and competence, low in both, or high in one dimension and low in the other. A group perceived as high in one dimension and low in the other is termed an ambivalent stereotype.

The stereotype content model has received considerable empirical support (see Cuddy et al., 2008, for a review). Of relevance to this chapter, the stereotype of older people falls into the ambivalent stereotype category, with respondents consistently evaluating older people as warm, but incompetent (Cuddy et al., 2005; Fiske et al., 2002). Other groups similarly identified as high warmth/low competence in the stereotype content model include those with physical disabilities, housewives, and individuals with developmental delays.

Cuddy et al. (2009) examined the generalizability of the stereotype content model across Western (individualist) and Asian (collectivist) cultures, with participants from one Western culture (Belgium) and three Asian cultures (Hong Kong, Japan, South Korea) considering older people as one of the groups rated. Results confirmed that the ambivalent stereotype of older people as more warm than competent was held by participants across Western and Asian cultures, just as it was by those in the U. S. studies. At the same time, where the warmth and competence judgments fell in the high warmth, low competence quadrant varied somewhat across the cultures. As the authors pointed out, their results demonstrate that some "overarching principles of bias are pancultural, while some manifestations are culturally idiosyncratic" (Cuddy et al., 2009, p. 25). Included in those elements more sensitive to cultural differences are the values placed on competition and status, as well as the specific contents of stereotypes.

Multiple Stereotypes and the Stereotype Content Model

The research supporting the stereotype content model suggested that an apt definition of the superordinate stereotype of older persons might be captured by the phrase "doddering, but dear" (Cuddy & Fiske, 2002, p. 3). In contrast, the superordinate category of older person discussed in the multiple stereotype literature was evaluatively neutral, possessing no distinctive traits other than old age (Hummert et al., 1994). Rather than negate evidence for multiple age stereotypes, however, the superordinate stereotype of old people as "doddering, but dear" provides necessary psychological and theoretical context for the highly differentiated, positive and negatively valenced stereotype subcategories identified earlier (Cuddy & Fiske, 2002).

A comparison of the methods used in these two lines of research provides insight into the hierarchical relationship of the stereotype content and multiple stereotype perspectives on age stereotypes. Investigations of the stereotype content model have asked participants to evaluate many different social groups, one of which was *elderly people*, on the dimensions of warmth, competence, competition, and status (Cuddy et al., 2005; Fiske et al., 2002). Participants' judgments represent comparative assessments at the group level which differentiate older people from the other groups on the targeted dimensions. The results reflect an overarching definition of the stereotype of older people on the key dimensions that it shares with stereotypes of other groups.

In contrast, the multiple stereotype research has focused on perceptions of older people as a group, not in comparison to other groups, but in an attempt to identify the full range of perceptions associated with people in that social category. The methods involved collecting characteristics participants associated with the social category *older people*, and examining how they grouped those characteristics when thinking about types of older people. This task yielded a broad range of positive and negative characteristics, including traits indicative of warmth or its lack and competence or its lack, and several stereotypes or prototypes of older people (see Table 16.1). These results do not contradict the stereotype content model, but confirm that ambivalence is inherent in age stereotypes and provide evidence of the complexity subsumed under the overarching stereotype of older people as "doddering, but dear" (Cuddy & Fiske, 2002).

THE AGE STEREOTYPING PROCESS

As the prior discussion has illustrated, age stereotypes are cognitive schemas that vary in valence and are hierarchically organized. While reflecting shared beliefs about older people, they also are sensitive to individual experience derived from position in the life span. However, age stereotypes are not static cognitive structures. Rather they are resources that are called forth as organizing frameworks to inform person perception and social interaction (Ashmore & Del Boca, 1981; Cuddy & Fiske, 2002; Hummert, 1999; Leyens et al., 1994; Operario & Fiske, 2004). Research on the age stereotyping process focuses on the ways in which age stereotypes become salient, engender attitudes, and influence behaviors. This research is grounded in three established social psychological principles. First, stereotypes consist of beliefs regarding the probability that persons in the category have certain characteristics, while attitudes represent evaluative responses to persons with those characteristics and influence behaviors toward those persons (Fishbein & Azjen, 1975). Second, stereotypes affect attitudes and behaviors only when they are relevant to social goals (Gilbert & Hixon, 1991); that is, they must be salient. Third, stereotypes can become salient outside conscious awareness, affecting attitudes and behaviors implicitly or automatically (Greenwald & Banaji, 1995).

Activating Age Stereotypes: Stereotype Salience, Attitudes, and Behaviors

Reviews of the research on age attitudes have consistently found that negative attitudes toward older persons predominate over positive attitudes (Crockett & Hummert, 1987; Hess, 2006; Hummert, 1999; Kite & Wagner, 2002), a conclusion confirmed by meta-analytic studies (Gordon & Arvey, 2004; Kite & Johnson, 1988; Kite et al., 2005). While this may be consistent with the relative number of negative and positive age stereotypes and stereotype traits identified in the stereotype literature reviewed in the previous section, the reviews and meta-analyses reveal that research design can contribute to the salience of age stereotypes in attitude studies. Specifically, Kite et al. (2005) reported significantly larger effect sizes for target age on attitude judgments and behaviors/behavioral intentions from studies that used within-subjects designs (attitude $d = 0.39$, $n = 44$; behavior $d = 0.51$, $n = 12$ studies) than from those that used between-subjects designs (attitude $d = 0.10$, $n = 56$ studies; behavior $d = 0.02$, $n = 17$ studies). These results suggest that direct comparisons of targets of different ages make age the focus of judgments, especially when participants are presented with little distinguishing information about the targets other than their ages. Laboratory settings too appear to increase the salience of age relative to field settings, perhaps because field settings include a wealth of contextual factors that minimize focus on age differences. Gordon and Arvey (2004) found significantly larger effect sizes for target age resulting from laboratory ($d = 0.19$, $n = 33$ studies) than field studies ($d = 0.10$, $n = 8$ studies).

Individual characteristics, particularly chronological age, may also be related to susceptibility to the influence of age stereotypes on attitude judgments. As noted in the discussion of the nature of age stereotypes, stereotype schemas appear to reflect both ingroup-outgroup or social identity processes and developmental processes (Brewer & Lui, 1984; Hummert et al., 1994). Chasteen (2005) examined how these two processes operated jointly to affect young and older participants' evaluations of their own and the other age group. She expected that in comparison to young participants, older participants would show less ingroup favoritism and outgroup derogation, consistent with their having been members of the young age group in the past. Results supported this hypothesis, demonstrating that age differences may be less salient in the judgments of older adults than young adults.

Research has also examined the factors in the social situation that increase the salience of negative as opposed to positive age stereotypes. Those factors include physical features signaling advanced old age such as facial aging, vocal indicators of age, and slow gait (Hummert et al., 1997, 1999; Montepare & Zebrowitz, 1993; Ryan & Capadano, 1978); settings associated with old age such as a nursing home or hospital (Hummert et al., 1998); and behaviors consistent with negative stereotypes such as forgetting, rambling talk, being inactive, and so on (Erber, 1989; Erber et al., 1997; Greenlee et al., 2007; Ruscher & Hurley, 2000; see Hess, 2006, for a review).

Some of these studies have tested the hypothesis that older individuals may be less susceptible than young people to information about others that implicates negative age stereotypes, due to the complex and highly differentiated age stereotype schemas held by older individuals and their greater tendency to see similarities between their age group and the young age group (Chasteen, 2005; Hummert et al., 1994). This hypothesis has received partial support, with older participants at times judging older targets less harshly and at other times more harshly than young participants. For example, older participants evaluated memory failures as less serious for an older target than did young participants (Erber, 1989), but were less sympathetic than young participants toward a forgetful older target living a stereotypically "old" lifestyle (Erber et al., 1997). The black sheep effect (Marques et al., 1988) offers a plausible explanation for the latter results. The black sheep effect occurs when group members derogate ingroup members whose characteristics threaten positive perceptions of the group. Hummert et al. (1997) found similar evidence of the black sheep effect in a study of age stereotyping based on facial cues to age. In that research, despite general agreement across young, middle-aged, and older participants on the association of positive age stereotypes with looking young-old (i.e., in one's 60s) and negative stereotypes with looking old-old (i.e., in one's 80s or 90s), the older participants were significantly more likely than those in the other two age groups to choose negative stereotypes for the old-old targets.

Other research suggests that these seemingly conflicting patterns show that older persons, more than younger ones, weigh the relevance of information to the type of judgment required in their assessments of other older adults. As a result, they are more discriminating in applying negative age stereotypes than are younger participants when the descriptive information is not relevant. For example, older and middle-aged individuals are less likely than young people to associate age-related communication problems and to use a patronizing communication style with older targets possessing stereotypically negative age traits that do not carry clear communicative implications (Hummert et al., 1995, 1998).

Lineweaver et al. (2009) tested this hypothesis in relation to the well-established evidence that participants of all ages agree that memory will decline with increasing age (Lineweaver & Hertzog, 1998; Ryan & Kwong See, 1993). Noting that the prior research had collected judgments only of a typical person, Lineweaver et al. (2009) presented young, middle-aged, and older participants with descriptions of 11 target individuals, 6 described with positive traits and 5 with negative traits of age stereotypes from Hummert et al. (1994). Participants evaluated the memory of each target at each decade of adult life from age 20 through age 90. Results revealed the same pattern of memory decline with advancing age reported in prior research, but also showed that judgments of the targets varied according to their traits. Participants predicted the least memory decline for positive targets with memory relevant traits, and the most decline for negative targets with memory relevant traits. In comparison to young and middle-aged participants, older participants showed greater sensitivity to the relevance of the traits to memory functioning, indicating that memory decline would begin later in life but would then fall more precipitously, especially for the negative targets with memory relevant traits.

These studies indicate that age stereotypes lead to negative attitudes and biased behavior toward older persons more often than not, even from members of the older age group. Situational cues and target characteristics that make positive age stereotypes salient serve to moderate negative attitudes and biased behaviors rather than to eliminate them. This evidence is consistent with the implications of the stereotype content model for behavior toward older persons, as proposed by Cuddy et al. (2007, 2008) in the Behavior from Intergroup Affect and Stereotypes (BIAS) map. According to the BIAS map, pity, a negative emotion, should be the predominant affective response to the ambivalent stereotype of older people as warm but incompetent. In turn, this emotional response should lead to active helping behavior or, alternative passive harm (e.g., benign neglect).

This pattern of affect and behavior has been investigated extensively in studies of communication with older persons as conceptualized under the communicative predicament of aging model (CPA; Ryan et al., 1986). In brief, tests of the CPA model have demonstrated that communicators accommodate to stereotypical expectations about age-related communication deficits by adopting a patronizing style of talk to older targets; that is, speaking more loudly and more slowly, using simpler words, and so on, than normal (see Giles and Gasiorek, Chapter 15, this volume for additional discussion; Hummert et al., 2004). Paradoxically those who are the recipients or observers of such communication may evaluate it negatively, while the intentions of the speakers are presumably to communicate effectively by using accommodations that will be helpful to older listeners (Hummert et al., 2004). Given the online processing demands of engaging in communication, it is unlikely that communicators consciously retrieve and consider age stereotypes in choosing accommodations to older listeners. Rather, patronizing communication may be one example of the way in which age stereotypes operate at an implicit level to exert an automatic or unconscious influence on behavior (Hummert, 1999).

Implicit Processes in Age Stereotyping

Greenwald and Banaji (1995) described the ways in which social cognitions, including stereotypes, work implicitly (i.e., outside conscious awareness and control) to affect perceptions of oneself and others. They defined implicit stereotypes as "the introspectively unidentified (or inaccurately identified) traces of past experience that mediate attributions of qualities to members of a social category" (p. 15). Using the implicit association test (IAT), Greenwald and colleagues (1998; Greenwald & Nosek, 2001) have demonstrated that unconscious or automatic evaluations indicate attitudes reflecting racial and gender biases, even when explicit measures of those attitudes show no bias.

Perdue and Gurtman (1990) conducted the first study of implicit age attitudes using a lexical decision task involving a list of positive and negative traits. Young participants made judgments about whether target items were words or nonwords after subliminal priming of either young or old age categories. Results provided evidence of automatic negative attitudes toward the old in comparison to the young: Participants responded more quickly to negative traits following the old prime, but more quickly to positive traits following the young prime.

Implicit attitudes toward young and older people have also been investigated using Greenwald et al.'s (1998) IAT (Hummert et al., 2002; Nosek et al., 2007). This assessment involves comparing two sets of response times: (1) the time required to pair photos of older people with good/pleasant objects and photos of young people with bad/unpleasant objects, and

(2) the time required to pair photos of young people with good/pleasant objects and photos of older people with bad/unpleasant objects. Results showed that both young and older participants complete the latter task significantly faster than the former, indicating that implicit attitudes favor the young over the old and are similar across age groups. Nosek et al. (2007) reviewed age attitude data collected on the IAT Web site from over 350,000 participants between 2000 and 2006. They reported that of the 17 topics and groups on which implicit data were collected, implicit age attitude exhibited the strongest IAT effect: Over 80% of the participants showed the implicit preference for young people over older people and only 6% showed an implicit preference for older people over young people. Further, Nosek et al. (2007) found substantial cross-cultural agreement in the strength of implicit age attitudes favoring the young over the old across participants from Asia, Europe, Australia, and North America.

Explicit measures of age attitudes in the Hummert et al. (2002) and Nosek et al. (2007) studies were only weakly correlated with the implicit attitudes and showed no consistent pattern of age differences: Hummert et al. (2002) found that young people were more positive toward the old than the young on the explicit measures, whereas Nosek et al. (2007) found a weak bias toward young people over old people across the participant age range.

Note that none of these studies (Hummert et al., 2002; Nosek et al., 2007; Perdue & Gurtman, 1990) tested the strength of implicit age stereotypes, but the strength of implicit age attitudes or the affective response to age categories. Research on implicit age stereotypes confirms the coexistence of positive and negative stereotypes, but also provides insight into the observed primacy of negative evaluations in the implicit attitude research (Chasteen et al., 2002; Krings, 2004; Wentura & Brandstädter, 2003).

Chasteen et al. (2002) employed Perdue and Gurtman's (1990) lexical decision task to investigate the strength of implicit age stereotypes of young and old people held by young and older participants. To ensure that they were assessing age stereotypes and not attitudes, they employed a list of 22 stereotypical old traits and 22 stereotypical young traits, with an equal number of positive and negative traits in each group. Both young and older participants responded more quickly to stereotypical old traits (both positive and negative) following the old than the young prime, whereas they responded more quickly to stereotypical young traits (both positive and negative) following the young prime than the old prime. In addition, those in both age groups responded more quickly to old than to young traits not only following the old prime, but also following the young prime. The authors concluded that these results provide evidence for implicit positive and negative stereotypes of both young and older people and agreement across age groups on the nature of those implicit stereotypes, but also show that the implicit stereotypes of older people are more accessible or stronger than those of young people.

Wentura and Brandstädter (2003) also used semantic priming and a lexical decision task to test the relative accessibility of positive and negative age stereotypes, but employed sentences about a young or old woman to prime age stereotypes rather than single words. They argued that the sentence prime reflected better the application of stereotypes in person perception than the single word prime. Participants were younger and older women. Target words for the lexical decision were either semantically related to the sentence prime and representative of negative (e.g., lonely, forgetful, helpless) or positive (e.g., composed, experienced, proud) age stereotypes, or they were unrelated words of equal valence (e.g., embarrassed, friendly). Response times indicated that the older women showed activation of both positive and negative age stereotypes, whereas young women only exhibited activation of negative stereotypes.

While these two studies confirm the coexistence of positive and negative age stereotypes, they do not address why implicit attitudes are predominantly negative. One explanation investigated by Krings (2004) is that negative stereotypes are more susceptible than positive stereotypes to automatic activation processes. She investigated this hypothesis in three experiments using a process dissociation procedure. In the first two experiments, young participants evaluated the valence of traits in two lists, one purportedly describing older adults and one describing young adults. They then completed two unexpected recognition tasks on lists that included some old, young, and new traits. In the first recognition task, they were to identify the traits that they had previously rated in either list. In the second, they were to identify only the traits that they had rated on the older adult list (Experiment 1) or on the young adult list (Experiment 2). Hit and error rates for positive and negative traits on these two tasks were analyzed to identify automatic and controlled memory processes. When the recognition focus was on traits of older adults in Experiment 1, the automatic process measure revealed the expected bias toward negative age traits over positive age traits, while the controlled process measure showed more influence on recognition of positive than negative age traits. When the recall focus was shifted to traits of young adults in Experiment 2, automatic and controlled processes equally influenced recognition of positive and negative age traits. The third experiment confirmed that the bias toward negative age stereotypes in automatic processing held for older women.

In sum, with one exception (Chasteen et al., 2002) these studies show that negative implicit stereotypes of older people are more accessible than are positive stereotypes. As a result, negative stereotypes are more likely to be automatically activated in social perception than are positive stereotypes and therefore to influence attitudes and behaviors. Together the research on implicit attitudes and stereotypes is consistent with a developmental process whereby key aspects of age stereotypes are internalized early in life. Although age stereotypes include positive as well as negative perceptions and may become more differentiated and complex over time, the early negative associations with aging appear to retain their prominence in the schemas of older individuals. To the extent that age stereotypes operate implicitly, they can lead to stereotype-consistent behavior or self-stereotyping by older people (Levy, 2003, 2009).

SELF-STEREOTYPING AND ITS EFFECTS

Self-stereotyping is defined as the unconscious or automatic assimilation to behaviors consistent with stereotypes of one's group (Levy, 2003; Wheeler & Petty, 2001). This assimilation may be cued by elements in the environment of which an individual is unaware, and may reflect positive as well as negative stereotypes of the group. For instance, Levy (1996) used subliminal priming to activate negative (e.g., Alzheimer's, decline, dependent, forgets, confused) or positive (e.g., wise, alert, sage, accomplished, insightful) age stereotypes in older and younger participants. Participants also completed five memory measures both before and after the priming manipulation. Evidence of both positive and negative self-stereotyping by older participants was found for four of the five memory measures, with participants exposed to the positive age stereotypes outperforming those exposed to the negative age stereotypes. Further, as predicted by Levy (1996), priming had no significant effect on the memory performance of young participants, emphasizing that self-stereotyping occurs when the group membership is relevant.

Hess et al. (2004) confirmed the validity of these findings in two experiments involving young and older participants. In both studies, implicit priming of age stereotypes affected the recall of older participants but not younger ones, with implicit positive primes resulting in significantly better recall by the older participants than implicit negative primes. In other experiments, Levy and coinvestigators demonstrated implicit self-stereotyping effects on older participants' handwriting, preference for end-of-life interventions, and gait, with priming of negative stereotypes associated with shakier handwriting, lower preference for life-saving interventions, and slower gait following exposure to negative primes than positive primes (see Levy, 2003, 2009, for reviews).

Implicit priming has not always produced a consistent pattern of effects, however, perhaps because the stereotype activated was not relevant to performance on the outcome measure (Stein et al., 2002). Levy and Leifheit-Limson (2009) examined the question of the match between the stereotype domain primed and the task in a 2 (stereotype valence) $\times$ 2 (stereotype domain: physical/cognitive) design. Older participants were randomly assigned to one of the four stereotype prime conditions. All completed post-prime assessments on a physical task measuring balance and a photo recall memory task. While those exposed to positive primes showed better performance on both tasks relative to the negative prime groups, the effects of positive valence were significantly stronger when the domain primed matched the task than when it did not. Negative priming, regardless of domain, had a similar detrimental impact on performance of the physical and memory tasks, suggesting that negative stereotypes have more general consequences for behavior of older persons than do positive stereotypes.

Self-Stereotyping and Stereotype Threat

Stereotype threat (Steele et al., 2002) occurs when situational factors activate group stereotypes in members of low status groups, inducing assimilation to the stereotypes or self-stereotyping behavior. Thus stereotype threat involves explicit rather than implicit activation of stereotypes. In contrast to the automatic assimilation to group stereotypes associated with implicit self-stereotyping, stereotypic behavior resulting from stereotype threat is thought to be mediated by the anxiety associated with the fear of confirming the stereotype and its personal consequences for the individual.

The strong association of poor memory with age stereotypes and the numerous cognitive aging studies demonstrating that young people have better memory than older people led Hess and colleagues to investigate stereotype threat effects on the memory performance of older individuals (Hess et al., 2003; Hess & Hinson, 2006). Test instructions were used to induce stereotype threat in these studies. For example, Hess et al. (2003) had participants read information about memory and aging research presented as newspaper articles that documented older adults' poorer memory in comparison to young adults (high threat-negative age stereotype activation) or older adults' better memory than young adults (low threat-positive age stereotype activation). Analysis of a subsequent trait recognition task confirmed that the manipulation served to activate age stereotypes as intended. Stereotype threat effects on the memory of older participants were documented in these and other studies, with older participants in high threat conditions showing poorer recall than those in low threat and control conditions, and young participants exhibiting equivalent recall across threat conditions (see Hess, 2006, for a review).

Critically, this line of research has gone beyond documenting stereotype threat effects on memory to examining the situational factors that serve to reduce or increase those effects, as well as those characteristics that affect individual susceptibility to stereotype threat. Results indicate that providing information that deemphasizes or contradicts negative age stereotypes about memory can decrease stereotype threat (Andreoletti & Lachman, 2004; Hess et al., 2003, 2004, but see Chasteen et al., 2005), as can situational adjustments such as introducing positive intergenerational contact (Abrams et al., 2006). Hess et al. (2009a) found that simply removing time constraints on response to a recognition memory test eliminated stereotype threat effects on older participants. Further, those with no time constraints were more confident in the accuracy of their responses than those required to perform the task within a limited time. This information is both practically relevant for designing test environments that facilitate optimal performance by older individuals, and theoretically important in indicating that stereotype threat may operate in the retrieval process by reducing confidence in one's memory. Individual characteristics which increase susceptibility to stereotype threat include the personal importance placed on memory ability (Hess et al., 2003) and perceived age stigma (Hess et al., 2009b; Kang & Chasteen, 2009a, 2009b).

Cultural differences in aging stereotypes may also be a factor in older participants' assimilation to age stereotypes about memory (Levy & Langer, 1994; Yoon et al., 2000). Levy and Langer (1994) examined this question in a study involving young and older participants from the U.S. mainstream culture, and from two cultures that presumably share more positive views of aging than the mainstream U.S. culture: the U.S. deaf community and the PRC. Analysis supported the prediction that the positive views of aging would be lowest in the U.S. hearing sample, followed by the U.S. deaf sample, and highest in the Chinese sample. Also as predicted, culture and age interacted to affect memory performance. Young participants in all cultures had higher memory scores than older participants from those cultures, but their performance was similar across the cultures. In contrast, older participants' memory performance varied across the cultures consistent with the pattern of views on aging: the older Chinese participants had the best memory performance, followed by the older U.S. deaf participants, followed by the older U. S. hearing participants. Path analyses provided further support: The relationship between positive views of aging and memory performance of older participants was fully mediated by culture (Chinese and U.S. deaf combined vs. U.S. hearing), but not for the young participants.

Note that in this discussion the term self-stereotyping has been used to describe behaviors in response to stereotype threat. Stereotype threat and self-stereotyping have often been conceptualized as distinct processes, with stereotype threat presumed to require explicit stereotype activation and mediation via anxiety, and self-stereotyping occurring only under conditions of implicit stereotype activation (Wheeler & Petty, 2001). O'Brien and Hummert (2006) conducted an experiment to examine the validity of this proposition in the context of aging in which group boundaries are at times ambiguous. Participants were adults in late middle-age (58–62) who first completed implicit (IAT) and explicit measures of age identity (Hummert et al., 2002) and an anxiety pretest. After a distractor task, participants were randomly assigned to stereotype threat (performance comparison to that of young adults), self-stereotyping (performance comparison to that of adults age 70 and older), and control (no comparison group) conditions prior to completing memory tests and an anxiety posttest. Consistent with a self-stereotyping hypothesis, those who thought their memory results would be compared to those of older adults, a group known for poor memory performance, recalled fewer words than those in the stereotype threat and control groups. Further this effect was not mediated by anxiety, but modified by implicit (but not explicit) age identity, with only those participants in the old comparison group who were less strongly identified with youth showing the self-stereotyping effect. Implicit age identity did not affect the recall of those in the young comparison and control groups.

Hess et al. (2009a) pointed out that it is often difficult to distinguish whether stereotype threat or self-stereotyping processes are operative, since both can result in similar assimilation to age stereotypes. In most cases, but not all, the evidence favors one process over the other. The O'Brien and Hummert (2006) results may provide evidence that stereotype threat and self-stereotyping processes can work jointly to produce assimilation to age stereotypes: Both the young and old comparisons constituted explicit stereotype activation consistent with stereotype threat, but implicit processes associated with self-stereotyping contributed to which condition led to assimilation to the activated stereotype.

Self-Stereotyping and Health

Research by Levy and colleagues suggests that the strength and valence of individuals' self-perceptions about aging and age stereotypes can have long-term effects on health outcomes (Levy et al., 2002a; Levy et al., 2002b; Levy et al., 2009). Analysis of data from a subset of participants in the Ohio Longitudinal Study of Aging and Retirement (OLSAR) showed that from 1977 to 1995 self-reported functional health declined significantly more for those who held more negative self-perceptions about aging at baseline than for those whose self-perceptions were more positive

(Levy et al., 2002a). Perceived control partially mediated the relationship between aging self-perceptions and health. Wurm et al. (2008) found similar beneficial effects of positive perceptions of aging on the self-reported health of middle-aged and older participants in the longitudinal German Ageing Study, even for those participants who had experienced a serious health event between baseline and the second round of data collection six years later.

Importantly, examination of mortality data from the OLSAR sample revealed that having more positive aging self-perceptions not only predicted self-reported functional health, but also longevity (Levy et al., 2002b). Okamoto and Tanaka (2004) reported similar effects of a positive view of one's own aging (i.e., in this case, subjective usefulness) on longevity of older participants in a Japanese longitudinal study. These results have led to an interest in identifying the pathways through which aging self-perceptions may affect physical health. Cardiovascular stress induced by negative age perceptions may be one such pathway. In experiments using implicit priming, both White and African American older adults primed with negative age stereotypes exhibited increased cardiovascular stress responses to subsequent cognitive tasks in comparison to baseline cardiovascular levels, whereas those primed with positive age stereotypes did not (Levy et al., 2000, 2008). Similar effects have been found in a clinical setting in which age stereotypes have been activated explicitly using a stereotype threat paradigm (Auman et al., 2005).

Levy et al. (2009) found additional evidence for the relationship between individually held stereotypes and cardiovascular health in a sample from the Baltimore Longitudinal Study of Aging. The sample included individuals who were aged 49 or younger and had never suffered a cardiovascular event (e.g., angina, stroke, myocardial infarction) at baseline in 1968. Data on outcomes from 1968 to 2007 revealed that those who held more negative age stereotypes at baseline were significantly more likely to experience a cardiovascular event at some point over the next 38 years, and that those with more negative stereotypes were more likely than those with more positive stereotypes to suffer a cardiovascular event at each point in time. Consistent with these results, a clinical study of 62 patients who experienced an acute myocardial infarction showed that those with more positive age stereotypes had significantly better recovery over a 7-month period than those with more negative age stereotypes (Levy et al., 2006). In both studies, the age stereotype effects remained after controlling for covariates such as age, comorbidities, race and, education.

In sum, the self-stereotyping studies reveal that age stereotypes not only affect behaviors of older persons on cognitive and behavioral measures, but also have significant long-term effects on health outcomes. Levy (2009) has proposed the theory of stereotype embodiment to explain the multiple ways in which age stereotypes affect the functioning of older individuals. She suggests that the process begins with the internalization of cultural age stereotypes early in life and leads to self-stereotyping behaviors as the stereotypes become increasingly self-relevant over the life course.

CONCLUSIONS

The research reviewed in this chapter illustrates the multifaceted nature of age stereotypes and the complexity of the age stereotyping process. Age stereotypes appear to be widely shared across cultures despite some variation in the emphasis on specific aspects of aging. Unfortunately the shared stereotypes are more negative than positive in valence, even within East Asian cultures with a strong tradition of respect for elders. The research provides evidence that implicit or explicit activation of these negative stereotypes can have profound detrimental effects on the performance and health status of older individuals, creating a negative feedback cycle as conceptualized by Rodin and Langer (1980). Considered in isolation, these conclusions offer little hope for reducing negative age stereotypes and their effects on older persons.

Examination of the full range of the studies reviewed provides a more hopeful perspective, however. Meta-analyses by Kite et al. (2005) and Gordon and Arvey (2004) reported less age bias in more current research than in earlier studies. The most recent research on self-stereotyping and stereotype threat has begun to identify those situational factors and individual characteristics that reduce susceptibility to self-stereotyping, whether through implicit or explicit processes. Further, the evidence is growing that positive stereotypes are not only an integral part of stereotype schemas, but also can function in the self-stereotyping process to facilitate the performance and functional health of older individuals.

Future research in several areas will help to move our understanding of age stereotypes and the age stereotyping process forward. First, additional attention to the processes through which age stereotypes, aging self-perceptions, and age identities are formed and transformed over time will help to clarify how the developmental process leads to individual differences in the strength of positive and negative age stereotypes (Hummert et al., 2002; O'Brien & Hummert, 2006). Additional focus on the middle-aged years, for instance, may reveal how transitions from youth to middle-age to old age are incorporated into age stereotypes and self-perceptions.

Second, continuing to examine the situational factors that can reduce stereotype threat effects and increase positive self-stereotyping can provide insights into how environments and institutional practices (e.g., physician interview and testing protocols) can be structured to ensure optimal performance by older individuals (Hess, 2006, Hess et al., 2009a).

Third, an increased focus on individual differences that increase susceptibility to negative self-stereotyping will help to identify those persons most at risk, and also suggest interventions to reduce their susceptibility. Two promising candidates for additional research are age identity and sensitivity to perceived age bias (Garstka et al., 2004; Hess et al., 2009b; Kang & Chasteen, 2009a; O'Brien & Hummert, 2006). Kang and Chasteen (2009b) have developed the age-based rejection sensitivity questionnaire to support additional research on the role of perceived age stigma in the experience of stereotype threat. Characteristics such as these may affect the coping behavior of older individuals when faced with negative stereotypes or age discrimination in applied settings such as the workplace (Maurer et al., 2008; Posthuma & Campion, 2009).

Fourth, although a relationship between age stereotypes, aging self-perceptions, and health function has been established through the work of Levy and colleagues (2002a, 2006, 2009), the mechanisms underlying that relationship require further study. Some mediators of the relationship between aging self-perceptions and health have emerged, including perceived control (Levy et al., 2002a), will to live (Levy et al., 2002b), cardiovascular stress (Auman et al., 2005; Levy et al., 2000, 2008), and health behaviors (Levy & Myers, 2004), but others such as social support may also be important to health maintenance in old age. In addition determining which mediators are most influenced by self-perceptions may suggest interventions to reduce the impact of negative self-perceptions on the health of older individuals.

Finally, cross-cultural age stereotype research has largely focused on comparisons between East Asian and Western cultures (U.S., Canada, Western Europe, etc.). Little is known about age stereotypes held by those in Eastern Europe, Africa, and South America. The research to date would suggest that the stereotypes will be substantially the same as in Western and East Asian cultures. However, religious and demographic factors in these regions may affect age stereotypes and the relative status of and competition between age groups. For example, the decimation of the young adult and middle-aged population by HIV/AIDS in sub-Saharan Africa may redefine what constitutes old age within those cultures, as well as create new role expectations for older people.

This review demonstrates that understanding the nature of age stereotypes and the age stereotyping process, both as it affects attitudes and behaviors toward others and self-perceptions, is integral to the study of psychology and aging. Advances in the areas identified will not only contribute to psychological theory about age stereotypes, but also lead to an improved experience of aging – on both social and physical levels – for adults across the life span.

REFERENCES

Abrams, D., Eller, A., & Bryant, J. (2006). An age apart: The effects of intergenerational contact and stereotype threat on performance and intergroup bias. *Psychology and Aging, 21*, 691–702.

All Politics. (1996). The debates '96: 1984 presidential debates. *All Politics — CNN TIME*. Retrieved from http://www-cgi.cnn.com/ALLPOLITICS/1996/debates/history/1984/

Andreoletti, C., & Lachman, M. E. (2004). Susceptibility and resilience to memory aging stereotypes: Education matters more than age. *Experimental Aging Research, 30*, 129–148.

Ashmore, R. D., & Del Boca, F. K. (1981). Conceptual approaches to stereotypes and stereotyping. In D. L. Hamilton (Ed.), *Cognitive processes in stereotyping and intergroup behavior* (pp. 1–35). Hillsdale, NJ: Lawrence Erlbaum Associates.

Auman, C., Bosworth, H. B., & Hess, T. M. (2005). Effect of health-related stereotypes on physiological responses of hypertensive middle-aged and older men. *Journals of Gerontology: Psychological Sciences, 60B*, P3–P10.

Boduroglu, A., Yoon, C., Luo, T., & Park, D. C. (2006). Age-related stereotypes: A comparison of American and Chinese cultures. *Gerontology, 52*, 324–333.

Brewer, M., Dull, V., & Lui, L. (1981). Perceptions of the elderly: Stereotypes as prototypes. *Journal of Personality and Social Psychology, 41*, 656–670.

Brewer, M., & Lui, L. (1984). Categorization of the elderly by the elderly. *Personality and Social Psychology Bulletin, 10*, 585–595.

Chasteen, A. L. (2005). Seeing eye-to-eye: Do intergroup biases operate similarly for younger and older adults? *International Journal of Aging & Human Development, 61*, 123–139.

Chasteen, A. L., Bhattacharyya, S., Horhota, M., Tam, R., & Hasher, L. (2005). How feelings of stereotype threat influence older adults' memory performance. *Experimental Aging Research, 31*, 235–260.

Chasteen, A. L., Schwarz, N., & Park, D. C. (2002). The activation of aging stereotypes in younger and older adults. *Journals of Gerontology, 57B*, P540–P547.

Crockett, W. H., & Hummert, M. L. (1987). Perceptions of aging and the elderly. *Annual Review of Gerontology and Geriatrics, 7*, 217–241.

Cuddy, A. J. C., & Fiske, S. T. (2002). Doddering but dear: Process, content, and function in stereotyping of elder persons. In T. D. Nelson (Ed.), *Ageism: Stereotyping and prejudice against older persons* (pp. 3–26). Cambridge, MA: The MIT Press.

Cuddy, A. J. C., Fiske, S. T., & Glick, P. (2008). Warmth and competence on universal dimensions of social perception. The Stereotype Content Model and the BIAS map. In M.P. Zanna (Ed.) *Advances in experimental social psychology, 40,* 62–149.

Cuddy, A. J. C., Fiske, S. T., & Glick, P. (2007). The BIAS map: Behaviors from intergroup affect and stereotypes. *Journal of Personality and Social Psychology, 92,* 631–648.

Cuddy, A. J. C., Fiske, S. T., Kwan, V. S. Y., Glick, P., Demoulin, S., Leyens, J.-P., et al. (2009). Stereotype content model across cultures: Towards universal similarities and some differences. *British Journal of Social Psychology, 48,* 1–33.

Cuddy, A. J. C., Norton, M. I., & Fiske, S. T. (2005). This old stereotype: The pervasiveness and persistence of the elderly stereotype. *Journal of Social Issues, 61,* 267–285.

Erber, J. T. (1989). Young and older adults' appraisal of memory failures in young and older adults target persons. Does age matter? *Journals of Gerontology: Psychological Sciences, 44,* P170–P175.

Erber, J. T., Szuchman, L., & Prager, I. G. (1997). Forgetful but forgiven: How age and life style affect perceptions of memory failure. *Journals of Gerontology: Psychological Sciences, 52B,* P303–P307.

Fishbein, M., & Azjen, I. (1975). *Belief, attitude, intention and behavior: An introduction to theory and research.* Reading, MA: Addison-Wesley.

Fiske, S. T., Cuddy, A. J. C., & Glick, P. (2007). Universal dimensions of social cognition: Warmth and competence. *Trends in Cognitive Sciences, 11,* 77–83.

Fiske, S. T., Cuddy, A. J. C., Glick, P., & Xu, J. (2002). A model of (often mixed) stereotype content: Competence and warmth respectively follow from perceived status and competition. *Journal of Personality and Social Psychology, 82,* 878–902.

Garstka, T. A., Schmitt, M., Branscombe, N. R., & Hummert, M. L. (2004). How young and older adults differ in their responses to perceived age discrimination. *Psychology and Aging, 19,* 326–335.

Gilbert, D. T., & Hixon, J. G. (1991). The trouble of thinking: Activation and application of stereotypic beliefs. *Journal of Personality Social Psychology, 60,* 509–517.

Goodman, E. (2008, March 28). McCain's senior moment. *The Boston Globe.* Retrieved from http://www.boston.com/new/nation/articles/2008/03/28/mccains_senior_moment/.

Gordon, R. A., & Arvey, R. D. (2004). Age bias in laboratory and field settings: A meta-analytic investigation. *Journal of Applied Social Psychology, 34,* 468–492.

Greenlee, I., Webb, H., Hall, B., & Manley, A. (2007). Curmudgeon or golden-ager? Reported exercise participation influences the perception of older adults. *Journal of Sport & Exercise Psychology, 29,* 333–347.

Greenwald, A. G., & Banaji, M. R. (1995). Implicit social cognition: Attitudes, self-esteem, and stereotypes. *Psychological Review, 102,* 4–27.

Greenwald, A. G., McGhee, D. E., & Schwartz, J. L. K. (1998). Measuring individual differences in implicit cognition: The implicit association test. *Journal of Personality and Social Psychology, 74,* 1464–1480.

Greenwald, A. G., & Nosek, B. A. (2001). Health of the Implicit Association Test at age 3. *Zeitschrift für Experimentelle Psychologie, 48,* 85–93.

Harwood, J., Giles, H., McCann, R. M., Cai, D., Somera, L. P., Ng, S. H., et al. (2001). Older adults' trait ratings of three age-groups around the Pacific Rim. *Journal of Cross-Cultural Gerontology, 16,* 157–171.

Harwood, J., Giles, H., Ota, H., Pierson, H. D., Gallois, C., Ng, S. H., et al. (1996). College students' trait ratings of three age groups around the Pacific Rim. *Journal of Cross-Cultural Gerontology, 11,* 307–317.

Heckhausen, J., Dixon, R. A., & Baltes, P. B. (1989). Gains and losses in development throughout adulthood as perceived by different adult age groups. *Developmental Psychology, 25,* 109–121.

Hess, T. M. (2006). Attitudes toward aging and their effects on behavior. In J. E. Birren & K. W. Schaie (Eds.), *Handbook of the psychology of aging* (pp. 379–406). Burlington, MA: Elsevier Academic Press.

Hess, T. M., Auman, C., Colcombe, S. J., & Rahhal, T. A. (2003). The impact of stereotype threat on age differences in memory performance. *Journals of Gerontology: Series B: Psychological Sciences & Social Sciences, 58B,* P3–P11.

Hess, T. M., Emery, L., & Queen, T. L. (2009a). Task demands moderate stereotype threat effects on memory performance. *Journals of Gerontology: Psychological Sciences, 64B,* P482–P486.

Hess, T. M., & Hinson, J. T. (2006). Age-related variation in the influences of aging stereotypes on memory in adulthood. *Psychology and Aging, 21,* 621–625.

Hess, T. M., Hinson, J. T., & Hodges, E. A. (2009b). Moderators of and mechanisms underlying stereotype threat effects on older adults' memory performance. *Experimental Aging Research, 35,* 153–177.

Hess, T. M., Hinson, J. T., & Statham, J. A. (2004). Explicit and implicit stereotype activation effects on memory: Do age and awareness moderate the impact of priming? *Psychology and Aging, 19,* 495–505.

Ho, D. Y. F. (1994). Filial piety, authoritarian moralism, and cognitive conservatism in Chinese society. *Genetic, Social, & General Psychology Monograph, 129,* 349–365.

Hummert, M. L. (1999). A social cognitive perspective on age stereotypes. In T. M. Hess & F. Blanchard-Fields (Eds.), *Social cognition and aging* (pp. 175–195). New York: Academic Press.

Hummert, M. L., Garstka, T. A., O'Brien, L. T., Greenwald,

A. G., & Mellott, D. S. (2002). Using the Implicit Association Test to measure age differences in implicit social cognitions. *Psychology and Aging, 17*, 482–495.

Hummert, M. L., Garstka, T. A., Ryan, E. B., & Bonnesen, J. L. (2004). The role of age stereotypes in interpersonal communication. In J. F. Nussbaum & J. Coupland (Eds.), *Handbook of communication and aging research* (2nd ed., pp. 91–115). Hillsdale, NJ: Lawrence Erlbaum.

Hummert, M. L., Garstka, T. A., & Shaner, J. L. (1995). Beliefs about language performance: Adults' perceptions about self and elderly targets. *Journal of Language and Social Psychology, 14*, 235–259.

Hummert, M. L., Garstka, T. A., & Shaner, J. L. (1997). Stereotyping of older adults: The role of target facial cues and perceiver characteristics. *Psychology and Aging, 12*, 107–114.

Hummert, M. L., Garstka, T. A., Shaner, J. L., & Strahm, S. (1994). Stereotypes of the elderly held by young, middle-aged, and elderly adults. *Journals of Gerontology: Psychological Sciences, 49*, P240–P249.

Hummert, M. L., Mazloff, D. C., & Henry, C. (1999). Vocal characteristics of older adults and stereotyping. *Journal of Nonverbal Behavior, 23*, 111–132.

Hummert, M. L., Shaner, J. L., Garstka, T. A., & Henry, C. (1998). Communication with older adults: The influence of age stereotypes, context, and communicator age. *Human Communication Research, 25*, 124–151.

Jin, Y.-S., Ryan, E. B., & Anas, A. P. (2001). Korean beliefs about everyday memory and aging for self and others. *International Journal of Aging & Human Development, 52*, 103–113.

Kang, S. K., & Chasteen, A. L. (2009a). The moderating role of age-group identification and perceived threat on stereotype threat among older adults. *International Journal of Aging & Human Development, 69*, 201–220.

Kang, S. K., & Chasteen, A. L. (2009b). The development and validation of the age-based rejection sensitivity questionnaire. *The Gerontologist, 49*, 303–316.

Kite, M. E., & Johnson, B. T. (1988). Attitudes toward older and younger adults: A meta-analysis. *Psychology and Aging, 3*, 233–244.

Kite, M. E., Stockdale, G. D., Whitley, B. E., Jr., & Johnson, B. T. (2005). Attitudes toward younger and older adults: An updated meta-analytic review. *Journal of Social Issues, 61*, 241–266.

Kite, M. E., & Wagner, L. S. (2002). Attitudes toward older adults. In T. D. Nelson (Ed.), *Stereotyping and prejudice against older persons* (pp. 129–161). Cambridge, MA: MIT Press.

Krings, F. (2004). Automatic and controlled influences of association with age on memory. *Swiss Journal of Psychology, 63*, 247–259.

Levy, B. (1996). Improving memory in old age through implicit self-stereotyping. *Journal of Personality and Social Psychology, 71*, 1092–1107.

Levy, B. R. (2003). Mind matters: Cognitive and physical effects of aging self-stereotypes. *Journals of Gerontology: Psychological Sciences, 58B*, P203–P211.

Levy, B. (2009). Stereotype embodiment: A psychosocial approach to aging. *Current Directions in Psychological Science, 18*, 332–336.

Levy, B., Hausdorf, J., Hencke, R., & Wei, J. Y. (2000). Reducing cardiovascular stress with positive self-stereotypes of aging. *Journals of Gerontology: Psychological Sciences, 55B*, P205–P213.

Levy, B., & Langer, E. (1994). Aging free from negative stereotypes: Successful memory among the American deaf and in China. *Journal of Personality and Social Psychology, 66*, 935–943.

Levy, B. R., & Leifheit-Limson, E. (2009). The stereotype-matching effect: Greater influence on functioning when age stereotypes correspond to outcomes. *Psychology and Aging, 24*, 230–233.

Levy, B. R., & Myers, L. M. (2004). Preventive health behaviors influenced by self-perceptions of aging. *Preventive Medicine, 39*, 625–629.

Levy, B. R., Ryall, A. L., Pilver, C. E., Sheridan, P. L., Wei, J. Y., & Hausdorff, J. M. (2008). Influence of African American elders' age stereotypes on their cardiovascular response to stress. *Anxiety, Stress & Coping: An International Journal, 21*, 85–93.

Levy, B. R., Slade, M. D., & Kasl, S. V. (2002a). Longitudinal benefit of positive self-perceptions of aging on functional health. *Journals of Gerontology: Series B: Psychological Sciences and Social Sciences, 57B*, P409–P417.

Levy, B. R., Slade, M. D., Kunkel, S. R., & Kasl, S. V. (2002b). Longevity increased by positive self-perceptions of aging. *Journal of Personality and Social Psychology, 83*, 261–270.

Levy, B. R., Slade, M. D., May, J., & Caracciolo, E. A. (2006). Physical recovery after acute myocardial infarction: Positive age self-stereotypes as a resource. *International Journal of Aging & Human Development, 62*, 285–301.

Levy, B. R., Zonderman, A. B., Slade, M. D., & Ferrucci, L. (2009). Age stereotypes held earlier in life predict cardiovascular events in later life. *Psychological Science, 20*, 296–298.

Leyens, J-P., Yzerbyt, V., & Schadron, G. (1994). *Stereotypes and social cognition*. London: Sage.

Lineweaver, T. T., Berger, A. K., & Hertzog, C. (2009). Expectations about memory change across the life span are impacted by aging stereotypes. *Psychology and Aging, 24*, 169–176.

Lineweaver, T. T., & Hertzog, C. (1998). Adults' efficacy and control beliefs regarding memory and aging: Separating general from personal beliefs. *Aging, Neuropsychology, and Cognition, 5*, 264–296.

Linville, P. W. (1982). The complexity-extremity effect and age-based stereotyping. *Journal of Personality and Social Psychology, 42*, 193–211.

Liu, J. H., Ng, S. H., Loong, C., Gee, S., & Weatherall, A. (2003). Cultural stereotypes and social representations of elders from Chinese and European perspectives. *Journal of Cross-Cultural Gerontology, 18*, 149–168.

Marques, J. M., Yzerbyt, V. Y., & Leyens, J-P. (1988). The black-sheep effect: Extremity of judgments towards ingroup members as a function of ingroup identification. *European Journal of Social Psychology, 18*, 1–16.

Maurer, T. J., Barbeite, F. G., Weiss, E. M., & Lippstreu, M. (2008). New measures of stereotypical beliefs about older workers' ability and desire for development: Exploration among employees age 40 and over. *Journal of Managerial Psychology, 23*, 395–418.

Montepare, J. M., & Zebrowitz, L. A. (1993). A cross-cultural comparison of impressions created by age-related variations in gait. *Journal of Nonverbal Behavior, 17*, 55–68.

Nagourney, A. (2008, June 15). Age becomes the new race and gender. *The New York Times*. Retrieved from http://www.nytimes.com/.

Nelson, T. D. (Ed.), (2002). *Ageism: Stereotyping and prejudice against older persons*. Cambridge, MA: The MIT Press.

Nosek, B. A., Smyth, F. L., Hansen, J. J., Devos, T., Lindner, N. M., Ranganath, K. A., et al. (2007). Pervasiveness and correlates of implicit attitudes and stereotypes. *European Review of Social Psychology, 18*, 36–88.

O'Brien, L., & Hummert, M. L. (2006). Memory performance of late middle-aged adults: Contrasting self-stereotyping and stereotype threat accounts of assimilation to age stereotypes. *Social Cognition, 24*, 338–358.

Okamoto, K., & Tanaka, Y. (2004). Subjective usefulness and 6-year mortality risks among elderly persons in Japan. *Journals of Gerontology: Psychological Sciences, 59B*, P246–P249.

Operario, D., & Fiske, S. T. (2004). Stereotypes: Content, structures, processes, and context. In M. B. Brewer & M. Hewstone (Eds.), *Social cognition* (pp. 120–141). Malden, MA: Blackwell.

Perdue, C. W., & Gurtman, M. B. (1990). Evidence for the automaticity of ageism. *Journal of Experimental Social Psychology, 26*, 199–216.

Posthuma, R. A., & Campion, M. A. (2009). Age stereotypes in the workplace: Common stereotypes, moderators and future research directions. *Journal of Management, 35*, 158–188.

Rodin, J., & Langer, E. J. (1980). Aging labels: The decline of control and the fall of self-esteem. *Journal of Social Issues, 36*, 12–29.

Rosch, E. H. (1978). Principles of categorization. In E. Rosch & B. Lloyd (Eds.), *Cognition and categorization* (pp. 27–48). Hillsdale, NJ: Erlbaum Associates.

Ruscher, J. B., & Hurley, M. M. (2000). Off-target verbosity evokes negative stereotypes of older adults. *Journal of Language and Social Psychology, 19*, 139–147.

Ryan, E. B., & Capadano, H. L. (1978). Age perceptions and evaluative reactions toward adult speakers. *Journals of Gerontology, 33*, 98–102.

Ryan, E. B., Giles, H., Bartolucci, G., & Henwood, K. (1986). Psycholinguistic and social psychological components of communication by and with the elderly. *Language and Communication, 6*, 1–24.

Ryan, E. B., & Kwong See, S. (1993). Age-based beliefs about memory change for self and others across adulthood. *Journal of Gerontology: Psychological Sciences, 48*, P199–P201.

Schmidt, D. F., & Boland, S. M. (1986). The structure of impressions of older adults: Evidence for multiple stereotypes. *Psychology and Aging, 1*, 255–260.

Steele, C. M., Spencer, S. J., & Aronson, J. (2002). Contending with group image: The psychology of stereotype and social identity threat. In M. P. Zanna (Ed.), *Advances in Experimental Social Psychology, 34* (pp. 379–440). New York: Academic Press.

Stein, R., Blanchard-Fields, F., & Hertzog, C. (2002). The effects of age-stereotyping priming on the memory performance of older adults. *Experimental Aging Research, 28*, 169–181.

Walsh, K. T. (2008, May 9). A dust-up over the McCain age issue. *U.S. News & World Report*. Retrieved from http://www.usnews.com/.

Wentura, D., & Brandtstädter, J. (2003). Age stereotypes in younger and older women: Analyses of accommodative shifts with a sentence-priming task. *Experimental Psychology, 50*, 16–26.

Wheeler, S. C., & Petty, R. E. (2001). The effects of stereotype activation on behavior: A review of possible mechanisms. *Psychological Bulletin, 127*, 797–826.

Wurm, S., Tomasik, M. J., & Tesch-Römer, C. (2008). Serious health events and their impact on changes in subjective health and life satisfaction: The role of age and a positive view on ageing. *European Journal of Ageing, 5*, 117–127.

Yoon, C., Hasher, L., Feinberg, F., Rahhal, T. A., & Winocur, G. (2000). Cross-cultural differences in memory: The role of culture-based stereotypes of aging. *Psychology and Aging, 15*, 694–704.

Yun, R. J., & Lachman, M. E. (2006). Perceptions of aging in two cultures: Korean and American views on old age. *Journal of Cross-Cultural Gerontology, 21*, 55–70.

Zhang, Y. B., Hummert, M. L., & Garstka, T. A. (2002). Stereotype traits of older adults generated by young, middle-aged, and older Chinese participants. *Hallym International Journal of Aging, 4*, 119–140.

Chapter | 17 |

Aging in the Work Context

Catherine E. Bowen, Martin G. Noack, Ursula M. Staudinger

Jacobs Center on Lifelong Learning and Institutional Development, Jacobs University Bremen, Bremen, Germany

CHAPTER CONTENTS

Introduction 263
The Process of Aging in the Work Context 263
Work as an Important Developmental Context: the Effect of Work Experiences on Adult Development 264
Work and Cognitive Development 264
Work and Personality Development 265
Personality Growth and Adjustment 266
Work Experiences and Personality Adjustment 266
Work Experiences and Personality Growth 266
Aging and Work Outcomes 267
Fostering Positive Relationships Between Aging and Work: Further Training, Attitudes Toward Older Workers 268
Further Training 268
Attitudes Toward Older Workers 268
The Transition into and after Retirement 269
Retirement and Health 270
Post-Retirement Activities: Volunteering 271
Conclusions and Future Directions 272
References 272

INTRODUCTION

In this chapter, we discuss the interplay between work and the psychological aspects of aging. There are of course many ways in which people can "work," that is, be productive, in terms of their intellectual, emotional, and motivational outputs (cf. Staudinger, 1996, 2008). We focus specifically on work in the form of paid employment and to a lesser extent on post-retirement volunteering. The influence of the employment context on adult development (e.g., cognition, personality) has received increasing attention as one of the major contextual influences of adult life. Reciprocally, the relationship between age or aging, respectively, and employment outcomes (i.e., productivity) has increased in importance for companies and policy makers in light of falling birth rates and lengthened life spans.

THE PROCESS OF AGING IN THE WORK CONTEXT

As lifespan psychologists, we take the view that aging is a lifelong process that does not suddenly begin (or end) at any particular age. Also, the aging process is *multidirectional* as well as *multidimensional*. In contrast to traditional conceptualizations of aging which conceive of human development as characterized by gains and advances in functioning up to a certain age and then by losses, we take the view that development at all times — including adulthood and even into old age — is characterized by *selective age-related adaptation* (Baltes, 1987). Individuals select (consciously or not), where to direct and invest their resources, within the various constraints posed by biology as well as their social environment. Please note that "selection" refers not only to conscious decisions such as whether or not to work or which career to pursue, but also how resources are invested within any given context. Here we consider not only resource investment in outcomes like task performance but also the wider notion of *psychological productivity* (Staudinger, 1996, 2008), which turns our attention to the whole of an individual's intellectual and emotional, as well as motivational outputs. According to this framework, intellectual productivity refers to problem solving, creating and

DOI: 10.1016/B978-0-12-380882-0.00017-6

sharing ideas, and giving advice. Emotional productivity consists of the ways that people contribute to their own and other's emotional well-being; for example, through their vitality, lust for life, and good humor even in the face of difficult life circumstances (i.e., resilience), or through their capacity for comforting and sympathizing with others. Motivational productivity consists of the ways that people inspire others, for instance, by being a role model or offering support to others in the attainment of their goals. In addition to different forms of productivity, different returns or currencies of productivity can also be distinguished. Money is the return most broadly discussed in our society but other returns such as subjective well-being, motivating others, and increasing social connectedness are crucially important but are less easily measurable. Acknowledging this wider psychological notion of productivity and providing for contexts that facilitate its different facets may represent an important contribution to developing a society for all ages.

How people direct their resources (again, consciously or not) results in selective gains, maintenance in some selected domains, and losses in others. As the effects of individual "choice" and varying contexts accumulate across adulthood (e.g., cumulative advantages and disadvantages, Dannefer, 2003), it is perhaps not surprising that between-person variability on any number of outcomes tends to *increase* across adulthood until very old age (Nelson & Dannefer, 1992). In other words, chronological age becomes less and less informative with increasing age (e.g., Staudinger & Kocka, 2010). While historically much of the research on work and age has focused on cross-sectional comparisons between age groups, to describe "older workers" as a homogenous social group can be misleading given the increasing diversity of age trajectories. Furthermore, there is no dichotomy between "older" and "younger" workers (see also Kessler et al., in press). Therefore, one of the aims of this chapter is to consider the work-related research alongside theories and research on the *aging process* as continuous, multidimensional, and multidirectional. By taking a lifespan view, we would like to emphasize that how people age is — within biologically set limits — malleable and not determined.

WORK AS AN IMPORTANT DEVELOPMENTAL CONTEXT: THE EFFECT OF WORK EXPERIENCES ON ADULT DEVELOPMENT

Work and Cognitive Development

Much research has been devoted to understanding the role of the work context — specifically, the degree of cognitive stimulation adults encounter within their work environments — in predicting concurrent and later patterns of cognitive functioning. Overwhelmingly, the most common hypothesis informing research on the relationship between the work context and cognitive development is some derivation of the use-it-or-lose-it or the disuse hypothesis (Denney, 1984). According to this theory, changes in cognition typically observed with increasing age are at least in part caused by disuse of certain skills and abilities. Earlier considerations of the use-it-or-lose-it/disuse hypothesis typically did not differentiate between the need to practice skills to maintain competence from the need to be continuously faced with new, optimally discrepant cognitive challenges to support cognitive development throughout adulthood and old age (lack of new challenge hypothesis). This latter aspect has received more attention in more recent work that also incorporates the neurophysiological level.

Biologically speaking, these two aspects of the hypotheses; that is, disuse and the lack of new challenges, are consistent with human and animal studies showing that exposure to complex, mental challenges resulting from activity engagement and environmental conditions can stimulate changes in the brain that are beneficial for cognitive functioning — specifically, the generation of new dendritic branches and more synapses (e.g., van Praag et al., 2000). These processes create more "cognitive reserve," which enhances the brain's ability to compensate for age-related decline (e.g., Kramer et al., 2004). According to the scaffolding model of cognitive functioning (e.g., Park & Reuter-Lorenz, 2009), the brain adaptively uses compensatory scaffolding (finding alternative pathways, building new pathways) in response to challenge (when the "normal" pathway is blocked). While this process is not unique to any particular age, as the number of "neural insults" increases as the result of the biological aging process (e.g., brain volume shrinks, loss of dopaminergic receptors), scaffolding processes become more important for maintaining cognitive functioning toward later phases of the life span.

Despite the intuitive appeal of the use-it-or-lose-it/optimal challenge hypotheses, this literature has been criticized on the basis of methodological concerns that render many of the findings inconclusive (e.g., Ghisletta et al., 2006; Salthouse, 2006). For instance, support for the use-it-or-lose-it/optimal challenge hypotheses has typically been based on cross-sectional studies that cannot appropriately distinguish between the selection effects that attract more able people to more stimulating activities and environments from any causal effects of cognitive stimulation on cognitive functioning. Furthermore, many studies have failed to account for important covariates such as gender, socioeconomic status, and health (see Salthouse, 2006 for a review of the problems in this literature).

Recent analyses have made more conclusive suggestions about possible causal links between cognitive stimulation at work and cognitive development. Building on their seminal work, Schooler and colleagues used structural equation modeling on longitudinal data to demonstrate that the self-directedness of work (a combined measure of job complexity, routinization, and the closeness of supervision) affected intellectual functioning 20 years later more than intellectual functioning affected self-directedness (these analyses were controlled for age, gender, race, and education; Schooler et al., 2004). Analysis of data from approximately 1000 World War II veterans revealed that higher levels of intellectual demands and human interaction at work (retrospectively assessed) were associated with higher cognitive status after controlling for early adulthood intelligence, age, and education (Potter et al., 2007). Interestingly, results suggested that there was an aptitude by context interaction such that individuals with lower initial intelligence in young adulthood derived greater benefit from intellectually demanding work. Longitudinal data from the Maastricht Aging Study indicated that older people (average age 61, range 50–85 years) with mentally demanding jobs (currently or formerly) had lower risks of developing cognitive impairment three years later (1.5% vs. 4% for individuals with high and low mental work demands, respectively). This relation was independent of intellectual abilities at baseline as well as age, sex, education, smoking, physical activity, alcohol, depression, family history of dementia, and disease (Bosma et al., 2003). Similarly, a study of Swedish twins found that the work complexity of an individual's predominant lifetime occupation, and in particular, the complexity of the work with other people and with data (as opposed to things), predicted the incidence of dementia and Alzheimer's disease (AD) among adults aged 65 to 100 controlling for age, gender, and education (Andel et al., 2005). While the precise causal pathways responsible for the relationship between cognitive stimulation in the work context and cognitive development remain unclear, overall evidence suggests that intellectual engagement and cognitive stimulation, which can be fostered by a cognitively stimulating work context, does indeed promote more successful cognitive aging (see also Hertzog et al., 2009).

In consideration of the biological mechanisms thought to underlie the disuse and optimal challenge hypotheses, we would like to suggest that distinguishing between novel processing and other kinds of cognitive stimulation may be useful in teasing out the different mechanisms behind any possible effect of cognitive stimulation (at work) and cognitive development. In short, practice seems to help prevent the need for scaffolding (Park & Reuter-Lorenz, 2009), whereas optimal levels of mental challenge support better scaffolding. Likewise, it would seem that more complex jobs with regard to the skills practiced may support the maintenance of a wider range of already established pathways (i.e., crystallized abilities), whereas it is particularly the encountering of *novel situations* (at different levels of complexity) – at work and in general – that supports the maintenance of fluid abilities across adulthood (cf. Sternberg, 1985). In tentative support of this argument, the results of a 6-year longitudinal study of older adults (mean age 68.5 years, SD = 7.61), found that novel information processing was one of the few engagement domains (as opposed to engagement in, e.g., social or passive information processing activities) that significantly predicted less longitudinal decline in one indicator of cognitive speed (semantic decision) (Bielak et al. 2007).[1] In addition, retrospective self-reported novelty-seeking behavior (sample items: learning a new skill, getting a new experience) was negatively associated with the development of AD relative to a control group after controlling for education, occupational status, gender, age, and ethnicity (Fritsch et al., 2005). The novelty perspective may also explain why the complexity of social interactions encountered on the job, which may be related to a higher likelihood of continuously encountering novel aspects, seems to play a particularly important role in cognitive development relative to other aspects of complexity (e.g., motor skills, work with data; Andel et al., 2005; Finkel et al., 2009; Kröger et al., 2008).

Work and Personality Development

In contrast to the hypothesis that personality past young adulthood is "set like plaster" (Costa & McCrae, 1994, 2006), an increasing number of studies have demonstrated that personality continues to develop across adulthood and even into old age (e.g., Donnellan & Lucas, 2008; Roberts & Mroczek, 2008; Roberts et al., 2006a; Staudinger, 2005). The work domain is thought to be one driver of adult personality change as adults learn and adapt to the demands of working life (e.g., Hogan & Roberts, 2004; Roberts et al., 2005; Schooler et al., 2004). The work context socializes adults by demanding certain behaviors and characteristics, for example, conscientiously completing tasks, attuning to others' needs and limiting social conflict. Over time these behaviors and characteristics become automatic and can subsequently "spill over" into other life domains. The extent to which an individual invests in his or her work role is thought to moderate the extent to which these socialization effects take place (cf. Ryff & Essex, 1992). In addition to a socialization effect, a selection effect also seems to play a role. The very characteristics that attract

[1]Note though, that examples of novel information processing included completing income tax forms or playing bridge. It is questionable how "novel" this kind of processing actually is. While the brain must handle new *data* in such situations, the metacognitive structure of the task stays the same.

certain people to certain jobs (or particular contexts more generally) are the same characteristics most likely to change over time; for example, people who are more open to start with also tend to prefer jobs that are related to the encounter of continuously new situations, and thus increase in openness over time (e.g., Roberts & Robins, 2004). Importantly, the role of the work context as a driver of personality development tempers exclusively biological explanations of adult personality change (e.g., McCrae et al., 1999).

Personality Growth and Adjustment

When considering adult personality change, we have found it helpful to distinguish between two trajectories of positive personality development, that is, personality adjustment and personality growth (Staudinger & Bowen, 2010; Staudinger & Kessler, 2009; Staudinger et al., 2005; Staudinger & Kunzmann, 2005). *Personality adjustment* refers to successful adaptation to contextual demands arising from history-graded, age-graded, and idiosyncratic developmental contexts (Staudinger & Kessler, 2009). Indicators of personality adjustment include subjective well-being as well as the indicators of social adaptability like the Big Five (Costa & McCrae, 1992) traits neuroticism/emotional stability, conscientiousness, and agreeableness. Noting that positive personality development has other dimensions that are not captured by positive feelings or everyday competence, we have defined *personality growth* to involve advances in self and world insight and increases in the complexity of emotion regulation (degree of affective differentiation, tolerance of the coactivation of positive and negative emotions) as well as the motivation to optimize not only one's own well-being, but also that of others (cf. Staudinger & Kessler, 2009). All three components need to be simultaneously realized for personality growth to occur. An important correlate and/or antecedent of personality growth is the Big Five dimension of openness to new experience indicating an individual's interest to pursue the kind of novel, challenging contexts that increase the likelihood to be confronted with new experiences, which in turn are prone to challenge extant insights into self and life. Loevinger's (1997) measure of ego development is a performance indicator of personality growth.

Work Experiences and Personality Adjustment

Many indicators of personality adjustment have been related to work experiences. Earlier research demonstrated that working and succeeding in work robustly leads to increases in adjustment-related personality dimensions such as self-confidence, norm adherence, independence, and responsibility (Clausen & Gilens, 1990; Elder, 1969; Kohn & Schooler, 1978; Roberts, 1997). More recent longitudinal findings have also shown that increases in work satisfaction are associated with increases in measures of emotional stability (Roberts & Chapman, 2000; Roberts et al., 2003; Scollon & Diener, 2006). Two recent studies by Roberts and colleagues (2003, 2006b) have linked increases in personality adjustment in young adulthood to investment in and rewards from the work context. Job satisfaction, social status, and financial reward as well as the degree to which individuals reported investing in their jobs moderated the degree to which typical developmental patterns in indicators of personality adjustment took place between ages 18 and 26. For example, young adults in jobs that provided higher status, more satisfaction, and more financial security decreased faster in neuroticism and increased faster in communal positive emotionality (cf. agreeableness; Roberts et al., 2003). In contrast, young adults who invested less in their work role tended to *increase* in neuroticism and maintain initial levels of constraint (cf. conscientiousness), *contrary* to typical developmental patterns in young adulthood (Roberts et al., 2006b). Although only young adults participated in the two studies previously cited, we find the results relevant as aging is a *lifelong process* that does not suddenly begin after one has reached advanced age.

Control beliefs are important predictors of adjustment across the life span, including health (e.g., Chapter 11, this volume). The degree of freedom with which an employee is allowed to self-determine his or her job content or approach (i.e., job autonomy and work control) has important influences on more global control beliefs (Huyck, 1991; Kivett et al., 1977; Kohn & Schooler, 1973; Wickrama et al., 2008). Longitudinal analysis of middle-aged men indicated that changes in work control affected changes in personal control, which in turn predicted self-reported health ten years later — independent from baseline levels of work control and global personal control (Wickrama et al., 2008). Low work control has been directly associated with indicators of (lacking) adjustment such as depression (Mausner-Dorsch & Eaton, 2000) as well as physical health (Wickrama et al., 2005).

Work Experiences and Personality Growth

Generally, the development of personality growth has received much less attention than personality adjustment, a pattern likewise reflected in the work literature. In a rare study that investigated the relationship between the work context and personality growth, women's ego development over time was associated with uninterrupted, successful work experiences (Helson & Roberts, 1994). Some studies have investigated work and the development of general wisdom. General wisdom has been defined as an expertise in the fundamental pragmatics of life permitting exceptional insight and judgment involving complex and uncertain matters of the human condition including its developmental and contextual variability, plasticity, and limitations (e.g., Baltes & Staudinger, 2000). Contextual conditions thought to facilitate the development of general wisdom include extensive exposure to and experience with a wide range of human conditions and mentor-guided practice in dealing with difficult life issues (Charness, 1989; Salthouse, 1991, see also Staudinger et al., 2006). With some exceptions (e.g., theologian, judge, clinical psychologist), such conditions are not characteristic of most work contexts. In two cross-sectional studies, clinical psychologists displayed higher levels of general wisdom-related performance than comparison groups from nonsocial service academic professions (Smith et al., 1994; Staudinger et al., 1992). Still, it is important to note that advances in general wisdom (i.e., world-insight) may not necessarily correlate with advances in *personal wisdom* (i.e., self-insight), which is more relevant for our discussion of personality growth (cf. Mickler & Staudinger, 2008).

Trajectories of personality growth in recent cohorts tend to stagnate after young adulthood (Staudinger & Bowen, 2010; Staudinger & Kessler, 2009). However, we underline that the developmental trajectories we currently observe are in part the product of the contexts in which current cohorts are aging. Theoretically, more universally applicable features (as opposed to the stringent contextual characteristics described in the previous paragraph) of the workplace could also facilitate personality growth. For example, positions with supervising responsibilities may be conducive to above-average confrontation with dilemma situations that need to be resolved. Changing work contexts across the life span such that novel experiences are a continuous part of the work life (irrespective of the level of qualification) may foster the reconsideration of earlier life experiences. In addition, contextual demands to critically consider alternative viewpoints – for instance, within diverse work teams – may stimulate a broadening of self- and world-insight (cf. Staudinger & Bowen, 2010). In particular, the workplace has the potential to provide an arena for intergenerational interactions that under certain conditions can stimulate personality growth. Experimental research has shown that interactions between older and younger adults in which older adults share their expertise can stimulate advances in indicators of personality growth (i.e., emotional complexity), as well as improve older adults' fluid cognitive functioning (Kessler & Staudinger, 2007).

AGING AND WORK OUTCOMES

Demographic changes including the rising median age of workers and the need to increase the proportion of older workers in the labor force have stimulated many studies on the relationship between age and various work outcomes such as performance. Within the organizational literature, researchers distinguish between task performance and "non-core" dimensions of work performance such as attendance, innovation, and helping behaviors (i.e., *organizational citizenship behavior*). On the one hand, the well-documented decreases in fluid cognitive abilities and physical strength have given rise to concerns about the ability of older adults to maintain task performance. On the other hand, it has often been argued that older workers' greater experience can improve performance or at least compensate for age-related declines in some areas of functioning.

A recent meta-analysis of 380 studies found that age was largely unrelated to core task performance as indicated by supervisor-ratings, self-ratings, and objective measures (Ng & Feldman, 2008). Indeed, a wide range of research supports the idea that older adults can successfully compensate for decrements in cognitive mechanics by drawing on pragmatic resources (e.g., Bäckman & Dixon, 1992). This idea is supported by the results of a recent study of manufacturing employees, which demonstrated that the negative effect of age was canceled out by a positive effect of job tenure on objective task performance as indicated by the number of errors (in this study the authors controlled for the selectivity bias of early exit from the labor force; Börsch-Supan & Weiss, 2007).

On an individual level, the relationship between age and task performance is likely mediated by many factors. In particular, the extent to which task performance is affected by age seems to be mediated by occupational demands on fluid abilities, job-related knowledge, motivation, and physical strength (e.g., Kanfer & Ackermann, 2004; Warr, 2001). All else held equal, age has little and most likely even positive effects on job performance within occupations that depend more on crystallized abilities and social demands (e.g., salesperson, teacher), which are normatively stable well into old age, rather than within occupations that depend more upon more fluid abilities (e.g., air traffic controller) or physical abilities (e.g., manual laborer; Skirbekk, 2008). Indeed, professional experience, in the sense of practice (see above) does not seem to compensate for age-related changes in the cognitive mechanics. For instance, practice as an architect or as a graphic designer did not appear to transfer to a compensation of age-related declines in spatial visualization and visual memory performance, respectively (Lindenberger et al., 1993; Salthouse, 1991). Age decrements tend to be smaller when more complex cognitive processes can be supported by environmental cues and aids, such as personal memos and computer programs that remind people of the appropriate steps to be taken to tackle a problem (Warr, 2001).

As opposed to the overall null relationship between age and task performance, age has generally been positively associated with a range of work-related outcomes beneficial for employers (Ng & Feldman, 2008). Specifically, age was related to increased attendance, safety performance, and organizational citizenship behaviors (e.g., helping colleagues, not complaining about trivial matters, trying to improve group performance) and negatively associated with counterproductive work behaviors (e.g., workplace aggression, substance use, tardiness). Interestingly, the relationship between age and organizational citizenship behaviors was stronger in longitudinal studies than in cross-sectional studies, indicating that developmental effects and not only cohort differences underlie the relationship (Ng & Feldman, 2008). As organizational citizenship behaviors seems to benefit group and organizational effectiveness (Podsakoff et al., 2000), the positive correlation between age and organizational citizenship behaviors represents one potential benefit of employing older workers.

The research reviewed in this section underlines the importance of considering multiple dimensions of what is considered "productive" performance. Overall, older workers' productivity can be expected to reveal itself in a contribution to the whole group in the form of experience passed on to others and contribution to a less-stressful and supportive climate, rather than individual task performance (e.g., Kessler et al., in press). Still, we emphasize that group-level trends (old vs. young) say little about how *individuals* — given the increasing variability in developmental trajectories with increasing age — will age within individual work contexts.

FOSTERING POSITIVE RELATIONSHIPS BETWEEN AGING AND WORK: FURTHER TRAINING, ATTITUDES TOWARD OLDER WORKERS

Two factors have been particularly prominent in the recent literature concerning factors that moderate the ability of societies, companies, and individuals to foster positive relationships between aging and the work context: further training and attitudes toward older workers.

Further Training

Lifelong learning and thereby bolstering participation rates in further education has been offered as one solution to the challenge posed by an aging workforce. Intervention research has shown that adults of all ages can benefit from training in terms of increased levels of cognitive functioning (e.g., Ball et al., 2002). Indeed, a representative, 24-year longitudinal study of American men revealed a positive association between participation in post-educational training of any kind and cognitive functioning (Short Portable Mental Status Questionnaire) in older adulthood, independent of the respondent's formal education, race, age, income, occupational status (blue/white collar), and health (Wight et al., 2002). This study suggested that further training can have a compensatory effect: In old age, those with initially low levels of formal education who received subsequent training had comparable levels of cognitive functioning as those with the highest initial levels of formal education. Training also has positive effects for firms. It has also been associated with higher organizational commitment and job satisfaction (Mikkelsen et al., 1999) as well as productivity increases on the industry and firm levels (Dearden et al., 2005; Zwick, 2002).

Further training can help ameliorate and prevent employees' (especially older employees') knowledge from becoming outdated. This may be especially important for updating employees' technological skills. Technology clearly has become an integral part of the workplace, but age has been found to be negatively related to both technology use and breadth of computer use (e.g., Czaja et al., 2006). In this study, technology use was mediated by self-efficacy and anxiety, signaling that training, particularly with regard to technology, needs to focus on building confidence in addition to skill.

Current rates of participation in adult education vary widely across the Organisation for Economic Co-operation and Development (OECD) member countries (e.g., from <10% to over 35%; OECD, 2009a). Importantly, in all countries, the most qualified adults participate in more training than the less qualified. This indicates a pattern of accumulated disadvantage (e.g., Dannefer, 2003), such that those with fewer educational qualifications also subsequently participate less in the learning activities, which could potentially compensate for initially lower qualifications (cf. Wight et al., 2002). Furthermore, the discrepancy between the participation rates of older relative to younger employees has been the focus of much attention. Sweden is the only country in the OECD in which 55 to 64 year olds participate in as much training as 25 to 34 year olds (OECD, 2009a). In most other countries, the participation rates of older working age adults are well below half that of younger working age adults. Multiple factors are thought to underlie the age discrepancies, including ageist attitudes of managers who make training decisions and older workers' attitudes (e.g., reduced self-efficacy, reduced motivation), as well as higher costs and reduced incentives for both the firm and the older employee to invest in further training (e.g., Wooden et al., 2001) .

Attitudes Toward Older Workers

Despite a lack of evidence that age is systematically and generally related to job performance (e.g., Ng & Feldman, 2008), older workers continue to face negative attitudes (e.g., Gordon & Arvey, 2004). Often just as workers are entering the zenith of their careers, they are already considered less flexible, less energetic, and at greater health risk as well as slower, less creative, and disinterested in training, but also more reliable and loyal (see Posthuma & Campion, 2009 for a review of age stereotypes in the workplace). Negative attitudes about older workers are thought to affect recruitment patterns as well as promotion and training decisions.

The endorsement of such attitudes appears to vary somewhat between countries. An international survey of 6,320 private sector employers in 21 countries indicated that there were considerable differences between countries in the age at which an employee was considered old, ranging from 44 years in Turkey to 60.4 years in Japan (Harper et al., 2006). Interestingly, these differences were unrelated to the population's median age, despite appearances given the two countries cited. Employers were asked to compare older and younger workers on a range of stereotypical characteristics (e.g., loyal, flexible, technologically oriented). On the whole, employers did not generally regard older employees less positively than younger workers, although employers did indeed tend to assign individual traits to either older (e.g., reliable, loyal) or younger workers (e.g., flexible, quick learners). Still, there was variation between countries: Employers' age attitudes were most positive in the UK and the United States (interestingly two countries with strong anti-age discrimination laws that may result in a stronger social desirability bias), and most negative in Turkey and Saudi Arabia.

Age stereotypes do not only vary between societies. Initial evidence from work on *age climate* – a construct capturing organization-specific age stereotypes – found that companies differed significantly with regard to how older employees within the company were regarded (Noack & Staudinger, 2010a). Age climate is assessed by asking respondents to indicate the extent to which adjectives related to work-related age stereotypes (e.g., productive, flexible, reliable) correspond with the image of older employees in their company. Responses are averaged to create an indicator of how favorably older employees are regarded within the company. The differences between companies' age climates concurred with differences in their personnel, knowledge, and health management practices regarding older workers. For example, in production companies with a more favorable age climate, older workers were hired directly from the labor market, tended to participate frequently in further education, and were offered preventive health training. On the individual level, more positive perceptions of the company's age climate coincided with higher levels of affective organizational commitment — indicating the emotional attachment to, identification with, and involvement in the organization — among the company's older workers (Noack et al., 2010c) as well as lower turnover intentions among employees of all ages (Bowen & Staudinger, 2010). Furthermore, for workers age 40 and above, less positive perceptions of the age climate went along with lower self-reported work ability (Noack & Staudinger, 2010b).

Creating work environments that optimize work and developmental outcomes necessitates an *integrated* age management strategy that includes simultaneous attention to relevant issues like further training and age attitudes, alongside dynamic personnel practices that are cognizant of the fact that individuals' abilities, interests, and needs change over the course of their career. Because aging is a continuous, lifelong process, companies need to create work environments that support human development across the life span, as opposed to beginning interventions only once an employee has reached the age of 45 or 50 (Staudinger, 2007; Staudinger et al., 2008). For example, to most effectively use further training as a mechanism to buffer or compensate for cognitive decline, training should not be restricted to higher ages, although this is probably currently and for some years to come the life period that needs the most attention, given the rather low participation of over 55 years olds relative to younger adults (OECD, 2009a). Rather, training should become an integral part of (working) life *across* the life span, so that individuals do not fall out of the education loop. Indeed, previous further training predicts current participation in future training (e.g., Maurer et al., 2003). Likewise, fostering positive images of aging as well as a sense of internal control over attaining positive developmental outcomes needs to begin early on in the life span.

THE TRANSITION INTO AND AFTER RETIREMENT

Given the many ways in which working contributes to adult development, retirement (i.e., exit from the paid work context) also deserves some attention in our discussion of work and aging. Importantly, retirement is a transitional process as opposed to a sudden change in life. The process begins with thoughts about retirement, the development of a desire to retire, later followed by the decision and finally the actual act of retirement (Beehr, 1986).

Beginning in midlife, employees begin to place more emphasis on intrinsic rewards from work, such as a feeling of accomplishment, of learning and experiencing new things, and of doing something worthwhile (Penner et al., 2002). In a survey by the American Association of Retired Persons (AARP), 84% of older employees (45–74 years) indicated a desire to work even if they were financially set for life, and 69% said they planned to work into their retirement years

(Montenegro et al., 2002). Older employees' reasons for continuing to work are wide ranging, including not only extrinsic benefits such as increased financial security and health care benefits, but also enjoyment and a sense of purpose as well as social participation (Hedge et al., 2006).

Older adults are increasingly seeking some sort of bridge employment that allows for gradual (as opposed to sudden) transition out of the work context. On the individual level, age and stress experienced at pre-retirement jobs seem to be predictive of choosing full retirement over bridge employment (Gobeski & Beehr, 2009). Full retirement can offer an escape from unpleasant work roles (e.g., Barnes-Farrell, 2003). Higher levels of education and better health led older workers to decide for continued involvement in paid work (Wang et al., 2008). While most employees who plan to work after retirement hope to build on their accumulated expertise by remaining in a line of work that is similar to their current occupation (Hedge et al., 2006), more than half of the retirees who take bridge jobs change occupation and/or industry, often accepting reduced wages and status in return for the flexibility of a bridge job (e.g., Feldman, 1994; Shultz, 2003). Whether an older worker seeks bridge employment in the same or a new line of work depends on the costs and benefits associated with that line of work. When intrinsic job characteristics, like autonomy, task identity, task significance, feedback, and skill variety were high in his or her previous line of work, the likelihood for continuing in a job similar to the career job was also high (Gobeski & Beehr, 2009). In contrast, higher job-related strain was predictive of taking a non-career bridge job.

Company policies can affect the retirement process. For instance, corporate restructuring and downsizing by means of buyouts and layoffs has resulted in many older workers tending to retire earlier from their long-tenure, career jobs. Companies can also influence the retirement transition by providing roles and opportunities for older workers seeking bridge employment. For instance, companies can retain retired employees as internal consultants. Some companies recruit their retiring managers into a filial enterprise that provides consulting service at a high level (Deller et al., 2008). Other companies create alumni-networks and thus keep in touch with their retirees, which creates a similar potential for back-recruiting (cf. Staudinger et al., 2008). As one of the motives underlying post-retirement activities seems to be generativity (Deller et al., 2009), offering retiring employees the position of a mentor for incoming members of the company is just one of many ways how retirees can contribute to the work context.

Societal policies also affect the retirement process. For example, before recent retirement policy changes, the German federal government set strong incentives for companies to lay off their older employees, or rather, to send them into early retirement by heavily subsidizing their severance pay. Even as recently as 2005, Germany spent 0.06% of its gross domestic product on early retirement programs with 1 in 450 workers in early retirement (OECD, 2009b). Furthermore, German policy creates a disincentive for older adults to continue working past pension eligibility, since a large proportion of any earned salary is deducted from state pension benefits. The situation is quite different in the United States, where there are no public incentives for early retirement. These policy differences are reflected in changes of the labor force participation rates of 55 to 64 year olds in the two countries. In both countries, the labor force participation of the above 55 year olds increased continuously from 1994 to 2008. However, the changes were much more pronounced among older men (53.1 to 67.2%) and women (28.3 to 50.6%) in Germany relative to the older men (65.5 to 70.4%) and women (48.9 to 59.1%) in the United States, where participation rates were already initially much higher (OECD, 2009b).

Retirement and Health

An important question regarding the transition into retirement regards its potential impact on physical and mental health (see Wurm et al., 2009 for a comprehensive review on the topic). With regard to physical health, empirical findings from longitudinal studies suggest that retirement per se neither harms nor benefits health (e.g., Ekerdt et al., 1983; Mein et al., 2003; Van Solinge, 2007). Pre-retirement unemployment, in comparison, was found to have significantly negative effects on physical health of participants in the Health and Retirement Study (Gallo et al., 2006). Similarly, there does not appear to be a straightforward relationship between retirement and indicators of mental health. Retirement has been found to be related to fewer depressive symptoms in some studies (e.g., Reitzes et al., 1996), while other studies found that the reduction of depressive symptoms was limited to only individuals retiring from highly prestigious positions (e.g., Mein et al., 2003) or found that retirement weakly increased depressive symptoms (James & Spiro, 2006). Generally, bridge employment has been found to be predictive of both retirement satisfaction and psychological well-being (Kim & Feldman, 2000).

Retirement may entail certain losses in terms of, for example, income, social interactions, status, and structure as well as meaning in life (cf. Havighurst et al., 1968). But retirement may also entail new opportunities, freedom, and independence after hierarchy, time demands, and other work-related strains cease (cf. Rosenmayr, 1983). The extent to which retirement *individually* represents losses and gains would seem to correspond with any potential changes in overall physical and mental health. Indeed, a study using data from the German Socioeconomic Panel and growth mixture modeling identified three distinct trajectories of life satisfaction experienced during the retirement transition (Pinquart & Schindler, 2007). For most people, retirement predicted a small increase in life satisfaction. The second trajectory was characterized by an increase in life satisfaction immediately following retirement, against the backdrop of a relatively strong overall decline in life satisfaction in the years prior to and following retirement. This trajectory was particularly characteristic of retirees who had been unemployed immediately prior to retirement. The third trajectory was characterized by immediate post-retirement decline followed by a slow recovery. Relative to the first, most common trajectory, people in the latter two classes had fewer resources (e.g., socioeconomic status, physical health, married) for adapting to retirement. Interestingly, it seems that individuals may have a limited ability to predict their well-being after leaving work. In one study, older employees included in early retirement schemes initially tended to anticipate retirement as a reward. After one year, however, the majority of early retirees wanted to return to work, mostly in a part-time position and with more freedom in working arrangements (Aleksandrowicz et al., 2009).

In sum, there does not appear to be any general causal relationship between retirement and either physical or mental health. The effect of retirement on health seems to greatly depend upon individual preferences and pre-retirement working conditions as well as the individual's ability and resources to adapt to the new life stage. Changes in social status, social engagement, meaning in life, financial security, and even physical activity (Berger et al., 2005; Slingerland et al., 2007) may accompany the retirement process and probably to a great extent explain any effect of retirement on health. It is therefore critical in considerations of the effect of retirement on health to take into account post-retirement opportunities as well as individual resources (e.g., health, social network, openness to new experience) that can help people to mitigate any potential negative changes as well as profit from new opportunities that may accompany the retirement process.

Post-Retirement Activities: Volunteering

In recent years, more and more older adults have been participating in volunteer activities. For instance, in Germany, participation in volunteer activities rose from 31% in 1999 to 37% in 2004 among 60 to 69 year olds (Gensicke et al., 2005). In Germany, the main areas of voluntary engagement for individuals age 60 and above are sports (e.g., trainer), religion (e.g., organizer of charity events), care-taking (of very young and old-old non-family members), structured leisure time activities (e.g., organizer of excursions for senior citizens), and culture (e.g., manager or conductor of a choir) (Gensicke et al., 2005). Between 1999 to 2004, the areas of older adults' voluntary engagement became more diversified with a small but rapidly increasing participation also in other areas like citizens' initiatives, nature protection groups, politics, and labor unions. Still, volunteer participation rates vary widely between countries. In Europe, data from the second wave of the Survey for Health, Aging, and Retirement in Europe (SHARE) revealed that participation rates among individuals age 50 and above ranged between approximately 2 and 25% (Hank & Erlinghagen, 2009). Many more respondents had been engaged in volunteer activities during the month preceding the interview in Northern European countries as compared to Southern and Eastern European countries. This finding was interpreted to be consistent with differences between the welfare state regimes of these countries that seem to offer different incentives and opportunities for civic engagement (Hank & Stuck, 2008).

Data from the Berlin Aging Study (BASE) showed that post-retirement social participation is cumulative (e.g., Bukov et al., 2002) and demonstrates a high degree of continuity across the life span (e.g., Hank & Stuck, 2008; Maas & Staudinger, 2009). Individuals who volunteered during adolescence and early adulthood had a significantly higher likelihood to also volunteer as retirees. Educational and occupational resources predict the intensity of social engagement, over and above gender differences. In addition, age (i.e., being younger than 75), current health status, and having a stable partnership also seem to predict social engagement (Erlinghagen & Hank, 2006). Caro (2009) illustrated that for older adults — especially for the highly educated Baby Boomers — to contribute substantial amounts of their time to volunteering they might need specific opportunities that draw upon their individual experience and skills. Thus, systematic recruitment, placement, and training of volunteers may be helpful to fully profit from retiring workers' potentials and to provide older adults with meaningful roles in their post-retirement life.

Importantly, volunteering has been found to have positive consequences for older individuals. For example, volunteer work was significantly and positively related to quality of life in retirement and to retirement satisfaction (Kim & Feldman, 2000). Similarly, longitudinal data from the United States has shown that for individuals aged 60 years and older, volunteering was associated with higher levels of well-being (Morrow-Howell et al., 2003). In another study using U.S. panel data, a moderate amount of volunteering (about two hours per week) had a protective effect regarding older adults' self-reported health (Luoh & Herzog, 2002). In this longitudinal study based on a representative sample of older adults, the authors controlled for potential selectivity effects into volunteer activities by assessing objective health status at baseline.

A bi-directional relationship between health and volunteering emerged: While earlier self-reported health affected later volunteering activities, volunteering also reciprocally positively affected later health status. Such positive effects have been traced back to increases in self-esteem, strengthening of social networks and purpose in life (Morrow-Howell et al., 2003). In a recent experimental study, we demonstrated that older adult volunteers who participated in competence training as part of their volunteering activities, and also reported above median internal control beliefs, demonstrated continuous increases in openness to experience over a period of 15 months, in contrast to nonvolunteers as well as volunteers who did not receive the competence training (Mühlig-Versen & Staudinger, 2010). These results show that volunteering, in combination with certain internal resources (e.g., internal control, strategies to master the situation), can reverse the typical adulthood pattern of decreasing openness to new experience — an indicator of personality growth as previously described.

CONCLUSIONS AND FUTURE DIRECTIONS

In this chapter we have reviewed evidence that for better or worse, work experiences are one important source for adult development. Most of the evidence presented has referred to work in the sense of paid employment and to some extent to work in the sense of volunteering, although many of the mechanisms and trends we have described are also more generally applicable to other forms of productive activity. We have also reviewed evidence that older workers and adult development can positively contribute to the work domain. This view becomes particularly apparent when one considers "productivity" in a wider sense, both within the work context (e.g., Ng & Feldman, 2008) as well as a notion of psychological productivity (Staudinger, 1996, 2008).

In line with a contextualistic perspective (cf. Baltes et al., 1980), we would like to emphasize that development — as we currently observe it — is not set in stone. The impressive plasticity of human development and aging needs to be taken seriously with regard to the construction of the work context and contexts more generally. Optimizing developmental outcomes — within the work and volunteer contexts, or in any context more generally — can be aided by taking a lifespan view of development as opposed to focusing only on older adults. More systematic intervention knowledge is needed to be in a position to construct work environments such that they not only prevent the exhaustion of an individual's productivity but also develop and foster it across the life span. Of course, work is necessary to afford our living. But work (or activity to use a more neutral notion) also is one of the prime sources of meaning and well-being in an individual's life. A society of longer lives may develop its potential to the fullest only if it succeeds in creating work contexts that support continued development into later adulthood.

REFERENCES

Aleksandrowicz, P., Fasang, A., Schömann, K., & Staudinger, U. M. (2009). Die Bedeutung der Arbeit beim vorzeitigen Ausscheiden aus dem Arbeitsleben [The meaning of work during early retirement]. *Zeitschrift für Gerontologie und Geriatrie, 11*, 1–6.

Andel, R., Crowe, M., Pedersen, N. L., Mortimer, J. A., Crimmins, E., Johansson, B., et al. (2005). Complexity of work and risk of Alzheimer's Disease: A population-based study of Swedish twins. *Journals of Gerontology: Psychological Sciences, 60B*, P251–P258.

Bäckman, L., & Dixon, R. A. (1992). Psychological compensation: A theoretical framework. *Psychological Bulletin, 112*, 259–283.

Ball, K., Berch, D. B., Helmers, K. F., Jobe, J. B., Leveck, M. D., Marsiske, M., et al. (2002). Effects of cognitive training interventions with older adults: A randomized controlled trial. *Journal of the American Medical Association, 288*(18), 2271–2281.

Baltes, P. B. (1987). Theoretical propositions of life span developmental psychology: On the dynamics between growth and decline. *Developmental Psychology, 23*, 611–626.

Baltes, P. B., & Staudinger, U. M. (2000). Wisdom. A metaheuristic (pragmatic) to orchestrate mind and virtue toward excellence. *American Psychologist, 55*(1), 122–136.

Baltes, P. B., Reese, H. W., & Lipsitt, L. P. (1980). Life-span developmental psychology. *Annual Review of Psychology, 31*, 65–110.

Barnes-Farrell, J. L. (2003). Beyond health and wealth: Attitudinal and other influences on retirement decision-making. In G. A. Adams & T. A. Beehr (Eds.), *Retirement: Reasons, processes, and results* (pp. 159–187). New York: Springer.

Beehr, T. A. (1986). The process of retirement: A review and recommendations for future investigation. *Personnel Psychology, 39*, 31–55.

Berger, U., Der, G., Mutrie, N., & Hannah, M. K. (2005). The impact of retirement on physical activity. *Ageing and Society, 25*(2), 181–195.

Bielak, A. A. M., Hughes, T. F., Small, B. J., & Dixon, R. A. (2007). It's never too late to engage in lifestyle activities: Significant concurrent but not change relationships between lifestyle activities and cognitive speed. *Journals of Gerontology: Psychological Sciences and Social Sciences, 62B*, 331–339.

Börsch-Supan, A., & Weiss, M. (2007). Productivity and the age composition of work teams: Evidence from the assembly line. Report for the Mannheim Research Institute of the Economics of Aging. Accessed on Jan 5, 2009 from http://www.mea.uni-mannheim.de/publications/meadp_148-07.pdf.

Bosma, H., van Boxtel, M. P. J., Ponds, R. W. H. M., Houx, P. J., Burdorf, A., & Jolles, J. (2003). Mental work demands protect against cognitive impairment: MAAS Prospective Cohort Study. *Experimental Aging Research, 29*, 33–45.

Bowen, C. E., & Staudinger, U. M. (2010). Do I have a future here? Images of Aging in the workplace and employee turnover intentions. Manuscript in preparation.

Bukov, A., Maas, I., & Lampert, T. (2002). Social participation in very old age: Cross-sectional and longitudinal findings from BASE. *Journals of Gerontology: Psychological Sciences, 57B*(6), P510–P517.

Caro, F. G. (2009). Productive aging and volunteering in the United States — Conceptual, political, empirical, and policy issues. In A. Börsch-Supan, M. Erlinghagen, K. Hank, H. Jürges, & G. G. Wagner (Eds.), *Produktivität in alternden Gesellschaften* (Altern in Deutschland Bd. 4). Nova Acta Leopoldina NF Bd. 102, Nr. 366 (pp. 131–142). Stuttgart: Wissenschaftliche Verlagsanstalt.

Charness, N. (1989). Expertise in chess and bridge. In D. Klahr & K. Kotovsky (Eds.), *Complex information processing: The impact of Herbert A. Simon* (pp. 183–289). Hillsdale, NJ: Erlbaum.

Clausen, J. A., & Gilens, M. (1990). Personality and labor force participation across the life course: A longitudinal study of women's careers. *Sociological Forum, 5*, 595–618.

Costa, P. T., & McCrae, R. R. (1994). Set like plaster? Evidence for the stability of adult personality. In T. F. Heatherton & J. L. Weinberger (Eds.), *Can personality change?* (pp. 21–40). Washington, DC: American Psychological Association.

Costa, P. T., Jr., & McCrae, R. R. (2006). Age changes in personality and their origins: Comment on Roberts, Walton, and Viechtbauer (2006). *Psychological Bulletin, 132*, 28–30.

Costa, P. T., & McCrae, R. R. (1992). *NEO PI-R. Professional manual.* Odessa, FL: Psychological Assessment Resources, Inc.

Czaja, S. J., Charness, N., Fisk, A. D., Hertzog, C., Nair, S. N., Rogers, W. A., et al. (2006). Factors predicting the use of technology: Findings from the Center for Research and Education on Aging and Technology Enhancement (CREATE). *Psychology and Aging, 21*(2), 333–352.

Dannefer, D. (2003). Cumulative advantage/disadvantage and the life course: Cross-fertilizing age and social science theory. *Journals of Gerontology Series B: Psychological Sciences and Social Sciences, 58*, 327–337.

Dearden, L., Reed, H., & Van Reenen, J. (2005). The impact of training on productivity and wages: Evidence from British panel data. Discussion Paper No. 674. Centre for Economic Performance, London. Retrieved January 5, 2009, from http://cep.lse.ac.uk/pubs/download/dp0674.pdf.

Deller, J., Kern, S., Hausmann, E., & Diederichs, Y. (2008). *Personalmanagement im demografischen Wandel: Ein Handbuch für den Veränderungsprozess* [Personnel management during demographic change: A handbook for the change process]. Heidelberg: Springer.

Deller, J., Liedtke, P. M., & Maxin, L. M. (2009). Old-age security and silver workers: An empirical survey identifies challenges for companies, insurers and society. *The Geneva Papers, 34*, 137–157.

Denney, N. W. (1984). A model of cognitive development across the life span. *Developmental Review, 4*, 171–191.

Donnellan, M. B., & Lucas, R. E. (2008). Age differences in the Big Five across the life span: Evidence from two national samples. *Psychology and Aging, 23*, 558–566.

Ekerdt, D. J., Baden, L., Bossé, R., & Dibbs, E. (1983). The effect of retirement on physical health. *American Journal of Public Health, 73*(7), 779–783.

Elder, G. H. (1969). Occupational mobility: Life patterns, and personality. *Journal of Health and Social Behavior, 10*, 308–323.

Erlinghagen, M., & Hank, K. (2006). The participation of older Europeans in volunteer work. *Ageing & Society, 26*, 567–584.

Feldman, D. C. (1994). The decision to retire early: A review and conceptualization. *Academy of Management Review, 19*, 285–311.

Finkel, D., Andel, R., Gatz, M., & Pedersen, N. L. (2009). The role of occupational complexity in trajectories of cognitive aging before and after retirement. *Psychology and Aging, 24*(3), 563–573.

Fritsch, T., Debanne, S. M., Smyth, K. A., Petot, G., & Friedland, R. P. (2005). Participation in "novelty seeking" leisure activities and Alzheimer's Disease. *Journals of Geriatric Psychology and Neurology, 18*(3), 134–141.

Gallo, W. T., Teng, H. M., Falba, T. A., Kasl, S. V., Krumholz, H. M., & Bradley, E. H. (2006). The impact of late career job loss on myocardial infarction and stroke: A 10 year follow up using the health and retirement survey. *Occupational and Environmental Medicine, 63*(10), 683–687.

Gensicke, T., Picot, S., & Geiss, S. (Eds.), (2005). *Freiwilliges Engagement in Deutschland: Empirische Studien zum Bürgerschaftlichen Engagement* [Voluntary engagement in Germany: Empirical studies of civil engagement]. Wiesbaden: VS Verlag für Sozialwissenschaften.

Ghisletta, P., Bickel, J.-F., & Lövdén, M. (2006). Does activity engagement protect against cognitive decline in old age? Methodological and analytical considerations. *Journals of Gerontology Series B: Psychological Sciences, 61B*(5), 253–261.

Gobeski, K. T., & Beehr, T. A. (2009). How retirees work: Predictors of different types of bridge employment. *Journal of Organizational Behavior, 30,* 401–425.

Gordon, R. A., & Arvey, R. D. (2004). Age bias in laboratory and field settings: A meta-analytic investigation. *Journal of Applied Social Psychology, 34*(3), 468–492.

Hank, K., & Erlinghagen, M. (2009). Dynamics of volunteering in older Europeans. *The Gerontologist, 50*(2), 170–178.

Hank, K., & Stuck, S. (2008). Volunteer work, informal help, and care among the 50+ in Europe: Further evidence for 'linked' productive activities at older ages. *Social Science Research, 37,* 1280–1291.

Harper, S., Khan, H. T. A., Saxena, A., & Leeson, G. (2006). Attitudes and practices of employers towards ageing workers: Evidence from a global survey on the future of retirement. *Ageing Horizons, 5,* 31–41.

Havighurst, R. J., Neugarten, B. L., & Tobin, S. S. (1968). Disengagement and patterns of aging. In B. L. Neugarten (Ed.), *Middle age and aging: A reader in social psychology* (pp. 223–237). Chicago: University of Chicago Press.

Hedge, J. W., Borman, W. C., & Lammlein, S. E. (2006). *The aging workforce: Realities, myths, and implications for organizations.* Washington, DC: American Psychological Association.

Helson, R., & Roberts, B. W. (1994). Ego development and personality change in adulthood. *Journal of Personality and Social Psychology, 66,* 911–920.

Hertzog, C., Kramer, A. F., Wilson, R. S., & Lindenberger, U. (2009). Enrichment effects on adult cognitive development. *Psychological Science in the Public Interest, 9*(1), 1–65.

Hogan, R., & Roberts, B. W. (2004). A socioanalytic model of maturity. *Journal of Career Assessment, 12,* 207–217.

Huyck, M. H. (1991). Predicates of personal control among middle-aged and young-old men and women in middle America. *International Journal of Human Development, 32*(4), 261–275.

James, J. B., & Spiro, A. (2006). The impact of work on the psychological well-being of older Americans. In J. B. James, & P. Wink (Eds.), *Annual review of gerontology and geriatrics: Vol. 26* (pp. 153–173). New York: Springer.

Kanfer, R., & Ackerman, P. L. (2004). Aging, adult development and work motivation. *Academy of Management Review, 29*(3), 440–458.

Kessler, E.-M., Kruse, A., & Staudinger, U. M. Produktivität durch eine lebenslauforientierte Konzeption von Altern in Unternehmen [Productivity in organizations from a lifespan perspective on aging]. In A. Kruse (Ed.), *Potentiale des Alters.* Akademische Verlagsgesellschaft, Heidelberg, in press.

Kessler, E.-M., & Staudinger, U. M. (2007). Intergenerational potential: Effects of social interaction between older adults and adolescents. *Psychology and Aging, 22*(4), 690–704.

Kim, S., & Feldman, D. C. (2000). Working in retirement: The antecedents of bridge employment and its consequences for quality of life in retirement. *The Academy of Management Journal, 43*(6), 1195–1210.

Kivett, V. R., Watson, J. A., & Busch, J. C. (1977). The relative importance of physical psychological and social variables to locus of control orientation in middle age. *Journals of Gerontology, 32*(2), 203–210.

Kohn, M. L., & Schooler, C. (1973). Occupational experience and psychological functioning: An assessment of reciprocal effects. *American Sociological Review, 34,* 97–118.

Kohn, M. L., & Schooler, C. (1978). The reciprocal effects of the substantive complexity of work and intellectual flexibility: A longitudinal assessment. *American Journal of Sociology, 84,* 24–52.

Kramer, A. F., Bherer, L., Colcombe, S., Dong, W., & Greenough, W. T. (2004). Influence of structured and unstructured environments on cognitive and brain plasticity during aging. *The Journals of Gerontology Series A: Biological Sciences and Medical Sciences, 59,* 940–957.

Kröger, E., Andel, R., Lindsay, J., Benounissa, Z., Verreault, R., & Laurin, D. (2008). Is complexity of work associated with risk of dementia or Alzheimer's disease? The Canadian Study of Health and Aging. *American Journal of Epidemiology, 167,* 820–830.

Lindenberger, U., Kliegl, R., & Baltes, P. B. (1993). Professional expertise does not eliminate negative age differences in imagery-based memory performance during adulthood. *Psychology and Aging, 7,* 585–593.

Loevinger, J. (1997). Stages of personality development. In R. Hogan, J. Johnson, & S. Briggs (Eds.), *Handbook of personality psychology.* San Diego: Academic Press.

Luoh, M.-C., & Herzog, A. R. (2002). Individual consequences of volunteer and paid work in old age: Health and mortality. *Journal of Health and Social Behavior, 43*(4), 490–509.

Maas, I., & Staudinger, U. M. (2009). Lebensverlauf und Altern: Kontinuität und Diskontinuität der gesellschftlichen Beteiligung, des Lebensinvestments und ökonomischer Ressourcen [The lifecourse and aging: Continuity and discontinuity of social pariticipation, life investments and economic resources]. In U. Lindenberg, S. J. K. Mayer, & P. B. Baltes (Eds.), *Die Berliner Altersstudie* (3rd ed.). Berlin: Akademie Verlag.

Maurer, T. M., Weiss, E. M., & Barbeite, F. G. (2003). A model of involvement in work-related learning and development activity: The effects of individual, situational, motivational, and age variables. *Journal of Applied Psychology, 88*(4), 707–724.

Mausner-Dorsch, H., & Eaton, W. W. (2000). Psychosocial work environment and depression: Epidemiologic assessment of the demand-control model. *American Journal of Public Health, 90,* 1765–1770.

McCrae, R. R., Costa, P. T., Lima, M. P., Simoes, A., Ostendorf, F., Anglitner, A., et al. (1999). Age differences in personality across the adult lifespan: Parallels in five cultures. *Developmental Psychology, 35,* 466–477.

Mein, G., Martikainen, P., Hemingway, H., Stansfeld, S., & Marmot, M. (2003). Is retirement good or bad for mental and physical health functioning? Whitehall II longitudinal study of civil servants. *Journal of Epidemiology and Community Health, 57*(1), 46–49.

Mickler, C., & Staudinger, U. M. (2008). Personal wisdom: Validation and age-related differences of a performance measure. *Psychology and Aging, 23*(4), 787–799.

Mikkelsen, A., Saksvik, P. Ö., Eriksen, H., & Ursin, H. (1999). The impact of learning opportunities and decision authority on occupational health. *Work and Stress, 13,* 20–31.

Montenegro, X., Fisher, L., & Remez, S. (2002, September). *Staying ahead of the curve: The AARP work and career study – A national survey conducted for AARP by RogerASW.* Washington, DC: AARP Knowledge Management.

Morrow-Howell, N., Hinterlong, J., Rozario, P. A., & Tang, F. (2003). Effects of volunteering on the well-being of older adults. *Journals of Gerontology: Social Sciences, 58B*(3), 137–145.

Mühlig-Verson, A., & Staudinger, U. M. (2010). Can openness to experience be promoted in older adulthood? Manuscript in preparation.

Nelson, E. A., & Dannefer, D. (1992). Aged heterogeneity: Fact or fiction? The fate of diversity in gerontological research. *The Gerontologist, 32,* 17–23.

Ng, T. W. H., & Feldman, D. C. (2008). The relationship of age to ten dimensions of job performance. *Journal of Applied Psychology, 93*(2), 392–423.

Noack, C. M. G., & Staudinger, U. M. (2010a). *Assessing successful aging workforce management: Organizational age climate.* Manuscript submitted for publication.

Noack, C. M. G., & Staudinger, U. M. (2010b). *Psychological age climate and successful aging in the workplace: Adaptiveness of selection, optimization, and compensation strategy use under constrained external resources.* Unpublished manuscript.

Noack, C. M. G., Baltes, B. B., & Staudinger, U. M. (2010c). Age stereotypes in organizations: Associations with work-related outcomes. Manuscript submitted for publication.

Organisation for Economic Co-operation and Development [OECD] (2009a). *Education at a glance 2008* [Data file]. Paris: OECD. Retrieved January 6, 2010 from ww.oecd.org/edu/eag2008.

OECD. (2009b). *Employment Outlook.* Paris: OECD.

Park, D. C., & Reuter-Lorenz, P. (2009). The adaptive brain: Aging and neuorcognitive scaffolding. *Annual Review of Psychology, 60,* 173–196.

Penner, R. G., Perun, P., & Steuerle, E. (2002). *Legal and institutional impediments to partial retirement and part-time work by older workers.* Washington, DC: Urban Institute.

Pinquart, M., & Schindler, I. (2007). Changes of life satisfaction in the transition to retirement: A latent class approach. *Psychology and Aging, 22*(3), 442–455.

Podsakoff, P. M., MacKenzie, S. B., Paine, J. B., & Bachrach, D. G. (2000). Organizational citizenship behaviors: A critical review of the theoretical and empirical literature and suggestions for future research. *Journal of Management, 26,* 513–563.

Posthuma, R. A., & Campion, M. A. (2009). Age stereotypes in the workplace: Common stereotypes, moderators, and future research directions. *Journal of Management, 35*(1), 158–188.

Potter, G. G., Helms, M. J., & Plassman, B. L. (2007). Associations of job demands and intelligence with cognitive performance among men in late life [Abstract]. *Neurology, 70*(19), 1803–1808.

Reitzes, D. C., Mutran, E. J., & Fernandez, M. E. (1996). Does retirement hurt well-being? Factors influencing self-esteem and depression among retirees and workers. *Gerontologist, 36,* 649–656.

Roberts, B. W., & Mroczek, D. (2008). Personality trait change in adulthood. *Current Directions in Psychological Science, 17*(1), 3135.

Roberts, B. W., & Robins, R. W. (2004). A longitudinal study of person-environment fit and personality development. *Journal of Personality, 72,* 89–110.

Roberts, B. W., Walton, K. E., & Viechtbauer, W. (2006a). Patterns of mean-level change in personality traits across the life course: A meta-analysis of longitudinal studies. *Psychological Bulletin, 132*(1), 1–25.

Roberts, B. W. (1997). Plaster or plasticity: Are adult work experiences associated with personality change in women? *Journal of Personality, 65*(2), 205–232.

Roberts, B. W., & Chapman, C. N. (2000). Change in dispositional well-being and its relation to role quality: A 30-year longitudinal study. *Journal of Research in Personality, 34,* 26–41.

Roberts, B. W., Caspi, A., & Moffitt, T. E. (2003). Work experiences and personality development in young adulthood. *Journal of Personality and Social Psychology, 84*(3), 582–593.

Roberts, B. W., Walton, K. E., Bogg, T., & Caspi, A. (2006b). De-investment in work and non-normative personality trait change in young adulthood. *European Journal of Personality, 20,* 461–474.

Roberts, B. W., Wood, D., & Smith, J. L. (2005). Examining five-factor theory and social investment perspectives on personality trait development. *Journal of Research in Personality, 39,* 166–184.

Rosenmayr, L. (1983). *Die späte Freiheit: Das Alter – ein Stück bewußt gelebten Lebens* [Late freedom: Old age – a period of deliberately lived life]. Berlin: Severin & Siedler.

Ryff, C. D., & Essex, M. J. (1992). The interpretation of life experience and well-being: The sample case of relocation. *Psychology and Aging, 7*, 507–517.

Salthouse, T. A. (2006). Mental exercise and mental aging: Evaluating the validity of the 'Use It or Lose It' hypothesis. *Perspectives on Psychological Science, 1*(1), 68–87.

Salthouse, T. A. (1991). *Theoretical perspectives on cognitive aging.* Hillsdale, NJ: Erlbaum.

Schooler, C., Mulatu, M. S., & Oates, G. (2004). Occupational self-direction, intellectual functioning, and self-directed orientation in older workers: Findings and implications for individuals and societies. *American Journal of Sociology, 110*(1), 161–197.

Scollon, C. N., & Diener, E. (2006). Love, work, and changes in extraversion and neuroticism over time. *Journal of Personality and Social Psychology, 91*(6), 1152–1165.

Shultz, K. S. (2003). Bridge employment: Work after retirement. In G. A. Adams & T. A. Beehr (Eds.), *Retirement: Reasons, processes, and results* (pp. 214–241). New York: Springer.

Skirbekk, V. (2008). Age and productivity capacity: Descriptions, causes and policy options. *Ageing Horizons, 8*, 4–12.

Slingerland, A. S., van Lenthe, F. J., Jukema, J. W., Kamphuis, C. B. M., Looman, C., Giskes, K., et al. (2007). Aging, retirement, and changes in physical activity: Prospective cohort findings from the GLOBE study. *American Journal of Epidemiology, 165*(12), 1356–1363.

Smith, J., Staudinger, U. M., & Baltes, P. B. (1994). Occupational settings facilitating wisdom-related knowledge: The sample case of clinical psychologists. *Journal of Consulting and Clinical Psychology, 62*, 989–999.

Staudinger, U. M., & Bowen, C. E. (2010). Lifespan perspectives on positive personality development. In A. Freund & M. Lamb (Eds.), *Handbook of lifespan development.* Volume II, Hoboken, NJ: John Wiley & Sons, Ltd.

Staudinger, U. M., & Kessler, E.-M. (2009). Adjustment and growth: Two trajectories of positive personality development across adulthood. In M. C. Smith & N. DeFrates-Densch (Eds.), *Handbook of research on adult learning and development* (pp. 241–268). New York and London: Routledge.

Staudinger, U. M., & Kocha, J. (2010). Aging in Germany English Edition (2010). More Years, More Life. Translation of the Recommendations of the Joint Academy Initiative on Aging "Genomene Jahre". (Altern in Deutschland Bd. 9) Nova Acta Leopoldina N.F.Bd. 107, Nr. 371. Stuttgart: Wissenschaftliche Verlagsgesellschaft.

Staudinger, U. M. (1996). Psychologische Produktivität und Selbstentfaltung im Alter [Psychological productivity and self-development in old age]. In M. M. Baltes & L. Montada (Eds.), *Produktivität und Altern [Productivity and old age]* (pp. 344–373). Hamburg: Campus Verlag.

Staudinger, U. M. (2007). Dynamisches Personal-management als eine Antwort auf den demographischen Wandel [Dynamic personnel management as an answer to demographic change]. In *Demographischer Wandel als unternehmerische Herausforderung [Demographic change as an organizational challenge].* Report from the 60th German Conference on Business Administration (pp. 35–48). Stuttgart: Schäffer-Poeschel.

Staudinger, U. M. (2008). Produktives Leben im Alter [Productive living in advanced age]. In F. Petermann, & W. Schneider (Eds.), *Enzyklopädie der Psychologie [Encyclopedia of Psychology]: Vol. 7* (pp. 885–915). Göttingen: Hogrefe.

Staudinger, U. M., & Kunzmann, U. (2005). Positive adult personality development: Adjustment and/or growth? *European Psychologist, 10*(4), 320–329.

Staudinger, U. M., Dörner, J., & Mickler, C. (2005). Wisdom and Personality. In R. Sternberg & J. Jordan (Eds.), *Handbook of wisdom.* New York: Cambridge University Press.

Staudinger, U. M., Kessler, E.-M., & Dörner, J. (2006). Wisdom in social context. In K. W. Schaie & L. Carstensen (Eds.), *Social Structures, aging, and self-regulation in the elderly* (pp. 33–54). New York: Springer.

Staudinger, U. M., Roßnagel, C., & Voelpel, S. (2008). Strategische Personalentwicklung und demographischer Wandel: Eine interdisziplinäre Perspektive [Strategic personnel development and demographic development: An interdisciplinary perspective]. In K. Schwuchow & J. Gutmann (Eds.), *Jahrbuch Personalentwicklung 2008 - Ausbildung, Weiterbildung, Management Development* [Yearbook of Personnel Development 2008: Education, Further training and Mangement Development] (pp. 295–304). München: Luchterhand.

Staudinger, U. M., Smith, J., & Baltes, P. B. (1992). Wisdom-related knowledge in a life review task: Age differences and the role of professional specialization. *Psychology and Aging, 7*, 271–281.

Staudinger, U. M. (2005). Personality and aging. In M. Johnson, V. L. Bengtson, P. G. Coleman, & T. Kirkwood (Eds.), *Handbook of age and ageing* (pp. 237–244). Cambridge, UK: Cambridge University Press.

Sternberg, R. J. (1985). Human intelligence: The model is the message. *Science, 230*, 1111–1118.

Van Praag, H., Kempermann, G., & Gage, F. H. (2000). Neural consequences of environmental enrichment. *Nature Reviews Neuroscience, 1*, 191–198.

Van Solinge, H. (2007). Health change in retirement. A longitudinal study among older workers in the Netherlands. *Research on Aging, 29*(3), 225–256.

Wang, M., Zhan, Y., Liu, S., & Shultz, K. S. (2008). Antecedents of bridge employment: A longitudinal investigation. *Journal of Applied Psychology, 93*(4), 818–830.

Warr, P. (2001). Age and work behavior: Physical attributes, cognitive abilities, knowledge, personality traits and motives. *International Review of Industrial and Organizational Psychology, 16*, 1–36.

Wickrama, K. A. S., Lorenz, F. O., Fang, S. A., Abraham, W. T., & Elder, G. H., Jr. (2005). Gendered trajectories of work control and health outcomes in the middle years: A perspective from the rural Midwest. *Journal of Health and Social Behavior, 38*, 363–375.

Wickrama, K. A. S., Surjadi, F. F., Lorenz, F. O., & Elder, G. H., Jr. (2008). The influence of work control trajectories on men's mental and physical health during the middle years: Mediatrional role of personal control. *Journals of Gerontology: Social Sciences, 63B*, 135–145.

Wight, R. G., Aneshensel, C. S., & Seeman, T. E. (2002). Educational attainment, continued learning experience, and cognitive functioning among older men. *Journal of Aging and Health, 14*, 211–236.

Wooden, M. W., VandenHeuvel, A., Cully, M., & Curtain, R. (2001). Barriers to training for older workers and possible policy solutions. Report for the National Institute of Labour Studies, Australia. Accessed February 11, 2010 from http://www.dest.gov.au/archive/iae/documents/olderworkers/olderworkers.htm.

Wurm, S., Engstler, H., & Tesch-Römer, C. (2009). Ruhestand und Gesundheit [Retirement and health]. In K. Kochsiek (Ed.), *Altern und Gesundheit* (Altern in Deutschland Bd. 7). Nova Acta Leopoldina NF Bd. 105, Nr. 363. Stuttgart: Wissenschaftliche Verlagsanstalt.

Zwick, T. (2002). Training and firm productivity: Panel evidence for Germany (Research Paper No. 23). Oxford: ESRC Centre on Skills, Knowledge and Organisational Performance (SKOPE). Retrieved January 5, 2009, from ftp://ftp.zew.de/pub/zew-docs/dp/dpskope.pdf.

Chapter | 18 |

Wisdom, Age, and Well-Being

Monika Ardelt
Department of Sociology and Criminology & Law, University of Florida, Gainesville, Florida, USA

CHAPTER CONTENTS

Introduction 279
Definition of an Elusive Concept 279
Western Definitions of Wisdom 280
Western Implicit Wisdom Theories 280
Western Explicit Wisdom Theories 280
Eastern Definitions of Wisdom 281
Eastern Implicit Wisdom Theories 281
Eastern Explicit Wisdom Theories 282
Culturally Inclusive Explicit Definitions of Wisdom 282
Aging and Wisdom 282
Hypothetical Associations between Age and Wisdom 282
Empirical Associations between Age and Wisdom 283
Wisdom and Well-Being 285
Summary and Future Directions of Wisdom Research 287
References 288

INTRODUCTION

Do people grow wiser with age and what are the benefits of wisdom in the later years of life? Are wise older people more content and better able to cope with the adversities of old age than elders who failed to grow wiser with age? How exactly does wisdom develop and which factors foster or thwart the emergence of later life wisdom? Those are some of the questions wisdom researchers have tried to answer during the past three decades, starting with the most important question about the essential elements and characteristics of wisdom.

DEFINITION OF AN ELUSIVE CONCEPT

What exactly is wisdom? Wisdom appears to be a virtue that is valued highly by most, although it is possible that the meaning of wisdom varies from person to person. In fact, since antiquity, philosophers have tried to define this elusive concept. For example, the ancient Greek philosopher Plato (428–348 BC), a student of Socrates (470–399 BC), defined wisdom as an understanding of the physical and social world and the ultimate meaning of life. In the Platonic dialogues, wisdom can refer to *sophia,* the pursuit of timeless and universal truths through contemplation; *phronesis* or practical wisdom, prudent actions that resist the desires of the passions and the deception of the senses; or *episteme,* knowledge of the nature of things and the underlying principles governing their relationships (Robinson, 1990). The development of wisdom was thought to require rational thinking, sustained reflection on experiences, and deliberate efforts to overcome subjectivity (sensory distortions) and prejudices (Osbeck & Robinson, 2005). Plato and his student Aristotle (384–322 BC) regarded wisdom as one of the most basic human virtues (Birren & Svensson, 2005). According to Aristotle, wisdom requires self-knowledge and self-insight and leads to "… *eudaimonia,* that condition of flourishing and completeness that constitutes true and enduring joy" (Robinson, 1990, p. 16).

The attempt to define wisdom continues until this day (see, for example, the *Defining Wisdom Project* of the University of Chicago http://wisdomresearch.org/). Most contemporary wisdom researchers differentiate between lay people's definitions of wisdom (implicit wisdom theories) and wisdom researchers' definitions of wisdom (explicit wisdom theories). Furthermore, Western definitions of wisdom can differ from

DOI: 10.1016/B978-0-12-380882-0.00018-8

Eastern wisdom definitions (Sternberg & Jordan, 2005). However, all definitions describe wisdom as a multifaceted construct consisting of a variation of the following elements: cognitive ability and insight, reflectivity, compassionate concern for the welfare of others, and equanimity.

WESTERN DEFINITIONS OF WISDOM

Many of the earlier contemporary empirical wisdom research consisted of studies that attempted to summarize and synthesize laypeople's implicit theories of wisdom (Clayton & Birren, 1980; Holliday & Chandler, 1986; Sternberg, 1985). Parallel to this effort, however, other researchers developed their own explicit wisdom theories (Kekes, 1983; Sternberg, 1990). Most prominent was probably the research group at the Max Planck Institute of Berlin, led by Paul Baltes, which defined wisdom as expert knowledge related to life planning, life management, and life review (Baltes & Smith, 1990; Baltes et al., 1990; Smith et al., 1989).

Western Implicit Wisdom Theories

In their groundbreaking research on wisdom, Clayton and Birren (1980) asked young (M = 21 years), middle-aged (M = 49 years), and older (M = 70 years) adults to rate the similarity of the words "wise," "aged," "myself," and 12 wisdom characteristics generated from an earlier study. A multidimensional scaling analysis of the similarities between all nonredundant word pairs resulted in three dimensions, indicating that participants perceived wisdom as an integration of cognitive ability (knowledgeable, experienced, intelligent, pragmatic, and observant), reflectivity (introspective and intuitive), and compassionate concern for others and equanimity (understanding, empathetic, peaceful, and gentle). Another interesting finding was that older participants did not perceive a closer similarity between the word pairs "myself" and "wise" than the middle-aged and younger participants, but middle-aged and younger participants rated the similarity between "wise" and the words "aged" and "experienced" as closer than older participants. This suggests that older participants did not feel wiser than younger participants and also might have had some doubt that wisdom can be gained with age and experience. Instead, they placed the words "understanding" and "empathetic" closer to "wise" than the younger study participants, emphasizing the importance of a compassionate concern for others in wisdom.

A slightly different but similar approach was used by Holliday and Chandler (1986) to elicit the implicit wisdom theories of young (M = 22 years), middle-aged (M = 43 years), and older adults (M = 70 years). They first asked participants in those three age groups to describe wisdom, yielding 79 distinct wisdom attributes. Another group of young (M = 22 years), middle-aged (M = 42 years), and older adults (M = 71 years) then rated the salience of those attributes for prototypical wise people on a scale ranging from 1 (almost never true of wise people) to 7 (almost always true of wise people). There was substantial inter-rater agreement within each age cohort and between age cohorts on the characteristics of prototypical wise people. A subsequent principal component analysis of the 79 ratings produced five factors, consisting of two primarily reflective factors (e.g., has learned from experience, sees things within a larger context, observant/perceptive, considers all options in a situation, reflective), a predominantly cognitive factor (e.g., understands/evaluates information, well-read, intelligent, knowledgeable), and two factors combining compassionate concern for others with equanimity (e.g., fair, a good listener, patient, nonjudgmental, quiet).

Sternberg (1985) also asked laypersons and professors in various fields to give a description of the ideal wise person in general or in their respective profession. The obtained wisdom descriptors were subsequently given to a second group of laypersons and professor who rated them on a scale ranging from 1 (behavior extremely uncharacteristic for a wise person in general/in my profession) to 9 (behavior extremely characteristic). The average ratings of the wisdom descriptors did not differ significantly between laypersons and the various occupations. The 40 highest ranked wisdom descriptors were then sorted by college students into similarity piles. A non-metric multidimensional scaling analysis of these arrangements indicated six wisdom dimensions, with one dimension describing cognitive abilities (e.g., has the unique ability to look at a problem or situation and solve it, has a logical mind, is good at distinguishing between correct and incorrect answers), one dimension referring to reflectivity and concern for others (e.g., listens to all sides of an issue, considers advice, displays concern for others, is fair), and the remaining four dimensions consisting of a combination of cognitive abilities, insight, and reflectivity (e.g., can offer solutions that are on the side of right and truth, is able to see through things — read between the lines, learns from other people's mistakes, changes mind on basis of experience, has good judgment at all times).

Taken together, studies on implicit wisdom theories suggest that people in the West define wisdom as a combination of cognitive ability, insight, reflective attitude, compassionate concern for others, and equanimity (Bluck & Glück, 2005).

Western Explicit Wisdom Theories

In comparison to implicit wisdom theories of laypeople, explicit wisdom theories of wisdom researchers seem to vary to a greater degree. At one end of the spectrum, wisdom is primarily defined as a cognitive construct with special emphasis on the knowledge that wisdom conveys in order to lead a life that is good for oneself, others, and society as a whole. For example, the *Berlin Wisdom Paradigm* describes wisdom as knowledge and expertise in life planning, life management, and life review and in the meaning and conduct of life (Baltes & Staudinger, 2000; Staudinger, 1999; Staudinger et al.,1998). Sternberg's (1998) balance theory of wisdom similarly states that wisdom is applied tacit knowledge, mediated by values, to achieve a common good by balancing intrapersonal, interpersonal, and extrapersonal interests. For Brugman (2000), wisdom is knowledge and expertise in coping with the cognitive, emotional, and behavioral aspects of uncertainty that life inherently entails. Meacham (1990), however, cautioned that too much knowledge might actually lead to a loss of wisdom due to overconfidence and, therefore, needs to be counterbalanced by doubting to result in wisdom.

Other wisdom researchers focus more on the reflective element of wisdom. For example, according to Kekes (1983), descriptive knowledge is insufficient for wisdom to emerge. Descriptive knowledge gives information about facts (e.g., all humans are mortal), but wisdom is the reflective understanding of the deeper meaning of descriptive knowledge for one's own life (e.g., What does aging and mortality mean in the context of my own life?). Similarly, McKee and Barber (1999) defined wisdom as seeing through the illusion of superficial knowledge or beliefs by reflecting on the deeper meaning of things to perceive reality as it truly is.

A third group of wisdom researchers emphasizes the transformational aspects of wisdom. For example, Achenbaum and Orwoll (1991) define wisdom as the transformation of intrapersonal, interpersonal, and transpersonal experiences in the domains of cognition, personality, and conation. This results in self-knowledge (intrapersonal), understanding (interpersonal), and the recognition of the limits of knowledge and understanding (transpersonal) in the cognitive domain, self-development (intrapersonal), empathy (interpersonal), and self-transcendence (transpersonal) in the personality domain, and integrity (intrapersonal), mature relationships (interpersonal), and philosophical/spiritual commitments (transpersonal) in the conative domain. For Levenson et al. (2005), wisdom is equivalent to self-transcendence, which arises through a process leading from self-knowledge and detachment from external definitions of the self to an increased sense of connectedness with past and future generations, similar to the process of gerotranscendence in old age (Tornstam, 2005).

Although there is still no general agreement among wisdom researchers about what the essential characteristics of wisdom are (Ardelt, 2004; Ardelt & Jacobs, 2009; Baltes & Smith, 2008), many concur that wisdom is a multidimensional construct that contains cognitive, reflective, interpersonal, and conative components (Ardelt, 2000b; Blanchard-Fields & Norris, 1995; Clayton & Birren, 1980; Kekes, 1995; Sternberg, 1990; Sternberg & Jordan, 2005; Takahashi & Overton, 2002).

EASTERN DEFINITIONS OF WISDOM

Eastern definitions of wisdom are not completely different from Western wisdom definitions, but the relative importance of the various dimensions and aspects of wisdom tend to differ between Western and Eastern approaches.

Eastern Implicit Wisdom Theories

Unlike studies on Western implicit theories of wisdom, research on Eastern implicit wisdom theories is relatively rare. However, studies generally find that Eastern laypersons tend to emphasize the interpersonal element of wisdom more than Western laypersons (Takahashi & Overton, 2005). For example, in Takahashi and Bordia's (2000) multidimensional scaling analysis, Indian and Japanese undergraduate students tended to rate the word "wise" as more similar to "discreet" than to "experienced" and "knowledgeable." By contrast, American and Australian students tended to rate "wise" to be most similar to "experienced" and "knowledgeable." Furthermore, Western and Indian students ranked "wise" and "knowledgeable" as the most desirable characteristics of an ideal self, whereas Japanese students ranked "wise" and "discreet" as the most desirable characteristics. Yang (2001) asked Taiwanese Chinese adults from various age groups to rate the salience of 100 behavioral attributes of "a wise person." An explorative factor analysis revealed that the Taiwanese Chinese respondents tended to perceive wisdom as a combination of cognitive ability (competencies and knowledge), reflectivity (openness and profundity), and compassionate concern for others (benevolence and compassion) together with modesty and unobtrusiveness.

Hence, similar to Western implicit wisdom theories, Eastern implicit theories also emphasize that wisdom is a multifaceted construct consisting of cognitive ability and insight, reflectivity, and compassionate concern for others. Yet, in contrast to Western implicit wisdom theories, laypersons in the East also appear to give equal importance to social unobtrusiveness in their definitions of wisdom.

Eastern Explicit Wisdom Theories

There are almost no Eastern explicit theories of wisdom in the contemporary wisdom literature. An exception is Jeste and Vahia's (2008) explicit wisdom theory, which is derived from a content analysis of the Bhagavad-Gita, a sacred ancient text of Hindu philosophy. Based on the Bhagavad-Gita, Jeste and Vahia define wisdom as knowledge of life, emotional regulation, control over desires, decisiveness, love of God, duty and work, self-contentedness, yoga or integration of personality, compassion/sacrifice, and insight/humility.

CULTURALLY INCLUSIVE EXPLICIT DEFINITIONS OF WISDOM

Takahashi and Overton (2005) suggested that wisdom definitions should avoid cultural egocentrism and instead consist of the broadest and most culturally inclusive descriptions of this concept. To this end, Takahashi and Overton (2002) defined wisdom as a combination of two wisdom modes: the cognitive analytical mode (knowledge database and abstract reasoning abilities), which is dominant in Western wisdom theories, and the reflective and compassionate synthetic mode (reflective understanding, emotional empathy, and emotional regulation), which is prominent in Eastern wisdom theories.

Guided by Clayton and Birren's (1980) studies on Western implicit wisdom theories, I define wisdom as an integration of cognitive, reflective, and affective (compassionate) characteristics (Ardelt, 1997, 2000b, 2003, 2004; Ardelt & Jacobs, 2009). The *cognitive dimension* in this three-dimensional wisdom model refers to a desire to know the truth and to reach a deep and thorough understanding of life, with particular emphasis on its intra- and interpersonal aspects (Ardelt, 2000b; Blanchard-Fields & Norris, 1995; Kekes, 1983; Osbeck & Robinson, 2005). This necessitates a knowledge and acceptance of the positive and negative aspects of human nature, of the inherent limits of knowledge, and of life's unpredictability and uncertainty. To obtain such insight into life and the human condition requires reflective thinking to "see through illusion" (McKee & Barber, 1999) and transcend one's subjectivity and projections, which is the tendency to blame other people and circumstances for one's own faults and failures (Bradley, 1978; Sherwood, 1981). Hence, the *reflective wisdom dimension* describes the ability to perceive phenomena and events from multiple perspectives and to engage in self-examination to develop self-awareness and self-insight. Individuals who have overcome their subjectivity and projections are more likely to take responsibility for their actions and also can see reality more clearly, which allows them to acknowledge their own faults and weaknesses. This is likely to make them more humble, decrease their self-centeredness, and increase their understanding of life in general and the human condition in particular (Csikszentmihalyi & Rathunde, 1990; Kekes, 1995; Levitt, 1999; Taranto, 1989). A reduced self-centeredness, in turn, tends to result in compassionate love and concern for the welfare of others, which defines the *affective dimension of wisdom* (Achenbaum & Orwoll, 1991; Clayton & Birren, 1980; Csikszentmihalyi & Rathunde, 1990; Holliday & Chandler, 1986; Kramer, 1990; Levitt, 1999; Orwoll & Achenbaum, 1993). This conceptualization of wisdom as an integration of cognitive, reflective, and affective dimensions has the advantage of being relatively parsimonious, while preserving the major elements of both Western and Eastern implicit and explicit wisdom theories (Blanchard-Fields & Norris, 1995; Levitt, 1999; Sternberg, 1990; Sternberg & Jordan, 2005; Takahashi & Bordia, 2000).

AGING AND WISDOM

What is the relation between age and wisdom? Do people grow wiser with age, stay the same after adolescence, or even decrease in wisdom after childhood due to the vicissitudes of life? To answer those questions, the theoretical literature on age and wisdom will first be reviewed before presenting the existing empirical evidence.

Hypothetical Associations between Age and Wisdom

Sternberg (2005) described five generalized views or hypothetical models that might explain the relation between age and wisdom. First, according to the "received" view, wisdom develops in old age after a spiritual awakening or reawakening. In Erikson's stage model of human development (Erikson, 1963, 1982; Erikson et al., 1986), wisdom is the virtue that results from the successful resolution of the last developmental crisis, integrity versus despair, which consists of reconciliation with one's past and the acceptance of the finitude of life. Retired adults might also have more time than adults with demanding occupations and dependent children to engage in reflective activities, such as contemplation and self-examination, which foster self-knowledge and self-insight and might lead to a deeper understanding of life, greater sympathy and compassion for others, and an acceptance of the inevitable losses of old age, including death (Ardelt, 2000b; Moody, 1986). Second, similar to "fluid intelligence" or the ability to process new information efficiently and apply knowledge in novel ways, wisdom might increase during adolescence and young adulthood, remain relatively stable during early and middle adulthood, and start to decline in late middle adulthood. Third, wisdom might follow the trajectory of "crystallized intelligence" or accumulated knowledge and skills, steadily increasing with age until the end of life or until disease processes impede its growth. Fourth, wisdom might increase until middle or late middle adulthood similar to crystallized intelligence but decrease in the later years of life due to a decline in fluid intelligence that cannot be counterbalanced by a growth in crystallized intelligence. Fifth, wisdom might continually deteriorate with age due to the vicissitudes of life and the resulting imbalance between certainty and uncertainty, which might either lead to self-centered overconfidence or a self-defeating loss of meaning (Meacham, 1990).

Except for the view that wisdom is "received" in old age through a spiritual (re-)awakening, all other models presume that wisdom starts to develop during the early years of life. Richardson and Pasupathi (2005) speculated that an increase in wisdom during adolescence and young adulthood might be due to normative intellectual and personality development. Intellectual development leads to greater cognitive abilities, such as abstract reasoning and reflective thinking (Piaget, 1952), and it is during adolescence and young adulthood that the accumulated stock of crystallized knowledge is transmitted to the next generation through formal and informal educational training (Ardelt, 2004). Furthermore, personality development during adolescence and young adulthood entails greater openness to new experiences (Caspi et al., 2005; McCrae et al., 2002), the recognition and acceptance of uncertainty (Sorrentino et al., 1990), perspective taking and moral reasoning (Colby et al., 1994; Gurucharri & Selman, 1982), and ego-development (Cohn, 1998; Loevinger, 1998; Loevinger et al., 1985). However, because most adolescents have not yet reached a mature understanding of life and others, it is possible that only knowledge related to wisdom but not wise behavior or wisdom per se accumulates during the early years of life (Richardson & Pasupathi, 2005).

Theoretical models on the presumed association between age and wisdom tend to ignore the variations in individuals' paths to wisdom across the life course (Sternberg, 2005). Wisdom researchers generally agree that growth in wisdom in adulthood is unlikely to be normative (Ardelt, 1997; Assmann, 1994; Jordan, 2005; Staudinger, 1999). Rather, wisdom might develop differently for different people, increasing for some, remaining stable for others, and even declining under certain circumstances. Not age by itself but social conditions, family relationships, educational opportunities, career paths, specific life experiences, individual motivations, and habits of approaching the world are likely to promote or thwart the attainment of wisdom across the life course (Ardelt & Jacobs, 2009; Baltes & Staudinger, 2000). For example, openness to experience and the ability to reflect on experience might be essential prerequisites for the acquisition of wisdom (Csikszentmihalyi & Nakamura, 2005).

Yet, if the development of wisdom requires the right motivation and effort, the association between age and wisdom should at least *potentially* be positive, particularly for individuals who have dedicated their lives to the pursuit of wisdom, are willing and capable to learn from the experiences in their lives, and become more mature and integrated in the process (Ardelt, 2004; Kramer, 1990; Taranto, 1989). As Kekes (1983, p. 286) succinctly argued, "one can be old and foolish, but a wise man is likely to be old, simply because such growth takes time."

Empirical Associations between Age and Wisdom

Which of the theoretical models on the association between age and wisdom is supported by empirical research? Not surprisingly, the answer depends to some degree on the definition, operationalization, and measurement of this elusive concept.

The Berlin Wisdom Paradigm assesses wisdom by asking participants to "think aloud" about hypothetical life problems in the area of life review, life planning, or life management (Baltes & Staudinger, 2000; Smith & Baltes, 1990). The transcribed responses are then rated by independent coders on five criteria that assess the cognitive expertise and knowledge aspects of wisdom regarding judgment and advice about fundamental life matters: rich factual knowledge, rich procedural and strategic knowledge, knowledge about the contexts of life and how these change over time, knowledge that considers the relativism of values and life goals, and knowledge about the fundamental uncertainties of life and the management of uncertainty (Baltes & Smith, 2008). Wisdom, or more precisely general wisdom-related knowledge, is measured as the average of the five wisdom criteria (Kunzmann & Baltes, 2005).

In cross-sectional studies, general wisdom-related knowledge was positively related to age in adolescence and young adulthood up to the age of about 24 years but then remained stable with a suggested decline after the age of 80 (Baltes et al., 1995; Pasupathi et al., 2001; Staudinger, 1999). Similarly, older clinical psychologists between 65 and 82 years of age did not tend to receive significantly higher ratings on the wisdom tasks than younger clinical psychologists between 25 and 37 years of age (Smith et al., 1994; Staudinger et al., 1992). Yet, age was positively, albeit weakly, correlated with wisdom-related knowledge for participants between the ages of 20 and 87 who scored above the median level on moral reasoning (Kohlberg & Puka, 1994), whereas it was unrelated to wisdom-related knowledge for participants below the median level on moral reasoning (Pasupathi & Staudinger, 2001). Hence, the pathway to wisdom-related knowledge appears to follow Sternberg's (2005) "fluid intelligence" view for the general population and the crystallized intelligence view for individuals with a possibly greater motivation to develop wisdom as indicated by superior performances on moral reasoning tasks.

Not only general wisdom-related knowledge but also expertise in uncertainty (acknowledgement of uncertainty, emotional stability despite uncertainty, and the ability to act in the face of uncertainty) as assessed by Brugman's (2000) Epistemic Cognition Questionnaire (ECQ15) was unrelated to age in adulthood. There were no significant differences in ECQ15 scores between groups of young (20 to 36 years; $M = 23$ years), middle-aged (44 to 54 years; $M = 50$ years), and older (64 to 93 years; $M = 77$ years) participants.

Similarly, the non-cognitive components of wisdom, such as critical life experiences, reflectiveness/reminiscence, emotional regulation, openness to experience, and humor, as measured by Webster's (2003, 2007) Self-Assessed Wisdom Scale (SAWS) appear to be unrelated to age. Age was not significantly correlated with the SAWS in a study of adults between the ages of 22 and 78 ($M = 53$ years) and a later study of participants between the ages of 17 and 92 ($M = 43$ years). This is somewhat surprising because research has shown that critical life experiences, an inclination for reminiscence and life review, emotional regulation, and the use of humor to cope with life events tend to increase with age (Blanchard-Fields, 2009; Charles & Carstensen, 2010; Glück et al., 2005; Thorson & Powell, 1996), although openness to experience tends to decline in later life (Caspi et al., 2005).

Similarly, age was unrelated to the transformational aspect of wisdom, as measured by Levenson et al's. (2005) Adult Self-Transcendence Inventory (ASTI), in a sample of adults ranging in age from 18 to 73 years ($M = 34$ years). Even though the transcendence of the self probably takes a long time, only few individuals might be motivated and willing to engage in this process, which could explain the absence of an age effect (Staudinger & Kunzmann, 2005).

Yet, a different developmental trajectory might exist for other measures of wisdom. Takahashi and Overton (2002) assessed wisdom as a combination of knowledge database and abstract reasoning ability (the cognitive analytic wisdom mode) and reflective understanding, emotional empathy, and emotional regulation (the reflective and compassionate synthetic wisdom mode). Both older American adults and Japanese adults ($M = 70$ years) tended to score significantly higher on those wisdom components (except for emotional regulation) than did middle-aged adults ($M = 45$ years). A study comparing current undergraduate college students (mean age category = 21 years) with older adults ranging in age from 52 to 87 years ($M = 71$ years) revealed that college-educated older adults tended to score significantly higher on a self-administered Three-Dimensional Wisdom Scale (3D-WS), which measured the cognitive, reflective, and affective (compassionate) dimensions of wisdom (Ardelt, 2003), than current college students. However, older adults without a college degree had significantly lower average scores on the 3D-WS than either younger or older college-educated adults, suggesting that age alone cannot explain the emergence of wisdom (Ardelt, in press). Those studies support the crystallized intelligence view and even the "received" view, particularly for those individuals who have the opportunity, support, and motivation to acquire wisdom, as indicated, for example, by the attainment of a higher educational degree, openness to experience, and the desire to grow psychologically. In fact, prior longitudinal studies have shown that socioeconomic status, openness to experience, and psychological mindedness in early adulthood were positively related to wisdom in the later years of life (Ardelt, 1998; Wink & Dillon, 2003; Wink & Helson, 1997).

Because cross-sectional studies cannot distinguish between age, period, and cohort effects, they are not sufficient to reveal the relation between age and wisdom. Unfortunately, longitudinal research that investigates growth in wisdom over time is exceedingly rare. However, a longitudinal study following the development of wisdom-related performance in regard to the reflective recognition and understanding of the limits and uncertainty of human knowledge as measured by the Reflective Judgment Interview (RJI) showed that average scores on the RJI tended to increase from age 16 to 20 and from age 20 to 24. From age 28 to 32, increases in RJI scores occurred only for a minority of respondents, but many of the highly educated study participants already scored at or near the top of the RJI scale at the age of 28 (Kitchener & Brenner, 1990; Kitchener et al., 1989). Yet, longitudinal research by Wink and Helson (1997) found that practical wisdom (measured by self-reported cognitive, reflective, and mature adjectives from the Adjective Check List) tended to increase also later in life, from age 27 to age 52, and that those increases were on average even more profound for clinical psychologists who might have had a stronger motivation to develop psychologically and grow in wisdom, supporting the crystallized intelligence view of aging and wisdom.

The majority of the empirical research seems to suggest that wisdom does indeed increase with age in adolescence and early adulthood. Yet in adulthood, its development appears to be facilitated by favorable social conditions, educational opportunities, and a motivation to grow in wisdom. If this is the case, could interventions be implemented that might make people wiser? Staudinger and Baltes (1996) found that giving study participants the opportunity to reflect on a hypothetical life problem before responding to it, by either discussing the problem with a significant other and then thinking about it or by having imaginary conversations about the problem with persons whose opinion they valued, significantly increased their wisdom-related knowledge compared to the standard condition of no reflection. This increase in wisdom-related knowledge was even more pronounced among older adults (45 to 70 years; $M = 57$ years) than among younger participants (20 to 44 years; $M = 30$ years). Similarly, asking younger (20 to 31 years; $M = 25$ years) and older (59 to 71 years; $M = 64$ years) participants to visualize how people in different parts of the world live and solve certain life problems before the wisdom tasks were presented tended to have a positive effect on wisdom-related knowledge related to the relativism of values and life goals and the contexts of life for both age groups (Böhmig-Krumhaar et al., 2002). Those interventions suggest that wisdom-related knowledge can be increased when people are encouraged to perceive a life problem from multiple perspectives and thereby activate the reflective component of wisdom.

Finally, intergenerational volunteer programs that train older adults to serve as mentors and tutors for elementary school children might not only stimulate and promote the wisdom of elders through a reflection on prior knowledge and experience, an enhancement of interpersonal and intergenerational skills, and a concern for the welfare of future generations, but also foster wisdom development in children by providing them with wise role models (Parisi et al., 2009).

WISDOM AND WELL-BEING

What are the benefits of being wise in adulthood and old age? In general, wisdom researchers believe that the wise know "the art of living" or how to live a life that is good for oneself, good for others, and good for the whole society (Baltes & Staudinger, 2000; Csikszentmihalyi & Nakamura, 2005; Kekes, 1995; Kramer, 2000; Kupperman, 2005; Sternberg, 1998). Hence, wise individuals should feel in control of their lives, be satisfied and content, and give back to society (Ardelt, 2000b; Assmann, 1994; Bianchi, 1994; Clayton, 1982; Erikson, 1982; Vaillant, 2002). Moreover, as Csikszentmihalyi and Nakamura (2005) argue, the pursuit and attainment of wisdom might be intrinsically rewarding and accompanied by feelings of joy and serenity through the transcendence of self-centeredness. However, it might also be that wisdom has its price by increasing awareness of the vicissitudes of life and the negative aspects of human nature, which might have a deteriorating impact on life satisfaction (Staudinger et al., 2005).

The empirical evidence is again mixed, depending on the definition, operationalization, and measurement of wisdom and the characteristics of the sample. It appears that studies, which operationalize wisdom in primarily cognitive terms and/or use samples of highly privileged individuals, are less likely to find a significant association between wisdom and well-being than studies that assess wisdom as a combination of cognition, reflection, and compassionate concern for others in more diverse samples. For example, in a sample of German adults between the ages of 19 and 87 years ($M = 45$ years), cognitive wisdom-related knowledge, as measured by the Berlin Wisdom Paradigm, was unrelated to indicators of psychological well-being from the Ryff Inventory of Psychological Well-Being (Ryff, 1989), such as autonomy, environmental mastery, positive relations, purpose in life, and self-acceptance (Staudinger et al., 1997). Similarly, practical wisdom (assessed by cognitive, reflective, and mature adjectives from the Adjective Check List) and transcendent wisdom (ratings of respondents' examples of their own wisdom) were not associated with life satisfaction or marital satisfaction in a sample of college-educated adults around the age of 52 (Wink & Helson, 1997). In another sample of highly educated older adults in The Netherlands ranging in age from 64 to 93 years ($M = 74$ years), expertise in uncertainty, as assessed by Brugman's (2000) ECQ15, was also uncorrelated with life satisfaction. Yet, the ECQ15 was positively associated with life satisfaction in an educational diverse sample of middle-aged (44 to 54 years; $M = 50$ years) and older (77 to 90 years; $M = 83$ years) Dutch participants (Brugman, 2000).

Wisdom, assessed by cognitive and reflective items from the California Q-Sort (Block, 1971), was positively related to well-being from personal growth and generativity (characterized as giving, protective, sympathetic, warm, socially perceptive, and having broad interests) but not well-being from positive relations in a sample of predominantly White adults, ranging in age from the late 60s to the late 70s (Wink & Dillon, 2003). However, in prior studies of the elderly parents of the above participants ($M = 68$ years for mothers and 70 years for fathers), which also used the California Q-Sort together with Haan's Ego Rating Scale (Haan, 1969) to measure the cognitive, reflective, but also affective (compassionate) components of wisdom, wisdom was related to greater life satisfaction (Ardelt, 1997) and, for the mothers, to more positive family relations in old age as well (Ardelt, 2000a).

Similarly, in a sample of White men ranging in age from 77 to 86 years ($M = 80$ years), wisdom, assessed by cognitive, reflective, and affective (compassionate) items from the Gallup Wellsprings of a Positive Life Survey, was positively associated with life satisfaction, general adjustment to aging, and marital happiness (Ardelt & Vaillant, 2007). In a community sample of primarily older White adults (39 to 96 years; $M = 64$ years), wisdom, as measured by the cognitive, reflective, and affective (compassionate) dimensions of the 3D-WS, was positively correlated with life satisfaction (Le, in press). In a different community sample of White and African American adults between the ages of 52 and 87 years ($M = 71$ years), the 3D-WS was positively correlated with general well-being, mastery, and a sense of purpose in life and negatively associated with depressive symptoms, death avoidance, and death anxiety (Ardelt, 2003). Finally, in a sample of middle-aged (36 to 59 years; $M = 45$ years) and older (age >65; $M = 70$ years) American and Japanese adults, reflective understanding, emotional empathy, and emotional regulation (the reflective and compassionate synthetic wisdom mode) as well as knowledge database and abstract reasoning (the cognitive analytical wisdom mode) were positively correlated with life satisfaction (Takahashi & Overton, 2002).

It is not completely clear at this point whether the contradictory empirical findings are due to different measures of wisdom and well-being, the diversity of the samples, the age of the respondents, or a combination of those three factors. Unfortunately, studies vary widely in their assessment of wisdom and well-being, which makes a direct comparison between the various studies difficult. The Berlin Wisdom Paradigm, for example, assesses general wisdom-related knowledge rather than personal wisdom (Staudinger et al., 2005), which might explain the insignificant associations between general wisdom-related knowledge and indicators of personal psychological well-being (Staudinger et al., 1997).

It also appears that studies, whose definition and assessment of wisdom include the element of "compassionate concern for others," are more likely to find a significant association between wisdom and well-being than studies that primarily operationalize wisdom as a cognitive and/or reflective construct. Another possibility is that the association between personal wisdom and well-being is stronger for people with less social and economic power, such as women, minorities, and older adults, who might have fewer resources to find fulfillment and satisfaction in the external world. Although disadvantaged groups, such as women and minorities, do not seem to be wiser in old age than more privileged populations (Ardelt, 2003, 2009; Smith & Baltes, 1990; Takahashi & Overton, 2002; Wink & Dillon, 2003), it is worth noting that the only two studies that did not show a significant correlation between personal wisdom and measures of satisfaction (Brugman, 2000; Wink & Helson, 1997) consisted of highly educated middle-aged and older adults who probably belonged to the majority population. Hence, wisdom might have an insignificant effect on well-being among individuals who are able to derive satisfaction from their objective life situation, such as their good health, high income, and supportive social relationships. However, personal wisdom might result in a greater sense of well-being if external circumstances are less than ideal or start to deteriorate in old age (Ardelt, 2000b; Bianchi, 1994; Clayton, 1982; Kekes, 1995; Kramer, 2000).

In this regard, wisdom might be similar to religiosity, which also tends to sustain life meaning and well-being in old age even under conditions of failing health, widowhood, and the approach of death (Ardelt & Koenig, 2009; McFadden, 2000; Neill & Kahn, 1999; Wong, 1998). Yet, as prior research has shown, there are differences between wisdom and religiosity, although some wise individuals might be deeply spiritual.

In a study of European American and Vietnamese American adults of primarily middle-aged and older adults, belonging to a religious/spiritual community and the frequency of mystical experiences (e.g., loss of sense of self, feeling of oneness) were positively related to transcendent wisdom (self-knowledge, detachment, integration, and self-transcendence) but not to general wisdom-related knowledge. Moreover, religious/spiritual institutional and private practices were unrelated to transcendent wisdom and wisdom-related knowledge (Le, 2008). Similarly, in a study of older adults ranging in age from 56 to 88 years ($M = 73$ years), wisdom, measured by the cognitive, reflective, and affective (compassionate) dimensions of the 3D-WS, was unrelated to an intrinsic religious orientation and even negatively correlated with an extrinsic religious orientation (Ardelt, 2008b). According to Allport and Ross (1967), intrinsically religious people are committed to a religious/spiritual life, whereas extrinsically religious people use their religion for extrinsic purposes, such as enhancing their standing in the community, seeking companionship and social support, or finding solace in times of hardship. However, the three elders who scored the highest on the affective dimension of wisdom and relatively high on the cognitive and reflective dimensions of wisdom were deeply religious and strongly committed to their spiritual lives. They experienced spiritual growth throughout life through the development of humility, gratitude, and inner-centered guidance, which they expressed through a commitment to love and help others (Ardelt, 2008b). Wink and Dillon (2003) found that spirituality (noninstitutionalized religion or nontradition-centered beliefs and practices) but not religiousness (institutionalized or tradition-centered religious beliefs and practices) in late middle adulthood (50s to early 60s) and late adulthood (late 60s to late 70s) was significantly associated with greater cognitive/reflective wisdom in late adulthood. Those studies suggest that wisdom is unrelated to traditional religiosity but might resemble the equally elusive concept of spirituality, particularly if it is defined as transcendence rather than knowledge or if its operationalization includes a compassionate concern for the welfare of others.

SUMMARY AND FUTURE DIRECTIONS OF WISDOM RESEARCH

Although a uniform definition of wisdom does not exist, there is a general consensus among wisdom researchers and the general public that wisdom entails (a) cognitive knowledge, understanding, and insight, (b) reflective thought and an integration of one's own perspective and self-interests with that of others, (c) compassionate concern for the welfare of others, and (d) equanimity. It is less clear what the essential elements are to operationalize and measure the multifaceted construct of wisdom, which explains the variety of approaches in the assessment of wisdom. Yet despite the diversity in measurement, cross-sectional and longitudinal studies suggest that wisdom characteristics tend to increase in adolescence and early adulthood for individuals in general but then might require a supportive social environment, educational opportunities, or a strong motivation for psychosocial growth to develop further. Average trends, however, are likely to obscure the inter-individual variability in the association between age and wisdom. Future research should therefore investigate under which circumstances wisdom grows, remains stable, or declines with age.

Similarly, despite the differences in measurement, personal wisdom in the later years of life tends to be positively related to subjective and psychological well-being, except in samples of highly educated and privileged middle-aged and older adults. This suggests that wisdom might be less related to the well-being of individuals who have the economic and social resources to fulfill their material and social needs, even though educational opportunities might also foster the development of wisdom. Yet, it is not clear whether the educational system contributes directly to a growth in wisdom or whether individuals who pursue a higher degree are also more motivated to acquire wisdom.

Is it possible to cultivate the development of wisdom early in life to reap the benefits of well-being in the later years? Although research in this area is sparse, it appears that a social context that encourages reflectivity, openness, and a compassionate concern for others promotes greater wisdom and wisdom-related knowledge (Böhmig-Krumhaar et al., 2002; Parisi et al., 2009; Staudinger & Baltes, 1996). Evidence also suggests that family members, such as parents and particularly grandparents, can act as mentors and role models who give sage advice to the younger generation (Ardelt, 2008a).

Furthermore, there is some debate in the wisdom literature whether wisdom can be taught in schools (Ferrari & Potworowski, 2008; Reznitskaya & Sternberg, 2004; Sternberg, 2001) or universities (Brown, 2004). At present, schools and universities teach primarily knowledge and cognitive skills, which are not sufficient for wisdom to emerge (Jax, 2005; Sternberg, 2001). Instead, to grow in wisdom, students should be taught the importance of being open to new experiences, which appears to be a robust correlate and predictor of diverse assessments of wisdom both cross-sectionally (Kramer, 2000; Le, in press; Levenson et al., 2005; Staudinger et al., 1998) and longitudinally (Helson & Srivastava, 2002; Wink & Helson, 1997). Moreover, the promotion of certain virtues in schools, such as authenticity, curiosity, bravery, gratitude, and love, might also cultivate the emergence of wisdom (Park & Peterson, 2008). In fact, studies of high school students, adolescents, and adults have shown that wisdom tends to be positively related to pro-social and other-enhancing virtues and negatively correlated with hedonistic and self-enhancing virtues (Bailey & Russell, 2008; Kunzmann & Baltes, 2003; Webster, 2010). Future research should explore the possibility of teaching wisdom in schools and universities in greater depth and the long-term consequences of such a "wisdom curriculum."

Apart from schools, religion and certain spiritual practices might foster the development of wisdom through a transformation of personality in the direction of greater self-transcendence (Ferrari, 2008). Indeed, the vast majority of religious teachings in the world encourage the acquisition of wisdom, even though the prescribed paths to wisdom might differ (Birren & Svensson, 2005; Kupperman, 2005; Takahashi, 2000; Takahashi & Overton, 2005). Yet, wise people are not necessarily religious and religious individuals are not necessarily wise. Hence, it would be interesting to examine the role of religion and spirituality in the development of wisdom in future studies.

Finally, what are the benefits of cultivating wisdom for society at large? Although the development of wisdom appears to be beneficial for individuals of all age groups, it might be particularly important in old age when people are confronted by physical and social decline and their own mortality. Yet, the later years of life might also provide a unique opportunity to grow in wisdom through reduced social obligations, a confrontation with existential questions of meaning, and the greater availability of free time to pursue self-development and engage in volunteer activities to promote the welfare of others (Ardelt, 2000b; Moody, 1986; Parisi et al., 2009). Moreover, because wise people care about ethics, morality, and the well-being of present and future generations, wise elders might become the social consciousness of the nation by being unafraid to speak truth to power (Kupperman, 2005). Hence, rather than being a burden to younger generations, wise elders might become a valuable asset for a more just and caring future society.

REFERENCES

Achenbaum, A. W., & Orwoll, L. (1991). Becoming wise: A psycho-gerontological interpretation of the Book of Job. *International Journal of Aging and Human Development, 32*(1), 21–39.

Allport, G. W., & Ross, J. M. (1967). Personal religious orientation and prejudice. *Journal of Personality and Social Psychology, 5*(4), 432–443.

Ardelt, M. (1997). Wisdom and life satisfaction in old age. *Journals of Gerontology: Psychological Sciences, 52B*(1), P15–P27.

Ardelt, M. (1998). Social crisis and individual growth: The long-term effects of the Great Depression. *Journal of Aging Studies, 12*(3), 291–314.

Ardelt, M. (2000a). Antecedents and effects of wisdom in old age: A longitudinal perspective on aging well. *Research on Aging, 22*(4), 360–394.

Ardelt, M. (2000b). Intellectual versus wisdom-related knowledge: The case for a different kind of learning in the later years of life. *Educational Gerontology: An International Journal of Research and Practice, 26*(8), 771–789.

Ardelt, M. (2003). Development and empirical assessment of a three-dimensional wisdom scale. *Research on Aging, 25*(3), 275–324.

Ardelt, M. (2004). Wisdom as expert knowledge system: A critical review of a contemporary operationalization of an ancient concept. *Human Development, 47*(5), 257–285.

Ardelt, M. (2008a). Being wise at any age. In S. J. Lopez (Ed.), *Positive Psychology: Exploring the Best in People: Vol. 1: Discovering Human Strengths* (pp. 81–108). Westport, CT: Praeger.

Ardelt, M. (2008b). Self-development through selflessness: The paradoxical process of growing wiser. In H. A. Wayment & J. J. Bauer (Eds.), *Transcending self-interest: Psychological explorations of the quiet ego* (pp. 221–233). Washington, DC: American Psychological Association.

Ardelt, M. (2009). How similar are wise men and women? A comparison across two age cohorts. *Research in Human Development, 6*(1), 9–26.

Ardelt, M. Are older adults wiser than college students? A comparison of two age cohorts. *Journal of Adult Development*, in press. doi: 10.1007/s10804-009-9088-5.

Ardelt, M., & Jacobs, S. (2009). Wisdom, integrity, and life satisfaction in very old age. In M. C. Smith (Ed.), *Handbook of research on adult learning and development* (pp. 732–760). New York: Routledge.

Ardelt, M., & Koenig, C. S. (2009). Differential roles of religious orientation on subjective well-being and death attitudes in old age: Mediation of spiritual activities and purpose in life. In A. L. Ai & M. Ardelt (Eds.), *Faith and well-being in later life: Linking theories with evidence in an interdisciplinary inquiry* (pp. 85–112). Hauppauge, NY: Nova Science.

Ardelt, M., & Vaillant, G. E. (2007, November 2007). *Wisdom as a cognitive, reflective, and affective three-dimensional personality characteristic.* Paper presented at the Gerontological Society of America Annual Meetings, San Francisco, CA.

Assmann, A. (1994). Wholesome knowledge: Concepts of wisdom in a historical and cross-cultural perspective. In D. L. Featherman, R. M. Lerner, & M. Perlmutter (Eds.), *Life-span development and behavior: Vol. 12* (pp. 187–224). Hillsdale, NJ: Lawrence Erlbaum.

Bailey, A., & Russell, K. C. (2008). Psycho-social benefits of a service-learning experience. *Journal of Unconventional Parks, Tourism & Recreation Research, 1*(1), 9–16.

Baltes, P. B., & Smith, J. (2008). The fascination of wisdom: Its nature, ontogeny, and function. *Perspectives on Psychological Science, 3*(1), 56–64.

Baltes, P. B., & Staudinger, U. M. (2000). Wisdom: A metaheuristic (pragmatic) to orchestrate mind and virtue toward excellence. *American Psychologist, 55*(1), 122–136.

Baltes, P. B., Staudinger, U. M., Maercker, A., & Smith, J. (1995). People nominated as wise: A comparative study of wisdom-related knowledge. *Psychology and Aging, 10*(2), 155–166.

Bianchi, E. C. (1994). *Elder wisdom. Crafting your own elderhood.* New York: Crossroad.

Birren, J. E., & Svensson, C. M. (2005). Wisdom in history. In R. J. Sternberg & J. Jordan (Eds.), *A handbook of wisdom. Psychological perspectives* (pp. 3–31). New York: Cambridge University Press.

Blanchard-Fields, F. (2009). Flexible and adaptive socio-emotional problem solving in adult development and aging. *Restorative Neurology and Neuroscience, 27*(5), 539–550.

Blanchard-Fields, F., & Norris, L. (1995). The development of wisdom. In M. A. Kimble, S. H. McFadden, J. W. Ellor, & J. J. Seeber (Eds.), *Aging, spirituality, and religion. A handbook* (pp. 102–118). Minneapolis, MN: Fortress Press.

Block, J. (1971). *Lives through time.* Berkeley, CA: Bancroft Books.

Bluck, S., & Glück, J. (2005). From the inside out: People's implicit theories of wisdom. In R. J. Sternberg & J. Jordan (Eds.), *A handbook of wisdom. Psychological perspectives* (pp. 84–109). New York: Cambridge University Press.

Böhmig-Krumhaar, S. A., Staudinger, U. M., & Baltes, P. B. (2002). Mehr Toleranz tut Not: Lässt sich wert-relativierendes Wissen und Urteilen mit Hilfe einer wissensaktivierenden Gedächtnisstrategie verbessern? (In search of more tolerance: Testing the facilitative effect of a knowledge-activating mnemonic strategy on value relativism). *Zeitschrift für Entwicklungspsychologie und Pädagogische Psychologie, 34*(1), 30–43.

Bradley, G. W. (1978). Self-serving biases in the attribution process: A reexamination of the fact or fiction question. *Journal of Personality and Social Psychology, 36*(1), 56–71.

Brown, S. C. (2004). Learning across the campus: How college facilitates the development of wisdom. *Journal of College Student Development, 45*(2), 134–148.

Brugman, G. M. (2000). *Wisdom: Source of narrative coherence and eudaimonia.* Delft, The Netherlands: Eburon.

Caspi, A., Roberts, B. W., & Shiner, R. L. (2005). Personality development: Stability and change. *Annual Review of Psychology, 56*, 453–483.

Charles, S. T., & Carstensen, L. L. (2010). Social and emotional aging. *Annual Review of Psychology, 61*, 383–409.

Clayton, V. P. (1982). Wisdom and intelligence: The nature and function of knowledge in the later years. *International Journal of Aging and Development, 15*(4), 315–323.

Clayton, V. P., & Birren, J. E. (1980). The development of wisdom across the life-span: A reexamination of an ancient topic. In P. B. Baltes, & O. G. Brim, Jr. (Eds.), *Life-span development and behavior: Vol. 3* (pp. 103–135). New York: Academic Press.

Cohn, L. D. (1998). Age trends in personality development: A quantitative review. In P. M. Westenberg, A. Blasi, & L. D. Cohn (Eds.), *Personality development: Theoretical, empirical, and clinical investigations of Loevinger's conception of ego development* (pp. 133–143). Mahwah, NJ: Lawrence Erlbaum.

Colby, A., Kohlberg, L., Gibbs, J., & Lieberman, M. (1994). A longitudinal study of moral judgment. In B. Puka (Ed.), *New research in moral development* (pp. 1–124). New York: Garland Publishing.

Csikszentmihalyi, M., & Nakamura, J. (2005). The role of emotions in the development of wisdom. In R. J. Sternberg & J. Jordan (Eds.), *A handbook of wisdom. Psychological perspectives* (pp. 220–242). New York: Cambridge University Press.

Csikszentmihalyi, M., & Rathunde, K. (1990). The psychology of wisdom: An evolutionary interpretation. In R. J. Sternberg (Ed.), *Wisdom: Its nature, origins, and development* (pp. 25–51). New York: Cambridge University Press.

Erikson, E. H. (1963). *Childhood and society.* New York: Norton.

Erikson, E. H. (1982). *The life cycle completed. A review.* New York: Norton.

Erikson, E. H., Erikson, J. M., & Kivnick, H. Q. (1986). *Vital involvement in old age: The experience of old age in our time.* New York: Norton.

Ferrari, M. (2008). Developing expert and transformative wisdom: Can either be taught in public schools? In M. Ferrari & G. Potworowski (Eds.), *Teaching for wisdom: Cross-cultural perspectives on fostering wisdom.* (pp. 207–222). New York, NY: Springer.

Ferrari, M., & Potworowski, G. (2008). *Teaching for wisdom: Cross-cultural perspectives on fostering wisdom.* New York, NY: Springer.

Glück, J., Bluck, S., Baron, J., & McAdams, D. P. (2005). The wisdom of experience: Autobiographical narratives across adulthood. *International Journal of Behavioral Development, 29*(3), 197–208.

Gurucharri, C., & Selman, R. L. (1982). The development of interpersonal understanding during childhood, preadolescence, and adolescence: A longitudinal follow-up study. *Child Development, 53*(4), 924–927.

Haan, N. (1969). A tripartite model of ego functioning: Values and clinical research applications. *Journal of Nervous and Mental Diseases, 148*(1), 14–30.

Helson, R., & Srivastava, S. (2002). Creative and wise people: Similarities, differences and how they develop. *Personality and Social Psychology Bulletin, 28*(10), 1430–1440.

Holliday, S. G., & Chandler, M. J. (1986). *Wisdom: Explorations in adult competence.* Basel, New York: Karger.

Jax, C. (2005). No soul left behind: Paths to wisdom in American schools. *ReVision: A Journal of Consciousness and Transformation, 28*(1), 34–41.

Jeste, D. V., & Vahia, I. (2008). Comparison of the conceptualization of wisdom in ancient Indian literature with modern views: Focus on the Bhagavad Gita. *Psychiatry: Interpersonal and Biological Processes, 71*(3), 197–209.

Jordan, J. (2005). The quest for wisdom in adulthood: A psychological perspective. In R. J. Sternberg & J. Jordan (Eds.), *A handbook of wisdom. Psychological perspectives* (pp. 160–188). New York: Cambridge University Press.

Kekes, J. (1983). Wisdom. *American Philosophical Quarterly, 20*(3), 277–286.

Kekes, J. (1995). *Moral wisdom and good lives.* Ithaca, NY: Cornell University Press.

Kitchener, K. S., & Brenner, H. G. (1990). Wisdom and reflective judgment: Knowing in the face of uncertainty. In R. J. Sternberg (Ed.), *Wisdom: Its nature, origins, and development* (pp. 212–229). New York: Cambridge University Press.

Kitchener, K. S., King, P. M., Wood, P. K., & Davison, M. L. (1989). Sequentiality and consistency in the development of Reflective Judgment: A six-year longitudinal study. *Journal of Applied Developmental Psychology, 10*(1), 73–95.

Kohlberg, L., & Puka, B. (1994). *Kohlberg's original study of moral development.* New York: Garland Publishing.

Kramer, D. A. (1990). Conceptualizing wisdom: The primacy of affect-cognition relations. In R. J. Sternberg (Ed.), *Wisdom: Its nature, origins, and development* (pp. 279–313). New York: Cambridge University Press.

Kramer, D. A. (2000). Wisdom as a classical source of human strength: Conceptualization and empirical inquiry. *Journal of Social and Clinical Psychology, 19*(1), 83–101.

Kunzmann, U., & Baltes, P. B. (2003). Wisdom-related knowledge: Affective, motivational, and interpersonal correlates. *Personality and Social Psychology Bulletin, 29*(9), 1104–1119.

Kunzmann, U., & Baltes, P. B. (2005). The psychology of wisdom: Theoretical and empirical challenges. In R. J. Sternberg & J. Jordan (Eds.), *A handbook of wisdom. Psychological perspectives* (pp. 110–135). New York: Cambridge University Press.

Kupperman, J. J. (2005). Morality, ethics, and wisdom. In R. J. Sternberg & J. Jordan (Eds.), *A handbook of wisdom. Psychological perspectives* (pp. 245–271). New York: Cambridge University Press.

Le, T. N. (2008). Age differences in spirituality, mystical experiences and wisdom. *Ageing & Society, 28*, 383–411.

Le, T. N. Life satisfaction, openness value, self-transcendence, and wisdom. *Journal of Happiness Studies*, in press, doi:10.1007/S10902-010-9182-1.

Levenson, M. R., Jennings, P. A., Aldwin, C. M., & Shiraishi, R. W. (2005). Self-transcendence: Conceptualization and measurement. *International Journal of Aging & Human Development, 60*(2), 127–143.

Levitt, H. M. (1999). The development of wisdom: An analysis of Tibetan Buddhist experience. *Journal of Humanistic Psychology, 39*(2), 86–105.

Loevinger, J. (1998). Ego development in adolescence. In R. E. Muuss & H. D. Porton (Eds.), *Adolescent behavior and society: A book of readings* (5th ed.) (pp. 234–240). New York: McGraw-Hill.

Loevinger, J., Cohn, L. D., Bonneville, L. P., Redmore, C. D., Streich, D. D., & Sargent, M. (1985). Ego development in college. *Journal of Personality and Social Psychology, 48*(4), 947–962.

McCrae, R. R., Costa, P. T., Jr., Terracciano, A., Parker, W. D., Mills, C. J., De Fruyt, F., et al. (2002). Personality trait development from age 12 to age 18: Longitudinal, cross-sectional and cross-cultural analyses. *Journal of Personality and Social Psychology, 83*(6), 1456–1468.

McFadden, S. H. (2000). Religion and meaning in late life. In G. T. Reker & K. Chamberlain (Eds.), *Exploring existential meaning. Optimizing human development across the life span* (pp. 171–183). Thousand Oaks, CA: Sage.

McKee, P., & Barber, C. (1999). On defining wisdom. *International Journal of Aging and Human Development, 49*(2), 149–164.

Meacham, J. A. (1990). The loss of wisdom. In R. J. Sternberg (Ed.), *Wisdom: Its nature, origins, and development* (pp. 181–211). New York: Cambridge University Press.

Moody, H. R. (1986). Late life learning in the information society. In D. A. Peterson, J. E. Thornton, & J. E. Birren (Eds.), *Education and aging* (pp. 122–148). Englewood Cliffs, N.J: Prentice-Hall.

Neill, C. M., & Kahn, A. S. (1999). Role of personal spirituality and religious social activity on the life satisfaction of older widowed women. *Sex Roles, 40*(3–4), 319–329.

Orwoll, L., & Achenbaum, W. A. (1993). Gender and the development of wisdom. *Human Development, 36*, 274–296.

Osbeck, L. M., & Robinson, D. N. (2005). Philosophical theories of wisdom. In R. J. Sternberg & J. Jordan (Eds.), *A handbook of wisdom. Psychological perspectives* (pp. 61–83). New York: Cambridge University Press.

Parisi, J. M., Rebok, G. W., Carlson, M. C., Fried, L. P., Seeman, T. E., Tan, E. J., et al. (2009). Can the wisdom of aging be activated and make a difference societally? *Educational Gerontology, 35*, 867–879.

Park, N., & Peterson, C. (2008). The cultivation of character strengths. In M. Ferrari & G. Potworowski (Eds.), *Teaching for wisdom: Cross-cultural perspectives on fostering wisdom* (pp. 59–77). New York, NY: Springer.

Pasupathi, M., & Staudinger, U. M. (2001). Do advanced moral reasoners also show wisdom? Linking moral reasoning and wisdom-related knowledge and judgement. *International Journal of Behavioral Development, 25*(5), 401–415.

Pasupathi, M., Staudinger, U. M., & Baltes, P. B. (2001). Seeds of wisdom: Adolescents' knowledge and judgment about difficult life problems. *Developmental Psychology, 37*(3), 351–361.

Piaget, J. (1952). *The origins of intelligence in children*. Oxford, England: International Universities Press.

Reznitskaya, A., & Sternberg, R. J. (2004). Teaching students to make wise judgments: The "Teaching for Wisdom" program. In P. A. Linley & S. Joseph (Eds.), *Positive psychology in practice* (pp. 181–196). New York: Wiley.

Richardson, M. J., & Pasupathi, M. (2005). Young and growing wiser: Wisdom during adolescence and young adulthood. In R. J. Sternberg & J. Jordan (Eds.), *A handbook of wisdom. Psychological perspectives* (pp. 139–159). New York: Cambridge University Press.

Robinson, D. N. (1990). Wisdom through the ages. In R. J. Sternberg (Ed.), *Wisdom: Its nature, origins, and development* (pp. 13–24). New York: Cambridge University Press.

Ryff, C. D. (1989). Happiness is everything, or is it? Explorations on the meaning of psychological well-being. *Journal of Personality and Social Psychology, 57*(6), 1069–1081.

Sherwood, G. G. (1981). Self-serving biases in person perception: A reexamination of projection as a mechanism of defense. *Psychological Bulletin, 90*(3), 445–459.

Smith, J., & Baltes, P. B. (1990). Wisdom-related knowledge: Age/cohort differences in response to life-planning problems. *Developmental Psychology, 26*(3), 494–505.

Smith, J., Staudinger, U. M., & Baltes, P. B. (1994). Occupational settings facilitating wisdom-related knowledge: The sample case of clinical psychologists. *Journal of Consulting and Clinical Psychology, 62*(5), 989–999.

Sorrentino, R. M., Raynor, J. O., Zubek, J. M., & Short, J.-A. C. (1990). Personality functioning and change: Informational and affective influences on cognitive, moral, and social development. In E. T. Higgins & R. M. Sorrentino (Eds.), *Handbook of motivation and cognition: Foundations of social behavior: Vol. 2* (pp. 193–228). New York: Guilford Press.

Staudinger, U. M. (1999). Older and wiser? Integrating results on the relationship between age and wisdom-related performance. *International Journal of Behavioral Development, 23*(3), 641–664.

Staudinger, U. M., & Baltes, P. B. (1996). Interactive minds: A facilitative setting for wisdom-related performance. *Journal of*

Personality and Social Psychology, 71(4), 746–762.

Staudinger, U. M., Dörner, J., & Mickler, C. (2005). Wisdom and personality. In R. J. Sternberg & J. Jordan (Eds.), *A handbook of wisdom. Psychological perspectives* (pp. 191–219). New York: Cambridge University Press.

Staudinger, U. M., & Kunzmann, U. (2005). Positive adult personality development: Adjustment and/or growth? [Electronic Electronic; Print]. *European Psychologist, 10*(4), 320–329.

Staudinger, U. M., Lopez, D. F., & Baltes, P. B. (1997). The psychometric location of wisdom-related performance: Intelligence, personality, and more? *Personality and Social Psychology Bulletin, 23*(11), 1200–1214.

Staudinger, U. M., Maciel, A. G., Smith, J., & Baltes, P. B. (1998). What predicts wisdom-related performance? A first look at personality, intelligence, and facilitative experiential contexts. *European Journal of Personality, 12*(1), 1–17.

Staudinger, U. M., Smith, J., & Baltes, P. B. (1992). Wisdom-related knowledge in a life review task: Age differences and the role of professional specialization. *Psychology and Aging, 7*(2), 271–281.

Sternberg, R. J. (1985). Implicit theories of intelligence, creativity, and wisdom. *Journal of Personality and Social Psychology, 49*(3), 607–627.

Sternberg, R. J. (1998). A balance theory of wisdom. *Review of General Psychology, 2*(4), 347–365.

Sternberg, R. J. (2001). Why schools should teach for wisdom: The balance theory of wisdom in educational settings. *Educational Psychologist, 36*(4), 227–245.

Sternberg, R. J. (2005). Older but not wiser? The relationship between age and wisdom. *Ageing International, 30*(1), 5–26.

Sternberg, R. J. (Ed.), (1990). *Wisdom: Its nature, origins, and development.* New York: Cambridge University Press.

Sternberg, R. J., & Jordan, J. (Eds.), (2005). *A handbook of wisdom. Psychological perspectives.* New York: Cambridge University Press.

Takahashi, M. (2000). Toward a culturally inclusive understanding of wisdom: Historical roots in the East and West. *International Journal of Aging and Human Development, 51*(3), 217–230.

Takahashi, M., & Bordia, P. (2000). The concept of wisdom: A cross-cultural comparison. *International Journal of Psychology, 35*(1), 1–9.

Takahashi, M., & Overton, W. F. (2002). Wisdom: A culturally inclusive developmental perspective. *International Journal of Behavioral Development, 26*(3), 269–277.

Takahashi, M., & Overton, W. F. (2005). Cultural foundations of wisdom: An integrated developmental approach. In R. J. Sternberg & J. Jordan (Eds.), *A handbook of wisdom. Psychological perspectives* (pp. 32–60). New York: Cambridge University Press.

Taranto, M. A. (1989). Facets of wisdom: A theoretical synthesis. *International Journal of Aging and Human Development, 29*(1), 1–21.

Thorson, J. A., & Powell, F. C. (1996). Women, aging, and sense of humor. [Empirical Study]. *Humor: International Journal of Humor Research, 9*(2), 169–186.

Tornstam, L. (2005). *Gerotranscendence: A developmental theory of positive aging.* New York, NY: Springer Pub. Co.

Vaillant, G. E. (2002). *Aging well: Surprising guideposts to a happier life from the landmark Harvard Study of Adult Development.* Boston, MA: Little, Brown.

Webster, J. D. (2003). An exploratory analysis of a self-assessed wisdom scale. *Journal of Adult Development, 10*(1), 13–22.

Webster, J. D. (2007). Measuring the character strength of wisdom. *International Journal of Aging & Human Development, 65*(2), 163–183.

Webster, J. D. (2010). Wisdom and positive psychosocial values in young adulthood. *Journal of Adult Development,* 17(2), 70–80.

Wink, P., & Dillon, M. (2003). Religiousness, spirituality, and psychosocial functioning in late adulthood: Findings from a longitudinal study. *Psychology and Aging, 18*(4), 916–924.

Wink, P., & Helson, R. (1997). Practical and transcendent wisdom: Their nature and some longitudinal findings. *Journal of Adult Development, 4*(1), 1–15.

Wong, P. T. P. (1998). Spirituality, meaning, and successful aging. In P. T. P. Wong & P. S. Fry (Eds.), *The human quest for meaning: A handbook of psychological research and clinical applications* (pp. 359–394). Mahwah, NJ: Lawrence Erlbaum.

Yang, S.-Y. (2001). Conceptions of wisdom among Taiwanese Chinese. *Journal of Cross-Cultural Psychology, 32*(6), 662–680.

Part 4

Complex Behavioral Processes and Psychopathology of Aging

19 Emotional Experience and Regulation in Later Life *295*

20 Psychopathology, Bereavement, and Aging *311*

21 Assessment of Emotional and Personality Disorders in Older Adults *325*

22 Neuropsychological Assessment of the Dementias of Late Life *339*

23 Family Caregiving for Cognitively or Physically Frail Older Adults: Theory, Research, and Practice *353*

24 Decision Making Capacity *367*

Chapter | 19 |

Emotional Experience and Regulation in Later Life

Susan Turk Charles
School of Social Ecology, University of California, Irvine, Irvine, California, USA

CHAPTER CONTENTS

Introduction 295
Emotion and Emotion Regulation 296
Emotions Retain Basic Function and Structure Across Adulthood 296
Age and Losses in Multiple Domains Related to Emotional Experience 297
Age and Emotional Well-Being 298
Age Differences in Emotional Complexity 299
Understanding Emotion and Aging: Strength and Vulnerability Integration 299
Reasons for Age-Related Strengths in Emotion Regulation 300
Cognitive and Behavioral Strategies Related to Emotional Well-Being 301
Regulating Emotions in Social Contexts 301
Attention to and Appraisals of Positive and Negative Stimuli 302
Appraisals of Current and Past Emotional Experiences 302
Memory for Past Events 303
Potential Area of Vulnerability: Emotional Arousal 303
Threats to Emotional Well-Being 304
Early Experiences 304
Current Situations 305
Future Directions and Conclusions 305
References 306

INTRODUCTION

Current research on emotion and aging reflects a decade of theoretical and methodological innovation. Greater theoretical integration across subareas of psychology has resulted in new research directions in life-span psychology. For example, intersections between cognition and emotion reveal new insight into developmental processes (e.g., Carstensen & Mikels, 2005) as do studies focusing on social influences on adult developmental trajectories (e.g., Charles & Carstensen, 2009). The birth of social neuroscience has been accompanied by studies examining age differences in the neurobiological activity in response to emotional stimuli (Mather et al., 2004). Technological advances have provided easier and less invasive assessments of physiological processes (e.g., Hawkley et al., 2006; Uchino et al., 2005), and more economical and reliable methods to capture age differences in emotions experienced in daily life (Almeida, 2005). Advances in statistical software have enabled scientists to more easily model intra-individual variability in emotional experiences (Röcke et al., 2009), and to examine how physical and cognitive processes covary with emotional experiences across time (e.g., Chow et al., 2007).

Research amassed in the past decade provides a more ecological perspective of age differences in emotional experience, a greater awareness of the neurological processes involved when responding to emotional information, and a better understanding of the physiological correlates of emotional states. This chapter summarizes findings from this past decade. It begins with an overview of research indicating

DOI: 10.1016/B978-0-12-380882-0.00019-X

that emotions, at their core, retain their basic function and structure across adulthood (see review by Mather, 2004). Despite this consistency in structure and function, however, researchers have also documented age-related losses in reaction time and the accurate detection of emotional stimuli. After a brief discussion of these declines, this chapter presents literature suggesting that emotional well-being (defined as the relative difference between positive and negative affect) does not follow the same declining trajectory. Instead, older adults report similar if not higher levels of emotional well-being than do younger adults (e.g., Charles & Carstensen, 2007).

To explain potential mechanisms for this relatively positive trajectory of emotional experience, the theory of Strength and Vulnerability Integration (SAVI) is presented. This theory incorporates current findings and existing theories but also includes hypotheses that remain largely untested. SAVI posits that age-related gains occur alongside age-related losses in emotion-related processes. Specifically, strengths are found in the use of emotion regulation strategies, including how older adults direct their attention, appraise situations, and remember the past so that negative emotions are deemphasized and positive emotions increase in importance. Strengths in the use of emotion regulation strategies are countered by age-related vulnerabilities to emotion regulation, defined as reductions in physiological flexibility that create difficulties when people experience high levels of arousal. After reviewing this theory, this chapter concludes by pointing to areas where future research is needed in the ongoing study of emotion and aging.

EMOTION AND EMOTION REGULATION

Researchers differ in their definitions of emotion and emotion regulation. They agree that these terms represent complex and multifaceted phenomena, and perhaps the different definitions arise because researchers focus on different aspects of emotion. This chapter defines emotions as feeling states that vary in valence and intensity. They entail physiological activity and are associated with specific thoughts and behaviors. For example, annoyance, anger, and rage vary in intensity. Sadness and happiness vary in valence and also in the corresponding thoughts and behaviors associated with each emotional state. Emotions also influence subsequent physiological, cognitive, and behavioral activity. For example, happiness motivates exploration, whereas fear motivates avoidant behaviors (e.g., Fox & Reeb, 2008; Fredrickson, 2001). Emotion regulation is defined as any action (conscious or not) that either alters the valence and intensity of a current emotional experience or is initiated for the purpose of altering future emotional experiences. Emotion regulation strategies encompass a wide range of thoughts and behaviors. For example, identifying potentially caustic aspects of the environment and learning how best to avoid them is one emotion regulation strategy. Actions that reduce levels of distress are other very different emotion regulation strategies. Engaging in meditation or reappraising a situation to make it appear less caustic are two examples of how people might reduce levels of distress.

EMOTIONS RETAIN BASIC FUNCTION AND STRUCTURE ACROSS ADULTHOOD

Evolutionary theorists posit that emotions evolved over the millennia for functional purposes (Darwin, 1872). Internal emotional states direct actions to satisfy hunger, fight off or flee from invaders, successfully reproduce, and survive until offspring reach reproductive age. Emotional expression allows people to communicate information to others to further aid in group survival (Darwin, 1872). Differential Emotions Theory (DET) describes how evolution has shaped neurobiological processes related to emotions, positing that people are hardwired to experience basic, discrete emotions that motivate cognition and emotion, such as joy, anger, fear and surprise (Izard, 2007). DET describes how emotions unfold during infancy with distinct physiological, functional, phenomenological, and motivational properties that remain fairly stable across the life span. For example, the experience of anger creates the same pattern of neurochemical changes that leads to similar emotional experience in someone who is either 9 or 90 years old. Magai and her colleagues use this theory to explain findings showing that facial expression and subjective response to emotional stimuli are similar across the life span, even though motivations and abilities related to emotional experience change with age (see review by Magai, 2001; Magai et al., 2006).

Given that emotions are so fundamental to adaptive functioning, it may come as little surprise to find that the ability to experience emotions remains intact throughout adulthood. Adults of all ages report similar subjective responses to emotional stimuli, and the corresponding cognitive appraisals are consistent across age groups (e.g., Chipperfield et al., 2009; Tsai et al., 2000). Specific emotions are related to specific appraisals, and these relationships are observed across adults of all ages. For example, stories of loss lead to sadness for both younger and older adults, blocked goals elicit anger, and a sense of accomplishment engenders pride (Chipperfield et al., 2009). Emotions are reported with similar intensity across adult age groups in response to emotional videos or pictures

(Kunzmann & Grühn, 2005), in daily life as assessed by daily experience sampling techniques (Carstensen et al., 2000), and in the level of emotional reactivity in response to work- and home-related stressors (Neupert et al., 2007). Even clinical levels of anxiety and depression (severe emotional experiences that continue unabated across time and with such intensity that they impair daily functioning and the quality of daily life) are characterized by similar symptoms and feelings states among younger and older adults, although the frequency of certain symptoms may vary by age (Fiske et al., 2009; Wetherell & Stein, 2009). For example, feelings of guilt are more commonly observed among depressed younger adults, and fatigue is more often present in older adults with depression (see review by Fiske et al., 2009).

Researchers have also documented similar physiological and neural processes related to emotional experiences across different age groups. Emotional stimuli produce a similar pattern of physiological reactivity in both younger and older adults, including changes in heart rate, skin conductance levels, and body temperature (Phillips et al., 2008; Tsai et al., 2000). Within the profile of physiological activation, however, researchers have observed differences in the level of activation for different parameters (Levenson, 2000; Uchino et al., 2010). For example, increases in heart rate and changes in skin conductance levels are attenuated among older adults, but increases in systolic blood pressure are more pronounced among older adults compared to younger adults in response to stressors (see reviews by Levenson, 2000; Uchino et al., 2010).

The neural networks that are involved in processing emotional information are also similar across adult age groups (see review by Mather, 2004), although again the degree of activation observed in the brain in response to emotional stimuli is not always the same (LeClerc & Kensinger, 2008; St. Jacques et al., 2009). For example, when people are shown pictures of stigmatized individuals (Krendl et al., 2009), the areas of the brain involved in this activity (e.g., amygdala, left fusiform gyrus, ventromedial cortex) are the same for all age groups, although high functioning older adults show greater activation in some prefrontal cortex regions than do younger adults. Activation also varies by age when people are asked to identify facial expressions (Keightley et al., 2007). Findings indicate that older and younger adults show similar increases in the ventromedial prefrontal cortex and the lingual gyrus to emotional facial expressions, but older adults show decreased activity in the dorsal anterior cingulate in response to happy faces than do younger adults. Older adults also show a more distributed activation when viewing emotional facial expressions (both positive and negative) than do younger adults (Keightley et al., 2007). In another study where people viewed negative and positive images, older adults had greater activation in the amygdala for positive images, but less activation for negative images compared to younger adults (Mather et al., 2004).

Researchers have offered possible reasons why the degree of activation in various brain regions differs by age when people view emotional stimuli. These explanations include age-related increases in motivations to optimize emotional experience and thereby regulate their emotional experiences (see Mather et al., 2004), decreases in cognitive control that makes processing stimuli more difficult (see Krendl et al., 2009), or possibly a combination of these two factors that may lead to the recruitment of different brain regions. Studying age differences in patterns of activation, and finding underlying mechanisms to explain these patterns, are ongoing research aims in this area of emotion and aging.

Age and Losses in Multiple Domains Related to Emotional Experience

Similar neurological and physiological processes are involved when processing emotional stimuli across age groups, yet researchers find that older adults are sometimes less successful in this task than are younger adults. Both younger and older adults can accurately report whether a facial expression depicts a positive or a negative emotion, and older adults are sometimes more accurate at identifying expressions of disgust than are younger adults (Ruffman et al., 2008). The accuracy with which people correctly identify expressions of sadness, fear or anger, however, declines with age (e.g., Mill et al., 2009; Ruffman et al., 2008). This decline is gradual and begins around age 30 (Mill et al., 2009). Older adults are also worse at distinguishing between negative emotions expressed in speech (Laukka & Juslin, 2007; Mitchell, 2007; Paulmann et al., 2008) and in melodies (Laukka & Juslin, 2007). For example, one study asked participants to view a series of film clips depicting people being interrogated about a crime (Stanley & Blanchard-Fields, 2008). They were told that a quarter to three-fourths of these people were lying, and were asked to identify those lying versus those telling the truth. Older adults were worse at detecting deceit, although they performed equally well compared to younger adults when given only audio cues from which to base their judgments (Stanley & Blanchard-Fields, 2008). Researchers have attributed declines in the ability to identify emotional stimuli to neurological changes related to processing emotional material as opposed to sensory declines, such as poorer eyesight or worse hearing (e.g., Mitchell, 2007).

Declines are also evident in reaction time to emotional stimuli (e.g., Keightley et al., 2006). For example, one study assessed brain response to emotional pictures using event-related potentials (ERP; Wieser et al., 2006). Results indicate that the ERP of older adults, who averaged 66 years old, occurred after 220 ms, whereas younger adults, averaging around 32 years old, had an ERP response only 180 ms after picture onset.

A notable exception to age-related speed of processing declines comes from several studies examining detection of fear-related stimuli (LeClerc & Kensinger, 2008; Mather & Knight, 2006). Researchers have emphasized the importance of quickly detecting fear-related stimuli for survival purposes. So fundamental to survival, rapid detection of threatening stimuli is considered an automatic process that remains intact in later life (Mather & Knight, 2006). Findings from one study indicated that older adults were as adept at identifying facial expressions of fear in a crowd as were younger adults (Mather & Knight, 2006). Another study revealed that older adults are less accurate when judging the degree of threat expressed on faces than younger adults, but equally adept at judging the degree of danger portrayed by pictures of animals, activities, and environmental situations (Ruffman et al., 2006). Thus, reaction times in response to emotion-eliciting stimuli do occur, but fear may be one exception to the overall slowing in response to emotion-related stimuli.

Age and Emotional Well-Being

Do the declines mentioned above influence emotional well-being in daily life? To address this question, researchers often study positive and negative affective states, where the experience of positive emotions such as happiness, contentment, and joy are averaged to create a positive affect score, and the experience of negative emotions such as disgust, fear, and anger are averaged to create a negative affect score (e.g., Carstensen et al., 2000). These positive and negative states are important, as they direct approach or avoidance goals that regulate much of human behavior (Fredrickson, 2001). Negative emotions indicate a need to critically evaluate the situation to improve current circumstances, and positive emotions often signal contentment with the status quo or motivate exploratory behavior (e.g., Fredrickson, 2001). Moreover, higher levels of emotional well-being (i.e., assessed by the extent to which positive emotions are experienced to a greater degree than negative emotions, often calculated by difference scores between reports of positive and negative affect) correlate with and predict a number of positive outcomes in Western societies, including faster recovery from illness, better overall physical health, and stronger social relationships (Lyubomirsky et al., 2005).

A number of studies indicate that emotional well-being remains relatively stable over time. When changes are noted, they most often point to increased levels of emotional well-being across adulthood. For example, in both cross-sectional and longitudinal studies, older age is related to less frequent reports of negative affect and stable if not higher levels of positive affect (Carstensen et al., 2000; Charles et al., 2001). In cross-sectional studies, older adults report less worry (Basevitz et al., 2008) and less anger compared to younger adults (Phillips et al., 2006). They also report less anger when asked how they would respond to hypothetical scenarios or when recalling past negative experiences (Birditt & Fingerman, 2003; Löckenhoff et al., 2008). In addition, life satisfaction (an assessment that requires weighing positive and negative aspects of one's life to make an overall evaluation) increases over time among people from young to middle adulthood and peaks in the mid-60s (Mroczek & Spiro, 2005).

When examining age differences and patterns of change among people ranging from those in their mid-60s and older, findings are more mixed (see review by Charles & Carstensen, 2010). For example, one longitudinal study of older adults years found that depressive symptoms increased slightly across eight years (Davey et al., 2004), but another found relative stability in negative affect in very old age (Charles et al., 2001). Cross-sectional studies are also mixed, with some finding increases in negative affect and decreases in positive affect (Diener & Suh, 1998), and others finding decreases in negative affect (Kobau et al., 2004). Another study found that patterns of age differences in negative affect change based on whether researchers control for physical health status; without controlling for health problems, age is unrelated to increased negative affect (Kunzmann et al., 2000). When researchers control for physical health problems or examine physically healthy older adults, however, age is related to decreases in negative affect among successively older groups of people ranging from their 60s to their 90s (Charles et al., 2010; Kunzmann et al., 2000). In addition, negative affect even in the oldest age groups never decreases to levels observed among people in their 20s (e.g., Charles et al., 2001; Diener & Suh, 1998).

Studies examining age differences in positive affect among people over 65 years old are similarly mixed, with some finding age-related increases in positive affect until age 74 (Mroczek & Kolarz, 1998), and others documenting slight age-related decreases over time (Charles et al., 2001) or no differences between older adults ranging from their 60s to their early 90s (Charles et al., 2010). Together, age-related changes in emotional experiences after age 65 are not as consistent as changes throughout early and mid-adulthood. When changes are found, they are generally small in magnitude.

In contrast to findings examining the frequency of emotional experience in later life, studies of emotional arousal are less equivocal. Early views that older age leads to less intense emotional experiences have been dispelled by research using both daily sampling techniques and laboratory experiments (see review by

Charles & Carstensen, 2007). Older and younger adults report similar intensity levels for both positive and negative emotions over the course of the day (Carstensen et al., 2000), when recalling prior life events (Magai et al., 2006), and in response to emotion-eliciting film clips (Magai et al., 2006; Tsai et al., 2000). When age differences are noted, older adults often report higher intensity emotions than do younger adults (Charles, 2005; Kunzmann & Grühn, 2005). Thus, the ability to experience intense emotions remains intact across adulthood, and the frequency of emotional experiences points to less negative affect and stable levels of positive affect throughout most if not all of adulthood.

Age Differences in Emotional Complexity

In addition to studying age differences in levels of positive and negative affect or the relative difference between these two states, a growing number of studies are examining the frequency with which these two valenced states co-occur in daily life. Positive and negative affect are only moderately correlated with one another, are associated with different life events, motivate different goals, and show different age-related patterns across time (e.g., Charles et al., 2001; Fredrickson, 2001). Despite the unique qualities of positive and negative affect, researchers find that their interrelationships provide information that may be missed when studying each one on its own (e.g., Fredrickson & Losada, 2005; Reich et al., 2003). For example, the relative ratio of positive to negative affect experienced is a better measure of overall well-being and predicts positive psychological and social functioning better than studying each one separately (Fredrickson & Losada, 2004). According to the Dynamic Model of Affect, high levels of perceived stress and uncertainty without co-occurring positive emotional states leads to a narrowing of attention and cognitive capacity that is focused on immediate environmental demands (see review by Reich et al., 2003). Experiencing higher levels of positive emotions during stressful experiences, in contrast, signals greater cognitive complexity and faster recovery from the accompanying negative emotions (Reich et al., 2003).

Researchers have found that older adults commonly report the experience of both positive and negative affect (Ong et al., 2006), and some studies suggest that older adults experience these mixed emotional states more often than do younger adults (e.g., Carstensen et al., 2000). For example, older age is related to more complex, mixed emotional experiences in daily life (Carstensen et al., 2000) and when describing the emotions depicted in previously read scenarios (Löckenhoff et al., 2008). When examining co-occurring emotions within valence, older age is also associated with a greater heterogeneity, or mix, of negative emotions (such as both anger and disgust) as opposed to the experience of one dominant emotional state (Charles, 2005; Kliegel et al., 2007; but see Löckenhoff et al., 2008).

Age differences in emotional complexity are also reflected in facial expressions of older and younger adults; when recalling a past emotional event, older adults express more nuanced facial expressions that convey a mix of emotional experiences compared to younger adults (Magai et al., 2006). Rather than indicating an inability to accurately control their emotions, researchers posit that these more nuanced expressions reflect more mixed, complex, emotional experiences (Magai et al., 2006). And in further support that age differences in emotional expression do not represent declines, older adults are equally as adept as younger adults at either suppressing or amplifying their facial expressions in response to emotion-eliciting stimuli (Kunzmann et al., 2005).

Understanding Emotion and Aging: Strength and Vulnerability Integration

Reporting high levels of emotional well-being does not prove that older adults regulate their emotions more effectively. Higher levels of well-being with age (e.g., Mroczek & Kolarz, 1998) may result from people treating older adults with greater deference (e.g., Miller et al., 2009) or from older adults reporting fewer stressors in their lives (e.g., Charles et al., 2010). The input older adults receive from their social partners and from environmental demands may certainly play a role in their higher levels of well-being. People rarely, however, report low levels of negative affect when they are having difficulty regulating their emotions.

Researchers have studied possible actions on the part of older adults that may contribute to their high levels of emotional well-being. SAVI is a new life-span developmental theory about age and emotional experience that has been shaped by recent research and theoretical work (Charles & Carstensen, 2010; Charles & Piazza, 2009). According to SAVI, older age is related to strengths in the knowledge and use of emotion regulation strategies that result in maintained if not higher levels of emotional well-being. These age-related strengths are the result of time: time left in life motivates older adults to prioritize emotional well-being (as posited by socioemotional selectivity theory), and time lived provides older adults with greater knowledge about themselves and others that increase their ability to avoid distressing situations. When negative situations cannot be avoided, older adults use disengagement strategies that allow them to avoid prolonged exposure to these caustic experiences. By using emotion regulation strategies that allow them to avoid or quickly disengage from situations that create distress, they are able to maintain high levels of emotional well-being.

When older adults cannot avoid or reduce their exposure to negative situations, however, they will experience emotional distress. Although age-related changes in physiological functioning may aid emotion regulation by slowing the time to peak arousal during this reactivity, age-related changes will also create problems when downregulating emotional experience. Once people experience heightened physiological arousal, age-related vulnerabilities created by reduced physiological flexibility will lead to prolonged arousal and greater difficulty returning to baseline levels of affective well-being. Although physiological arousal and subjective experience have an imperfect relationship, they nonetheless inform one another. Thus, SAVI posits that older adults will experience fewer stressors than younger adults (Stawski et al., 2008), but they will be equally reactive to these events when they occur (e.g., Neupert et al., 2007; Stawski et al., 2008).

By integrating age-related strengths and vulnerabilities, researchers can predict when in the time course of emotional experience older adults will show improved well-being compared to younger adults, and when these age differences will attenuate or perhaps even reverse in direction. When people are not faced with an either real or perceived threat to their well-being, SAVI posits that older adults will report higher levels of emotional well-being than will younger adults. And, when initially confronted with a negative situation, older adults are more likely to engage in strategies that focus their attention away from the negative aspects of a situation. They are also more likely to engage in behaviors that enable them to disengage from the caustic event. If they cannot avoid prolonged exposure to these situations, however, older adults will be forced to attend to the situation and experience high levels of arousal. During this time, age differences will attenuate or perhaps even reserve in direction. Prolonged exposure is hypothesized to lead to worse outcomes for older rather than younger adults.

For many older adults, life is relatively predictable. They often have stable social networks (e.g., Lang, 2001) and retirement allows them more freedom to structure their time (Ginn & Fast, 2006; Rosenkoetter et al., 2001). In addition, people treat older adults more kindly than they do younger adults (Fingerman & Charles, 2010). For others, however, situations may arise over which they have little control and which create high levels of prolonged distress. SAVI discusses three chronic situations that increase in prevalence with age, that create high levels of distress, and over which people feel little control. These include neurological impairment, caregiving for a spouse with dementia, and chronic loneliness resulting from a lack of social belonging.

In contrast to these chronic stressors, acute experiences, by definition, are short-lived. As time from the event passes, SAVI posits that older adults will appraise and recall these events in a way that will once again enhance their well-being and lead to more positive emotion-related outcomes. Thus, age differences in emotional well-being will vary based on the time when it is captured — before, during, or after an emotional event. This theory grew from the findings of the past decade. Some of these findings are well-established empirically, but others need to be investigated to either confirm or amend SAVI, as discussed in the next section.

REASONS FOR AGE-RELATED STRENGTHS IN EMOTION REGULATION

Many theories and models of aging recognize strengths and vulnerabilities of aging. Strengths include a self-awareness that allows older adults to adapt to the losses that occur with age, which are discussed in detail in the model of selective optimization with compensation (Baltes & Baltes, 1990). According to this model, old age is associated with accumulated losses in social, mental, physical, and functional domains. Successful adaptation requires that people select areas in their life that they would like to maintain, areas chosen either by elective selection (e.g., choosing an activity for its enjoyment) or loss-based selection (e.g., needing to engage in physical therapy to preserve functioning after a stroke). People then work to optimize their abilities in this selected domain. For less important areas in their lives, they solicit help that allows them to compensate for their losses. This model makes no predictions about specific areas of optimization, but researchers have used this model to describe the gradual selection of emotion-related goals as people age (Baltes & Carstensen, 2003). Other adult life-span researchers also acknowledge the sophisticated adjustments people make in response to age-related losses to maintain well-being (Heckhausen et al., 2010; Rothermund & Brandtstädter, 2003). These motivational control theories emphasize the importance of recognizing when a goal is unattainable, and altering goals to compensate for these losses.

Another age-related strength in the ability to regulate emotions is the greater priority placed on maintaining emotional well-being. Socioemotional selectivity theory describes an age-related increase in the importance placed on emotion-related goals (Carstensen et al., 1999). This increased motivation leads to greater attention and focus on thoughts and behaviors that optimize emotional well-being. According to the theory, two overarching goals motivate much of human behavior: one encompasses information and knowledge gain, and the other includes emotional fulfillment and optimizing emotional well-being. The importance of goals is guided by a person's temporal horizons. When a person perceives a long, expansive future, information gain is prioritized above other goals. When time diminishes and people perceive a limited future, emotional goals assume priority. As people grow older, they gradually place increasing value on emotion-related goals.

Socioemotional selectivity theory posits that diminished temporal horizons shift motivational goals toward optimizing emotional well-being. Other theories and models have recognized yet another reason that older adults may grow adept at emotion regulation. Specifically, researchers have discussed the importance of time lived for accruing knowledge that enables older adults to regulate their emotions successfully (Blanchard-Fields, 2007; Hess & Aumann, 2001; Magai et al., 2006). According to this view, years of experience have provided older adults with knowledge about situations that lead to emotional distress and the behaviors necessary to avoid, or at least mitigate, these situations.

Cognitive and Behavioral Strategies Related to Emotional Well-Being

SAVI posits that older adults, bolstered by a motivation to optimize emotional well-being (as described by socioemotional theory) and capitalizing on their knowledge gained from years of experience, engage in thoughts and behaviors that enable them to regulate their emotions effectively (see review by Charles & Carstensen, 2010). A growing number of studies have examined age differences in thoughts and behaviors in response to emotional stimuli. Findings consistently point to age-related increases in actions and thoughts aimed at avoiding negative affect, such as directing attention toward positive and away from negative emotional stimuli (Isaacowitz et al., 2006), and appraising current and past emotional experiences as less distressing and more positive (e.g., Kennedy et al., 2004). These strategies encompass some of the most powerful emotion regulation strategies available, allowing people to maintain high levels of emotional well-being and avoiding the physiological arousal that accompanies strong emotional experiences (Gross, 1998).

Regulating Emotions in Social Contexts

Many emotion regulation strategies occur in the context of interpersonal relationships. Social relationships are strongly tied to physical health and emotional well-being (e.g., Rook et al., 2007). Although social relationships can be a source of joy and contentment, they also can be a source of distress. The most common daily stressors are interpersonal in nature (Almeida, 2005). Interpersonal stressors elicit high levels of emotional distress (e.g., Birditt et al., 2005), and they are strongly related to both emotional and physical well-being (e.g., Newsom et al., 2008).

Socioemotional selectivity theory posits that older adults place greater emphasis and importance on the emotions derived from social relationships than do younger adults (Carstensen, 2006; Carstensen et al., 1999). Older adults have smaller social networks than do younger adults, and researchers believe this decrease reflects active efforts on the part of older adults to remove social partners from whom they derive few emotional benefits (Lang, 2001; Lang & Carstensen, 2002). This decrease of more peripheral partners begins in middle-age, with declines beginning across the third and fourth decade of life (Carstensen, 1992). In contrast to the number of peripheral, less important social partners, the number of close friends and family members is similar across age groups (Lang, 2001). In addition, people report increasing emotional satisfaction with close friends and family members over time (Carstensen, 1992). When reporting the emotions experienced with family members across the course of the week, for instance, older adults report higher levels of positive emotions than do younger adults (Charles & Piazza, 2007).

Even when people experience tense interpersonal exchanges, older adults engage in behaviors that decrease the escalation of these situations to a greater extent than do younger adults (Blanchard-Fields, 2007). For example, younger adults are more likely to respond by engaging in an argument or confronting a person who is the source of the contention, whereas older adults are more likely to report that they disengage from these situations or that they wait until the situation has passed (Blanchard-Fields et al., 2007; Charles et al., 2001). More passive behaviors also appear to confer greater emotion regulation advantages with age. A study examining emotional reactivity in response to two types of interpersonal stressors – one where people engaged in an argument and another where people could have argued but decided to let the situation pass – revealed that older adults are less reactive to the avoided argument than the actual argument (Charles et al., 2009). When comparing across age, older age is related to less reactivity to the avoided argument, but younger, middle, and older adults are similarly reactive to the actual argument.

Evidence suggesting that older adults create more benign outcomes in otherwise tense situations is also found in studies of married couples (Carstensen et al., 1995; Seider et al., 2009; Story et al., 2007). In these studies, older and middle-aged couples are asked to discuss an area of contention in their relationship. Researchers then analyze age differences in expressive behaviors, comments, and physiological reactivity during these exchanges. Results indicate that older and middle-aged couples differ in how they express themselves to their spouses during these conflicts; specifically, older adults use more relationship "we" words, whereas middle-aged couples make more "I" comments (Seider et al., 2009). Researchers interpret the use of "we" as symptomatic of older adults adopting a more communal, relationship orientation than middle-aged adults, which is perhaps why greater use of "we" as opposed to "I" is associated with more positive emotions and less physiological arousal during these arguments. Older adults also express less negative affect and more affection than do middle-aged spouses even after controlling for levels of marital satisfaction (Carstensen et al., 1995). Thus, the actual arguments of older couples appear to be less negative than those of middle-aged couples.

ATTENTION TO AND APPRAISALS OF POSITIVE AND NEGATIVE STIMULI

The degree to which people attend to emotional stimuli predicts the strength of their emotional response (e.g., Scheier & Carver, 1977); for this reason, focusing attention away from negative and toward positive aspects of the environment is considered an effective emotion regulation strategy (Gross, 1998; 2001). Younger adults often show a bias for negative information, a bias not present among older adults (Isaacowitz, 2006). Studies indicate that older age is associated with a tendency to focus attention on more positive stimuli when presented choices between two expressive faces using a dot-probe task and when tracking eye gaze (Isaacowitz et al., 2006; Mather & Carstensen, 2003). Even after older and younger adults undergo a sadness induction, older adults are still more likely to direct their gaze toward the more positive facial expressions (Isaacowitz et al., 2008). The desire to disattend to negative information is illustrated in yet another study where younger and older adults imagine that they are overhearing negative comments directed at them (Charles & Carstensen, 2008). Unlike younger adults who are more likely to express a desire for more information, older adults express little interest in learning more about what motivated their remarks. Researchers interpret the fewer comments by older adults as efforts to distance themselves from the caustic situation (Charles & Carstensen, 2008).

Studies examining age differences in brain activity in response to emotional stimuli have confirmed the behavioral data described above (e.g., Wood & Kisley, 2006). When examining rapid processing of emotional information captured by evoked related potentials in the brain, younger adults have a higher amplitude response for negative emotional stimuli compared to positive stimuli, a negativity bias not present for older adults (Langeslag & van Strien, 2009; Wood & Kisley, 2006). Additional research indicates that brain activity in the amygdala (a region of the brain strongly tied to emotional experience) is more active after exposure to positive stimuli among older adults but equally active in response to both positive and negative stimuli for younger adults (Mather et al., 2004).

Researchers have referred to this age-related bias toward positive stimuli and away from negative stimuli as the "positivity effect" (Carstensen & Mikels, 2005; Charles et al., 2003). They emphasize that a positive bias is the default pattern for older adults. Because older adults place a higher priority on optimizing emotional experience (as posited by socioemotional selectivity theory), they engage in cognitive strategies that focus on more positive aspects of the environment. Allocating attention toward positive stimuli and away from negative stimuli represents one such cognitive strategy that enhances emotional well-being. Importantly, Carstensen and her colleagues (1999) posit that these different motivations lead to age differences in attention to positive and negative material. They further state that if older adults adopt the priorities of younger adults, or vice versa, age differences disappear (e.g., Carstensen & Mikels, 2005). For example, when older adults are instructed to focus on nonemotional goals, such as focusing on perceptual details or accuracy, they no longer show a positivity bias (e.g., Carstensen & Mikels, 2005).

Appraisals of Current and Past Emotional Experiences

Appraisal theorists posit that a person's perceptions of an event more accurately predict his or her emotional response than do objective indicators of the event (e.g., Lazarus, 1999). When first encountering a situation, people make initial evaluations about whether a situation poses harm, threat, or challenge to their well-being (e.g., Lazarus, 1999). When evaluating the stressors they encounter in their daily lives, younger adults rate them as more severe than do older adults, despite these stressors having similar severity levels when rated by objective coders (Almeida & Horn, 2004). For example, older adults are less likely to appraise a situation as being annoying or creating worry for others than are younger adults (Boeninger et al., 2009). Another study found that when middle-aged and older spouses recall how their spouse behaved during a prior disagreement, older adults recalled that their spouses expressed more positive emotions than did middle-aged couples (Story et al., 2007). Importantly, older adults rated their spouse's behavior more positively than did objective viewers, a bias not present in the recollections of the middle-aged spouses (Story et al., 2007).

Memory for Past Events

These more positive appraisals are reflected in the memories of older adults as well. Over time, for example, intensity of regret decreases for both younger and older adults, but this decrease is more pronounced for older adults (Bauer et al., 2008). Older adults remember their levels of loneliness, well-being, and physical health as being more positive and less negative than do their younger counterparts, a finding that remains even after controlling for their current ratings of these same psychosocial factors (Kennedy et al., 2004). In two diary studies, researchers also found that older adults recalled the events of the prior week more positively and less negatively than did younger adults (Ready et al., 2007). In these studies, participants reported the daily emotions they had reported every evening across a week (Ready et al., 2007). Later, they were asked to recall these experiences. Older adults remembered these emotions as more positive and less negative than they had reported during the week. In contrast, younger adults were more likely to report the emotions experienced in the prior week as more negative than what they had recorded in their nightly reports.

Potential Area of Vulnerability: Emotional Arousal

The research above overwhelmingly supports age-related strengths in the ability to engage in thoughts and behavior that promote emotional well-being. Will older adults, in general, always surpass the abilities of younger adults in studies examining reactions to emotional stimuli? SAVI predicts that age-related vulnerabilities in the ability to downregulate high levels of physiological arousal will lead to an attenuation or even a reversal of age-related trends when people experience prolonged, high intensity emotions. Fewer studies have addressed this question, and further research is needed to either support SAVI or demand its refinement.

Several studies have found that older age is related to less reactivity, not more, in response to emotion-eliciting stimuli (e.g., Labouvie-Vief et al., 2003; Tsai et al., 2000). For example, older age was related to less hemodynamic reactivity when people participated in a laboratory experiment where they relived experiences that elicited happiness, anger, fear, and sadness (Labouvie-Vief et al., 2003). When watching happy and sad emotion-eliciting film clips, older adults also displayed less physiological reactivity than did younger adults (Tsai et al., 2000). In another study examining age differences in response to videos eliciting sadness, however, older adults displayed higher levels of physiological reactivity than did younger adults (Kunzman & Grühn, 2005). Researchers suggest that perhaps one reason older age was related to greater reactivity in this study compared to prior studies is that the emotion-eliciting stimuli (e.g., bereavement and dementia) were more pertinent to the lives of older adults. Thus, older adults may experience lower levels of arousal in response to emotional stimuli in some of the prior studies because they differ in their appraisals and the perceived relevance of the stimuli.

Few studies have examined age differences in behaviors or emotional responses when people are experiencing high levels of arousal. One study examined the effects of high levels of physiological arousal on age differences on a subsequent stressful task (Mather et al., 2009). Prior to engaging in a simulating driving task, half of the younger and older participants underwent a physiologically stressful activity where they submerged one hand in ice cold water (referred to as the cold pressor task). Afterwards, they performed the driving task when circulating cortisol in response to the stress task was at its highest concentration. When comparing scores on the driving task, performance was similar across younger adults (regardless of whether they had engaged in the stress task) and older adults who did not undergo the stress task. Older adults who performed the driving task after the stress task, however, performed worse than all other groups. Thus, increases in cortisol had a negative influence on the performance of older adults but not younger adults.

Several other studies have found age-related increases in physiological reactivity in response to emotional stimuli and emotional events. For example, researchers find that older adults display an exaggerated startle response, as assessed by eye blink, to negative stimuli compared to younger adults (Langley et al., 2008; Smith et al., 2005). In a study examining older and younger adults involved in an active emotion-eliciting task where they had to perform before an evaluative audience, older age was related to higher systolic blood pressure reactivity in response (Uchino et al., 1999). A longitudinal study confirmed this age-related increase in reactivity in systolic blood pressure in response to a psychosocial stressor (Uchino et al., 2005). This pattern mirrors physiological reactivity in daily life, where again older age is related to greater blood pressure reactivity to daily hassles (Uchino et al., 2006).

Labouvie-Vief's (2003) Dynamic Integration Theory (DIT) offers a different interpretation for how levels of arousal will influence emotional functioning among older adults. DIT states that throughout childhood and up to middle adulthood, people develop increasingly complex representations and integrations of positive and negative affect. This higher order processing correlates strongly with other indicators of cognitive functioning, such as vocabulary tests and education level. In addition, this elaborative processing follows a curvilinear pattern based on the arousal of the emotional material – moderate levels of arousal allow for elaboration and enhanced processing, but high levels of arousal lead to decrease in the capacity to integrate positive and negative emotions. According to this theory, situations of high arousal are particularly difficult for older adults, because they have greater difficulty integrating positive and negative emotional information. In these taxing situations, people revert to a self-preserving strategy of optimizing their affective experience. Thus, these situations are posited to optimize emotional well-being in older adults. In a study that examined age differences when people performed the emotional Stroop task – a task where they must inhibit emotional information while they correctly identify the color or words — the performance of older adults was more impaired for highly arousing words than was the performance of younger adults (Wurm et al., 2004).

THREATS TO EMOTIONAL WELL-BEING

When comparing across age groups, older adults report similar if not higher levels of emotional well-being than do younger adults. In addition, longitudinal analyses indicate that negative affect decreases across middle-adulthood (e.g., Charles et al., 2001). Not all people, however, report high levels of emotional well-being, and not everyone reports lower levels of negative affect over time. Reasons for divergent trajectories of well-being are many. SAVI suggests that situations that are unpredictable, prolonged, and cause high levels of arousal are more prevalent in later life and may explain why a subset of older adults fair poorly in very old age. These are not the only reasons, however, that may explain why some people do not benefit from age-related increases in well-being (e.g., Mroczek & Spiro, 2005). Researchers have focused on personality types and life events that influence trajectories of well-being over time to understand the reasons why people deviate from normative patterns of change. Some life events are encountered less often with age, such as a job threat, unemployment, a ruminative cognitive style, or a recent problem with another person (Jorm et al., 2005). Other events, such as health problems, death of close friends and family members, and spousal caregiving increase in prevalence (Jorm et al., 2005; Langa et al., 2001). Unfortunately, many of these reasons include situations over which people have little control or may be events that happened earlier in life but continue to exert negative effects on well-being.

Early Experiences

Chronic circumstances experienced throughout life are believed to produce small psychological and physical insults that accumulate over time (e.g., Hawkley & Cacioppo, 2007). According to this view, exposure to negative situations results in a cascade of physiological and emotional responses that wear away at emotional and physical reserves. As a result, these negative experiences may have lasting consequences, some of which only reveal themselves when physical reserves decline with age.

Children are born with different temperaments that unfold into fairly stable personality traits in adulthood (McCrae et al., 2000). One personality trait most implicated in emotional distress is neuroticism. Neuroticism is a relatively stable personality trait characterized by emotional instability and tendencies to experience depression and anxiety. Research indicates that a lifetime of emotional instability may lead people to poorer emotional and physical outcomes in old age (e.g., Charles et al., 2008; Mroczek & Almeida, 2004). For example, early measures of neuroticism are related to increased prevalence of physical conditions in later life (Charles et al., 2008) and to all-cause mortality (Grossardt et al., 2009). In addition, neuroticism increases emotional reactivity to stressors, and this reactivity is more pronounced among older adults compared to younger adults (Mroczek & Almeida, 2004). Researchers posit that after years of heightened sensitivity to stressors, people with high levels of neuroticism become sensitized to negative events and therefore react more strongly to them (Mroczek & Almeida, 2004). This stance is consistent with longitudinal findings showing that people with high levels of neuroticism do not display age-related decreases in negative affect (Charles et al., 2001) or increases in life satisfaction (Mroczek & Spiro, 2005) enjoyed by their peers who score lower on this personality trait.

When researchers want to focus on environmental influences of emotional experiences in childhood, one fertile area is the parent-child relationship. Developmental psychologists have documented the link between parental behaviors on the physical and emotional well-being of their children (Repetti et al., 2002), but findings indicate that these effects persist into old age (e.g., Consedine & Magai, 2003). For example, older adults who recall more secure attachments with their parents in childhood report higher levels of positive emotions and lower levels of negative emotions in their daily lives compared to those reporting less secure attachments to childhood caregivers (Consedine & Magai, 2003). In addition, adults ranging from 25 to 74 years old who state that they received low levels of affection from their parents report higher levels of general emotional distress than adults who described having more affectionate parents (Shaw et al., 2004). Moreover, people whose childhoods were characterized by emotional neglect or adversity are more likely to feel emotionally isolated from others in old age (Korkeila et al., 2005; Wilson et al., 2006).

The wear and tear from years of chronic activation of stress, coupled with age-related declines in physical functioning, may explain why older adults often have stronger physiological correlates with emotion-related assessments than do younger adults. For example, researchers have found that older adults who are lonely show increased blood pressure and levels of hormones related to sympathetic activation in response to stress compared to their more socially connected peers (Cacioppo et al., 2002; Hawkley et al., 2006). Younger adults who are lonely, however, do not vary in health-related indicators from their less lonely peers. Researchers attribute the ties between loneliness and health-related outcomes among older adults to accrued impact of years living with feelings of loneliness and social isolation (Hawkley & Cacioppo, 2007). Living in a difficult marriage may also be a chronic situation that has greater repercussions on older than younger adults; low marital satisfaction is related to increased cortisol reactivity during a spousal interaction for older men but not middle-aged men (Heffner et al., 2004). Again, aggregated effects of an unhappy union may be responsible for these age-related findings.

Current Situations

Many older adults are surrounded by close family members, engage in intrinsically interesting activities, and have health conditions that are controlled through medication and health behaviors. A minority of older adults however, are experiencing negative life events over which they may feel little control and that are commonly associated with emotional distress. Unfortunately, three such situations increase in prevalence with age. These include physical health conditions that cause functional or cognitive impairment, spousal caregiving, and spousal bereavement. Each of these conditions has been related to high rates of depressive symptoms, anxiety, and overall emotional distress.

Physical health problems that include functional impairments and living with multiple chronic health impairments are both related to decreased life satisfaction and increased negative affect (e.g. Lucas, 2007; Piazza et al., 2007). Spousal bereavement is related to lower levels of life satisfaction that only return to pre-bereavement levels eight years later (Lucas et al., 2003). For some people faced with spousal bereavement, loneliness increases over time (Dykstra et al., 2005). Thus, although many older adults are living emotionally fulfilling lives marked by high levels of satisfaction and contentment, others face challenges to well-being that may partly reflect their exposure to uncontrollable and negative life events.

These situations may contribute to experiences of distress severe enough to receive clinical attention; although the prevalence rates of depression and anxiety are often lower among older adults than younger adults, half of the population of older adults diagnosed with clinical depression and those with Generalized Anxiety Disorder have no prior history of an affective disorder (Fiske et al., 2009; Wetherell & Stein, 2009). Researchers have speculated about the reasons for these new cases, with physical health conditions related to depression and cognitive declines and functional limitations among the strongest predictors of anxiety in later life (see review by Fiske et al., 2009; Wetherell & Stein, 2009).

FUTURE DIRECTIONS AND CONCLUSIONS

Recent research weaves a complex and rich story of emotion and aging. People report a gamut of emotional experiences across adulthood. Life events are associated with the same types of emotions for people across age groups: a marriage or birth is often associated with happiness, and an economic loss or physical illness often causes distress. Adults of all ages generally respond to distressing events using similar emotion regulation strategies. Older age, however, is related to decreases in several areas of emotional functioning. People are less accurate when decoding facial expressions and emotional tones in melodies. Their reactions times are slowed, and sometimes physiological reactivity is exaggerated in response to emotional stimuli.

Despite these losses, older adults report relatively high levels of emotional well-being. Researchers posit that they do so because they have acquired skills by which to navigate their environments. Older adults are less effective at decoding facial expressions, but they have acquired social expertise that allows them to navigate their social worlds effectively. Their social interactions include a greater proportion of people who are emotionally close to them and with whom they report higher levels of positive emotions. When confronted with negative situations, they quickly disengage from these situations in attempts to distance themselves from further emotional distress. As a result, physiological response to emotional arousal – sometimes associated with exaggerated responses among older adults compared to younger adults —can be avoided altogether.

Current findings provide information regarding age differences in emotional experience and also provide a roadmap for future research: studies are revealing age differences in neurobiological pathways, physiological reactivity, cognitive appraisals, and subjective responses. These studies include cutting edge research design methods and greater sensitivity to contextual factors that shape emotional experience. Future studies need to build on this research to continue confirming, or contradicting, current findings. Longitudinal studies will need to affirm or refine theories built largely from cross-sectional findings. Studies of neurological pathways and the mechanisms underlying age differences in the activation patterns of these pathways will further explain age differences in subjective experience.

SAVI represents a new theory that points to areas that are well-documented in the literature, as well as other areas in need of empirical research. A number of studies have outlined the strengths of aging where regulating emotions are concerned. For example, older adults more often focus their attention away from negative stimuli, and they remember experiences more positively than do younger adults. The potential role of physical vulnerabilities of aging, however, is an understudied area. More research is needed to examine age differences in response to highly arousing emotional situations both inside and outside of the laboratory. Future studies will need to examine age differences in both the arousal elicited by emotional stimuli as well as the effects of physiological arousal on other emotion-related outcomes. To this aim, the multiple components of emotional experience - physiological, subjective, cognitive, and behavioral responses - will need to be assessed before, during, and after the experience to capture the full time course of emotion regulation. Finally, older and younger adults often differ in baseline levels of positive and negative affect, and disentangling age differences in baseline levels of well-being as opposed to emotional reactivity to positive and negative events will be an important research aim.

With the findings garnered from recent efforts, scientists have reason to be optimistic about mental health and aging. Older adults face losses to emotional functioning — losses that also parallel age-related changes to brain structure and speed of processing on other cognitive tasks. At the same time, however, older adults appear to employ strategies that allow them to successfully navigate their environment to avoid many negative experiences. By understanding these processes, we can learn the strategies that help older adults and focus on disseminating our knowledge to older adults who are currently experiencing high levels of distress.

REFERENCES

Almeida, D. M. (2005). Resilience and vulnerability to daily stressors assessed via diary methods. *Current Directions in Psychological Science, 14,* 64–68.

Almeida, D. M., & Horn, M. C. (2004). Is daily life more stressful during middle adulthood? In O. G. Brim & C. D. Ryff (Eds.), *How healthy are we?: A national study of well-being at midlife* (pp. 425–451). Chicago: University of Chicago Press.

Baltes, P. B., & Baltes, M. M. (1990). Selective optimization with compensation. In P. B. Baltes & M. M. Baltes (Eds.), *Successful Aging: Perspectives from the Behavioral Sciences* (pp. 1–34). New York: Cambridge University Press.

Baltes, M. M., & Carstensen, L. L. (2003). The process of successful aging: Selection, optimization and compensation. In U. M. Staudinger & U. Lindenberger (Eds.), *Understanding human development: Dialogues with lifespan psychology* (pp. 81–104). Dordrecht, Netherlands: Kluwer Academic Publishers.

Basevitz, P., Pushkar, D., Dalton, C., Chaikelson, J., & Conway, M. (2008). Age-related differences in worry and related processes. *International Journal of Aging and Human Development, 66,* 283–305.

Bauer, I., Wrosch, C., & Jobin, J. (2008). I'm better off than most other people: The role of social comparisons for coping with regret in young adulthood and old age. *Psychology and Aging, 23,* 800–811.

Birditt, K. S., & Fingerman, K. L. (2003). Age and gender differences in adults' descriptions of emotional reactions to interpersonal problems. *Journals of Gerontology: Series B: Psychological Sciences & Social Sciences, 58B,* 237–245.

Birditt, K. S., Fingerman, K. L., & Almeida, D. M. (2005). Age differences in exposure and reactions to interpersonal tensions: A daily diary study. *Psychology and Aging, 20,* 330–340.

Blanchard-Fields, F. (2007). Everyday problem solving and emotion: An adult developmental perspective. *Current Directions in Psychological Science, 16,* 26–31.

Blanchard-Fields, F., Mienaltowski, A., & Seay, R. B. (2007). Age differences in everyday problem-solving effectiveness: Older adults select more effective strategies for interpersonal problems. *Journals of Gerontology: Psychological Science, 62,* P61–64.

Boeninger, D. K., Shiraishi, R. W., Aldwin, C. M., & Spiro, A. III. (2009). Why do older men report lower stress ratings? Findings from the Normative Aging Study. *International Journal of Aging & Human Development, 68,* 149–170.

Cacioppo, J. T., Hawkley, L. C., Crawford, L. E., Ernst, J. M., Burleson, M. H., Kowalewski, R. B., et al. (2002). Loneliness and health: Potential mechanisms. *Psychosomatic Medicine, 64,* 407–417.

Carstensen, L. L. (1992). Social and emotional patterns in adulthood: Support for socioemotional selectivity theory. *Psychology and Aging, 7,* 331–338.

Carstensen, L. L. (2006). The influence of a sense of time on human development. *Science, 312,* 1913–1915.

Carstensen, L. L., Gottman, J. M., & Levenson, R. W. (1995). Emotional behavior in long-term marriage. *Psychology & Aging, 10,* 140–149.

Carstensen, L. L., Isaacowitz, D. M., & Charles, S. T. (1999). Taking time seriously: A theory of socioemotional selectivity. *American Psychologist, 54*, 165–181.

Carstensen, L. L., & Mikels, J. A. (2005). At the intersection of emotion and cognition: Aging and the positivity effect. *Current Directions in Psychological Science, 14*, 117–121.

Carstensen, L. L., Pasupathi, M., Mayr, U., & Nesselroade, J. R. (2000). Emotional experience in everyday life across the adult life span. *Journal of Personality & Social Psychology, 79*, 644–655.

Charles, S. T., Mather, M., & Carstensen, L. L. (2003). Aging emotional memory: The forgettable nature of negative images for older adults. *Journal of Experimental Psychology: General, 132*, 310–324.

Charles, S. T. (2005). Viewing injustice: Age differences in emotional experience. *Psychology and Aging, 20*, 159–164.

Charles, S. T., & Carstensen, L. L. (2004). A life-span view of emotional functioning in adulthood and old age. In P. Costa (Ed.), *Advances in Cell Aging and Gerontology Series*. New York: Elsevier.

Charles, S. T., & Carstensen, L. L. (2007). Emotion regulation and aging. In J. J. Gross (Ed.), *Handbook of emotion regulation* (pp. 307–327). New York: Guilford Press.

Charles, S. T., & Carstensen, L. L. (2008). Unpleasant situations elicit different emotional responses in younger and older adults. *Psychology & Aging, 23*, 495–504.

Charles, S. T., & Carstensen, L. L. (2010). Social and emotional aspects of aging. *Annual Review of Psychology, 61*, 383–409.

Charles, S. T., Carstensen, L. L., & McFall, R. M. (2001). Problem-solving in the nursing home environment: Age and experience differences in emotional reactions and responses. *Journal of Clinical Geropsychology. Special Issue: Management of Behavioral Problems in Late Life–Therapeutic Approaches and Related Issues, 7*, 319–330.

Charles, S. T., Gatz, M., Kato, K., & Pedersen, N. L. (2008). Physical health twenty-five years later: The predictive ability of neuroticism. *Health Psychology, 27*, 369–378.

Charles, S. T., Luong, G., Almeida, D. M., Ryff, C., Sturm, M., & Love, G. (2010). Fewer ups and downs: Daily stressors mediate age differences in negative affect. *Journals of Gerontology Series B: Psychological Sciences and Social Sciences, 65*, 279–286.

Charles, S. T., & Piazza, J. R. (2007). Memories of social interactions: Age differences in emotional intensity. *Psychology and Aging, 22*, 300–309.

Charles, S. T, & Piazza, J. R. (2009). Age differences in affective well-being: Context matters. *Social & Personality Psychology Compass, 3*, 711–724.

Charles, S. T., Piazza, J. R., Luong, G., & Almeida, D. M. (2009). Now you see it, now you don't: Age differences in affective reactivity to social tensions. *Psychology & Aging, 24, 645–653.*

Charles, S. T., Reynolds, C. A., & Gatz, M. (2001). Age-related differences and change in positive and negative affect over 23 years. *Journal of Personality and Social Psychology, 80*, 136–151.

Chipperfield, J. G., Perry, R. P., Weiner, B., & Newall, N. E. (2009). Reported causal antecedents of discrete emotions in late life. *International Journal of Aging & Human Development, 68*, 215–241.

Chow, S.-M., Hamagami, F., & Nesselroade, J. R. (2007). Age differences in dynamical emotion-cognition linkages. *Psychology and Aging, 22*, 765–780.

Consedine, N., & Magai, C. (2003). Attachment and emotion experience in later life: The view from emotions theory. *Attachment & Human Development, 5*(2), 165–187.

Darwin, C. (1872). *The expression of the emotions in man and animals.* London, UK: Murray.

Davey, A., Halverson, C. F. J., Zonderman, A. B., & Costa, P. T., Jr. (2004). Change in depressive symptoms in the Baltimore Longitudinal Study of Aging. *Journals of Gerontology: Series B: Psychological Sciences and Social Sciences, 59*, 270–277.

Diener, E., & Suh, E. M. (1998). Subjective well-being and age: An international analysis. In K. W. Schaie & M. P. Lawton (Eds.), *Annual Review of Gerontology and Geriatrics, 17*, 304–324.

Dykstra, P. A., van Tilburg, T. G., & Gierveld, J. (2005). Changes in older adult loneliness. *Research on Aging, 27*, 725–747.

Fingerman, K. L., & Charles, S. T. (2010). It takes two to tango: Why old people have the best relationships. *Current Directions in Psychological Science, 18*, 172–176.

Fiske, A., Wetherell, J. L., & Gatz, M. (2009). Depression in older adults. *Annual Review of Clinical Psychology, 5*, 363–389.

Fox, N. A., & Reeb, B. C. (2008). Effects of early experience on the development of cerebral asymmetry and approach-withdrawal. In A. Elliot (Ed.), *Handbook of approach and voidance motivation* (pp. 25–49). New York: Psychology Press.

Fredrickson, B. L. (2001). The role of positive emotions in positive psychology: The broaden-and-build theory of positive emotions. *American Psychologist, 56*, 218–226.

Fredrickson, B. L., & Losada, M. F. (2005). Positive affect and the complex dynamics of human flourishing. *American Psychologist, 60*, 678–686.

Ginn, J., & Fast, J. (2006). Employment and social integration in midlife: Preferred and actual time use across welfare regime types. *Research on Aging, 28*, 669–690.

Gross, J. J. (1998). The emerging field of emotion regulation: An integrative review. *Review of General Psychology. Special New Directions in Research on Emotion, 2*, 271–299.

Grossardt, B. R., Bower, J. H., Geda, Y. E., Colligan, R. C., & Rocca, W. A. (2009). Pessimistic, anxious, and depressive personality traits predict all-cause mortality: The Mayo Clinic cohort study of personality and aging. *Psychosomatic Medicine, 71*, 491–500.

Hawkley, L. C., & Cacioppo, J. T. (2007). Aging and loneliness: Downhill quickly? *Current Directions in Psychological Science, 16*, 187–191.

Hawkley, L . C., Masi, C. M., Berry, J. D., & Cacioppo, J. T. (2006). Loneliness is a unique predictor of age-related differences in systolic blood pressure. *Psychology & Aging, 21*, 152–164.

Heckhausen, J. (2005). Competence and motivation in adulthood and old age: Making the most of changing capacities and resources. In A. J. Elliot & C. S. Dweck (Eds.), *Handbook of competence and motivation* (pp. 240–256). New York: Guilford.

Heckhausen, J., Wrosch, C., & Schulz, R. (2010). A motivational theory of lifespan development. *Psychological Review, 117*, 32–60.

Heffner, K. L., Kiecolt-Glaser, J. K., Loving, T. J., Glaser, R., & Malarkey, W. B. (2004). Spousal support satisfaction as a modifier of physiological responses to marital conflict in younger and older couples. *Journal of Behavioral Medicine, 27*, 233–254.

Hess, T. M., & Auman, C. (2001). Aging and social expertise: The impact of trait-diagnostic information on impressions of others. Psychology & *Aging, 16*, 497–510.

Isaacowitz, D. M. (2006). Motivated gaze: The view from the gazer. *Current Directions in Psychological Science, 15*, 68–72.

Isaacowitz, D. M., Toner, K., Goren, D., & Wilson, H . R. (2008). Looking while unhappy: Mood congruent gaze in young adults, positive gaze in older adults. *Psychological Science, 19*, 843–853.

Isaacowitz, D. M., Wadlinger, H. A., Goren, D., & Wilson, H. R. (2006). Is there an age-related positivity effect in visual attention? A comparison of two methodologies. *Emotion, 6*, 511–516.

Izard, C. E. (2007). Basic emotions, natural kinds, emotion schemas, and a new paradigm. *Perspectives on Psychological Science, 2*, 260–280.

Jorm, A. F., Windsor, T. D., Dear, K. B. G., Anstey, K. J., Christensen, H., & Rodgers, B. (2005). Age group differences in psychological distress: The role of psychosocial risk factors that vary with age. *Psychological Medicine, 35*, 1253–1263.

Keightley, M., Chiew, K., Winocur, G., & Grady, C. (2007). Age-related differences in brain activity underlying identification of emotional expression in faces. *Social Cognitive and Affective Neuroscience, 2*, 292–302.

Keightley, M. L., Winocur, G., Burianova, H., Hongwanishkul, D., & Grady, C. L. (2006). Age effects on social cognition: Faces tell a different story. *Psychology and Aging, 21*, 558–572.

Kennedy, Q., Mather, M., & Carstensen, L. L. (2004). The role of motivation in the age-related positivity effect in autobiographical memory. *Psychological Science, 15*, 208–214.

Kliegel, M., Jäger, T., & Phillips, L. H. (2007). Emotional development across adulthood: Differential age-related emotional reactivity and emotion regulation in a negative mood induction procedure. *International Journal of Aging and Human Development, 64*, 217–244.

Kobau, R., Safran, M. A., Zack, M. M., Moriarty, D. G., & Chapman, D. (2004). Sad, blue, or depressed days, health behaviors and health-related quality of life, Behavioral Risk Factor Surveillance System, 1995–2000. *Health Quality of Life Outcomes, 2*, 1–8.

Korkeila, K., Korkeila, J., Vahtera, J., Kivimaki, M., Kivela, S., Sillanmaki, L., et al. (2005). Childhood adversities, adult risk factors and depressiveness: A population study. *Social Psychiatry & Psychiatric Epidemiology, 40*, 700–706.

Krendl, A. C., Heatherton, T. F., & Kensinger, E. A. (2009). Aging minds twisting attitudes: An fMRI investigation of age differences in inhibiting prejudice. *Psychology & Aging, 24*, 530–541.

Kunzmann, U., & Grühn, D. (2005). Age differences in emotional reactivity: The sample case of sadness. *Psychology & Aging, 20*, 47–59.

Kunzmann, U., Kupperbusch, C. S., & Levenson, R. W. (2005). Behavioral inhibition and amplification during emotional arousal: A comparison of two age groups. *Psychology & Aging, 20*, 144–158.

Kunzmann, U., Little, T. D., & Smith, J. (2000). Is age-related stability of subjective well-being a paradox? cross-sectional and longitudinal evidence from the Berlin aging study. *Psychology & Aging, 15*, 511–526.

Labouvie-Vief, G. (2003). Dynamic Integration: Affect, cognition, and the self in adulthood. *Current Directions in Psychological Science, 12*, 201–206.

Labouvie-Vief, G., Lumley, M. A., Jain, E., & Heinze, H. (2003). Age and gender differences in cardiac reactivity and subjective emotion responses to emotional autobiographical memories. *Emotion, 3*, 115–126.

Lang, F. R. (2001). Regulation of social relationships in later adulthood. *Journals of Gerontology: Psychological Sciences, 56B*, P1–P6.

Lang, F. R., & Carstensen, L. L. (2002). Time counts: Future time perspective, goals and social relationships. *Psychology and Aging, 17*, 125–139.

Langa, K. M., Chernew, M. E., Kabeto, M. U., Herzog, A. R., Ofstedal, M. B., Willis, R. J., et al. (2001). National estimates of the quantity and cost of informal caregiving for the elderly with dementia. *Journal of General Internal Medicine, 16*, 770–778.

Langeslag, S. J. E., & Van Strien, J. W. (2009). Aging and emotional memory: The co-occurrence of neurophysiological and behavioral positivity effects. *Emotion, 9*, 369–377.

Langley, L. K., Rokke, P. D., Stark, A. C., Saville, A. L., Allen, J. L., & Bagne, A. G. (2008). The emotional blink: Adult age differences in visual attention to emotional information. *Psychology & Aging, 23*, 873–885.

Laukka, P., & Juslin, P. N. (2007). Similar patterns of age-related differences in emotion recognition from speech and music. *Motivation and Emotion, 31*, 182–191.

Lazarus, R. S. (1999). *Stress and emotion: A new synthesis.* New York: Springer.

Leclerc, C. M., & Kensinger, E. A. (2008). Effects of age on detection of emotional information. *Psychology & Aging, 23*, 209–215.

Levenson, R. W. (2000). Expressive, physiological, and subjective changes in emotion across adulthood. In S. H. Qualls & N. Abeles (Eds.), *Psychology and the aging revolution: How we adapt to longer life* (pp. 123–140). Washington, DC: American Psychological Association.

Löckenhoff, C. E., Costa, P. T., & Lane, R. D. (2008). Age differences in descriptions of emotional experience in oneself and others. *Journals of Gerontology: Psychological Sciences, 63,* P92–P99.

Lucas, R. E. (2007). Adaptation and the set-point model of subjective well-being: Does happiness change after major life events? *Current Directions in Psychological Science, 16,* 75–79.

Lucas, R. E., Clark, A. E., Georgellis, Y., & Diener, E. (2003). Reexamining adaptation and the set point model of happiness: Reactions to changes in marital status. *Journal of Personality and Social Psychology, 84,* 527–539.

Lyubomirsky, S., King, L., & Diener, E. (2005). The benefits of frequent positive affect: Does happiness lead to success? *Psychological Bulletin, 131,* 803–855.

Magai, C. (2001). Emotions over the lifespan. In J. E. Birren & K. W. Schaie (Eds.), *Handbook of the psychology of aging* (5th ed.) (pp. 310–344). San Diego, CA: Academic Press.

Magai, C., Consedine, N. S., Krivoshekova, Y. S., Kudadjie-Gyamfi, E., & McPherson, R. (2006). Emotion experience and expression across the adult life span: Insights from a multimodal assessment study. *Psychology & Aging, 21,* 303–317.

Mather, M. (2004). Aging and emotional memory. In D. Reisberg & P. Hertel (Eds.), *Memory and Emotion* (pp. 272–307). New York: Oxford University Press.

Mather, M., Canli, T., English, T., Whitfield, S., Wais, P., Ochsner, K., et al. (2004). Amygdala responses to emotionally valenced stimuli in older and younger adults. *Psychological Science, 15,* 259–263.

Mather, M., & Carstensen, L. L. (2003). Aging and attentional biases for emotional faces. *Psychological Science, 14,* 409–415.

Mather, M., & Carstensen, L. L. (2005). Aging and motivated cognition: The positivity effect in attention and memory. *Trends in Cognitive Sciences, 9, 496–502.*

Mather, M., Gorlick, M. A., & Lighthall, N. R. (2009). To brake or accelerate when the light turns yellow? Stress reduces older adults' risk taking in a driving game. *Psychological Science, 20,* 174–176.

Mather, M., & Carstensen, L. L. (2005). Aging and motivated cognition: The positivity effect in attention and memory. *Trends in Cognitive Sciences, 9, 496–502.*

Mather, M., & Knight, M. R. (2006). Angry faces get noticed quickly: Threat detection is not impaired among older adults. *Journals of Gerontology Series B: Psychological Sciences and Social Sciences, 61,* P54–P57.

McCrae, R. R., Costa, P. T., Ostendorf, F., Angleitner, A., Hrebickova, M., Avia, M. D., et al. (2000). Nature over nurture: Temperament, personality, and life span development. *Journal of Personality & Social Psychology, 78,* 173–186.

Mill, A., Allik, J., Realo, A., & Valk, R. (2009). Age-related differences in emotion recognition ability: A cross-sectional study. *Emotion, 9,* 619–630.

Miller, L. M., Charles, S. T., & Fingerman, K. L. (2009). Perceptions of social transgressions in adulthood: Does age make a difference? *Journals of Gerontology: Psychological Sciences, 64,* 551–559.

Mitchell, R. L. C. (2007). Age-related decline in the ability to decode emotional prosody: Primary or secondary phenomenon. *Cognition & Emotion, 21,* 1435–1454.

Mroczek, D. K., & Almeida, D. M. (2004). The effect of daily stress, personality, and age on daily negative affect. *Journal of Personality, 72,* 355–378.

Mroczek, D. K., & Kolarz, C. M. (1998). The effect of age on positive and negative affect: A developmental perspective on happiness. *Journal of Personality & Social Psychology, 75,* 1333–1349.

Mroczek, D. K., & Spiro, A. III. (2005). Change in life satisfaction over 20 during adulthood: Findings from the VA Normative Aging Study. *Journal of Personality and Social Psychology, 88,* 189–202.

Neupert, S., Almeida, D. M., & Charles, S. T. (2007). Age differences in reactivity to daily stressors: The role of personal control. *The Journals of Gerontology: Psychological Sciences, 62,* 216–225.

Newsom, J. T., Mahan, T. L., Rook, K. S., & Krause, N. (2008). Stable negative social exchanges and health. *Health Psychology, 27,* 78–86.

Ong, A. D., Bergeman, C. S., Bisconti, T. L., & Wallace, K. A. (2006). Psychological resilience, positive emotions, and successful adaptation to stress in later life. *Journal of Personality and Social Psychology, 91*(4), 730–749.

Paulmann, S., Pell, M. D., & Kotz, S. A. (2008). How aging affects the recognition of emotional speech. *Brain and Language, 104,* 262–269.

Phillips, L. H., Henry, J. D., Hosie, J. A., & Milne, A. B. (2006). Age, anger regulation and well-being. *Aging and Mental Health, 10,* 250–256.

Phillips, L. H., Henry, J. D., Hosie, J. A., & Milne, A. B. (2008). Effective regulation of the experience and expression of negative affect in old age. *Journal of Gerontology: Psychological Sciences, 63,* 138–145.

Piazza, J. R., Charles, S. T., & Almeida, D. M. (2007). Living with chronic health conditions: Age differences in affective well-being. *Journals of Gerontology: Psychological Sciences, 62B*(6), 313–321.

Ready, R. E., Weinberger, M., & Jones, K. (2007). How happy have you felt lately? A diary study of emotion recall in older and younger adults. *Cognition and Emotion, 21,* 728–757.

Reich, J. W., Zautra, A. J., & Davis, M. (2003). Dimensions of affect relationship: Models and their integrative implications. *Review of General Psychology, 7,* 66–83.

Repetti, R. L., Taylor, S. E., & Seeman, T. E. (2002). Risky families: Family social environments and the mental and physical health of offspring. *Psychological Bulletin, 128*(2), 230–366.

Röcke, C., Li, S., & Smith, J. (2009). Intraindividual variability in positive and negative affect over 45 days: Do old adults fluctuate less than young adults? *Psychology & Aging, 24*, 863–878.

Rook, K. S., Mavandadi, S., Sorkin, D. H., & Zettel, L. A. (2007). Optimizing social relationships as a resource for health and well-being in later life. In C. M. Aldwin, C. L. Park, & A. Spiro III, (Eds.), *Psychology of aging and health*. New York: Guilford.

Rosenkoetter, M. M., Garris, J. M., & Engdahl, R. A. (2001). Postretirement use of time: Implications for preretirement planning and postretirement management. *Activities, Adaptation & Aging, 25*, 1–18.

Rothermund, K., & Brandtstädter, J. (2003). Coping with deficits. and losses in later life: From compensatory action to accommodation. *Psychology and Aging, 18*, 896–905.

Ruffman, T., Henry, J. D., Livingstone, V., & Phillips, L. H. (2008). A meta-analytic review of emotion recognition and aging: Implications for neuropsychological models of aging. *Neuroscience and Biobehavioral Reviews, 32*, 863–881.

Ruffman, T., Sullivan, S., & Edge, N. (2006). Differences in the way older and younger adults rate threat in faces but not situations. *Journals of Gerontology, 61B*(4), 187–194.

Scheier, M. F., & Carver, C. S. (1977). Self-focused attention and the experience of emotion: Attraction, repulsion, elation, and depression. *Journals of Personality and Social Psychology, 35*, 625–636.

Schieman, S. (1999). Age and anger. *Journal of Health & Social Behavior, 40*, 273–289.

Seider, B. H., Hirschberger, G., Nelson, K. L., & Levenson, R. W. (2009). We can work it out: Age differences in relational pronouns, physiology, and behavior in marital conflict. *Psychology and Aging, 24*, 604–615.

Shaw, B., Krause, N., Chatters, L., Connell, C., & Ingersoll-Dayton, B. (2004). Emotional support from parents early in life, aging, and health. *Psychology and Aging, 19*(1), 4–12.

Smith, D. P., Hillman, C. H., & Duley, A. R. (2005). Influences of age on emotional reactivity during picture processing. *Journals of Gerontology: Series B: Psychological Sciences and Social Sciences, 60*, 49–56.

St. Jacques, P., Dolcos, F., & Cabeza, R. (2009). Effects of aging on functional connectivity of the amygdala during negative emotional evaluation: A network analysis of fMRI data. *Psychological Science, 20*, 74–84.

Stanley, J. T., & Blanchard-Fields, F. (2008). Challenges older adults face in detecting deceit: The role of emotion recognition. *Psychology and Aging, 23*, 24–32.

Stawski, R. S., Sliwinski, M. J., Almeida, D. M., & Smyth, J. M. (2008). Reported exposure and emotional reactivity to daily stressors: The roles of adult age and global perceived stress. *Psychology and Aging, 23*(1), 52–61.

Story, T. N., Berg, C. A., Smith, T. W., Beveridge, R., Henry, N. J. M., & Pearce, G. (2007). Age, marital satisfaction, and optimism as predictors of positive sentiment override in middle-aged and older married couples. *Psychology and Aging, 24*(4), 719–727.

Tsai, J. L., Levenson, R. W., & Carstensen, L. L. (2000). Autonomic, subjective, and expressive responses to emotional films in older and younger Chinese Americans and European Americans. *Psychology & Aging, 15*, 684–693.

Uchino, B. N., Holt-Lunstad, J., Bloor, L. E., & Campo, R. A. (2005). Aging and cardiovascular reactivity to stress: Longitudinal evidence for changes in stress reactivity. *Psychology and Aging, 20*, 134–143.

Uchino, B., Berg, C. A., Smith, T. S., Pearce, G., & Skinner, M. (2006). Age-related differences in ambulatory blood pressure during daily stress: Evidence for greater blood pressure reactions in older individuals. *Psychology and Aging, 21*, 231–239.

Uchino, B. N., Birmingham, W., & Berg, C. A. (2010). Are older adults less of more physiologically reactive? A meta-analysis of age-related differences in cardiovascular reactivity to laboratory tasks. *Journals of Gerontology: Psychological and Social Sciences, 65*, 152–164.

Uchino, B. N., Uno, D., Holt-Lunstad, J., & Flinders, J. B. (1999). Age-related differences in cardiovascular reactivity during acute psychological stress in men and women. *Journals of Gerontology: Series B: Psychological Sciences and Social Sciences, 54*, 339–346.

Wagner, B. M., Compas, B. E., & Howell, D. C. (1988). Daily and major life events: A test of an integrative model of psyho-social stress. *American Journal of Community Psychology, 166*(2), 189–205.

Wetherell, J. L., & Stein, M. B. (2009). Anxiety disorders (pp. 4040–4046). In B. J. Sadock, V. A. Sadock, & P. Ruiz (Eds.), *Kaplan & Sadock's comprehensive textbook of psychiatry: Vol. II* (9th ed.) (pp. 4040–4046). New York: Wolters Kluwer.

Wieser, M. J., Mühlberger, A., Kenntner-Mabiala, R., & Pauli, P. (2006). Is emotion processing affected by advancing age? An event-related brain potential study. *Brain Research, 1096*(1), 138–147.

Wilson, R. S., Krueger, K . R., Arnold, S. E., Barnes, L. L., Mendes de Leon, C. F., et al. (2006). Childhood adversity and psychosocial adjustment in old age. *American Journal of Geriatric Psychiatry, 14*, 307–315.

Wood, S., & Kisley, M. A. (2006). The negativity bias is eliminated in older adults: Age-related reduction in event-related brain potentials associated with evaluative categorization. *Psychology & Aging, 21*, 815–820.

Wurm, L. H., Labouvie-Vief, G., Aycock, J., Rebucal, K. A., & Koch, H. E. (2004). Performance in auditory and visual emotional Stroop tasks: A comparison of older and younger adults. *Psychology & Aging, 19*, 523–535.

Chapter | 20 |

Psychopathology, Bereavement, and Aging

Susan Krauss Whitbourne,[1] Suzanne Meeks[2]

[1]Department of Psychology, University of Massachusetts-Amherst, Amherst, Massachusetts, USA; [2]Department of Psychological and Brain Sciences, University of Louisville, Louisville, Kentucky, USA

CHAPTER CONTENTS

Introduction 311
A Life-Span Model of Risk and Protective Factors in Late-Life Psychopathology 311
Normal Aging Processes, Physical Health, and Psychopathology 313
Physical Illness and Life Events 313
Mood Disorders in Later Adulthood 313
Epidemiology of Unipolar Depression 313
Epidemiology of Bipolar Disorder 314
The Nature of Affective Symptoms in Older Adults 314
Risk and Protective Factors in Late-Life Depression 315
Physical Illness 315
Early Life Experiences 315
Psychosocial Risk Factors 315
Suicide 316
Anxiety Disorders in Later Adulthood 316
Epidemiology of Anxiety Disorders 316
The Nature of Anxiety Symptoms in Older Adults 316
Risk and Protective Factors in Late-Life Anxiety Disorders 316
Schizophrenia and Related Disorders 317
Psychotic Disorders Across the Life Course 317
Risk and Protective Factors in Late-Life Schizophrenia 317
Substance Abuse Disorders in Later Adulthood 317
Bereavement 318
Summary 319
References 320

INTRODUCTION

Psychopathology in later life occurs in the context of lifelong patterns of coping, social support, and connectedness, accumulated resources such as education and income, and characteristic late-life changes in physical health, cognition, and social relationships. This chapter presents a life-span perspective on psychopathology in late life, considering the interactions of specific manifestations of psychological disorders with the biopsychosocial and personal historical contexts within which they occur. We will focus on major clinical syndromes that fall within the categories of mood disorders, anxiety disorders, schizophrenia, and substance abuse disorders. We will also examine the role of bereavement as a common late life stressor.

A LIFE-SPAN MODEL OF RISK AND PROTECTIVE FACTORS IN LATE-LIFE PSYCHOPATHOLOGY

An understanding of psychopathology that first emerges in later adulthood must consider a different set of factors and influences than an understanding of psychopathology that has either intermittently or chronically been present for much of an individual's adult life. Researchers and clinicians do not necessarily consider life-long experiences when characterizing late-life psychopathology, but as we will show in this chapter, the life-span approach is vital to both diagnostic and treatment considerations. The importance of such an approach was recognized by contributors to an earlier edition of this *Handbook* (Gatz et al., 1996), when they proposed a "life span developmental diathesis-stress model" (p. 366) to examine

DOI: 10.1016/B978-0-12-380882-0.00020-6

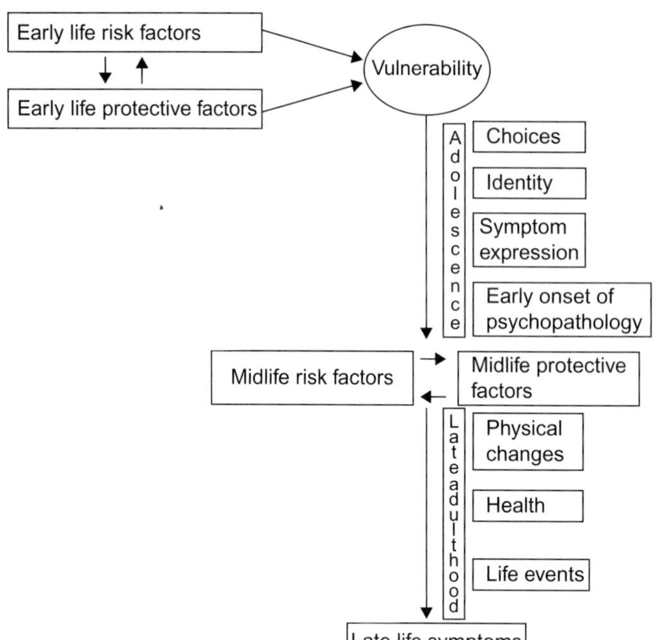

Figure 20.1 Life-span model of risk and protective factors in late-life psychopathology.

the interaction of life stressors and vulnerabilities over the life span. We expand on this model to recognize the influence not only of risk factors (stressors, genetic vulnerability), but also of protective factors, all of which interact across the life span.

As shown in Figure 20.1, a life-span model begins with a delineation of the risk and protective factors that characterize the individual's early years. Childhood risk factors include, at the most extreme, trauma such as parental death, serious illness, or abuse. Social conditions that involve deprivation, such as poverty, poor housing, malnutrition, and lack of access to educational resources provide another set of risk factors that affect not only the individual but also the individual's family, community, and culture. Biological risk factors include genetic predisposition, brain damage, and illness.

Not all individuals exposed to these risk factors will develop psychopathology; hence it is important to consider the interaction of these factors as the individual's life unfolds. Risk factors will have a different impact on the individual as they are balanced against protective factors that can have both moderating and mediating influences. Within the individual's social context, these protective factors can include a supportive family environment, access to educational opportunities, and average or above average household income.

During childhood, the balance of risk and protective factors will interact with subsequent events that serve to influence further experiences. As the individual develops into adolescence, these factors set the stage for how he or she will respond to events that may be thought of as in the realm of personal control. Decisions begin to be made that alter the subsequent path of life events such as choices of friends, subjects of study in school, recreational activities, and ultimately career. It is also at this time in life when personal identity begins to emerge and the individual begins to gain a sense of continuity over time. Also beginning in the late teen years and particularly by the early 20s, individuals who ultimately develop a major psychological disorder begin to experience the first signs of serious disturbance. The co-occurrence of these phenomena may prove to have ramifications for subsequent identity development as the individual's sense of self begins to form in relationship to being a person with a psychological disorder.

As life events unfold both in relation to the developing individual's identity and in the context of the risk and protective factors, further influences on the expression of the disorder may occur. Risk factors may increase if symptoms interfere with pursuit of education, a career, and long-term relationships as well as if the symptoms contribute to further adjustment difficulties or attempts to self-medicate. At the same time, effective treatments may help to avert negative sequelae. During the adult years, the individual's identity as a person with a psychological disorder can continue to have an impact on the further expression of symptoms, and on the acceptance of treatment. In later adulthood, the accumulation of physical changes, the balance of risk and protective factors, and the occurrence of life events continue to affect the nature of the individual's presenting symptoms.

Another course of development characterizes the individual whose first symptoms present in later life. Particular stressors in late life, such as bereavement, physical illness, relocation, financial hardship, or other family stressors may place the older individual at risk for late-life onset of particular psychological disorders. The onset of late-life schizophrenia and bipolar disorders in later life are rare, but individuals are known to develop depression, anxiety, and substance abuse for the first time in late life. Thus, our understanding and management of late-life psychopathology requires that an individual's prior history be taken into account to obtain a true life-span biopsychosocial perspective. Throughout this chapter, we will flesh out this model which we shall use as a basis for interpreting current research findings, suggesting avenues of future research, and providing a perspective for treatment.

NORMAL AGING PROCESSES, PHYSICAL HEALTH, AND PSYCHOPATHOLOGY

The stability and change of physical and cognitive abilities, emotional experience, and personality across the adult life span, reviewed in other chapters of this *Handbook*, provide the background for the development and experience of psychopathology in later life. To the extent that psychopathology in later life is different than psychopathology in other phases of adulthood, it is presumably because of the interplay among these normal aging processes, personal and environmental risk factors for late onset of mental disorders, and the natural history of mental disorders with onset in early adulthood. There are three ways in which normal aging processes may be related to late-life psychopathology. First, aging processes may be risk factors for the development, exacerbation, or relapse of psychopathology. Second, psychopathology may in turn be a risk factor for negative outcomes of aging processes such as physical health and cognition. Third, aging processes may influence the ways in which psychopathology is expressed and managed.

Physical Illness and Life Events

The number of and burden from physical illnesses, particularly chronic illnesses, increase with age (e.g., Baxter et al., 2009). People with severe mental illnesses also have a higher number of physical illnesses than those without such illnesses, a risk that increases with age (Jones & Meredith, 1996; Weber et al., 2009). Among older adults with mental illness, the association with physical illness is particularly strong for unipolar depression (Gierz & Jeste, 1993), a finding that has led to numerous studies examining whether physical illness is a risk factor for depression. Early longitudinal research suggested that physical health can predict both worsening of depressive symptoms and the onset of new depressive symptoms (Murrell & Meeks, 1991), but a direct effect of physical illness on depression has not always been supported (e.g., Zeiss et al., 1996). Turvey and colleagues (2009) demonstrated that illness indicators, functional impairment, and cognitive impairment all independently predicted change in depressive symptoms over two years in a large, nationally representative sample of U.S. elders. The prediction of changes in diagnosed depressive disorders was considerably weaker. These findings suggest that illness and disability might be considered common stressors in late life that increase distress for all older adults rather than being specific risk factors for the onset of mental illness in late life.

Prospective associations between increased symptoms and later life events suggest that mental illness symptoms, particularly in the long-term, may have at least as great an impact on life events as vice versa (e.g., Jackson et al., 2002). This relationship has clearly been demonstrated in the case of depressive symptoms that multiple studies relate to physical illness, disability, and sometimes mortality (e.g., Carbonare et al., 2009; Parmelee et al., 1992; Smalbrugge et al., 2006). Schizophrenia is a risk factor for multiple physical conditions even among younger adults (Weber et al., 2009), which may contribute to the higher mortality rate among people with schizophrenia. Presence of severe mental illness is also related to lower levels of positive health behaviors such as exercising and being a nonsmoker (Dickerson et al., 2006).

This brief review of the association between physical illness factors, life events, and mental illness illustrates that late-life events are likely related to increases or exacerbations in psychiatric symptoms, and that, conversely, psychiatric symptoms are risk factors for physical illnesses and negative life events. The intersection of later life events and psychiatric illness appears to be moderated by diagnosis, and protective factors of importance for older adults in general, such as social support and maintaining positive engagement in activities, are also important for individuals with mental illness. Thus, our understanding and treatment of late-life mental illness must be informed by an awareness of risk and protective factors that are common to all older adults.

MOOD DISORDERS IN LATER ADULTHOOD

Epidemiology of Unipolar Depression

Unipolar mood disorders in the DSM-IV-TR (American Psychiatric Association, 2000) include major depressive disorder and dysthymia. However, these categories do not fully capture the range of depressive syndromes presented to clinicians, who may see a variety of presentations of lesser severity, including minor depression (Kessler et al., 1997) and subsyndromal depression (Judd et al., 1994) as well as major depression in partial remission. These latter syndromes may be reflected in elevated symptom scores on self-report indices of depression. It is therefore important to note that epidemiological estimates of depression in late life vary according to the type of assessment used. It is equally important to note that prevalence estimates vary by setting or subpopulation of elders who are assessed, with higher prevalence estimates coming from medical or long-term care settings.

Epidemiological studies that have compared younger and older cohorts on depression prevalence consistently show lower prevalence of depressive disorders after the age of 65 (Ohayon, 2007); depression appears to peak in middle age and decline thereafter, although it is not clear whether this is an age or a cohort phenomenon. Some researchers have noted an increase of depressive symptoms (but not depressive disorders) in the very old (Murrell & Meeks, 1991; Newmann, 1989). As with other age groups, women have significantly higher prevalence rates than men, in the order of 50–60% (Steffens et al., 2000). Among older adults in community populations, point or one-month prevalence rates of major depression range from about 1 to 4% (Ohayon, 2007; Steffens et al., 2000; Trollor et al., 2007), as compared to community estimates of younger adults at about 6 to 8% (Gum et al., 2009). DSM-IV-TR-defined minor depression or dysthymia show lower rates in these studies (less than 1%), again lower than rates for younger adults (Judd et al., 1994). Studies that examine clinically significant depressive symptoms among community elders using cutoff scores based on self-report instruments generally show prevalence rates ranging from 15 to 30% (Anstey et al., 2007; Murrell & Meeks, 1991), greater than the cumulative rates of all depressive disorders identified in studies using diagnostic categories.

Depressive disorders and symptoms are significantly more prevalent in older adult populations with medical problems. The rate of depressive diagnoses in primary care was 5.8% in one large study of Medicare users (Crystal et al., 2003). Diagnosis rates in this naturalistic study were higher for non-Hispanic whites, suggesting that either there are differing rates in different ethnic groups in the United States, or disparities in identification and treatment. The latter explanation is supported by more deliberate sampling and assessment of minority elders (Kemp et al., 1987). In samples of people with chronic diseases, the rates are even higher, as are rates of depressive disorders in long-term care settings, where estimates of major depression range from 6 to 25% (Teresi et al., 2001), with minor or subsyndromal depression affecting 30–50% of individuals in long-term care (Jongenelis et al., 2004; Teresi et al., 2001).

Epidemiology of Bipolar Disorder

Data from representative community samples show lower rates of bipolar disorder in older adults (around 0.1%) than in the younger population (1.4% for young adults; 0.4% for middle-aged; Depp & Jeste, 2004; Robins & Regier, 1991). In their review, Depp and Jeste (2004) found that the proportion of older psychiatric patients in inpatient and emergency settings who were diagnosed with bipolar disorder was approximately the same as the proportions found in younger age groups (8–10%). This finding suggests that the factors that affect lower prevalence of bipolar disorder are probably similar to the factors affecting lower prevalence of other disorders, most probably a combination of excess mortality and cumulative improvement of some individuals over the life span (Meeks, 1999). Older adults with bipolar disorder admitted to the hospital may have longer inpatient stays due to comorbid medical problems, and are about four times as likely to be discharged to an institution as younger adults (Brown, 2001).

The likelihood of an individual experiencing a manic episode for the first time in old age is relatively low. The onset of a bipolar illness typically is in late adolescence or early adulthood, although there does appear to be a tendency for samples of older persons with bipolar disorder to report a later onset than younger samples (Depp & Jeste, 2004). When bipolar disorder develops late in adulthood, it appears to be related to a higher risk for cerebrovascular disease (Subramaniam et al., 2006).

The Nature of Affective Symptoms in Older Adults

The observed age differences in prevalence of depressive disorders have led to speculation about whether depression may manifest differently in late life, leading to poorer recognition and treatment. Early suggestions that depressed affect tended to be "masked" in older adults have not been strongly supported by empirical research (Murrell & Meeks, 1991), which suggests that dysphoria continues to be an important hallmark of depressive disorders across the life span. The overlap of depression and physical disease has led to speculation about whether focus on vegetative symptoms might lead to over diagnosis of depression among older medical patients, but when a formal diagnostic interview is used, classification does not appear to be influenced by whether or not somatic symptoms are included.

Similar conclusions can be drawn regarding the manifestation of mania and bipolar depression in later life. Depp and Jeste (2004) found little evidence that the character of episodes changes substantially over the life span, although they did note that there is a subgroup of older adults with bipolar disorder whose lifelong course is predominated by depressive illness and who have manic episodes only relatively late in life. Understanding an individual's lifelong pattern of episodes and treatment experiences therefore is critical for adequate treatment in late life.

RISK AND PROTECTIVE FACTORS IN LATE-LIFE DEPRESSION

The majority of research on unipolar depression prevalence in late life fails to distinguish between depressive disorders that were recurrences or continuations of disorders in early adulthood and those that occurred for the first time in late life. This is true also of the majority of research examining predictors of depressive episodes in late life. Major depression is a recurrent disorder for approximately 50% of adults who experience a single episode, and the majority of those who experience two or more episodes have a recurring course. Thus it seems obvious that occurrence of prior episodes of depression is one of the strongest predictors of risk for depression in later life. Once diagnosed, major, minor, and subsyndromal depression all have a tendency to be either chronic or intermittent in later life, with only about a third remitting after identification (Beekman et al., 2002). It is as yet unclear how we might distinguish individuals with short-term, remitting, depression in late life from those who will have a recurrent or chronic course, in terms of predictors, treatment response, or management. One might hypothesize that they are individuals who have not suffered depressive episodes earlier in their adult lives and therefore have developed more protective factors.

Physical Illness

Possible risk factors for late-life depression include a host of physical diseases and conditions, sensory impairments, disability, and cognitive changes. Much of this research is cross-sectional and fails to account for prior levels of depressive symptoms or history of depressive disorders. Nevertheless, the very high rates of depression in medical populations suggest that medical illness and physical disability are legitimate risk factors. A cross-sectional study comparing women with no prior history of major depression, those with early onset, and those with late-life onset (Sneed et al., 2007) showed poorer health in those with late onset, suggesting that medical illness may be a particular risk factor for those individuals without a prior history of depression. In samples with medical illness, pain, higher levels of disability, poorer self-rated health, a tendency to focus on negative experiences associated with aging and poorer social support appear to be risk factors for onset of depressive episodes (Brodaty et al., 2007; Weinberger et al., 2009; Weinberger & Whitbourne 2010) even controlling for initial levels of depression. There is some evidence that neurological abnormalities can be risk factors for chronicity in late-life depression (Alexopoulos et al., 2008). Executive function impairments also predict poor outcomes for depressive disorders in primary care (Bogner et al., 2007). Hypertension is also linked to the development of depressive symptoms, independent of a variety of stressors, associated physical conditions, cognitive impairment, and baseline disability (Garcia-Fabela et al., 2009).

Early Life Experiences

Age of onset predicts poor outcomes in bipolar disorder in late life (Meeks, 1999), perhaps due to a combination of genetic risk and early life disruption of development of important social and economic protective factors. Other early life characteristics and experiences continue to be predictive of risk for depressive disorders in late life. For example, several studies have linked the personality trait of neuroticism to late-life depression (Sneed et al., 2007; Steunenberg et al., 2009). Childhood trauma is also associated with late-life risk for depression (Pesonen et al., 2007), possibly moderated by alterations in the serotonin gene-linked promoter region (5-HTTLPR). Ritchie and her colleagues (2009) found that childhood adversity associated with 5-HTTLPR alterations predicted depression even accounting for proximal risk factors such as medical illness, widowhood, and vascular disorder. This study nicely illustrated the importance of a life-span perspective on late-life disorder, suggesting that early life experiences may affect outcomes many years later not only through the psychosocial consequences but also by interacting with genetic predisposing factors to influence the ways in which the brain responds to stressful situations.

Psychosocial Risk Factors

Psychosocial issues such as caregiving, bereavement, loneliness, and stressful life events have also been associated with risk for depressive disorders in later adulthood (Bruce, 2002).

An investigation of caregivers in the United States Health and Retirement Study identified a relationship between urinary incontinence in the wife and depressive symptoms in the husband (Fultz et al., 2005). In one study covering a 10-year period, older adults who used ineffective coping methods, such as avoidance, were more likely to develop symptoms of depression compared with their age peers who attempted to handle their problems through direct, problem-focused coping methods (Holahan et al., 2005). Within older adults already diagnosed with depression, social support and self-efficacy can be important protective factors that can predict functional outcomes (e.g., Sirey et al., 2008).

Suicide

Suicide is associated with affective disorders for individuals of all ages. Older adults, particularly men, have among the highest rates of suicide in the United States (Bharucha & Satlin, 1997). In the Established Populations for Epidemiologic Studies of the Elderly (EPESE), predictors of suicide included depressive symptoms, perceived physical health, quality of sleep, and absence of a confidant (Turvey et al., 2002). Among primary care patients with depression, anxiety, or at-risk alcohol ethnic differences were found Asian Americans having particularly high risk and African Americans relatively low risk compared to other groups (Bartels et al., 2002). Medical burden and hopelessness also add to severity of depression to predict suicide completion (Conwell et al., 2000; Fiske et al., 2008). The presence of firearms is a particular risk factor for older men (Conwell et al., 2000). Since a large number of older adults who have committed suicide have had contact with primary care providers, primary care has become a target for prevention of late-life suicides (Bruce et al., 2004). As with risk factors for affective disorders in general, understanding the risk for suicide in late life requires examination of a confluence of early and late-life genetic, psychosocial, and physical factors.

ANXIETY DISORDERS IN LATER ADULTHOOD

Epidemiology of Anxiety Disorders

There is less information on anxiety disorders in late life than is available regarding mood disorders. Data from the National Comorbidity Study Replication suggest that the 12-month prevalence of any anxiety disorder is markedly lower among adults over the age of 65 (7.0% as compared to 20.7% in young adults and 18.7% in adults aged 45–64). As with younger adults, the most prevalent anxiety disorder among older adults is specific phobia (4.7%), followed by social phobia (2.3%), and generalized anxiety disorder (GAD; 1.2%) (Gum et al., 2009). Women in this national sample were almost five times as likely to have a DSM-IV anxiety disorder than men. Data from an Australian population study showed lower prevalence rates (1.7% for any anxiety disorder), and GAD had the highest prevalence (0.9%), however specific phobias were not included in this study (Trollor et al., 2007). Women in the Australian sample were about twice as likely to be suffering from GAD and OCD, but there were no significant sex differences for the other disorders studied. The low rates of GAD in both of these national samples may reflect rates of "pure" GAD; that is, GAD that does not co-occur with major depression and GAD occurring in individuals with major depression may be four times as high (Flint, 2005).

The Nature of Anxiety Symptoms in Older Adults

Anxiety and depression are commonly comorbid in older adults as they are with younger cohorts (King-Kallimanis et al., 2009). This observed comorbidity has led to extensive research on younger adults concerning the conceptual and practical differentiation of anxiety and mood disorders. Analyses of the overlap of these disorders examine models that differentiate anxiety and depression factors such as positive and negative affect plus arousal or fear (Mineka et al., 1998; Watson, 2005). In these models, anxiety and depression are differentiated by the presence of low positive affect in depression and high arousal or fear in anxiety. However, among older adults depression and anxiety are more difficult to differentiate (Meeks et al., 2003). The ability to replicate measurement models of anxiety and depression may vary according to the types of instruments used to measure the constructs. Measurement of subclinical symptoms may also reveal differences by age that are less apparent once anxiety symptoms reach diagnostic significance. For example, older adults in a community sample had fewer social situations in which they experienced significant anxiety than younger adults, but older and younger participants who scored in the clinical range on a self-report assessment of social anxiety differed very little in symptom expression (Gretarsdottir et al., 2004). Similarly, clinical features of panic were comparable between younger and older adults (Depp et al., 2005). In sum, there is little evidence that anxiety symptoms are significantly different in older versus younger adults, but they may be more difficult to distinguish from depression.

Risk and Protective Factors in Late-Life Anxiety Disorders

Given the overlap between anxiety and depression in late life, risk factors for anxiety are similar to those for depression, although they have been much less studied. These factors include shared genetic risk (Kendler et al., 2007), particularly between GAD and depression. In the National Comorbidity Study sample, correlates of anxiety disorder other than gender included a number of comorbid chronic medical conditions, being unmarried or divorced, and having less than high school education (Gum et al., 2009).

Cognitive impairment appears to be a major risk factor for anxiety in late life (Seignourel et al., 2008). The symptom overlap between anxiety and dementia has confounded researchers interested in understanding this risk factor. Seignourel and colleagues (2008) concluded that anxiety could be differentiated from agitation but not conclusively from depression among samples of elders with dementia. Older Hispanic and Asian adults may be at higher risk for anxiety in dementia (Seignourel et al., 2008). Anxiety appears to be higher among individuals suffering from vascular as compared to Alzheimer's type dementia (Seignourel et al., 2008), suggesting that anxiety in dementia is related to the vascular risk for depression in late life.

SCHIZOPHRENIA AND RELATED DISORDERS

Psychotic Disorders Across the Life Course

It is estimated that schizophrenia has a lifetime prevalence of about 1%, with a peak prevalence at 1.5% for the 30 to 44 age group and 0.3% in people older than 65 years (Keith et al., 1991). In part the apparent decrease in older age groups reflects the higher risk of mortality for people with this disorder. Reflecting the higher life expectancy of women, there is a crossover in the gender distribution of the disorder, with a higher prevalence of schizophrenia among older women than older men (Meeks, 2000). People with schizophrenia and related disorders comprise a large proportion of admissions to psychiatric hospitals (24–40%), demonstrating that many older adults with schizophrenia continue to suffer illness episodes into late life. Further, hospital stays tend to be longer for older adults, perhaps because of complications related to medical comorbidity (McAlpine & Cohen, 2003).

In the large majority of people who develop schizophrenia, the onset occurs prior to the age of 40, although the onset in women is about 5 years later than that of men. Approximately 20 to 25% of people who develop schizophrenia improve to the point of complete remission, and at the other end of the spectrum, 10% remain chronically impaired. Among the remaining 50 to 70%, the disorder shows a varying course with gradual improvements in social functioning and a reduction of psychotic symptoms (Meeks, 2000). Some individuals can achieve very significant recovery after many years of being chronically impaired, including being able to work, drive a car, and live independently in their own homes (Palmer et al., 2002). As part of the recovery process, older adults with schizophrenia may develop coping skills that allow them to manage their symptoms as they accept their illness (Solano & Whitbourne, 2001).

Despite the favorable outcomes achieved by some, there are serious ramifications of having had the disorder at some point in life. The association with other illnesses, suicide, or substance abuse mean that a person with schizophrenia faces serious threats to health and excess mortality throughout the adult years (Ruschena et al., 1998). Depression, poorer cognitive functioning, and social isolation are additional complications (Graham et al., 2002). Furthermore, the symptoms of schizophrenia can lead to significant disruptions in everyday life as well as greater likelihood of negative life events (Patterson et al., 1997).

Risk and Protective Factors in Late-Life Schizophrenia

The many long-term follow-up studies of schizophrenia that have been carried out since the early twentieth century have consistently shown heterogeneous course patterns for the disorder. Although manifestations of schizophrenia persist into late life, approximately 50% manage to make sufficient social and vocational recovery to "reclaim their lives." Women, those with later onset, and those with more paranoid and fewer negative symptoms show better outcomes. Harding and Cohen (2003) have argued that these predictors, with the exception of negative symptoms, weaken over time. Meeks and Murrell (1997) found that age was predictive of better adjustment, although about 80% of their sample of severely mentally ill middle-aged and older adults had experienced significant symptoms in the previous four months. The combination of psychosis and affective symptoms predicted the poorest outcomes.

Although schizophrenia rarely has an onset later than the early- to mid-40s, there is anecdotal and research support for the occurrence of psychotic disorders that first emerge after the age of 60. These are generally not considered to be "schizophrenias," but rather some other phenotype of psychotic disorder, the risk factors for which may include sensory deficits, comorbid dementia and delirium, social isolation, or substance abuse. Thus the diagnosis and treatment of late-life psychosis requires the consideration of prior psychiatric and medical history (Desai et al., 2003).

SUBSTANCE ABUSE DISORDERS IN LATER ADULTHOOD

In 2008, illicit drugs were used by an estimated 20.1 million persons 12 years and older, representing

8% of the population (Substance Abuse and Mental Health Services Administration, 2009). The majority of adults who abuse or are dependent on alcohol or illicit drugs are in their late teens and early 20s. Very small percentages of adults 40 and older report abusing or being dependent on either illicit drugs or alcohol. Nevertheless researchers predict that the higher lifetime patterns of illicit drug use among Baby Boomers will lead to an increase in the prevalence of illicit drug use in adults 50 and older by the year 2020 (Colliver et al., 2006).

Older adults are particularly at risk for abuse of prescription drugs, as 36% of the medications used in the United States are taken by adults over the age of 65 years. Estimates place the potential of prescription drug abuse among older adults in outpatient treatment as ranging from 5 to 33%, with an estimated abuse rate (among women) at 11%. Further estimates are that the risk of abuse will rise dramatically between now and the year 2020 (Simoni-Wastila & Yang, 2006).

Attention has only recently been drawn to the problems of older drinkers. In part, this is because there is selective survival of people who do not use alcohol. The people who used alcohol to excess are no longer in the population by the time they reach their 60s and 70s. By the time they reach the age of 70, they have either become abstinent or died from excessive alcohol use or from related high-risk behaviors such as smoking (Vaillant, 2003). Estimates are that 2 to 5% of men and 1% of women over 65 abuse substances (Abeles et al., 1997) and that 1 to 2% of men and 0.3% of women over 65 are alcohol abusers (Grant et al., 1995), although these rates vary substantially by gender, ethnicity, education, and other behavioral risk factors (Satre et al., 2007).

In contrast to the under-65 population, among those over 65 the prevalence rates of alcohol abuse are higher for African Americans. Hispanic females over 65 have the lowest rates of alcohol abuse. In the future, it is estimated that rates of alcohol abuse will increase significantly with the aging of the current cohort of Baby Boomers, who have higher rates of alcohol consumption than previous generations (Department of Health and Human Services, 1999).

Symptoms of alcohol dependence are thought to be present in as many as 14% of older adults who receive medical attention in hospitals and emergency rooms. It is also estimated that alcohol use is relatively prevalent in settings in which only older adults live, such as nursing homes and retirement communities. The risks of alcohol abuse among this population are considerable, ranging from cirrhosis of the liver to heightened rate of injury through hip fractures and motor vehicle accidents. Alcohol may also interact with the effects of prescription medications, potentially limiting their effectiveness. Even without a change in drinking patterns, an older person may experience difficulties associated with physiological changes that affect tolerance. Long-term alcohol use may also lead to changes in the frontal lobes and cerebellum, exacerbating the effects of normal aging on cognitive and motor functioning (Oscar-Berman & Marinkovic, 2007). In severe and prolonged alcohol abuse, dementia can develop, leading to permanent memory loss and early death.

BEREAVEMENT

Many of the above risk and protective factors combine to influence the older adult's response to the death of a spouse, widely regarded as one of the most stressful events of life. For example, in a study of bereaved spouses that controlled for prior dysphoria, bereavement was a stronger risk factor for depression among those who had no such history than among those who did (Bruce et al., 1990). Among the many ramifications of widowhood are loss of an attachment figure, interruption of the plans and hopes invested in the relationship, and construction of a new identity in accordance with the reality of being single (Field et al., 1999). Older adults who are widowed are at higher risk of developing depression as well as anxiety disorders (Onrust & Cuijpers, 2006).

Widows and widowers may experience symptoms such as sensing the presence, dreaming about, and having hallucinations or illusions of seeing or hearing the deceased (Lindstrom, 1995; LoConto, 1998). These feelings of grief over the loss of the spouse may persist for as long as two and a half years (Ott & Lueger, 2002). Indeed, although not necessarily considered a sign of psychopathology, widows may continue to think about the spouse and even have "conversations" with the deceased on a weekly basis for as long as 35 years or more (Carnelley et al., 2006). Individuals working with bereaved older adults must be able to distinguish between these normative responses to grief and more pathological developments.

Whether an older adult who is experiencing bereavement ultimately develops psychopathology reflects the mutual intersection of a number of risk and protective factors (Mancini & Bonanno, 2009). One set of factors has to do with the bereaved individual's personality. A major prospective study of over 200 individuals who were tested before they became widowed, and followed for 18 months after they became widowed, identified 5 patterns of bereavement: common grief, chronic grief, chronic depression, improvement during bereavement, and resilience (Bonanno et al., 2002). In common grief, the individual experiences an initial increase in depression that diminishes over time. This pattern is actually relatively infrequent. More likely to occur is resilient grief, in which the bereaved shows little or no distress following the loss. Two additional patterns distinguish grief from depression. In chronic grief, the individual experiences high levels of both depression and grief within six months after the loss, and the grief does not subside over time. In chronic depression, the bereaved suffers from high levels of depression prior to and after the loss.

Bonanno and his co-investigators (2002) examined the coping resources, interpersonal dependency, personality traits (based on the Five Factor Model), religiosity, world views, and social support of the widows. People with high levels of interpersonal dependency (including dependence on their spouses) who showed the pattern of resilience were most accepting of death and were more likely to agree with the notion that the world is "just" (i.e., that people "get" what they "deserve"). Studies such as these underscore the notion that bereavement is not a unitary process and that there are multiple factors influencing reactions to the loss of a spouse.

Age is another individual difference factor predicting reactions to widowhood. It is well established that younger widows suffer more negative consequences of widowhood, including more severe deterioration of health and higher mortality rates (M. Stroebe et al., 1981; W. Stroebe & Stroebe, 1987). One reason for the differing effects of widowhood on younger and older spouses may be the expectedness of the death. Older spouses are more prepared for the death of the partner, a fact that is particularly true for women, who are likely to be younger than their husbands. However, being able to anticipate the death is not necessarily the key factor in accounting for the age difference in reactions to widowhood. Anticipatory grief may heighten rather than reduce the grief that follows the spouse's death (Gilliland & Fleming, 1998). When their bereavement follows an anticipated death, younger widows may benefit somewhat more from the forewarning given to them compared to older widows because the younger widows have more resources for managing the stress of prolonged caregiving.

Difficult emotional responses may follow the death of a spouse due to illnesses such as cancer and Alzheimer's disease that involved marked physical and mental deterioration and placed extensive burden on the caregivers (Ferrario et al., 2004). Relief from the pressures of caregiving can lead to alleviation of symptoms of depression and stress present during the spouse's dying months or years (Bonanno et al., 2004).

Men appear to experience greater stress following the death of their wives than women upon the death of their husbands (M. Stroebe, 2001). Widowers are at greater mortality risk within the first 6 months after bereavement than are widows, with a mortality rate estimated in one study to be 12 times higher for men than women for those over 75 years of age (Gallagher-Thompson et al., 1993). This sex difference in reactions to bereavement does not appear to be due simply to the greater social support that women experience as widows (W. Stroebe et al., 1999). Men are more likely to remarry, but women are more likely to form new friendships, particularly with neighbors (Lamme et al., 1996). It is possible that social support plays a greater role in the adaptation of women to widowhood, but for men (particularly current cohorts) a more relevant factor for men is the lack of availability of practical support in performing household tasks (Gass, 1989). In addition, widowers are more likely to engage in higher rates of alcohol consumption. They have also suffered the loss of their most important confidante who, in addition, had monitored her husband's health status (Stroebe et al., 2007).

SUMMARY

We have applied a life-span perspective to understanding the nature of the major psychological disorders in later life, focusing on differentiation by when in the life course symptoms are first expressed and on summarizing research evidence on risk and protective factors as these evolve over the life course. Most existing data on aging and psychopathology do not, however, take a life course perspective but instead describe prevalence data and associated symptoms without the backdrop of the individual's past and present life experiences. Even studies that take into account psychiatric history do not often examine this history in the context of the rest of the individual's personality, self-concept, or social context.

To gain a fuller appreciation of the strengths and the vulnerabilities of older adults being evaluated for psychological disorders, psychologists working with these populations, both as researchers and as clinicians, should instead place the individual against a chronological backdrop that regards the expression of symptoms as a reflection of the multiple intersecting factors impinging on the individual at any one point in time that may have changed from the past and may change in the future. Rarely do we have the luxury, in clinical settings, of longitudinal data against which to evaluate the older adult. Thus, adequate assessment should include a thorough history-taking, the use of informants, and the use of multiple data sources from a variety of disciplines. Research on late-life psychopathology could be greatly strengthened by assessment of early life risk and protective factors, recognizing that prospective studies are not necessarily sufficient to capture the lifelong advantages or disadvantages individuals bring to old age. These advantages and disadvantages, which at the individual level are integral to the individual's identity, at the group level may provide us with tools that can optimize both functional and psychological well-being.

The epidemiological data surveyed in this chapter suggest that proportionally fewer older adults suffer from psychopathology than younger adults. This lower prevalence is no doubt at least partially explained by differential mortality, but also suggests that older adults may bring coping strategies to the task of coping with mental illness that younger people have not yet developed. Understanding, and capitalizing on, such strategies will allow us to think about treatment of disorders in late life not only in terms of remission of symptoms, but also in terms of maximizing quality of life. The majority of older adults maintain high levels of subjective well-being, even in the face of serious health problems and physical limitations. Those who suffer symptoms of mental illness should also be evaluated with the goal of restoring or optimizing well-being and independence.

REFERENCES

Abeles, N., Cooley, S., Deitch, I., Harper, M. S., Hinrichsen, G., Lopez, M., et al. (1997). *What practitioners should know about working with older adults*. Washington DC: American Psychological Association.

Alexopoulos, G. S., Murphy, C. F., Gunning-Dixon, F. M., Latoussakis, V., Kanellopoulos, D., Klimstra, S., et al. (2008). Microstructural white matter abnormalities and remission of geriatric depression. *American Journal of Psychiatry, 165*, 238–244.

American Psychiatric Association. (2000). *DSM-IV: Diagnostic and statistical manual of mental disorders text revision*. Washington DC: American Psychiatric Association.

Anstey, K. J., von Sanden, C., Sargent-Cox, K., & Luszcz, M. A. (2007). Prevalence and risk factors for depression in a longitudinal, population-based study including individuals in the community and residential care. *American Journal of Geriatric Psychiatry, 15*, 497–505.

Bartels, S. J., Coakley, E., Oxman, T. E., Constantion, G., Oslin, D., Chen, H., et al. (2002). Suicidal and death ideation in older primary care patients with depression, anxiety, and at-risk alcohol use. *American Journal of Geriatric Psychiatry, 10*, 417–427.

Baxter, J. D., Samnaliev, M., & Clark, R. (2009). The quality of asthma care among adults with substance-related disorders and adults with mental illness. *Psychiatric Services, 60*, 1–43.

Beekman, A. T. F., Geerlings, S. W., Deeg, D. J. H., Smit, J. H., Schoevers, R. S., deBeurs, E., et al. (2002). The natural history of late-life depression. A 6-year prospective study in the community. *Archives of General Psychiatry, 59*, 605–611.

Bogner, H. R., Bruce, M. L., Reynolds, C. F., III, Mulsant, B. H., Cary, M. S., Morales, K., et al. (2007). The effects of memory, attention, and executive dysfunction on outcomes of depression in a primary care intervention trial: The PROSPECT study. *International Journal of Geriatric Psychiatry, 22*, 922–929.

Bonanno, G. A., Wortman, C. B., Lehman, D. R., Tweed, R. G., Haring, M., Sonnega, J., et al. (2002). Resilience to loss and chronic grief: A prospective study from preloss to 18-months postloss. *Journal of Personality & Social Psychology, 83*, 1150–1164.

Bonanno, G. A., Wortman, C. B., & Nesse, R. M. (2004). Prospective patterns of resilience and maladjustment during widowhood. *Psychology and Aging, 19*, 260–271.

Brodaty, H., Withall, A., Altendorf, A., & Sachdev, P. S. (2007). Rates of depression at 3 and 15 months poststroke and their relationship with cognitive decline: The Sydney Stroke Study. *American Journal of Geriatric Psychology, 15*, 477–486.

Brown, S. (2001). Variations in utilization and cost of inpatient psychiatric services among adults in Maryland. *Psychiatric Services, 52*, 841–843.

Bruce, M. L. (2002). Psychosocial risk factors for depressive disorders in late life. *Biological Psychiatry, 52*, 175–184.

Bruce, M. L., Kim, K., Leaf, P. J., & Jacobs, S. (1990). Depressive episodes and dysphoria resulting from conjugal bereavement in a prospective community sample. *American Journal of Psychiatry, 147*, 608–611.

Bruce, M. L., Ten Have, T. R., Reynolds, C. F., III, Katz, I. R., Schulberg, H. C., Mulsant, B. H., et al. (2004). Reducing suicidal ideation and depressive symptoms in depressed older primary care patients. A randomized controlled trial. *Journal of the American Medical Association, 291*, 1081–1091.

Carbonare, L. D., Maggi, S., Noale, M., Giannini, S., Rozzini, R., Lo Cascio, V., et al. (2009). Physical disability and depressive symptomatology in an elderly population: A complex relationship. The Italian Longitudinal Study on Aging (ILSA). *American Journal of Geriatric Psychiatry, 17*, 144–154.

Carnelley, K. B., Wortman, C. B., Bolger, N., & Burke, C. T. (2006). The time course of grief reactions to spousal loss: Evidence from a national probability sample. *Journal of Personality and Social Psychology, 91*, 476–492.

Colliver, J. D., Compton, W. M., Gfroerer, J. C., & Condon, T. (2006). Projecting drug use among aging baby boomers in 2020. *Annals of Epidemiology, 16*, 257–265.

Conwell, Y., Lyness, J. M., Duberstein, P. R., Cox, C., Seidlitz, L., DiGiorgio, A., et al. (2000). Completed suicide among older patients in primary care practices: A controlled study. *Journal of the American Geriatric Society, 48*, 23–29.

Crystal, S., Sambamoorthi, U., Walkup, J. T., & Akincigil, A.

(2003). Diagnosis and treatment of depression in the elderly Medicare population: Predictors, disparities, and trends. *Journal of the American Geriatrics Society, 51*, 1718–1728.

Department of Health and Human Services (1999). *Mental health: A report of the Surgeon General.* Bethesda MD: U.S. Public Health Service.

Depp, C. A., & Jeste, D. V. (2004). Bipolar disorder in older adults: a critical review. *Bipolar Disorders, 6*, 343–367.

Depp, C. A., Woodruff-Borden, J., Meeks, S., Gretarsdottir, E. S., & Dekngger, N. (2005). The phenomenology of non-clinical panic in older adults in comparison to younger adults. *Anxiety Disorders, 19*, 503–519.

Desai, A. K., Grossberg, G. T., & Cohen, C. I. (2003). Differential diagnosis of psychotic disorders in the elderly. In *Schizophrenia into later life: Treatment, research, and policy* (pp. 55–75). Washington, DC: American Psychiatric Association.

Dickerson, F. B., Brown, C. H., Daumit, G. L., LiJuan, F., Goldberg, R. W., Wohlheiter, K., et al. (2006). Health status of individuals with serious mental illness. *Schizophrenia Bulletin, 32*, 584–589.

Ferrario, S. R., Cardillo, V., Vicario, F., Balzarini, E., & Zotti, A. M. (2004). Advanced cancer at home: Caregiving and bereavement. *Palliative Medicine, 18*, 129–136.

Field, N. P., Nichols, C., Holen, A., & Horowitz, M. J. (1999). The relation of continuing attachment to adjustment in conjugal bereavement. *Journal of Consulting & Clinical Psychology, 67*, 212–218.

Fiske, A., O'Riley, A. A., & Widoe, R. K. (2008). Physical health and suicide in late life: An evaluative review. *Clinical Gerontologist, 31*, 31–50.

Flint, A. J. (2005). Generalised anxiety disorder in elderly patients: Epidemiology, diagnosis and treatment options. *Drugs and Aging, 22*, 101–114.

Fultz, N. H., Jenkins, K. R., Ostbye, T., Taylor, D. H. J., Kabeto, M. U., & Langa, K. M. (2005). The impact of own and spouse's urinary incontinence on depressive symptoms. *Social Science & Medicine, 60*, 2537–2548.

Gallagher-Thompson, D., Futterman, A., Farberow, N., Thompson, L. W., & Peterson, J. (1993). The impact of spousal bereavement on older widows and widowers. In M. S. Stroebe, W. Stroebe, & R. O. Hansson (Eds.), *Handbook of bereavement*. Cambridge: Cambridge University Press.

Garcia-Fabela, L., Melano-Carranza, E., Aguilar-Navarro, S., Garcia-Lara, J. M., Gutierrez-Robledo, L. M., & Avila-Funes, J. A. (2009). Hypertension as a risk factor for developing depressive symptoms among community-dwelling elders. *Revista de Investigacion Clinica, 61*, 274–280.

Gass, K. A. (1989). Appraisal, coping, and resources: Markers associated with the health of aged widows and widowers. In D. A. Lund (Ed.), *Older bereaved spouses: Research and practical applications* (pp. 79–94). New York: Hemisphere.

Gatz, M., Kasl-Godley, J. E., & Karel, M. (1996). Aging and mental disorders. In J. E. Birren & K. W. Schaie (Eds.), *Handbook of the psychology of aging* (6th ed.) (pp. 365–382). New York: Academic Press.

Gierz, M., & Jeste, D. V. (1993). Physical comorbidity in elderly Veterans Affairs patients with schizophrenia and depression. *American Journal of Geriatric Psychiatry, 1*, 165–170.

Gilliland, G., & Fleming, S. (1998). A comparison of spousal anticipatory grief and conventional grief. *Death Studies, 22*, 541–569.

Graham, C., Arthur, A., & Howard, R. (2002). The social functioning of older adults with schizophrenia. *Aging and Mental Health, 6*, 149–152.

Grant, B. S., Harford, T. C., Dawson, D. A., Chou, P., Dufour, M., & Pickering, R. (1995). Prevalence of DSM-IV alcohol abuse and dependece, United States, 1992. *Alcohol Health and Research World, 18*, 243–248.

Gretarsdottir, E. S., Woodruff-Borden, J., Meeks, S., & Depp, C. A. (2004). Social anxiety in older adults: Phenomenology, prevalence, and measurement. *Behaviour Research and Therapy, 42*, 459–475.

Gum, A. M., King-Kallimanis, B., & Kohn, R. (2009). Prevalence of mood, anxiety, and substance-abuse disorders for older Americans in the National Comorbidity Survey-Replication. *American Journal of Geriatric Psychiatry, 17*, 782–792.

Harding, C. M., & Cohen, C. I. (2003). Changes in schizophrenia across time. Paradoxes, patterns, and predictors. In *Schizophrenia into later life: Treatment, research, and policy* (pp. 19–41). Washington, DC: American Psychiatric Association.

Holahan, C. J., Moos, R. H., Holahan, C. K., Brennan, P. L., & Schutte, K. K. (2005). Stress generation, avoidance coping, and depressive Symptoms: A 10-Year model. *Journal of Consulting and Clinical Psychology, 73*, 658–666.

Jackson, E. S., Meeks, S., & Vititoe, E. (2002). Life events, distress, functioning, and short-term symptom change in a diagnostically diverse, middle-aged and older adult sample of people with severe mental illness. *Journal of Mental Health and Aging, 8*, 59–87.

Jones, C. J., & Meredith, W. (1996). Patterns of personality change across the life span. *Psychology and Aging, 11*, 57–67.

Jongenelis, K., Pot, A. M., Eisses, A. M. H., Beekman, A. T. F., Kluiter, H., & Ribbe, M. W. (2004). Prevalence and risk indicators of depression in elderly nursing home patients: the AGED study. *Journal of Affective Disorders, 83*, 135–142.

Judd, L. L., Rapaport, M. H., Paulus, M. P., & Brown, J. L. (1994). Subsyndromal symptomatic depression: a new mood disorder? *Journal of Clinical Psychiatry, 55*(Suppl.), 18–28.

Keith, S. J., Regier, D. A., & Rae, D. S. (1991). Schizophrenic disorders. In L. N. Robins & D. A. Regier (Eds.), *Psychiatric disorders in America* (pp. 33–52). New York: Free Press.

Kemp, B. J., Staples, F., & Lopez-Aqueres, W. (1987). Epidemiology of depression and dysphoria in an elderly Hispanic population: Prevalence and correlates. *Journal of the American Geriatrics Society, 35*, 920–926.

Kendler, K. S., Gardner, C. O., Gatz, M., & Pedersen, N. L. (2007). The sources of co-morbidity between major depression and generalized anxiety disorder in a Swedish national twin sample. *Psychological Medicine, 37*, 453–462.

Kessler, R. C., Zhao, S., Blazer, D. G., & Swartz, M. (1997). Prevalence, correlates, and course of minor depression and major depression in the national comorbidity survey. *Journal of Affective Disorders, 45*, 19–30.

King-Kallimanis, B., Gum, A. M., & Kohn, R. (2009). Comorbidity of depressive and anxiety disorders for older Americans in the National Comorbidity Survey-Replication. *American Journal of Geriatric Psychiatry, 17*, 782–792.

Lamme, S., Dykstra, P. A., & Broese Van Groenou, M. I. (1996). Rebuilding the network: New relationships in widowhood. *Personal Relationships, 3*, 337–349.

Lindstrom, T. C. (1995). Experiencing the presence of the dead: Discrepancies in "the sensing experience" and their psychological concomitants. *Omega — Journal of Death & Dying, 31*, 11–21.

LoConto, D. G. (1998). Death and dreams: A sociological approach to grieving and identity. *Omega — Journal of Death & Dying, 37*, 171–185.

McAlpine, D. D., & Cohen, C. I. (2003). Patterns of care for persons 65 years and older with schizophrenia. In *Schizophrenia into later life: Treatment, research, and policy* (pp. 3–17). Washington, DC: American Psychiatric Association.

Mancini, A. D., & Bonanno, G. A. (2009). Predictors and parameters of residence of loss: Toward on individual differences model. *Journal of Personality, 77*, 1805–1832.

Meeks, S. (1999). Bipolar disorder in the latter half of life: Symptom presentation, global functioning, and age of onset. *Journal of Affective Disorders, 52*, 161–167.

Meeks, S. (2000). Schizophrenia and related disorders. In S. K. Whitbourne (Ed.), *Psychopathology in later life* (pp. 189–215). New York: Wiley.

Meeks, S., & Murrell, S. A. (1997). Mental illness in late life: Socioeconomic conditions, psychiatric symptoms, and adjustment of long-term sufferers. *Psychology and Aging, 12*, 296–308.

Meeks, S., Woodruff-Borden, J., & Depp, C. A. (2003). Structural differentiation of self-reported depression and anxiety in late life. *Journal of Anxiety Disorders, 17*, 627–646.

Mineka, S., Watson, D., & Clark, L. A. (1998). Comorbidity of anxiety and unipolar mood disorders. *Annual Review of Psychology, 49*, 377–412.

Murrell, S. A., & Meeks, S. (1991). Depressive symptoms in older adults: Predispositions, resources, and life experiences. In K. W. Schaie (Ed.), *Annual Review of Gerontology and Geriatrics* (pp. 261–286). New York: Springer.

Newmann, J. P. (1989). Aging and depression. *Psychology and Aging, 4*, 150–165.

Ohayon, M. M. (2007). Epidemiology of depression and its treatment in the general population. *Journal of Psychiatric Research, 41*, 207–213.

Onrust, S. A., & Cuijpers, P. (2006). Mood and anxiety disorders in widowhood: A systematic review. *Aging and Mental Health, 10*, 327–334.

Oscar-Berman, M., & Marinkovic, K. (2007). Alcohol: Effects on neurobehavioral functions and the brain. *Neuropsychology Review, 17*, 239–257.

Ott, C. H., & Lueger, R. J. (2002). Patterns of change in mental health status during the first two years of spousal bereavement. *Death Studies, 26*, 387–411.

Palmer, B. W., Heaton, R. K., Gladsjo, J. A., Evans, J. D., Patterson, T. L., Golshan, S., et al. (2002). Heterogeneity in functional status among older outpatients with schizophrenia: employment history, living situation, and driving. *Schizophrenia Research, 55*, 205–215.

Parmelee, P. A., Katz, I. R., & Lawton, M. P. (1992). Depression and mortality among institutionalized aged. *Journals of Gerontology, 47*, P3–P10.

Patterson, T. L., Shaw, W., Semple, S. J., Moscona, S., Harris, M. J., Kaplan, R. M., et al. (1997). Health-related quality of life in older patients with schizophrenia and other psychoses: relationships among psychosocial and psychiatric factors. *International Journal of Geriatric Psychiatry, 12*, 452–461.

Pesonen, A., Raikkonen, K., Heinonen, K., Kajantie, E., Forsen, T., & Eriksson, J. G. (2007). Depressive symptoms in adults separated from their parents as children: A natural experiment during World War II. *American Journal of Epidemiology, 166*, 1126–1133.

Ritchie, K., Jaussent, I., Stewart, R., Dupuy, A., Courtet, P., Ancelin, L., et al. (2009). Association of adverse childhood environment and 5-HTTLPR genotype with late-life depression. *Journal of Clinical Psychiatry, 70*, 1281–1288.

Robins, L. R., & Regier, D. A. (1991). *Psychiatric disorders in America*. New York: Free Press.

Ruschena, D., Mullen, P. E., Burgess, P., Cordner, S. M., Barry-Walsh, J., Drummer, O. H., et al. (1998). Sudden death in psychiatric patients. *British Journal of Psychiatry, 172*, 331–336.

Satre, D. D., Gordon, N. P., & Weisner, C. (2007). Alcohol consumption, medical conditions, and health behavior in older adults. *American Journal of Health Behavior, 31*, 238–248.

Seignourel, P. J., Kunik, M. E., Snow, L., Wilson, N., & Stanley, M. A. (2008). Anxiety in dementia: A critical review. *Clinical Psychology Review, 28*, 1071–1082.

Simoni-Wastila, L., & Yang, H. K. (2006). Psychoactive drug abuse in older adults. *American Journal of Geriatric Pharmacotherapy, 4*, 380–394.

Sirey, M. P., Raue, P. J., & Alexopoulos, G. S. (2008). Impact of social support and self-efficacy on functioning in depressed older adults with chronic obstructive pulmonary disease. *International*

Journal of COPD, 3, 713–718.

Smalbrugge, M., Jongenelis, L., Pot, A. M., Eefsting, J. A., Ribbe, M. W., & Beekman, A. T. F. (2006). Incidence and outcome of depressive symptoms in nursing home patients in the Netherlands. *American Journal of Geriatric Psychiatry, 14*, 1069–1076.

Sneed, J. R., Kasen, S., & Cohen, P. (2007). Early-life risk factors for late-onset depression. *International Journal of Geriatric Psychiatry, 22*, 663–667.

Solano, N. H., & Whitbourne, S. K. (2001). Coping with schizophrenia: Patterns in later adulthood. *International Journal of Aging and Human Development, 53*, 1–10.

Steffens, D. C., Skoog, I., Norton, M. C., Hart, A. D., Tschanz, J. T., Plassman, B. L., et al. (2000). Prevalence of depression and its treatment in an elderly population: The Cache County Study. *Archives of General Psychiatry, 57*, 601–607.

Steunenberg, B., Beekman, A. T., Deeg, D. J., & Kerkhof, A. J. (2009). Personality predicts recurrence of late-life depression. *Journal of Affective Disorders* doi: S0165-0327(09)0035-4[pii]10.1016/j.jad.2009.08.002.

Stroebe, M. (2001). Gender differences in adjustment to bereavement: An empirical and theoretical review. *Review of General Psychology, 5*, 62–83.

Stroebe, M., Schut, H., & Stroebe, W. (2007). Health outcomes of bereavement. *Lancet, 370*, 1960–1973.

Stroebe, M. S., Stroebe, W., Gergen, K. J., & Gergen, M. (1981). The broken heart: Reality or myth. *Omega, 12*, 87–105.

Stroebe, W., & Stroebe, M. S. (1987). *Bereavement and health: The psychological and physical consequences of partner loss*. Cambridge, England: Cambridge University Press.

Stroebe, W., Stroebe, M. S., & Abakoumkin, G. (1999). Does differential social support cause sex differences in bereavement outcome? *Journal of Community & Applied Social Psychology, 9*, 1–12.

Subramaniam, H., Dennis, M. S., & Byrne, E. J. (2006). The role of vascular risk factors in late onset bipolar disorder. *International Journal of Geriatric Psychiatry, 22*, 733–737.

Substance Abuse and Mental Health Services Administration. (2009). Results from the 2008 National Survey on Drug Use and Health: National Findings Retreived from http://www.oas.samhsa.gov/NSDUH/2k8NSDUH/2k8results.cfm#Ch2.

Teresi, J., Abrams, R., Homes, D., Ramirez, M., & Eimicke, J. (2001). Prevalence of depression and depression recognition in nursing homes. *Social Psychiatry and Psychiatric Epidemiology, 36*, 613–620.

Trollor, J. N., Anderson, T. M., Sachdev, P. S., Brodaty, H., & Andrews, G. (2007). Prevalence of mental disorders in the elderly: The Australian National Mental Health and Well-Being Survey. *American Journal of Geriatric Psychiatry, 15*, 455–466.

Turvey, C., Conwell, Y., Jones, M. P., Phillips, C., Simonsick, E. M., Pearson, J. L., et al. (2002). Risk factors for late-life suicide: A prospective, community-based study. *American Journal of Geriatric Psychiatry, 10*, 398–406.

Turvey, C., Schultz, S. K., Beglinger, L., & Klein, D. M. (2009). A longitudinal community-based study of chronic illness, cognitive and physical function, and depression. *American Journal of Geriatric Psychiatry, 17*, 632–641.

Vaillant, G. E. (2003). A 60-year follow-up of alcoholic men. *Addiction, 98*, 1043–1051.

Watson, D. (2005). Rethinking the mood and anxiety disorders: A quantitative hierarchical model for DSM-V. *Journal of Abnormal Psychology, 114*, 522–536.

Weber, N. S., Cowan, D. N., Millikan, A. M., & Niebuhr, D. W. (2009). Psychiatric and general medical conditions comorbid with schizophrenia in the National Hospital Discharge Survey. *Psychiatric Services, 60*, 1059–1067.

Weinberger, M. I., Raue, P. J., Meyers, B. S., & Bruce, M. L. (2009). Predictors of new onset depression in medically ill, disabled older adults at 1 year follow-up. *American Journal of Geriatric Psychiatry, 17*, 802–809.

Weinberger, M.I., Whitbourne, S.K. (2010). Depressive symptoms, self-reported physical functioning, and identity in community-dwelling older adults. *Aging International.* doi: 10.1007/s12126-010-9053-4.

Zeiss, A. M., Lewinsohn, P. M., Rohde, P., & Seeley, J. R. (1996). Relationship of physical disease and functional impairment to depression in older people. *Psychology and Aging, 11*, 572–581.

Chapter 21

Assessment of Emotional and Personality Disorders in Older Adults

Barry A. Edelstein,[1] Daniel L. Segal[2]

[1]Department of Psychology, West Virginia University, Morgantown, West Virginia, USA; [2]Department of Psychology, University of Colorado, Colorado Springs, USA

CHAPTER CONTENTS

Introduction	**325**
Multimethod Assessment	**325**
General Classification Issues	**326**
Assessment of Emotional Disorders: Depression and Anxiety	**326**
Anxiety	328
Assessment of Personality Disorders	**329**
Personality Stability Versus Change Across the Life Span	**330**
The Impact of Aging on the Experience and Presentation of PDs in Later Life	**331**
Measures of Personality Disorders	**331**
Psychometric Considerations	331
Self-Report Inventories	332
Semi-Structured Interviews	333
A Specialized Measure: The Gerontological Personality Disorders Scale	333
Conclusions	**333**
References	**334**

INTRODUCTION

The assessment of mental disorders in older adults is often daunting, and is typically quite challenging for a variety of reasons ranging from methodological and definitional to age-related practical issues. This chapter has two principal goals. First, we consider methodological and classification issues regarding the assessment of older adults. Second, we review some of the more commonly used instruments for the examination of emotional and personality disorders among older adults.

MULTIMETHOD ASSESSMENT

Emotions and personalities are multidimensional constructs that require appropriate measures for each dimension. For example, the emotion of anxiety can be conceptualized as having three principal dimensions: physiological, cognitive, and overt behavioral. Each of these requires a different method of measurement, and each provides information that is not necessarily congruent with information obtained from another dimension. For example, one could report extreme anxiety in the presence of an anxiety-arousing stimulus, yet one's overt behavior could belie the experience of anxiety. A comprehensive assessment of anxiety would likely incorporate three methods of measurement: physiological recording, self-report of cognitions, and direct observation of overt behavior. No single method of assessment is consistently superior to any other in cognitively intact individuals. The use of multiple methods has been strongly recommended at least as far back as the publication of the classic article by Campbell and Fiske (1959) on the multitrait-multimethod approach to the establishment of construct validity. This approach has been echoed by more recent authors (e.g., Eid & Diener, 2006; Haynes & O'Brien, 2000) as a means to ensure accurate, reliable, and valid information. The shortcomings of any one method can often be avoided to some degree by using two or more assessment methods.

DOI: 10.1016/B978-0-12-380882-0.00021-8

The self-report method is perhaps the most frequently employed assessment method (e.g., questionnaires, interviews, checklists), particularly for the assessment of emotions and personality. In addition, the self-report method is arguably the most likely to yield questionable results when used with older adults with substantial age-related changes in cognitive skills (e.g., working memory, attention). Moreover, older adults with significant cognitive impairment may deny memory loss and the presence of other symptoms (Feher et al., 1992). Even the self-reports of older adults without serious psychopathology can be influenced by age related sensory deficits. Self-report instruments are also susceptible to more subtle influences when used with older adults. For example, Schwarz (1999) noted that the self-reports of older adults can be influenced by question format, question context, and the specific wording of questions. In addition, older adults are more likely than younger adults to underreport symptoms of psychological distress, report more intense affect than younger adults when discussing past experiences (Alea et al., 2004), and minimize or deny symptoms (Blazer, 2009).

A variety of other factors can contribute to the inaccuracies of self-reported information among older adults. These might include, for example, physical and mental health status, affective responses to acute illness, changes from previous levels of physical functioning occurring during hospitalization, and the presence of acute or chronic cognitive impairment (Sager et al., 1992). In summary, self-report can be a very rich source of information when used with older adults, but one must be vigilant for the potential influences of normative and non-normative age-related factors that can influence the reliability and validity of older adult self-report. If there is reason to believe that the self-report method would be compromised, greater emphasis should be placed on other methods (e.g., direct observation, rating scales, reports by others).

GENERAL CLASSIFICATION ISSUES

Diagnosis of emotional and personality disorders can be challenging in part because of inadequacies of the DSM-IV-TR criteria for these disorders. There appear to be age-related differences in the presentation and prevalence of various disorders. Jeste et al. (2005) have cogently argued for the need for age-appropriate diagnostic criteria. In addition to the differences in symptom presentation, symptoms of affective and anxiety disorders that do not reach the threshold for diagnosis (i.e., subsyndromal symptoms) nonetheless can distressing and disabling (e.g., Broadhead et al., 1990; Hybels et al., 2001; Wetherell et al., 2003). Moreover, the prevalence of these symptoms can increase with age (Judd et al., 2002). Other problems with diagnosis arise from the comorbidity of psychiatric disorders (e.g., depression) with physical disorders, some of which were previously discussed. The diagnostic challenge arises with the symptom overlap of psychiatric disorders and physical illness and the difficulty of sorting out the symptoms of the underlying physical illness, psychiatric symptoms that represent responses to the illness, and the symptoms of the psychiatric disorder that are unrelated to the physical illness (Jeste et al., 2005).

In recent years several authors have argued for dimensional approaches to mental disorders, including depression (e.g., Shankman & Klein, 2002), personality disorders (Widiger et al., 2009), and anxiety and mood disorders (e.g., Brown & Barlow, 2009). Brown and Barlow argued for an approach to conceptualizing psychopathology that is empirically based and that incorporates common dimensions of the emotional disorders as an alternative to disorder-specific diagnostic criteria. This approach might well address the two different age-related diagnostic issues. The first issue is one of a mismatch between the nature of the current criterion symptoms of anxiety and mood disorders and the constellation of symptoms presented by older adults. An empirically based approach that incorporates older adults may well address that issue. The second issue is that older adults who do not meet criteria for anxiety and mood disorders often experience the burden and disability of these disorders. Many of these older adults may well benefit from treatment but do not meet diagnostic criteria for the needed treatment. A dimensional system, such as that proposed by Widiger et al. (2009) could provide a more balanced representation of the adaptive and maladaptive personality traits of older adults and avoid some of the pitfalls of the current categorical diagnostic system. A more formal discussion of the merits of dimensional approaches is beyond the scope of this chapter. The interested reader is referred to Smith and Oltmanns (2009).

ASSESSMENT OF EMOTIONAL DISORDERS: DEPRESSION AND ANXIETY

The prevalence of major depression in community-dwelling older adults is between 1 and 4% (see review by Blazer, 2003). The prevalence of major depression increases as one moves from the community to primary care settings, where the prevalence ranges from 5 to 10% (Lyness et al., 2002; Schulberg et al., 1998). The prevalence of major depression increases to 10 to 12% among hospitalized older adults (Koenig et al., 1988) and to 12.4 to 14.4% among long-term care residents (Parmalee et al., 1989; Teresi et al., 2001).

Clinically significant symptoms of depression, which do not meet criteria for diagnosis, range from 8 to 16% among community-dwelling older adults (Blazer, 2003). Interestingly, the prevalence of symptoms of depression remain relatively stable from mid-life into older adulthood (Blazer, 2003).

Several age-related diagnostic issues impact the assessment of late-life depression. First, older adults often present a different array or profile of symptoms than younger adults (Caine et al., 1994; Fiske & O'Riley, 2008). For example, depressed older adults are less likely than younger adults to report suicidal ideation, guilt, and dysphoria (Fiske & O'Riley, 2008). Older adults are more likely to report hopelessness and helplessness (Christensen et al., 1999), somatic symptoms and psychomotor retardation (Gallo et al., 1994), and weight loss and loss of appetite (Blazer et al., 1987). A second issue revolves around the question of whether somatic symptoms should be considered among the diagnostic criteria for depression among older adults (Norris et al., 1995), many of whom suffer from chronic diseases. This issue is due, in part, to the overlap of symptoms of physical disease and somatic symptoms of depression (e.g., low energy, sleep disturbance, diminished appetite and sexual drive). There is recent evidence that suggests that changes in appetite and sexual drive may not be indicative of late-life depression, but the remaining somatic symptoms are (Nguyen & Zonderman, 2006; Norris et al., 2004). Third, symptoms of depression that do not meet criteria for a DSM diagnosis (subsyndromal depression) are associated with psychosocial and functional impairment similar to that associated with major depression (Beekman et al., 1995; Hybels et al., 2001; Lavretsky et al., 2004). Thus, the categorical nature of the diagnostic system can preclude treatment of some older adults whose symptoms are significant but do not reach the diagnosis threshold.

Numerous assessment instruments have been developed for the assessment of depression; however, few have been developed specifically for older adults. Although several of the depression assessment instruments that were developed with young adults have psychometric support for their use with older adults, the content validity of these measures with older adults remains unsettled in light of the question of whether somatic symptoms should be included (as previously discussed). In this section we will briefly review the more popular of the depression assessment instruments that have psychometric support. A more extensive review of more instruments can be found in Edelstein et al. (in press).

The Geriatric Depression Scale (GDS; Yesavage et al., 1983) is a 30-item self-report inventory that was developed specifically for older adults. It includes a dichotomous item response format (yes–no) that is assumed to be more easily used by older adults than instruments using Likert-type or Guttman rating scales. Somatic symptoms are not assessed, which some view as a strength because of the increased likelihood of physical disease among older adults whereas others (Norris et al., 1995) question the prudence of removing all somatic symptoms. Total scores range from 0 to 30, with recommended cutoff scores ranging from 10 to 16. This wide range appears to be due to the varying levels of sensitivity and specificity sought by the investigators, and the variety of populations with which the research was conducted (Fiske et al., 1998; Fiske & O'Riley, 2008). Kieffer and Reese (2002) found an average reliability coefficient of 0.85 across 338 studies. Yesavage et al. (1983) found a convergent validity coefficient of 0.71. Reliability and validity estimates are available across a wide range of populations (e.g., medically ill outpatients, hospitalized older adults, nursing home residents, cognitively impaired individuals, psychiatric patients). A short form of the GDS (Lesher & Berryhill, 1994) also is available. These authors reported a strong internal consistency coefficient ($r = 0.88$) and a strong correlation ($r = 0.89$) between the 30-item and 15-item forms. Sensitivity and specificity for the two forms is similar across a variety of populations.

The GDS has psychometric support for its use with individuals with mild to moderate dementia (Feher et al., 1992). Individuals with more severe dementia are likely better assessed with an instrument created specifically for use with severely cognitively impaired individuals, as discussed later. Overall, the GDS is a reasonable depression screening measure that has a short form that can be easily administered as a self-report instrument or presented orally.

The Center for Epidemiologic Studies Depression Scale (CES-D; Radloff, 1977) is a 20-item self-report inventory with a 4-point (0 to 3) Likert-type scale that is used to rate the frequency of symptoms over a one-week period. Total scores range from 0 to 60. The recommended cutoff score for depression is 16 or higher. Strong internal consistency estimates have been reported for community-dwelling older adults (0.82; Lewinsohn et al., 1997), and older medical inpatients (0.86; Schein & Koenig, 1997). Criterion validity is strong for community-dwelling older adults with major depression, with a weighted sensitivity of 100% and specificity of 88% using DSM diagnostic criteria (Beekman et al., 1997). A 10-item short form of the CES-D (Andresen et al., 1994) compares favorably with the original version in terms of reliability and validity when used with older adults. The recommended cutoff for this form is 10. The CES-D appears to be another reasonable depression screening instrument with a short form. The only potentially significant disadvantage when used with cognitively impaired individuals is that the instrument requires recall of the frequency of symptoms experienced over a one-week period.

The Beck Depression Inventory-II (BDI-II; Beck et al., 1996) is a 21-item self-report inventory that uses a

Guttman scale. Individual item scores range from 0 to 3, with a total score ranging from 0 to 63. Cutoff scores range from 10 to 13 for minimal depression, to 29 or higher for severe depression. This second edition of the BDI was developed to better represent the current DSM criteria for Major Depressive Disorder. Although this instrument was not developed specifically for older adults, older adults were included in the normative sample. As with the earlier version, the BDI-II has strong support for its reliability (e.g., Segal et al., 2008; Steer et al., 2000), with internal consistency estimates ranging from 0.86 for community-dwelling older adults (Segal et al., 2008) to 0.90 for psychiatric inpatients (Steer et al., 2000). Support for its factorial validity (Steer et al., 2000) and convergent validity (Segal et al., 2008) is strong, with validity coefficients ranging from 0.59 to 0.69. Overall, the BDI-II is a good screening instrument for depression. The only potential shortcoming is its Guttman response scale, which may be challenging for moderate to severely cognitively impaired older adults.

The Hamilton Rating Scale for Depression (HRSD; Hamilton, 1960, 1967), although often considered the "gold standard" of depression assessment instruments, has been soundly criticized as conceptually and psychometrically flawed (Bagby et al., 2004). Nevertheless, it continues to be widely used, perhaps for the lack of a suitable alternative. The HRSD is a clinician rated inventory that has appeared in various forms, with the number of items ranging from 17 to 28. Each behaviorally anchored item is rated on a 3- or 5-point scale. The extracted 17-item version is perhaps the most frequently used, and has good psychometric support with medically ill older adults (Rapp et al., 1990). Validity coefficients range from 0.68 to 0.84 with older adult samples (Edelstein et al., in press). Relatively weak inter-rater reliability of the HRSD has been an issue for quite some time, which resulted in the development of a structured interview guide (SIGH-D; Williams, 1988). Although some researchers continued to report inadequate reliability even with the structured guide (Pachana et al., 1994), a recent study with older adults yielded a stronger inter-rater reliability coefficient (r = 0.90; Korner et al., 2006). The HRSD has been used both as a screening and a diagnostic instrument. It is valuable as a screening instrument because it does not have the response demands of self-report inventories. However, the inter-rater reliability of the HRSD remains questionable.

The Cornell Scale for Depression in Dementia (CS; Alexopoulos et al., 1988) is a 19-item clinician rating scale developed for use with dementia patients. Items are rated on a 0- to 2-point scale of severity, with total scores ranging from 0 to 38. Administration involves two steps. The first step involves the patient's caregiver providing information via a semi-structured interview, which addresses the patient's behavior during the previous week, whereas the second step involves interviewing the individual using the same items. Internal consistency estimates range from 0.36 to 0.84, inter-rater reliability estimates range from 0.65 to 0.86, and correlations are also good between the CS and both the GDS (0.82) and the HRSD (0.82; Korner et al., 2006). As with the BDI, this instrument is best used as a screening measure or as a measure of the level of depression for someone previously diagnosed. The CS appears to be one of only two measures developed for the assessment of depression in dementia and has the strongest psychometric support of the two.

Anxiety

Prevalence rates for anxiety disorders among older adults range from 1 to 15% (Bryant et al., 2007). Anxiety disorders are the most common psychiatric disorders of older adults, although the prevalence is greater among younger adults (Kessler et al., 2005; Regier et al., 1988). Phobic disorder (Regier et al., 1988) and generalized anxiety disorder (Beekman et al., 1999) are the two most common anxiety disorders of older adults. As with depression, anxiety symptoms are relatively common among older adults, and even subsyndromal symptoms of anxiety can significantly impact an individual's quality of life (Kogan & Edelstein, 2004; Wetherell et al., 2003).

There are several age-related concerns about the current DSM diagnostic criteria for anxiety disorders when applied to older adults. First, there is evidence that older adults may experience anxiety differently than younger adults, in part due to age-related changes in physiology (Lau et al., 2001). However, one of only two studies to experimentally induce anxiety in older adults (Teachman & Gordon, 2009) found no age differences between young and older undiagnosed adults with regard to reported subjective anxiety, perceived heart rate, bodily sensations, thoughts regarding a loss of control, or actual heart rate. Because most older adults suffer from at least one chronic health problem, the question remains as to whether some of the somatic symptoms of anxiety should be included among the diagnostic criteria for anxiety disorders. Second, current anxiety assessment instruments may not be content valid for older adults, which has led to the development of instruments that are content valid (e.g., Kogan & Edelstein, 2004; Pachana et al., 2007; Wisocki et al., 1986). Third, as previously noted, significant symptoms of anxiety that do not reach the threshold for a psychiatric diagnosis can be distressing and disabling.

Several anxiety assessment instruments have been used with older adults, some of which were developed specifically for use with older adults. We begin with descriptions of the older adult measures and then consider those that were developed with younger adults and have psychometric support for use with older adults. As with the depression instruments, we will discuss only the most commonly used measures. The interested reader is referred to Edelstein et al. (2008) for a more extensive review.

The Fear Survey Schedule-II-OA (Kogan & Edelstein, 2004) is a 22-item self-report fear survey that was developed to be content valid for older adults, whose fears often differ from those of young adults. Ratings of fear severity and impairment with everyday activities are obtained. Internal consistency estimates range from 0.90 to 0.92, and preliminary convergent validity coefficients range from 0.40 to 0.47 with criterion instruments measuring anxiety more broadly. This is the only fear survey that is content valid for older adults.

The Geriatric Anxiety Inventory (GAD) (Pachana et al., 2007) is a 20-item self-report inventory that employs a dichotomous response format and requires symptom recall over a one-week period. Internal consistency is strong (alpha = 0.91 to 0.93), and sensitivity for GAD is quite reasonable for a more general measure of anxiety (sensitivity = 0.75; specificity = 0.84). The number of items pertaining to worry suggests that this measure is perhaps a better measure of GAD than general anxiety, although the preliminary psychometric support suggests it is a good anxiety screening instrument for older adults.

The Worry Scale (WS; Wisocki et al., 1986) is a 35-item self-report measure of worry that examines the content of worries. Support for its convergent validity is reasonably good (r = 0.57 to 0.73), as are measures of internal consistency (alpha = 0.79 to 0.93). This is the only content valid measure of older adult worry content.

The Geriatric Anxiety Scale (GAS; Segal et al., in press) is a newly developed 30-item self-report measure used to screen for anxiety symptoms among older adults. Individuals are asked to indicate how often they have experienced each symptom in the last week, answering on a 4-point likert scale (0-3) GAS items were derived from the broad range of anxiety disorder symptoms in the DSM-IV, and includes three subscales: somatic symptoms, cognitive symptoms, and affective symptoms. The GAS total score is based on the first 25 items. The additional 5 content items are used clinically and they do not load on the total score. The GAS demonstrated high internal consistency and strong evidence of validity in community and clinical samples of older adults (Segal et al., in press).

The Beck Anxiety Inventory (BAI; Beck et al., 1988) is a 21-item self-report inventory that employs a 4-point rating scale (0–3) for the extent to which anxiety symptoms bothered the individual during the previous week. Total scores range from 0 to 63. Internal consistency estimates range from 0.90 to 0.92, and convergent validity coefficients range from 0.47 to 0.73. The BAI is a good overall measure of anxiety, although the inclusion of somatic items may cause an overestimation of anxiety among older adults with medical illnesses (Wetherell & Gatz, 2005).

The Penn State Worry Questionnaire (PSWQ; Meyer et al., 1990) is a popular 16-item inventory that examines the frequency and intensity of worry symptoms using a 5-point Likert-type scale. Total scores range from 16 to 80. The PSWQ was developed for use with young adults, but there is considerable evidence to support its psychometric properties with older adults. Internal consistency estimates range from 0.86 to 0.93. Convergent validity coefficients range from 0.45 to 0.55. The PSWQ is a good measure of the experience of worry, rather than its content.

The State-Trait Anxiety Inventory (STAI; Spielberger, 1983) is a 20-item self-report inventory with two forms. One form measures trait anxiety and the other measures state anxiety. The state version employs a 4-point Likert-type rating scale, ranging from "not at all" to "very much," and addresses how the individual feels at the moment. The trait version employs a 4-point Likert-type rating scale, ranging from "almost never" to "almost always." Although the STAI was developed for young adults, several studies with older adults provide support for the convergent validity (e.g., Kabacoff et al., 1997; Stanley et al., 1996). Validity coefficients for the STAI state version range from 0.38 to 0.46, whereas coefficients for the trait version range from 0.47 to 0.57. Internal consistency estimates range from 0.79 to 0.90 for the trait version and from 0.85 to 0.92 for the state version. Recommended use is with community-dwelling adults. One caveat is that the content validity of this instrument has not been explored with older adults.

In conclusion, the assessment of older adult depression and anxiety continues to be supported through the development of assessment instruments designed specifically for older adults. Nevertheless, many instruments designed for use with younger adults apparently continue to be used without apparent concern for their psychometric properties with older adults. In addition, diagnostic issues regarding the use of the current DSM remain salient and will continue to be sources of concern until the age-related diagnostic criteria issues and the shortcomings of a categorical diagnostic system are satisfactorily addressed.

ASSESSMENT OF PERSONALITY DISORDERS

Personality disorders (PDs) are defined as longstanding and long-lasting maladaptive patterns of inner experiences and behaviors that seriously impair an individual's ability to perform adequately in a variety of settings (American Psychiatric Association, 2000). Key features of PDs include their early onset (typically by adolescence or early adulthood), stability, inflexibility, pervasiveness, and chronicity (although individual symptoms and the overall severity may wax and wane), intrapsychic and interpersonal focus, and that the symptoms must lead to functional impairment or personal distress. Although this definition of requires an onset no later than early adulthood, many individuals with a PD are not diagnosed or treated until later life (Segal et al., 2006).

The precise prevalence of PDs among older adults is a source of debate in the literature (e.g., Balsis et al., 2007, 2009; Zweig & Agronin, 2006), although it is clear that PDs are relatively common and affect all age groups. In their meta-analysis, Abrams and Horowitz (1996) reported an overall prevalence rate of 10% (with a range of 6 to 33%) for those over the age of 50. In their expanded meta-analysis (Abrams & Horowitz, 1999), the overall prevalence rate increased to 20%. The general trend suggested a decline in frequency and intensity of PD pathology with advancing age, at least for certain PDs. The exact cause for this decline is one of the most controversial topics in the literature on PDs in older adults (Molinari & Segal, 2011), and highlights several challenging methodological and diagnostic issues.

First, there are serious concerns raised about the *relevance* of many of the DSM diagnostic criteria to accurately detect the unique presentation of some PDs in the context of later life, commonly referred to as "geriatric variants" of the PDs (Segal et al., 2006). As is true for many forms of psychopathology, the diagnostic criteria for PDs were simply not designed with older people in mind (Agronin & Maletta, 2000; Balsis et al., 2009; Segal et al., 2006). About 25% of the diagnostic criteria for PDs lack content validity with older adults. For example, consider the criterion for schizoid PD: "Neither enjoys nor experiences sexual relations." This criterion may be valid among younger adults but seems poorly suited to older adults. It could be argued that among older adults this type of experience may have little to do with schizoid PD pathology but rather may reflect the lack of suitable sexual partners for many older widows or may be endorsed by those older adults with reduced sexual interest or performance due to physical illness. Likewise, the antisocial PD criterion - "Irritability and aggressiveness, as indicated by repeated physical fights or assaults," — may not apply to some frail older adults who, because of their reduced physical strength and stamina, are less likely to express their aggressive feelings in the form of physical assaults. In an empirical investigation of potential age bias using item analysis, Balsis and colleagues (2007) found evidence of age bias in 29% of the criteria for 7 PDs. In this study, some diagnostic criteria were differentially endorsed by younger and older adults with equivalent PD pathology, suggesting a measurement bias.

A second diagnostic issue is that PD pathology is often *overlooked* in older adults. This may occur if professionals hold pejorative, stereotypical views of older adults, seeing them as rigid, irritable, bitter, dependent, depressed, or organically impaired. Such derogatory perceptions may erroneously lead professionals to view some pathological behavior (reflecting PD traits) as normal for older patients. Under diagnosis may also occur if professionals focus on the more overt signs and symptoms of Axis I clinical disorders (e.g., depression, anxiety, dementia), which are often easier to identify and understand than the underlying PD (Molinari & Segal, 2011).

A third diagnostic problem is that the *context* of later life can obscure the identification of PDs. According to Zweig (2008), the differentiation of PD from co-occurring Axis I disorders (e.g., the state vs. trait problem) is challenging particularly when heightened irritability and interpersonal difficulties are related at least in part to mood changes due to a recent loss. The differentiation of PD from context-dependent roles and behaviors is also problematic. For example, poor adaptation to a changing role such as becoming overwhelmed after the death of a spouse may reflect the anxiety of an acute adjustment disorder rather than the emergence of a dependent PD (Zweig, 2008). Another contextual issue is that the differentiation of a PD from personality change due to a neurological or medical condition requires an exhaustive medical work-up. In geriatric settings, somatic presentations of PD are common, which can complicate the "teasing out" of true comorbid medical/cognitive problems from PD pathology (Zweig, 2008).

A fourth diagnostic issue is that *changing definitions* and conceptualizations of PDs across the versions of the DSM (Coolidge & Segal, 1998) have made longitudinal studies difficult if not impossible. As the DSM classification system has evolved, some PDs present in earlier versions of the manual were removed (e.g., inadequate personality; asthenic personality), others have been added over time (e.g., schizotypal personality; dependent personality), and yet others have been renamed and reconceptualized (e.g., borderline PD was previously called emotionally unstable PD) across versions of the DSM. Expected changes to the PD category in the upcoming DSM-V, likely reflecting some emphasis on dimensional ratings of PD traits, will certainly create continued challenges to any type of longitudinal study of PDs.

PERSONALITY STABILITY VERSUS CHANGE ACROSS THE LIFE SPAN

The field of personality psychology has struggled with the extent to which personality should be conceptualized as a set of enduring traits versus situationally influenced behaviors, especially patterns of coping with stress and distress. Apparently, personality traits (including adaptive and maladaptive ones) are both stable and adaptable across the life span, depending on how the issue is framed (Clark, 2009; Vaillant, 2002). Provocative data from Roberts and DelVecchio (2000) suggest that personality traits become even more stable in later life based on higher correlations of trait scores with follow-up scores 7 years later for older adults compared to children, college students, and 30 year olds. However, change is best viewed as an individual difference variable in and of itself. Thus, rank-order stability of major personality traits are relatively stable, but some individuals certainly do change whereas others do not. Obviously, models of personality serve as a backdrop for models of disorders. Thus, general stability in personality traits could be construed as a backdrop for PDs, which are also considered generally stable but not immutable, with shifting amounts of distress and dysfunction depending on contextual variables, especially stressors. According to Clark (2009), emerging models for the diagnosis of PDs focus on (1) the assessment of level of psychological and interpersonal dysfunction and its acute manifestations (e.g., psychiatric symptoms such as depression, anxiety, suicidality) and (2) a description of the person's personality traits. Whereas symptoms may come and go over time, change in one's underlying personality traits would be expected to be less obvious and slower in nature.

THE IMPACT OF AGING ON THE EXPERIENCE AND PRESENTATION OF PDS IN LATER LIFE

The question of how PDs are affected by aging has been debated, but has lacked a research base on which to anchor a definitive answer. Some evidence points to a decline in expression of the symptoms associated with the cluster of disorders labeled *dramatic and erratic* (including borderline, histrionic, and narcissistic) in midlife with an increase in symptoms again in later life (Reich et al., 1988). Others suggest that the decline in dramatic PDs relates to increased mortality rates among severely impulsive and erratic individuals, a decrease in energy needed to maintain the high energy symptoms, and the poor fit of the current diagnostic criteria (Segal et al., 2006).

The stresses of old age are believed to *exacerbate* the expression of some PD symptoms, especially among vulnerable older adults whose usual forms of coping become outstripped by the environmental and psychological demands (Segal et al., 2006). Loss of control of the environment that is characteristic of the increasing dependency that comes with loss of mobility and declining resources among especially frail older adults can provoke anxiety that generates PD symptoms. However, the symptom criteria used by the DSM system include life circumstances that may be irrelevant to some older adults. For example, difficulties in the work environment and with residential family life may be less relevant because of the lower rate of participation in the work force and the tendency not to coreside with family members. Thus, the behavioral expressions of PDs in older adults may not match the template typically used to identify PDs in younger adults.

In some cases, there is an emergence of PD symptoms that were "hidden" earlier in life (Segal et al., 2006). For example, consider a highly dependent woman who was supported by a caring, perhaps dominating, spouse who did not mind making all of the decisions for the couple and essentially took care of his wife throughout much of their adult lives. Not until she struggled to take care of herself after becoming a widow would the extent of her "disorder" be recognized and perhaps diagnosed. While a theorized pattern for each of the PDs has been provided by Segal et al. (2006), empirical validation of the patterns is sorely needed.

The concept of heterotypic continuity may help one understand why the expression of PD traits may differ across the life span. In a nutshell, heterotypic continuity suggests that core psychological constructs remain constant throughout adulthood and later life, but the behavioral manifestations of the core constructs are expressed differently throughout the life cycle (e.g., Mroczek et al., 1999). For example, a core feature of antisocial PD is the failure to conform to social norms. Among younger adults, this core feature may be expressed by repeated physical fights. However, as we noted earlier, physical fighting is less likely among frail older adults who instead may express the core feature by repeated rule infractions in long-term care settings (Molinari & Segal, 2011). An example for borderline PD may involve the key feature regarding self-harm. In younger adults, this may be expressed as dramatic cutting, carving, or other blatant forms of self-mutilation whereas an older adult may present with more subtle self-harming behaviors such as intentional misuse of prescription medications or intentional failure to adhere to a rehabilitation regime. These important changes in the behavioral expressions of many PD features in later life highlight the need for revisions of the diagnostic criteria to more fully consider the late-life context (Balsis et al., 2009).

MEASURES OF PERSONALITY DISORDERS

Psychometric Considerations

As discussed earlier, the primary psychometric issues include reliability and validity. Because all of the standardized instruments used to measure specific PDs were developed for a younger population, there is no "gold standard" of diagnosis for PD in older adults. This fact, in conjunction with the problems of content validity of some PD diagnostic criteria, is cause for significant caution regarding the use of these instruments for the assessment of PDs in later life. Several self-report inventories and semi-structured interviews for PDs have been developed and validated primarily among diverse adult populations, the most prominent of which will be discussed in the next section with specific attention to their potential application to older adults.

Self-Report Inventories

The Coolidge Axis II Inventory (CATI; Coolidge, 2000) assesses the 10 standard DSM-IV PDs as well as passive-aggressive, depressive, sadistic, and self-defeating PDs. The CATI has been used in over 100 research publications and the psychometric properties appear strong among adult samples (Coolidge, 2000). The CATI includes three scales that may be particularly relevant to older adults: (1) a Personality Change Due to a General Medical Condition scale; (2) a Neuropsychological Dysfunction scale, with 3 subscales including language and speech dysfunction, memory and concentration difficulties, and neurosomatic complaints related to brain dysfunction; and (3) an Executive Functions of the Frontal Lobe scale with 3 subscales including poor planning, decision-making difficulty, and task incompletion. The CATI has been used successfully in studies with chronically mentally ill older adults (Coolidge et al., 2000) and community-dwelling older adults (Segal et al., 2001) providing some preliminary evidence for its validity with older respondents.

The Millon Clinical Multiaxial Inventory-III (MCMI-III; Millon et al., 1997) is a broad-band measure of personality pathology that includes 14 PD scales and 10 clinical syndromes scales (Axis-I related), which are all based on Millon's comprehensive theory of personality. The MCMI-III has been the focus of over several hundred research publications, it ranks among the most widely used testing instruments in clinical practice with adults, and it has a wealth of data supporting its psychometric properties (see review by Millon and Meagher, 2004). In general, age appears to have a minimal impact on the MCMI-III scales, with a slight tendency for scores to decrease with age for all scales except for the Histrionic, Narcissistic, and Compulsive PD scales in which scores tend to increase slightly (Haddy et al., 2005). Recently, Hyer et al. (2008) described the clinical utility of Millon's personality model and its assessment with older adults. Specific validation studies with older adults are spare, with the exception of one study that found modest convergence between the MCMI and the CATI among chronically mentally ill older inpatients (Silberman et al., 1997). Millon has no plans at present to develop an MCMI-IV.

The Personality Diagnostic Questionnaire-4+ (PDQ-4+; Hyler, 1994) assesses the 10 standard DSM-IV PDs as well as passive-aggressive PD and depressive PD (in Appendix B of DSM-IV). It has two validity scales: the Too Good scale measures underreporting of pathological personality traits whereas the Suspect Questionnaire scale detects lying and random responding. The PDQ is designed for use in both normal and clinical populations and provides dimensional and categorical scores for each PD. Regarding its psychometric properties, the primary concerns seems to be a high false positive rate and poor validity of the validity scales (Bagby & Farvolden, 2004). Like some prior studies with adult participants, one study with community-dwelling older adults (Segal et al., 1998) resulted in extremely high false positive rates for PDs. As such, it is inadvisable to use this measure with older adults, except perhaps to rule out PDs since it has a low false negative rate.

The Schedule for Nonadaptive and Adaptive Personality (SNAP-2; Clark et al., in press) evaluates trait dimensions or problem areas relevant to the understanding of personality pathology, and as such is not a direct measure of PDs per se. The measure includes 12 primary trait scales, which are subsumed into 3 broad temperament dimensions. The Negative Temperament dimension includes six scales: mistrust, manipulativeness, aggression, self-harm, eccentric perceptions, dependency. The Positive Temperament dimension includes three scales: exhibitionism, entitlement, and detachment. The Disinhibition Temperament dimension also includes three scales: impulsivity, propriety, and workaholism. The measure also includes seven validity scales. Among adults, the SNAP-2 yields predictable and meaningful relations with dimensional ratings of PDs (see Clark et al., in press), but studies with older adults are needed.

The Wisconsin Personality Disorders Inventory (WISPI-IV; Klein et al., 1993; Smith et al., 2003) is based on an interpersonal theory and approach to the PDs and assesses the 10 standard DSM-IV PDs as well as passive-aggressive PD. Scoring options include means, ipsatized, and normative scores for each of the 11 PD scales as well as a categorical diagnosis. Whereas the WISPI-IV has solid psychometric properties among adult respondents (Smith et al., 2003), like the SNAP-2, psychometric studies with older adults are noticeably lacking.

As we have noted, for each of these measures, specific validity studies with older adults are presently scarce. Whereas all of these measures have been used clinically with older adults, their uncertain reliability and validity are cause for some caution when interpreting the assessment data. These measures (with the exception of the SNAP-2) are also potentially problematic because they are essentially tied to the DSM diagnostic criteria which, as described earlier, may not necessarily capture the unique presentation of some PDs in later life. A typical application of these measures is that they are used by clinicians and researchers to *screen* for the presence of PDs or their features. Disorders that are elevated on the screening measure are then further examined through either a clinical interview or a semi-structured interview, where the context of aging can be more clearly elucidated.

Semi-Structured Interviews

The five most prominent semi-structured interviews for PDs will be reviewed in this section. The interviews are as follows: Structured Clinical Interview for DSM-IV Axis II Personality Disorders (First et al., 1997); Structured Interview for DSM-IV Personality (Pfohl et al., 1997); International Personality Disorder Examination (Loranger, 1999); Personality Disorder Interview-IV (Widiger et al., 1995); and Diagnostic Interview for DSM-IV Personality Disorders (Zanarini et al., 1996). Each of these instruments covers the 10 standard PDs in DSM-IV and has solid evidence for reliability and validity among diverse adult respondents (see the data provided in the manual for each measure). Most of these measures have been used in research studies with older adults providing some preliminary support for their utility. However, limited psychometric data are available for older adults, and because each of these measures adheres to the diagnostic criteria of the DSM-IV diagnostic system, they are limited by the potential problems of the system as it relates to later life. Clinically, each of these measures are lengthy to administer, which may overly burden the older patient.

A Specialized Measure: The Gerontological Personality Disorders Scale

To aid in the screening of PDs in later life, a brief specialized self-report measure called the Gerontological Personality Disorders Scale (GPS; Van Alphen et al., 2006) has recently been developed and preliminarily examined. Because the GPS includes items based on General Diagnostic Criteria for PDs in the DSM-IV-TR, it does not assess specific PDs. The GPS includes two subscales: Habitual behavior and Biographical information, both which have adequate internal consistency. Compared to a clinical diagnosis, the sensitivity and specificity of the GPS were both 69% indicating moderate diagnostic accuracy. Notably, an informant version of the GPS was not useful. Further validation of the GPS is warranted, especially in diverse samples of outpatient and inpatient older adults. Clearly, an elder-specific measure of individual PDs that takes into account the unique manifestations of PD pathology in the context of later life is certainly needed. It is also imperative that future editions of the DSM revise the PD diagnostic criteria to take into account the later life context (Agronin & Maletta, 2000; Balsis et al., 2009).

In conclusion, the assessment of PDs in later life remains challenging due to a number of methodological and conceptual issues. The fact remains, however, that PDs are commonly seen in clinical settings yet seldom formally identified (Molinari & Segal, 2011). A more accurate assessment of underlying PD traits and features in older clients is needed to facilitate effective interventions.

CONCLUSIONS

As this chapter has highlighted, the psychological assessment of older adults is fraught with multiple age-related factors that contribute to its complexity and resulting challenges. The assessment of emotional and personality disorders has advanced considerably in the past two decades through the design and development of assessment instruments for older adults, and through an appreciation of the many factors that can contribute to the performance of older adults. Nevertheless, the array of assessment instruments available with appropriate age-related psychometric properties pales in comparison to those available for young adults. The accumulation of older adult psychometric data on instruments developed for younger adults is likely not the best solution to this problem because of the limitations of the DSM-IV criteria for emotional and personality disorders when applied to older adults. Until the issue of age-related presentations of emotional and personality disorders is addressed, clinicians should be circumspect in their use of assessment instruments developed with young adults, and their application of the current diagnostic criteria. At the very least, clinicians might consider adopting a more dimensional approach to assessment that is more sensitive to the subsyndromal presentations of emotional disorders among older adults.

REFERENCES

Abrams, R. C., & Horowitz, S. V. (1996). Personality disorders after age 50: A meta-analysis. *Journal of Personality Disorders, 10*, 271–281.

Abrams, R. C., & Horowitz, S. V. (1999). Personality disorders after age 50: A meta-analytic review of the literature. In E. Rosowsky, R. C. Abrams, & R. A. Zweig (Eds.), *Personality disorders in older adults: Emerging issues in diagnosis and treatment* (pp. 55–68). Mahwah, NJ: Erlbaum.

Agronin, M. E., & Maletta, G. (2000). Personality disorders and later life: Understanding the gap in research. *American Journal of Geriatric Psychiatry, 8*, 4–18.

Alea, N., Bluck, S., & Semegon, A. B. (2004). Young and older adults' expression of emotional experience: Do autobiographical narratives tell a different story? *Journal of Adult Development, 11*, 235–250.

Alexopoulos, G. S., Abrams, R. C., Young, R. C., & Shamoian, C. A. (1988). Cornell Scale for Depression in Dementia. *Biological Psychiatry, 23*, 271–284.

American Psychiatric Association. (2000). *Diagnostic and statistical manual of mental disorders* (4th ed., text revision). Washington, DC: Author.

Andresen, E. M., Malmgren, J. A., Carter, W. B., & Patrick, D. L. (1994). Screening for depression in well older adults: Evaluation of a short-form of the CES-D. *American Journal of Preventive Medicine, 10*, 77–84.

Bagby, R. M., Ryder, A. G., Schuller, M. D., & Marshall, M. B. (2004). The Hamilton Depression Rating Scale: Has the gold standard become a lead weight? *American Journal of Psychiatry, 161*, 2163–2177.

Bagby, R. M., & Farvolden, P. (2004). The Personality Diagnostic Questionnaire-4 (PDQ-4). In M. Hilsenroth & D. L. Segal (Eds.), Personality assessment. Vol. 2 in M. Hersen (Ed.-in-Chief), *Comprehensive handbook of psychological assessment* (pp. 122–133). New York: Wiley.

Balsis, S., Gleason, M. E. J., Woods, C. M., & Oltmanns, T. F. (2007). An item response theory analysis of DSM-IV personality disorder criteria across younger and older age groups. *Psychology and Aging, 22*, 171–185.

Balsis, S., Segal, D. L., & Donahue, C. (2009). Revising the personality disorder diagnostic criteria for *Diagnostic and Statistical Manual of Mental Disorders (DSM-V)*: Consider the later life context. *American Journal of Orthopsychiatry, 79*, 452–460.

Beck, A. T., Epstein, N., Brown, G., & Steer, R. (1988). An inventory for measuring clinical anxiety: Psychometric properties. *Journal of Consulting and Clinical Psychology, 56*, 893–897.

Beck, A. T., Steer, R. A., & Brown, G. K. (1996). *Manual for the Beck Depression Inventory* (2nd ed.). San Antonio, TX: The Psychological Corporation.

Beekman, A. T. F., Bremmer, M. A., Deeg, D. J. H., Van Balkom, A. J. L. M., Smit, J. H., De Beurs, E., et al. (1999). Anxiety disorders in later life: A report from the longitudinal aging study Amsterdam. *International Journal of Geriatric Psychiatry, 13*(10), 717–726.

Beekman, A. T., Deeg, D. J., Van Limbeek, J., Braam, A. W., De Vries, M. Z., & Van Tilburg, W. (1997). Criterion validity of the Center for Epidemiologic Studies Depression Scale (CES-D): Results from a community-based sample of older subjects in The Netherlands. *Psychological Medicine, 27*, 231–235.

Beekman, A. T. F., Deeg, D. J. H., van Tilburg, T., Smit, J. H., Hooijer, C., & van Tilburg, W. (1995). Major and minor depression in later life: A study of prevalence and risk factors. *Journal of Affective Disorders, 36*, 65–75.

Blazer, D. G. (2003). Depression in late life: Review and commentary. *Journals of Gerontology: Medical Sciences, 58A*, 249–265.

Blazer, D. G. (2009). The psychiatric interview of older adults. In D. G. Blazer & D. C. Steffens (Eds.), *The American Psychiatric Publishing textbook of geriatric psychiatry* (4th ed.) (pp. 187–200). Arlington, VA: American Psychiatric Publishing.

Blazer, D., Bachar, J. R., & Hughes, D. C. (1987). Major depression with melancholia: A comparison of middle-aged and elderly adults. *Journal of the American Geriatrics Society, 35*, 927–932.

Broadhead, W. W., Blazer, D. G., George, L. K., & Tse, C. K. (1990). Depression, disability days, and days lost from work: A prospective epidemiologic survey. *Journal of the American Medical Association, 264*, 2524–2528.

Brown, T., & Barlow, D. (2009). A proposal for a dimensional classification system based on the shared features of the DSM-IV anxiety and mood disorders: Implications for assessment and treatment. *Psychological Assessment, 21*, 256–271.

Bryant, C., Jackson, H., & Ames, D. (2008). The prevalence of anxiety in older adults: Methodological issues and a review of the literature. *Journal of Affective Disorders, 109*, 233–250.

Caine, E. D., Lyness, J. M., King, D. A., & Connors, L. (1994). Clinical and etiological heterogeneity of mood disorders in elderly patients. In: L. S. Scneider, C. F. Reynolds, B. D. Lebowitz, & A. J. Friedhoff (Eds.), *Diagnosis and treatment of depression in late life: Results of the NIH Consensus Development Conference* (pp. 21–53). Washington, DC: American Psychiatric Press.

Campbell, D. T., & Fiske, D. W. (1959). Convergent and discriminant validation by the multitrait-multimethod matrix. *Psychological Bulletin, 56*, 81–105.

Christensen, H., Jorm, A. F., Mackinnon, A. J., Korten, A. E., Jacomb, P. A., Henderson, A. S., et al. (1999). Age differences in depression and anxiety symptoms: A structural equation modelling analysis of data from a general population sample. *Psychological Medicine, 29*, 325–339.

Clark, L. A. (2009). Stability and change in personality disorder.

Current Directions in Psychological Science, 18, 27–31.

Clark, L. A., Simms, L. J., Wu, K. D., & Casillas, A. *Schedule for Nonadaptive and Adaptive Personality (SNAP-2). Manual for administration, scoring, and interpretation*. Minneapolis, MN: University of Minnesota Press, (in press).

Coolidge, F. L., & Segal, D. L. (1998). Evolution of the personality disorder diagnosis in the Diagnostic and Statistical Manual of Mental Disorders. *Clinical Psychology Review, 18*, 585–599.

Coolidge, F. L. (2000). *Coolidge Axis II Inventory: Manual*. Colorado Springs, CO: Author.

Edelstein, B., Drozdick, L., & Ciliberti, C. Assessment of depression and bereavement in older adults. In P. Lichtenberg (Ed.), *Handbook on geriatric assessment* (2nd ed.). New York: Wiley, (in press).

Edelstein, B. A., Woodhead, E. L., Segal, D. L., Heisel, M. J., Bower, E. H., Lowery, A. J., et al. (2008). Older adults psychological assessment: Current instrument status and related considerations. *Clinical Gerontologist, 31*(3), 1–35.

Eid, M., & Diener, E. (2006). *Handbook of multimethod measurement in psychology*. Washington, DC: American Psychological Association.

Feher, E. P., Larrabee, G. J., & Crook, T. J. (1992). Factors attenuating the validity of the geriatric depression scale in a dementia population. *Journal of the American Geriatrics Society, 40*, 906–909.

First, M. B., Gibbon, M., Spitzer, R. L., Williams, J. B. W., & Benjamin, L. S. (1997). *Structured Clinical Interview for DSM-IV Axis II Personality Disorders (SCID-II)*. Washington, DC: American Psychiatric Press.

Fiske, A., & O'Riley. (2008). Depression in late life. In J. Hunsley & E. J. Marsh (Eds.), *A guide to assessments that work*. New York: Oxford University Press.

Fiske, A., Kasl-Godley, J. E., & Gatz, M. (1998). Mood disorders in late life. In B. Edelstein (Ed.), *Clinical geropsychology* (pp. 193–230). Oxford: Elsevier Science.

Gallo, J. J., Anthony, J. C., & Muthen, B. O. (1994). Age differences in the symptoms of depression: A latent trait analysis. *Journals of Gerontology: Psychological Sciences, 49*, P251–P264.

Haddy, C., Strack, S., & Choca, J. P. (2005). Linking personality disorders and clinical syndromes on the MCMI-III. *Journal of Personality Assessment, 84*, 193–204.

Hamilton, M. (1960). A rating scale for depression. *Journal of Neurology, Neurosurgery, and Psychiatry, 23*, 56–62.

Hamilton, M. (1967). Development of a rating scale for primary depressive illness. *British Journal of Social and Clinical Psychology, 6*, 278–296.

Haynes, S. N., & O'Brien, W. H. (2000). *Principles and practice of behavioral assessment*. New York: Plenum/Kluwer.

Hybels, C., Blazer, D., & Pieper, C. (2001). Toward a threshold for subthreshold depression: An analysis of correlates of depression by severity of symptoms using data from an elderly community survey. *The Gerontologist, 41*, 357–365.

Hyer, L., Molinari, V., Mills, W. L., & Yeager, C. (2008). Personological assessment and treatment of older adults. In T. Millon & C. Bloom (Eds.), *The Millon inventories: A practitioner's guide to personalized clinical assessment* (2nd ed.) (pp. 296–326). New York: Guilford.

Hyler, S. E. (1994). *Personality Diagnostic Questionnaire (4th edition*, PDQ-4+). New York: New York State Psychiatric Institute.

Jeste, D. V., Blazer, D. G., & First, M. (2005). Aging-related diagnostic variations: Need for diagnostic criteria appropriate for elderly psychiatric patients. *Biological Psychiatry, 58*, 265–271.

Judd, L. L., Schettler, P. J., & Akiskal, H. S. (2002). The prevalence, clinical relevance, and public health significance of subthreshold depressions. *Psychiatric Clinics of North America, 25*, 685–698.

Kabacoff, R. I., Segal, D. L., Hersen, M., & Van Hasselt, V. B. (1997). Psychometric properties and diagnostic utility of the Beck Anxiety Inventory and the State-Trait Anxiety Inventory with older adult psychiatric outpatients. *Journal of Anxiety Disorders, 11*, 33–47.

Kessler, R. C., Chiu, W. T., Demler, O., Merikangas, K. R., & Walters, E. E. (2005). Prevalence, severity, and comorbidity of 12-month DSM-IV disorders in the National Comorbidity Survey Replication. *Archives of General Psychiatry, 62*, 617–627.

Kieffer, K. M., & Reese, R. J. (2002). A reliability generalization study of the Geriatric Depression Scale. *Educational and Psychological Measurement, 62*, 969–994.

Klein, M. H., Benjamin, L. S., Rosenfeld, R., Treece, C., Husted, J., & Greist, J. H. (1993). The Wisconsin Personality Disorders Inventory: I. Development, Reliability, and Validity. *Journal of Personality Disorders, 7*, 285–303.

Koenig, H. G., Meador, K. G., Cohen, H. J., & Blazer, D. G. (1988). Depression in elderly hospitalized patients with medical illness. *Archives of Internal Medicine, 148*, 1929–1936.

Kogan, J., & Edelstein, B. (2004). Modification and psychometric examination of a self-report measure of fear in older adults. *Journal of Anxiety Disorders, 18*, 397–409.

Korner, A., Lauritzen, L., Abelskov, K., Gulmann, N., Brodersen, A. M., Wedervang-Jensen, T., et al. (2006). The Geriatric Depression Scale and the Cornell Scale for Depression in Dementia. A validity study. *Nordic Journal of Psychiatry, 60*, 360–364.

Lau, A., Edelstein, B., & Larkin, K. (2001). Psychophysiological responses of older adults: A critical review with implications for assessment of anxiety disorders. *Clinical Psychology Review, 21*, 609–630.

Lavretsky, H., Kurbanyan, K., & Kumar, A. (2004). The significance of subsyndromal depression in geriatrics. *Current Psychiatry Reports, 6*, 25–31.

Lesher, E. L., & Berryhill, J. S. (1994). Validation of the Geriatric Depression Scale-Short Form among inpatients. *Journal of Clinical Psychology, 50*, 256–260.

Lewinsohn, P. M., Seeley, J. R., Roberts, R. E., & Allen, N. B. (1997). Center for Epidemiologic

Studies Depression Scale (CES-D) as a screening instrument for depression among community-residing older adults. *Psychology and Aging, 12*, 277–287.

Loranger, A. W. (1999). *International Personality Disorder Examination. DSM-IV and ICD-10 Interviews*. Odessa, FL: Psychological Assessment Resources, Inc.

Lyness, J. M., Caine, E. D., King, D. A., Conwell, Y., Duberstein, P. R., & Cox, C. (2002). Depressive disorders and symptoms in older primary care patients: One-year outcomes. *American Journal of Geriatric Psychiatry, 10*, 275–282.

Meyer, T. J., Miller, M. L., Metzger, R. L., & Borkovec, T. D. (1990). Development and validation of the Penn State Worry Questionnaire. *Behavior Research and Therapy, 28*, 487–495.

Millon, T., & Meagher, S. E. (2004). The Millon Clinical Multiaxial Inventory-III (MCMI-III). In M. Hilsenroth & D. L. Segal (Eds.), Personality assessment. Volume 2 in M. Hersen (Ed.-in-Chief), *Comprehensive handbook of psychological assessment* (pp. 108–121). New York: Wiley.

Millon, T., Davis, R., & Millon, C. (1997). *MCMI-III manual* (2nd ed.). Minneapolis, MN: National Computer Systems.

Molinari, V., & Segal, D. L. (2011). Personality disorders: Description, etiology, and epidemiology. In M. Abou-Saleh, C. Katona, & A. Kumar (Eds.), *Principles and practice of geriatric psychiatry* (3rd ed.). New York: Wiley.

Mroczek, D. K., Hurt, S. W., & Berman, W. H. (1999). Conceptual and methodological issues in the assessment of personality disorders in older adults. In E. Rosowsky, R. C. Abrams, & R. A. Zweig (Eds.), *Personality disorders in older adults: Emerging issues in diagnosis and treatment* (pp. 135–150). Mahwah, NJ: Erlbaum.

Nguyen, H. T., & Zonderman, A. B. (2006). Relationship between age and aspects of depression: Consistency and reliability across two longitudinal studies. *Psychology and Aging, 21*, 119–126.

Norris, M. P., Arnau, R. C., Bramson, R., & Meagher, M. W. (2004). The efficacy of somatic symptoms in assessing depression in older primary care patients. *Clinical Gerontologist, 27*, 43–57.

Norris, M. P., Snow-Turek, A. L., & Blankenship, L. (1995). Somatic depressive symptoms in the elderly: Contribution or confound? *Journal of Clinical Geropsychology, 1*, 5–17.

Pachana, N. A., Burane, G. J., Siddle, H., Koloski, N., Harley, E., & Arnold, E. (2007). Development and validation of the Geriatric Anxiety Inventory. *International Psychogeriatrics, 19*, 103–114.

Pachana, N. A., Gallagher-Thompson, D., & Thompson, L. W. (1994). Assessment of depression. In M. P. Lawson & J. A. Teresi (Eds.), *Annual review of gerontology and geriatrics: focus on assessment techniques* (pp. 234–256). New York, NY: Springer.

Parmalee, P., Katz, I., & Lawton, M. (1989). Depression among institutionalized aged: Assessment and prevalence estimation. *Journals of Gerontology: Medical Science, 44*, M22–M29.

Pfohl, B., Blum, N., & Zimmerman, M. (1997). *Structured Interview for DSM-IV Personality (SIDP-IV)*. Arlington VA: American Psychiatric Publishing, Inc.

Radloff, L. S. (1977). The CES–D Scale: A self-report depression scale for research in the general population. *Applied Psychological Measurement, 1*, 385–401.

Rapp, S. R., Smith, S. S., & Britt, M. (1990). Identifying comorbid depression in elderly medical patients: Use of the extracted Hamilton Depression Rating Scale. *Psychological Assessment: A Journal of Consulting and Clinical Psychology, 2*, 243–247.

Reich, J., Nduaguba, M., & Yates, W. (1988). Age and sex distribution of DSM-III personality cluster traits in a community population. *Comprehensive Psychiatry, 29*, 298–303.

Regier, D. A., Boyd, J. H., Burke, J. D., Rae, D. S., Myers, J. K., Kramer, M., et al. (1988). One-month prevalence of mental disorders in the United States. *Archives of General Psychiatry, 45*, 977–986.

Roberts, B. W., & DelVecchio, W. F. (2000). The rank-order consistency of personality traits from childhood to old age: A quantitative review of longitudinal studies. *Psychological Bulletin, 126*, 3–25.

Sager, M. A., Dunham, N. C., Schwantes, A., Mecum, L., Halverson, K., & Harlowe, D. (1992). Measurement of activities of daily living in hospitalized elderly: A comparison of self-report and performance-based methods. *Journal of the American Geriatrics Society, 40*, 457–462.

Schein, R. L., & Koenig, H. G. (1997). The Center for Epidemiological Studies-Depression (CES–D) Scale: Assessment of depression in the medically ill elderly. *International Journal of Geriatric Psychiatry, 12*, 436–446.

Schulberg, H. C., Mulsant, B., Schulz, R., Rollman, B. L., Houck, P. R., & Reynolds, C. F. (1998). Characteristics and course of major depression in older primary care patients. *International Journal of Psychiatry in Medicine, 28*, 421–436.

Schwarz, N. (1999). Self-reports: How the questions shape the answers. *American Psychologist, 54*, 93–105.

Segal, D. L., Coolidge, F. L., & Rosowsky, E. (2006). *Personality disorders and older adults: Diagnosis, assessment, and treatment*. Hoboken, NJ: Wiley.

Segal, D. L., Coolidge, F. L., Cahill, B. S., & O'Riley, A. A. (2008). Psychometric properties of the Beck Depression Inventory-II (BDI-II) among community-dwelling older adults. *Behavior Modification, 32*, 3–20.

Segal, D. L., Hersen, M., Kabacoff, R. I., Falk, S. B., Van Hasselt, V. B., & Dorfman, K. (1998). Personality disorders and depression in community-dwelling older adults. *Journal of Mental Health and Aging, 4*, 171–182.

Segal, D. L., Hook, J. N., & Coolidge, F. L. (2001). Personality dysfunction, coping styles, and clinical symptoms in younger and older adults. *Journal of Clinical Geropsychology, 7*, 201–212.

Segal, D. L., June, A., Payne, M., Coolidge, F. L., & Yochim, B. Development and initial validation of a self-report assessment tool for anxiety among older adults: The Geriatric anxiety scale. *Journal of Anxiety Disorders* (in press).

Shankman, S., & Klein, D. (2002). Dimensional diagnosis of depression: Adding the dimension of course to severity and comparison to the DSM. *Comprehensive Psychiatry, 43*(6), 420–426.

Silberman, C. S., Roth, L., Segal, D. L., & Burns, W. (1997). Relationship between the Millon Clinical Multiaxial Inventory-II and Coolidge Axis II Inventory in chronically mentally ill older adults: A pilot study. *Journal of Clinical Psychology, 53*, 559–566.

Smith, G. T., & Oltmanns, T. F. (2009). Scientific advances in the diagnosis of psychopathology: Introduction to the Special Section. *Psychological Assessment, 21*, 241–242.

Smith, T. L., Klein, M. H., & Benjamin, L. S. (2003). Validation of the Wisconsin Personality Disorders Inventory IV with the SCID II. *Journal of Personality Disorders, 17*, 173–187.

Spielberger, C. D. (1983). *State-Trait Anxiety Inventory, Form Y.* Redwood City, CA: Mind Garden Inc.

Stanley, M., Beck, J. G., & Zebb, B. J. (1996). Psychometric properties of four anxiety measures in older adults. *Behaviour Research and Therapy, 34*, 827–838.

Steer, R. A., Rissmiller, D. J., & Beck, A. T. (2000). Use of the Beck Depression Inventory-II with depressed geriatric inpatients. *Behaviour Research and Therapy, 38*, 311–318.

Teachman, B. A. (2006). Aging and negative affect: The rise and fall and rise of anxiety and depression symptoms. *Psychology and Aging, 21*, 201–207.

Teachman, B. A., & Gordon, T. L. (2009). Age differences in anxious responding: Older and calmer, unless the trigger is physical. *Psychology and Aging, 24*, 703–714.

Teresi, J., Abrams, R., Holmes, D., Ramirez, M., & Eimicke, J. (2001). Prevalence of depression and depression recognition in nursing home. *Social Psychiatry and Psychiatric Epidemiology, 36*, 613–620.

Vaillant, G. E. (2002). *Aging well.* Boston: Little Brown and Company.

Van Alphen, S. P. J., Engelen, G. J. J. A., Kuin, Y., Hoijtink, H. J. A., & Derksen, J. J. L. (2006). A preliminary study of the diagnostic accuracy of the Gerontological Personality disorders Scale (GPS). *International Journal of Geriatric Psychiatry, 21*, 862–868.

Wetherell, J. L., & Gatz, M. (2005). The Beck Anxiety Inventory in older adults with generalized anxiety disorder. *Journal of Psychopathology and Behavioral Assessment, 27*, 17–24.

Wetherell, J. L., Le Roux, H., & Gatz, M. (2003). DSM-IV criteria for generalized anxiety disorder in older adults: Distinguishing the worried from the well. *Psychology and Aging, 18*, 622–627.

Widiger, T. A., Livesley, W. J., & Clark, L. W. (2009). An integrative dimensional classification of personality disorder. *Psychological Assessment, 21*, 243–255.

Widiger, T. A., Mangine, S., Corbitt, E. M., Ellis, C. G., & Thomas, G. V. (1995). *Personality Disorder Interview-IV. A semistructured interview for the assessment of personality disorders. Professional manual.* Odessa, FL: Psychological Assessment Resources.

Williams, J. B. (1988). A structured interview guide for the Hamilton Depression Rating Scale. *Archives of General Psychiatry, 45*, 742–747.

Wisocki, P. A., Handen, B., & Morse, C. K. (1986). The worry scale as a measure of anxiety among homebound and community active elderly. *The Behavior Therapist, 9*, 91–95.

Yesavage, J. A., Brink, T. L., Rose, T. L., Lum, O., Huang, V., Adey, M., et al. (1983). Development and validation of a geriatric depression screening scale: A preliminary report. *Journal of Psychiatric Research, 17*, 37–49.

Zanarini, M. C., Frankenburg, F. R., Sickel, A. E., & Yong, L. (1996). *The Diagnostic Interview for DSM-IV Personality Disorders (DIPD-IV).* Belmont, MA: McLean Hospital.

Zweig, R. A., & Agronin, M. E. (2006). Personality disorders in late life. In M. E. Agronin & G. J. Maletta (Eds.), *Principles and practice of geriatric psychiatry* (pp. 449–469). Philadelphia: Lippincott Williams & Wilkins.

Zweig, R. A. (2008). Personality disorder in older adults: Assessment challenges and strategies. *Professional Psychology: Research and Practice, 3*, 298–305.

Chapter | 22 |

Neuropsychological Assessment of the Dementias of Late Life

Stephanie A. Cosentino, Adam M. Brickman, Jennifer J. Manly

Gertrude H. Sergievsky Center, Taub Institute for Research on Alzheimer's Disease and the Aging Brain, and the Department of Neurology at Columbia University Medical Center, New York, USA

CHAPTER CONTENTS

Overview of the Neuropsychological Evaluation 339
Neuropsychological Evaluation of the Older Adult 340
Age-Associated Cognitive and Brain Changes 340
Dementias of Late Life 341
The Differential Diagnosis of Dementia 342
Memory 342
Attention and Processing Speed 342
Executive Functions 343
Language 343
Visuospatial Abilities 344
Metacognition 344
Applying Neuropsychological Assessment in Studies of Cognitive Aging 345
Specific Considerations in Assessing Dementia 345
Racial/Ethnic Background 346
Acculturation 346
Racial Socialization 346
Years of Education/Quality of Education/Literacy 346
Cognitive Reserve 347
Translation of English-Language Tests 347
Summary 347
References 348

OVERVIEW OF THE NEUROPSYCHOLOGICAL EVALUATION

Clinical neuropsychology is "an applied science that examines the impact of both normal and abnormal brain functioning on a broad range of cognitive, emotional, and behavioral functions" (American Academy of Clinical Neuropsychology Board of Directors, 2007), and is based on empirical data linking brain function and brain damage with performance on neuropsychological measures (Lezak et al., 2004). A typical clinical neuropsychological evaluation includes the multimodal assessment of cognitive domains including memory, attention, language, processing speed, executive function, visuospatial skills, and sensorimotor skills. Assessment of general intellectual function (Wechsler, 2008a) is also included in a typical test battery, as are measures of academic achievement, personality, and emotional function (American Academy of Clinical Neuropsychology Board of Directors, 2007; Lezak et al., 2004). Raw scores on neuropsychological tests are interpreted with the use of specific test norms (Mitrushina et al., 2005) that provide a best estimate of an individual's pre-morbid ability, or expected score, to which the current score can be compared (Heaton et al., 2001). The appropriate normative group is matched to the individual on demographic factors such as age, education, gender, and ethnicity, all of which have been shown to have significant effects on verbal and nonverbal neuropsychological test performance (Manly, 2001). Results from formal testing are integrated with medical records, including neuroimaging and other relevant medical data, and interpreted in the context of historical information

DOI: 10.1016/B978-0-12-380882-0.00022-X

gained from a clinical interview of the patient and a family member, friend, or caregiver.

NEUROPSYCHOLOGICAL EVALUATION OF THE OLDER ADULT

Neuropsychologists who work with older adults are most typically charged with the task of determining whether a pattern of test performance is indicative of a neurodegenerative disease. Several unique challenges emerge for the neuropsychologist in the context of aging, with one of the biggest challenges being the determination of whether a diagnosis is warranted at all. With advancing age comes unavoidable abatement of most biological systems. Certainly, the brain and its accompanying cognitive and intellectual abilities are not spared. But cognitive aging is heterogeneous. Some individuals experience a fairly global decline in cognition, while others show more subtle deficits in specific cognitive areas or even improvement in certain domains. As such, the distinction between "normal" and "pathological" can be difficult to establish, leading many authors to regard the terms "normal" or "healthy" cognitive aging as misnomers, and to focus instead on a continuum of neurobiological aging, comprising "optimal," "average," and "abnormal" ranges (Story & Attix, 2010).

AGE-ASSOCIATED COGNITIVE AND BRAIN CHANGES

The precise pattern of neuropsychological change associated with typical or average aging remains somewhat elusive, but the "Frontal Aging Hypothesis" (West, 2000) has enjoyed some popularity as a convenient although somewhat controversial scheme to summarize the extant literature. The idea that neuropsychological abilities mediated by the frontal lobes and their interconnectivity (i.e., executive functions such as mental set shifting or problem solving described in detail on page 343) show a relatively exaggerated pattern of decline in typical aging is based on myriad observations from neuroimaging and behavioral literatures. Arguing against the hypothesis, however, are studies demonstrating age-associated decline in non-frontal regions and their associated behaviors such as visuospatial performance (Golomb et al., 1993) and episodic memory (Kral, 1958), suggesting a more network-based theory of age-related changes (Greenwood, 2000).

Much of the decline and heterogeneity in cognitive aging can be attributed to structural brain changes that occur across the adult life span. Examination of gross volumetric changes on structural magnetic resonance imaging (MRI) generally supports an anterior-to-posterior gradient of age-associated atrophy with the prefrontal cortex particularly affected (DeCarli et al., 1994), followed by temporal lobes (Bartzokis et al., 2001), and relative sparing of the occipital lobes and primary sensory regions (Good et al., 2001). Typical age-related atrophy of frontal regions appears to mediate age-associated declines in executive function (Brickman & Buchsbaum, 2008), whereas distributed patterns of age-associated cortical atrophy are associated with more general age-related cognitive changes (Brickman et al., 2008). In terms of subcortical structures, Volume loss in the caudate and putamen partially mediates age-related changes in perceptual-motor skills and speed (Kennedy & Raz, 2005).

Loss of white matter microstructure, best visualized by diffusion tensor imaging, may be among the most pertinent changes in typical aging. Diffusion tensor studies have been unified in revealing decreasing anisotropy, a measure of coherence and orientation, in white matter across the adult life span (Sullivan & Pfefferbaum, 2006). Decline in white matter integrity within frontal-striatal circuitry, in particular, may be a major source of cognitive change in typical aging (Sullivan & Pfefferbaum, 2006). Small- and large-vessel cerebrovascular disease visualized radiologically as white matter hyperintensities and infarction is ubiquitous but highly variable among older, community-dwelling adults (Luchsinger et al., 2009). The accumulation of cerebrovascular disease with advancing age may not have obvious associated neurological signs or symptoms, but may accelerate a subtle downward trajectory of cognitive change. In fact, in our community-based studies of older adults, markers of cerebrovascular disease are among the strongest correlates of cognition in nondemented older adults (Brickman et al., 2009). Because cerebrovascular disease is so prevalent among older adults (indeed, lack of evidence of cerebrovascular disease is the exception; de Leeuw et al., 2001), it can be considered a typical feature of aging with tremendous potential influence on cognitive functioning. However, the role of cerebrovascular disease in cognitive aging is complicate by the fact that cerebrovascular disease and its antecedents are also risk factors for neurodegenerative diseases such as Alzheimer's disease and vascular dementia.

In summary, "typical" aging is accompanied by heterogeneous cognitive changes and differential rates of cognitive decline reflecting variable genetic and lifetime risk factors. The primary ways in which cognitive changes occurring in the course of typical aging are dissociated from those indicative of a degenerative disease are the severity of the changes as well as their impact on daily function. In the following section, we review the diagnosis of dementia, and describe the specific cognitive changes that characterize the various dementias of late life.

DEMENTIAS OF LATE LIFE

Most diagnostic criteria for dementia incorporate objective evidence of cognitive dysfunction accompanied by impairment in basic or instrumental activities of daily living. The term "dementia" does not refer to a specific disease, but rather is a general term used to describe a syndrome that could be the result of several different or overlapping pathologies. Table 22.1 presents the most common causes of dementia in the elderly, their pathological features, core symptoms and signs, and their most typical, early neuropsychological deficits. It should be noted that ongoing discoveries in the genetic

Table 22.1 Primary features of the dementias of late life

	PATHOLOGY	PRIMARY CLINICAL FEATURES	EARLY NEURO-PSYCHOLOGICAL DEFICITS
AD	Intraneuronal neurofibrillary tangles; accumulation of extracellular neuritic, amyloid plaques	Insidious onset of memory loss with gradual decline in global cognition	Delayed recall, recognition, and semantic knowledge; variable visuospatial and EF
VaD	Several large-vessel infarctions (i.e., multi-infarct dementia), and/or a single "strategic" infarct, and/or small vessel ischemic disease (i.e., Binswanger disease); often occurs with AD pathology	Abrupt onset that is contemporaneous with recognized vascular event; potential motor signs; stepwise or gradual decline	Recall and EF; other deficits depending on location and extent of vascular damage
PDD	Spread of Lewy bodies, a hallmark feature of PD, from subcortical to cortical areas	Diagnosis of PD (e.g., rigidity, tremor, and bradykinesia) with subsequent and gradual cognitive changes	EF, processing speed, and recall
DLB	Cortical Lewy bodies, often occurring with AD pathology	Progressive decline accompanied by fluctuating cognition, well-formed visual hallucinations, and/or parkinsonism; cognitive symptoms prior to or concurrent with parkinsonism	Recall, visuospatial, attention, and EF
FTD	Tauopathy OR Non-tauopathy (TDP-43, FUS, UPS, ni)	**Behavioral**: Loss of personal and social awareness, disinhibition, mental inflexibility, hyperorality; perseverative or stereotyped behavior; utilization behavior; blunted affect	EF, Recall
		PNFA: Non-fluent expression	Verbal fluency and other expressive language abilities
		SD: Empty but fluent speech with comprehension difficulties	Semantic knowledge and receptive language abilities
CBD	Tauopathy	**CBD**: Parkinsonism; alien hand syndrome; apraxia	Spatial abilities, language, and EF
PSP	Tauopathy	**PSP**: Loss of balance and falls; bradykinesia; ophthalmoplegia	EF, processing speed, recall; variable language

Note: EF = Executive functioning; AD = Alzheimer's disease; VaD = Vascular dementia; PDD = Parkinson's disease dementia; DLB = Dementia with Lewy bodies; FTD = Frontotemporal dementia; CBD = Corticobasal degeneration; PSP = Progressive supranuclear palsy; PNFA = Progressive non-fluent aphasia; SD = Semantic dementia. TDP = TAR DNA-Binding protein; FUS = Fused in sarcoma protein; UPS = Ubiquitin proteasome system; ni = No inclusions.

and molecular basis of FTD have resulted in shifting classification schemes over time. The information included in this table reflects the latest recommendations for classifying the various neuropathologic substrates of FTD.

THE DIFFERENTIAL DIAGNOSIS OF DEMENTIA

With the increased prevalence of dementia in late life, a primary role of the neuropsychologist working with an older adult is to determine if dementia is present, and if so, the most likely cause based on the *pattern* of cognitive impairment. From a diagnostic perspective, some of the most widely used measures of cognitive function in older adults are brief screening tests (Folstein et al., 1975) that are intended to maximize sensitivity for cognitive impairment. Such tests are useful in the broad classification of an individual as cognitively intact or impaired, but are not intended for use in differential diagnosis, a goal that warrants careful analysis of performance across cognitive domains. Performance profiles provide information regarding the regional distribution of neuropathology, and thus the likely etiology of cognitive and functional changes. Examination of cognitive profiles rather than absolute scores is especially relevant in the context of dementia, when the presence of global cognitive impairment after a certain point generally reduces scores across all tests. As noted above, the typical and earliest neuropsychological deficits in each dementia syndrome are presented in Table 22.1.

Here we provide an overview of how performance in each cognitive domain informs the differential diagnosis of dementia.

Memory

The diagnosis of dementia traditionally requires evidence of impairment in memory and at least one other cognitive domain (American Psychiatric Association, 1994), although it is important to note that these criteria are not fully relevant to all types of dementia (e.g., Frontotemporal Dementia (FTD), and are currently under revision. Nonetheless, with Alzheimer's disease (AD) being the most common cause of dementia, and episodic memory loss the earliest and most prominent symptom of AD (Storandt et al., 1984), rigorous assessment of episodic memory is a core component of a dementia evaluation. Measures of episodic memory generally include lists (Bushke, 1973), stories (R. M. Reitan & Wolfson, 1987), paired associates, or nonverbal information such as geometric figures (Meyers & Meyers, 1995). Of these, list learning tasks are generally considered to be the most sensitive to early memory changes given their organizational demands.

Typical list learning tasks involve repeated exposure (auditory or visual) to a list of words that may be semantically unrelated (Brandt, 1991) or that can be grouped into categories (Delis et al., 1987). By examining the profile of performance across the learning trials and delayed phases of the task, one can determine the precise nature and likely etiology of the memory impairment. A prototypical pattern of performance across learning trials for an individual with AD is generally characterized by limited recall and little improvement from the first to last trial, reflecting poor and inefficient new learning secondary to hippocampal dysfunction. Qualitative examination of recall performance is likely to reveal a recency rather than primacy effect (tendency to recall words from the end vs. the beginning of the list), reflecting relatively intact working memory but impaired long-term storage (Bayley et al., 2000). Most striking, however, is the disproportionately impaired recall of target information after a 20–40 minute delay, resulting from an inability to transfer new information into long-term memory. This primary storage deficit also results in difficulty discriminating target words from distracters on yes/no recognition testing, yielding a discriminability index near chance (Fine et al., 2008).

A number of non-Alzheimer's dementias such as FTD, Dementia with Lewy Bodies (DLB), Vascular Dementia (VaD), Parkinson's disease dementia (PDD), and Progressive Supranuclear Palsy (PSP) also have detrimental effects on memory performance. However, in contrast to AD, such conditions generally impact memory secondary to a *dysexecutive syndrome* characterized by poor or inefficient organization of the information to be remembered. A dysexecutive profile may reflect direct compromise to the prefrontal cortex (Listerud et al., 2009), or the indirect effects of damage to cholinergic projections from the basal forebrain (Lemstra et al., 2003), subcortical white matter pathways (Jokinen et al., 2009), or the basal ganglia (Sawamoto et al., 2007). Memory deficits resulting from a dysexecutive syndrome are generally dissociable from the pure amnestic deficit seen in AD. While both patterns of memory loss are typically characterized by lower than average immediate and delayed recall, non-AD groups tend to show less forgetting over time (high proportions of information retained from immediate to delay) and improved performance in the context of recognition testing (Hamilton et al., 2004). This improvement reflects the reduced demand on the organized search and spontaneous retrieval of information supported by prefrontal networks, and indicates that information was transferred successfully into long-term memory.

Attention and Processing Speed

The evaluation of attention (e.g., immediate auditory attention measured by Digit Span Forward) and processing speed (e.g., the ability to rapidly connect a series of numbers in Trail Making Test Part A) in any neuropsychological evaluation is important for interpreting performance on higher level tasks that build upon these fundamental skills. Early notable impairment in attention and processing speed would likely lead the clinician toward a non-AD diagnosis depending on the remainder of the clinical presentation. For example, fluctuating attention is characteristic of DLB (Metzler-Baddeley, 2007), inattention may be seen in FTD (Piquard et al., 2009) and slowed processing speed can reflect basal ganglia compromise in the case of PD (Sawamoto et al., 2002) or damage to subcortical white matter tracts secondary to cerebrovascular disease (Delano-Wood et al., 2008). Severely impaired attention and arousal, however, may raise concerns about delirium, particularly if the onset of cognitive difficulties was relatively recent and abrupt (Fong et al., 2009).

Executive Functions

This diverse set of higher order skills enables complex goal-directed behaviors, and includes but not limited to mental set shifting, inhibition, fluency, working memory, problem solving, strategy generation, and abstract reasoning. Although executive functions are in some respect a diverse and seemingly arbitrary grouping of skills, they are linked in two important ways. First, they are bound by a common theme, which is the ability to take an organized, novel, complex, or future-oriented approach to a task that is not bound by stimuli in the immediate environment or governed by a pre-potent or automatic response. Second, this broad grouping of higher order cognitive abilities appears to be mediated largely, although not solely, on frontal and frontal-subcortical circuitry (Alexander et al., 1986).

Several batteries have been designed to comprehensively measure a variety of executive abilities (e.g., Delis Kaplan Executive Function Scale (D-KEFS; Delis et al., 2001)) as well as to sample a range of executive abilities more briefly (Frontal Assessment Battery; Dubois et al., 2000). Frequently, however, neuropsychologists administer several separate tasks to examine the integrity of specific executive abilities. Trail Making Tests (R. Reitan, 1958) and card sorting tasks (Heaton, 1981) are often used to determine the ability to shift mental set, while measures such as the Stroop Test (Golden, 1978) assess inhibition of a pre-potent verbal response and susceptibility to interference. Fluency measures, including verbal and design fluency tasks, are also considered executive tasks (Delis et al., 2001) as they require the organized generation of novel information. Working memory, or the mental manipulation of information in short-term memory, can be assessed using backward span tasks (Wechsler, 2008a,b), although computerized measures of working memory are gaining popularity (Collie et al., 2003). Finally, verbal and nonverbal abstract reasoning tasks demonstrate an individual's ability to think flexibly about information in a manner that is not bound by the immediate semantic or perceptual properties of a stimulus (Similarities and Matrix Reasoning subtests of the Wechsler Adult Intelligence Scales; Wechsler, 2008a). In addition to looking at overall scores, qualitative examination of performance on these as well as nonexecutive measures can be highly informative. Specifically, perseverations, or repetitious responses when novel responses are appropriate, is a form of executive dysfunction (Luria, 1980).

At least one aspect of executive functioning is generally compromised in the context of most dementia syndromes, making it critical to evaluate the overall extent of executive dysfunction in relation to memory and other skills. For example, moderately impaired executive abilities in the context of severely impaired delayed recall and recognition would be highly consistent with a diagnosis of AD. In contrast, severely impaired executive abilities in the context of relatively spared delayed memory would argue more strongly for a non-AD dementia, depending on the remainder of the clinical presentation (e.g., FTD in the context of behavioral disturbance, DLB in the context of extrapyramidal signs, VaD in the context of vascular risk factors, PSP in the context of vertical gaze palsy and frequent falls). However, it should be noted that individuals with a frontal variant of AD (Johnson et al., 1999) may have profoundly impaired executive abilities early on (Woodward et al., 2009).

Language

Measures of confrontation naming (Kaplan et al., 1983), vocabulary (Wechsler, 2008b), fluency, comprehension, and repetition (Goodglass & Kaplan, 1983) are regularly included in dementia evaluations, as several of the dementia subtypes affect either some aspect of expressive (e.g., fluency) or receptive (e.g., comprehension) language abilities. In the absence of memory loss, a severe and progressive change in language, referred to as primary progressive aphasia (PPA), is most typically a sign of a non-AD dementia. One form of PPA, progressive non-fluent aphasia, is consistent with FTD, corticobasal degeneration (CBD), or PSP (Kertesz & McMonagle, 2009). A second form of PPA, semantic dementia (SD), characterized by fluent but empty speech with impaired comprehension, is generally reflective of FTD.

However, more subtle language deficits detectable on confrontation naming and verbal fluency tasks also offer particularly critical information in the differential diagnosis of dementia. Among other things, naming and fluency tasks provide information about the integrity of an individual's semantic knowledge, or general knowledge about the world including the verbal label for objects, which relies largely on anterior temporal lobe functioning (Simmons & Martin, 2009). Confrontation naming, most commonly measured by the Boston Naming Test (Kaplan et al., 1983), is an informative measure of semantic processing, requiring the patient to name a series of increasingly infrequent objects. Poor performance on this task, particularly in the context of high education, would be considered a typical symptom of mild AD given the disease's early impact on temporal regions.

Another key way in which semantic networks are assessed is through examination of category fluency in which patients are asked to rapidly name words included in a specified category, generally animals. High scores reflecting rapid access to category members presumably reflect efficient connections among the neural links that support word meaning and categorical structure. Verbal fluency tasks are multidimensional, however, and also require the quick and efficient organization and output of verbal information (thus their previous inclusion as an executive task). As such, evidence for a specific impairment in semantic knowledge rather than executive functioning comes from comparing category versus phonemic fluency in which the patient is asked to generate words beginning with a specific letter. As degradation to temporal networks differentially impacts categorical knowledge, a significant advantage of phonemic over category fluency is thought to reflect relatively preserved frontal versus temporal networks (Baldo et al., 2006; Lopez et al., 2000), and is considered to be a characteristic feature of the early AD cognitive profile. In contrast, equally impaired performance on both tasks, would suggest more prominent involvement of frontal subcortical networks (Rascovsky et al., 2002) that are important for both tasks. Such a profile would be more consistent with FTD, DLB, PD, and VaD. However, it is important to note that in the moderate stages of AD there is generally marked impairment on both fluency tasks, making disease severity a critical factor to consider when interpreting test results.

Visuospatial Abilities

A fourth key component of a dementia evaluation is the assessment of visuospatial skills, a cognitive domain that provides important information regarding the integrity of parietal networks (Black & Bernard, 1984). Visuospatial ability can be measured using tasks that involve perceptual organization, construction, copying, or free drawing (Freedman et al., 1994; Hooper, 1983; Meyers & Meyers, 1995; Wechsler, 2008b). Spatial disorientation is a commonly reported symptom in early AD and this deficit is often corroborated on formal examination of spatial skills requiring patients to copy models of three-dimensional drawings, or arrange blocks to create abstract geometric shapes. However, as language predominant or frontal variant AD may not impact spatial skills until later in the course of the illness, an absence of a spatial deficit does not preclude the diagnosis of AD.

If spatial deficits are judged to be relatively worse than memory deficits early in the course of cognitive decline, diagnoses such as DLB or CBD may be considered depending on the clinical history. Several studies have suggested that impaired visuospatial performance (Tiraboschi et al., 2006) and relatively spared recognition memory (Hamilton et al., 2004) points to the presence of DLB rather than AD. However, DLB can be difficult to distinguish from AD based on cognitive testing and clinical symptoms, in part reflecting the fact that individuals diagnosed with either condition frequently have pathological features of both disorders at autopsy (Lopez et al., 2000). Visuospatial deficits are also seen in the context of CBD, a condition that is given greater consideration in the presence of unilateral apraxia, language deficits, executive dysfunction and relatively preserved free recall (Murray et al., 2007). In contrast, there is some evidence that spatial skills are spared early in the course of FTD given the relative preservation of posterior brain regions (Rascovsky et al., 2002).

Metacognition

In addition to the primary cognitive skills previously discussed, consideration of an individual's metacognition (knowledge of one's own cognitive abilities) may provide important information in a dementia evaluation. A significant proportion of individuals in the early stages of AD, FTD, and other dementias have reduced awareness of cognitive and behavioral changes (Cosentino & Stern, 2005). Such individuals are generally identified only when brought to the clinic by family members, and tend to report minimal or no cognitive problems when queried in an interview. The absence of a memory complaint paired with significant deficits on objective testing, would be more consistent with a degenerative condition than with mood-related (e.g., anxiety or depression) memory impairment or normal age-associated memory loss. However, it is essential to understand that preserved awareness of memory loss *does not* argue against a diagnosis of dementia. Many individuals with dementia are acutely aware of their memory changes, and perform comparably to healthy adults on objective metacognitive testing (Cosentino et al., 2007).

In this section, we have tried to shed light on the manner in which neuropsychological performance is integrated and interpreted to determine the regional distribution of pathology in the brain, and thus the most likely etiology of cognitive changes. However, there are atypical presentations of each dementia syndrome, as well as pathological overlap of the various diseases, making it difficult to identify a single profile that characterizes each dementia syndrome. Moreover, differences that are noted in autopsy-confirmed studies contrasting dementia groups do not always apply to individual patients. With these qualifications in mind, we list the earliest and most typical neuropsychological deficits of each dementia syndrome in Table 22.1.

APPLYING NEUROPSYCHOLOGICAL ASSESSMENT IN STUDIES OF COGNITIVE AGING

We have reviewed the application of neuropsychological assessment of the older adult in the clinical setting. However, it should be noted that there is tremendous utility in the inclusion of neuropsychological measures in health research of older adults. Multiple large-scale epidemiologic studies of aging that focus on cardiovascular or other health conditions have incorporated neuropsychological measures, either in-person or telephone-based, into their assessment of function due to the powerful relationship of cognitive function with outcomes such as medical status, medication adherence, and mortality (Alves de Moraes et al., 2002; Grodstein et al., 2000; Herzog & Wallace, 1997; Howard et al., 2005; Kanaya et al., 2004; Langa et al., 2009; Plassman et al., 2007).

There are several conclusions that can be drawn from a review of these large-scale studies and others that use neuropsychological measures in research on aging and health. Researchers seeking to add neuropsychological measures to the assessment of older adults should consider recommendations for evaluation of multiple cognitive domains, not just memory and IQ (National Research Council & Committee on Future Directions for Cognitive Research on Aging, 2000). Other domains, including attention, speed, and language, may be sensitive to change over time, may decline early in the course of dementia, and may help differentiate dementia etiology, as is detailed earlier in this chapter. However, the advantages of assessing multiple cognitive domains conflict with the desire to shorten the length of time and burden of cognitive instruments. Promising responses to the pressure to reduce participant burden include the development of brief computer adaptive tests of cognitive ability (McArdle et al., 2009) and initiatives to develop brief domain-specific instruments that are co-normed, can be shared, and are uniform across different studies (Gershon et al., 2010).

Neuropsychological assessment in conjunction with a detailed history and physician evaluation can be used to determine the presence of dementia in research participants. However, an older adult contacted as part of an epidemiologic study may be in the early stages of dementia, but may have little awareness of cognitive/functional decline as described previously. As investigators choose their research-based diagnostic criteria for dementia, consideration should be given to the potential for such metacognitive impairment, as well as the cost-benefit ratio and cultural considerations (Malmstrom et al., 2009) of involving informants to ascertain information about participants' function relative to their previous abilities (Morris, 1993).

Not only are neuropsychological measures used to derive diagnoses of dementia, but they are also used to track change in cognitive function over time and to determine pre- vs. posttreatment change in clinical trials (Rosen et al., 1984). Use of neuropsychological tests as sensitive measures of change presents challenges that researchers are only beginning to grapple with in longitudinal studies of aging. While test batteries have been validated as sensitive and specific measures of impairment, they are not necessarily designed to be sensitive to subtle change over relatively short periods of time, for example, between annual evaluations. Practice, ceiling, and floor effects (Wang et al., 2008), and performance variability may all stand in the way of detecting subtle change over time (Collie et al., 2003; Wilson et al., 2006). However, many researchers are now embracing these effects to show that lack of short-term practice effects may be more sensitive to early or preclinical AD than traditional indicators such as word list memory (Darby et al., 2002; Duff et al., 2010).

A controversy that has arisen as a result of the increasing use of neuropsychological measures in studies of aging and health is the argument that cognition mediates the relationship between early life socioeconomic status and later life health (Gottfredson, 2004). The mechanism by which intelligence is purported to influence health is self-care, such that many activities that individuals must do to maintain health, such as monitoring and treating one's chronic disease, are too intellectually complex for many people to manage (Gottfredson & Deary, 2004). However, these theories have not yet addressed the construct validity of cognitive measures across diverse groups, nor have they properly accounted for the possibility of confounding (M. Glymour & Manly, 2008; M. M. Glymour et al., 2008).

SPECIFIC CONSIDERATIONS IN ASSESSING DEMENTIA

There are a number of factors that complicate the interpretation of neuropsychological performance in the clinic or in research settings, particularly in older adults, and are thus critical to consider in the diagnosis of dementia. Here we briefly review research on racial/ethnic background, acculturation, racial socialization, education, and cognitive reserve as they relate to neuropsychological test performance.

Racial/Ethnic Background

Few cognitive ability measures have been properly validated for use among ethnic minorities in the United States. Lack of such validation attenuates specificity of verbal and nonverbal neuropsychological tests, such that cognitively normal ethnic minorities are more likely to be misdiagnosed as impaired as compared to Whites, even when ethnic groups are matched on socioeconomic variables (Jacobs et al., 1997; Manly et al., 1998). These findings indicate that not all tasks are functionally equivalent (Helms, 1992). Although establishing local test norms for each ethnic group may help reduce misdiagnosis (Miller et al., 1997), there is also variability of educational and cultural experiences within ethnicity that should be considered. The implication of this work is that investigators should collect race and ethnicity data but not rely only on these variables when conducting research on cognitive aging. The variables for which race serves as a proxy, some of which are discussed next, account for significant variability between racial/ethnic groups but also within them, and should be explicitly measured.

Acculturation

Specification of experiential, attitudinal, or behavioral variables that distinguish those belonging to different ethnic groups, and that also vary among individuals within an ethnic group, may allow investigators to understand better the underlying reasons for the relationship between ethnic background and cognitive test performance (Helms, 1992). Previous studies have identified ideologies, beliefs, expectations, and attitudes as important components of acculturation, as well as cognitive and behavioral characteristics such as language and customs (Negy & Woods, 1992; Padilla, 1980). Although acculturation has traditionally been measured as language use and years in the country, these variables are most relevant among immigrant groups, and recently, several measures of acculturation have been developed for use among nonimmigrant groups (Landrine & Klonoff, 1994). Degree of acculturation in Hispanics has been linked to neuropsychological performance among college students (Arnold et al., 1994), and may be especially relevant among those with fewer than eight years of education (Artiola i Fortuny et al., 1998). Similarly, African American acculturation accounts for a significant amount of variance in verbal and nonverbal abilities after accounting for age, education, and gender (Manly et al., 2004).

Racial Socialization

Level of comfort and confidence during the test session may also vary among ethnic groups. The concept of stereotype threat has been described as a factor that may attenuate the performance of racial minorities on cognitive tests. Stereotype threat describes the effect of attention diverting from the task at hand to the concern that one's performance will confirm a negative stereotype about one's group. Steele and colleagues (1997, 1995) demonstrated that the introduction of stereotype threat among Black college students attenuated performance on difficult verbal GRE exam items compared to SAT score-matched Whites. Researchers have also shown that when gender differences in math ability were invoked, stereotype threat undermined women's math performance (Spencer et al., 1999) and that of White men (when comparisons to Asians were invoked) (Aronson et al., 1999). Aging and other experiential, social, and cultural variables are likely to modulate the salience of negative stereotypes differently among racial minorities; this should be examined in future work.

Years of Education/Quality of Education/Literacy

Educational experience has a notable influence on neuropsychological test performance (Heaton et al., 1986), as does literacy (Manly et al., 1999). Extreme differences in educational level are often found between ethnic minority and white elders (Bauman & Graf, 2003), and illiteracy rates in the United States are highest among people aged 65 and over, especially in ethnic minority elders (Kirsch et al., 1993). Thus, very low educational levels and poor literacy are highly relevant issues for the assessment of dementia using cognitive measures, particularly in ethnic minorities (Glymour & Manly, 2008; Manly et al., 2002, 2003; Weiss et al., 1995). Most typically, neuropsychologists address these issues by adjusting for educational experience or reading level, thus improving the specificity of the test. However, some researchers caution against controlling for such variables in studies of dementia because low education may itself be a risk factor for disease, as is discussed in the following section. While numerous prior research has documented the associations between education and other health outcomes, delineation of the pathways between early life educational setting and later life cognition are only now being examined (Richards & Sacker, 2003), partially because of the need for longitudinal data and the use of analytic techniques that avoid the confounding effects of potential common underlying causes of educational achievement and cognitive function (Glymour et al., 2008)

Cognitive Reserve

Multiple studies both in and outside the United States have shown that in comparison to older adults with relatively high levels of education, those with lower levels demonstrate more rapid cognitive and functional decline (see Stern, 2009 for review) and higher prevalence and incidence of dementia (reviewed in Manly & Mayeux, 2004; Stern, 2009). Differential cognitive trajectories have also been observed in the context of high versus low literacy such that more rapid decline is seen among older adults with low literacy (Manly et al., 2003). Cognitive reserve, or the brain's ability to cope with pathology, has been suggested as a mechanism for the link between educational experiences and risk of dementia and cognitive decline (Mortimer et al., 1988; Satz, 1993; Stern, 2002). That is, the factors that lead to, are afforded by, or are associated with higher literacy or educational attainment enhance the brain's ability to cope with pathology. The result is the delayed clinical onset of symptoms, despite levels of pathology in the brain that are comparable to individuals with lower literacy or educational attainment (Bennett et al., 2003; Stern et al., 1992). In line with this theory, although at first counterintuitive, highly educated individuals diagnosed with AD appear to have faster rates of cognitive decline (Stern et al., 1999; Teri et al., 1995; Unverzagt et al., 1998) and increased risk of mortality once diagnosed (Stern et al., 1995), suggesting that by the time clinical signs of dementia develop in this group, the level of brain pathology is relatively high. The indirect relationship between neuropathology and its clinical manifestations that is moderated by cognitive reserve certainly complicates the diagnosis of dementia. Although adjusting for variables such as education or literacy improves the specificity of diagnoses, these adjustments may obscure the association between background factors and risk for developing dementia. Longitudinal studies following individuals from a point prior to the onset of brain pathology and dementia are needed to better understand these complex issues.

Translation of English-Language Tests

Similar principles and cautions that apply to the adaptation of cognitive measures for use among older adults also apply to the translation and adaptation of neuropsychological tests into languages other than English. In other words, rather than relying only on a literal translation, significant adjustments to the content and administration steps of the test may need to occur to maintain construct validity when applied to people for whom English is not their first language. Literal translation may not produce items with comparable word frequency and/or salience in each culture, resulting in different difficulty levels (Sano et al., 1997; Teng et al., 1996). In addition, idiosyncrasies of different languages may introduce problems in equating certain tests. For example, Hispanics produce fewer animal exemplars in one minute than do Vietnamese, a discrepancy that can be explained by the fact that most animal names in Spanish are multisyllabic, while most animal names in Vietnamese are monosyllabic (Kempler et al., 1998). Moreover, investigators must be aware that the published norms for tests administered in English are not necessarily valid when tests are administered in another language (just as you would never apply norms for 25–35 year olds to an 85 year old for diagnostic purposes). Furthermore, researchers should not assume that tests or test norms can be applied to distinct populations simply because they share a language. For example, there is evidence that several instruments developed in Spanish-speaking countries may not be functionally or linguistically equivalent when used among Spanish speakers in the United States (Artiola i Fortuny et al., 1998). The accuracy of translated and adapted instruments should be checked following established guidelines (Artiola i Fortuny & Mullaney, 1997; Mungas et al., 1996). Researchers and clinicians must also develop standards to determine in which language bilinguals should be assessed (Rivera-Mindt et al., 2008).

SUMMARY

This chapter reviewed the utility and limitations of the neuropsychological assessment of dementia in older adults, and touched on the value of neuropsychological measures in research on cognitive aging and epidemiological studies of health among older adults. We refer the reader to several resources for more comprehensive and specific information on the use of neuropsychological tests among older adults (Green, 2000; Potter & Attix, 2005) and across the age spectrum (Mitrushina et al., 2005; Strauss et al., 2006). Continued research examining neuropsychological performance across autopsy-confirmed dementia groups will greatly facilitate our ability to draw diagnostic inferences from neuropsychological tests, and to identify those tests that are most useful in differential diagnosis. In addition, the collection and improvement of normative data across a variety of populations will enhance the specificity of our cognitive measures for detecting neurologically based cognitive impairment as opposed to culture-related factors. In closing, it should be noted that with an emerging emphasis on identifying AD and other dementias at the preclinical stage, the diagnostic criteria for dementia are shifting. As a result, the precise manner in which neuropsychological testing contributes to the diagnosis of dementia will certainly evolve and likely take on greater importance.

REFERENCES

Alexander, G. E., DeLong, M. R., & Strick, P. L. (1986). Parallel organization of functionally segregated circuits linking basal ganglia and cortex. *Annual Review of Neuroscience, 9*, 357–381.

Alves de Moraes, S., Szklo, M., Knopman, D., & Sato, R. (2002). The Relationship between Temporal Changes in Blood Pressure and Changes in Cognitive Function: Atherosclerosis Risk in Communities (ARIC) Study. *Preventive Medicine, 35*, 258–263.

American Academy of Clinical Neuropsychology Board of Directors. (2007). American Academy of Clinical Neuropsychology (AACN) Practice Guidelines for Neuropsychological Assessment and Consultation. *Clinical Neuropsychologist, 21*, 209–231.

American Psychiatric Association. (1994). *Diagnostic and Statistical Manual of Mental Disorders* (*Fourth ed.*). Washington DC: American Psychiatric Association.

Arnold, B. R., Montgomery, G. T., Castaneda, I., & Longoria, R. (1994). Acculturation and performance of Hispanics on selected Halstead-Reitan neuropsychological tests. *Assessment, 1*, 239–248.

Aronson, J., Lustina, M. J., Good, C., Keough, K., Steele, C. M., & Brown, J. (1999). When White men can't do math: Necessary and sufficient factors in stereotype threat. *Journal of Experimental and Social Psychology, 35*, 29–46.

Artiola i Fortuny, L., Heaton, R. K., & Hermosillo, D. (1998). Neuropsychological comparisons of Spanish-speaking participants from the U.S.-Mexico border region versus Spain. *Journal of the International Neuropsychological Society, 4*, 363–379.

Artiola i Fortuny, L., & Mullaney, H. (1997). Neuropsychology with Spanish speakers: Language use and proficiency issues for test development. *Journal of Clinical and Experimental Neuropsychology, 19*, 615–622.

Baldo, J. V., Schwartz, S., Wilkins, D., & Dronkers, N. F. (2006). Role of frontal versus temporal cortex in verbal fluency as revealed by voxel-based lesion symptom mapping. *Journal of the International Neuropsychological Society, 12*(6), 896–900.

Bartzokis, G., Beckson, M., Lu, P. H., Nuechterlein, K. H., Edwards, N., & Mintz, J. (2001). Age-related changes in frontal and temporal lobe volumes in men: a magnetic resonance imaging study. *Archives of General Psychiatry, 58*(5), 461–465.

Bauman, K. J., & Graf, N. L. (2003). *Educational Attainment: 2000*. (Brief No. C2KBR-24). Washington, DC. US Census Bureau.

Bayley, P. J., Salmon, D. P., Bondi, M. W., Bui, B. K., Olichney, J., Delis, D. C., et al. (2000). Comparison of the serial position effect in very mild Alzheimer's disease, mild Alzheimer's disease, and amnesia associated with electroconvulsive therapy. *Journal of the International Neuropsychological Society, 6*(3), 290–298.

Bennett, D. A., Wilson, R. S., Schneider, J. A., Evans, D. A., Mendes de Leon, C. F., Arnold, S. E., et al. (2003). Education modifies the relation of AD pathology to level of cognitive function in older persons. *Neurology, 60*(12), 1909–1915.

Black, F. W., & Bernard, B. A. (1984). Constructional apraxia as a function of lesion locus and size in patients with focal brain damage. *Cortex, 20*(1), 111–120.

Brandt, J. (1991). The Hopkins Verbal Learning Test: Development of a new memory test with six equivalent forms. *Clinical Neuropsychologist, 5*, 125–142.

Brickman, A. M., & Buchsbaum, M. S. (2008). Alzheimer's disease and normal aging: Neurostructures. In J. H. Byrne (Ed.), *Learning and memory: A comprehensive reference: Vol. 3* (pp. 601–621). New York: Elsevier.

Brickman, A. M., Habeck, C., Ramos, M. A., Scarmeas, N., & Stern, Y. (2008). A forward application of age associated gray and white matter networks. *Human Brain Mapping, 29*(10), 1139–1146.

Brickman, A. M., Muraskin, J., & Zimmerman, M. E. (2009). Structural neuroimaging in Alzheimer's disease: Do white matter hyperintensities matter? *Dialogues of Clinical Neuroscience, 11*(2), 181–190.

Bushke, H. (1973). Selective reminding for analysis of memory and learning. *Journal of Verbal Learning and Verbal Behavior, 12*, 543–550.

Collie, A., Maruff, P., Darby, D. G., & McStephen, M. (2003). The effects of practice on the cognitive test performance of neurologically normal individuals assessed at brief test-retest intervals. *Journal of the International Neuropsychological Society, 9*(03), 419–428.

Cosentino, S., Metcalfe, J., Butterfield, B., & Stern, Y. (2007). Objective metamemory testing captures awareness of deficit in Alzheimer's disease. *Cortex, 43*(7), 1004–1019.

Cosentino, S., & Stern, Y. (2005). Metacognitive theory and assessment in dementia: Do we recognize our areas of weakness?

Journal of the International Neuropsychological Society, 11(7), 910–919.

Darby, D., Maruff, P., Collie, A., & McStephen, M. (2002). Mild cognitive impairment can be detected by multiple assessments in a single day. *Neurology, 59*(7), 1042–1046.

de Leeuw, F. E., de Groot, J. C., Achten, E., Oudkerk, M., Ramos, L. M., Heijboer, R., et al. (2001). Prevalence of cerebral white matter lesions in elderly people: A population based magnetic resonance imaging study. The Rotterdam Scan Study. *Journal of Neurology Neurosurgery & Psychiatry, 70*(1), 9–14.

DeCarli, C., Murphy, D. G., Gillette, J. A., Haxby, J. V., Teichberg, D., Schapiro, M. B., et al. (1994). Lack of age-related differences in temporal lobe volume of very healthy adults. *American Journal of Neuroradiology, 15*(4), 689–696.

Delano-Wood, L., Abeles, N., Sacco, J. M., Wierenga, C. E., Horne, N. R., & Bozoki, A. (2008). Regional white matter pathology in mild cognitive impairment: differential influence of lesion type on neuropsychological functioning. *Stroke, 39*(3), 794–799.

Delis, D. C., Kramer, J. H., Kaplan, E., & Ober, B. A. (1987). *California Verbal Learning Test: Adult Version Manual.* San Antonio, TX: The Psychological Corporation.

Dubois, B., Slachevsky, A., Litvan, I., & Pillon, B. (2000). The FAB: A Frontal Assessment Battery at bedside. *Neurology, 55*(11), 1621–1626.

Duff, K., Beglinger, L. J., Moser, D. J., Paulsen, J. S., Schultz, S. K., & Arndt, S. (2010). Predicting Cognitive Change in Older Adults: The Relative Contribution of Practice Effects. *Archives of Clinical Neuropsychology, 25*(2), 81–88.

Fine, E. M., Delis, D. C., Wetter, S. R., Jacobson, M. W., Hamilton, J. M., Peavy, G., et al. (2008). Identifying the "source" of recognition memory deficits in patients with Huntington's disease or Alzheimer's disease: Evidence from the CVLT-II. *Journal of Clinical and Experimental Neuropsychology, 30*(4), 463–470.

Folstein, M. F., Folstein, S. E., & McHugh, P. R. (1975). "Mini-mental state." A practical method for grading the cognitive state of patients for the clinician. *Journal of Psychiatric Rewards, 12*(3), 189–198.

Fong, T. G., Tulebaev, S. R., & Inouye, S. K. (2009). Delirium in elderly adults: Diagnosis, prevention and treatment. *National Review of Neurology, 5*(4), 210–220.

Freedman, M., Leach, L., Kaplan, K., Winocur, G., Shulman, K. I., & Delis, D. (1994). *Clock drawing: A neuropsychological analysis.* New York: Oxford University Press.

Gershon, R. C., Cella, D., Fox, N. A., Havlik, R. J., Hendrie, H. C., & Wagster, M. V. (2010). Assessment of neurological and behavioural function: The NIH Toolbox. *The Lancet Neurology, 9*(2), 138–139.

Glymour, M., & Manly, J. (2008). Lifecourse social conditions and racial and ethnic patterns of cognitive aging. *Neuropsychology Review, 18*(3), 223–254.

Glymour, M. M., Kawachi, I., Jencks, C. S., & Berkman, L. F. (2008). Does childhood schooling affect old age memory or mental status? Using state schooling laws as natural experiments. *Journal of Epidemiology and Community Health, 62*(6), 532–537.

Golden, C. J. (1978). *Stroop Color and Word Test.* Chicago, IL: Stolting.

Golomb, J., de Leon, M. J., Kluger, A., George, A. E., Tarshish, C., & Ferris, S. H. (1993). Hippocampal atrophy in normal aging. An association with recent memory impairment. *Archives of Neurology, 50*(9), 967–973.

Good, C. D., Johnsrude, I. S., Ashburner, J., Henson, R. N., Friston, K. J., & Frackowiak, R. S. (2001). A voxel-based morphometric study of ageing in 465 normal adult human brains. *Neuroimage, 14*(1 Pt 1), 21–36.

Goodglass, H., & Kaplan, D. (1983). *The assessment of aphasia and related disorders* (2nd ed.). Philadelphia, PA: Lea & Febiger.

Gottfredson, L. S. (2004). Intelligence: Is it the epidemiologists' elusive "fundamental cause" of social class inequalities in health? *Journal of Personality and Social Psychology, 86*(1), 174–199.

Gottfredson, L. S., & Deary, I. J. (2004). Intelligence predicts health and longevity, but why? *Current Directions in Psychological Science, 13*(1), 1–4.

Green, J. (2000). *Neuropsychological evaluation of the older adult: A clinician's guidebook.* San Diego: Academic Press.

Greenwood, P. M. (2000). The frontal aging hypothesis evaluated. *Journal of the International Neuropsychological Society, 6*(6), 705–726.

Grodstein, F., Chen, J., Pollen, D. A., Albert, M. S., Wilson, R. S., Folstein, M. F., et al. (2000). Postmenopausal hormone therapy and cognitive function in healthy elderly women. *Journal of the American Geriatrics Society, 48*(7), 746–752.

Hamilton, J. M., Salmon, D. P., Galasko, D., Delis, D. C., Hansen, L. A., Masliah, E., et al. (2004). A comparison of episodic memory deficits in neuropathologically-confirmed dementia with Lewy bodies and Alzheimer's disease. *Journal of the International Neuropsychological Society, 10*(5), 689–697.

Heaton, R. K. (1981). *Wisconsin Card Sorting Test Manual.* Odessa, FL: Psychological Assessment Resources, Inc.

Heaton, R. K., Grant, I., Matthews, C. G., & Adams, K. M. (1986). Differences in neuropsychological test performance associated with age, education, and sex. In *Neuropsychological assessment of neuropsychiatric disorders* (Vol. 1, pp. 100–120). New York: Oxford University Press.

Heaton, R. K., Taylor, M., Manly, J., Tulsky, D., Chelune, G. J., Ivnik, I., et al. (2001). Demographic effects and demographically corrected norms with the WAIS-III and WMS-III. In *Clinical Interpretations of the WAIS-II and WMS-III* (pp. 181–210). San Diego, CA: Academic Press.

Helms, J. E. (1992). Why is there no study of cultural equivalence in standardized cognitive ability testing? *American Psychologist, 47*, 1083–1101.

Herzog, A. R., & Wallace, R. B. (1997). Measures of Cognitive Functioning in the AHEAD Study. *Journals of Gerontology:*

Psychological and Social Sciences, 52B (Special Issue), 37–48.

Hooper, H. E. (1983). *Hooper Visual Organization Test* (VOT). Los Angeles, CA: Western Psychological Services.

Howard, V. J., Cushman, M., Pulley, L., Gomez, C. R., Go, R. C., Prineas, R. J., et al. (2005). The reasons for geographic and racial differences in stroke study: Objectives and design. *Neuroepidemiology, 25*(3), 135–143.

Jacobs, D. M., Sano, M., Albert, S., Schofield, P., Dooneief, G., & Stern, Y. (1997). Cross-cultural neuropsychological assessment: A comparison of randomly selected, demographically matched cohorts of English- and Spanish-speaking older adults. *Journal of Clinical & Experimental Neuropsychology, 19*, 331–339.

Johnson, J. K., Head, E., Kim, R., Starr, A., & Cotman, C. W. (1999). Clinical and pathological evidence for a frontal variant of Alzheimer disease. *Archives of Neurology, 56*(10), 1233–1239.

Jokinen, H., Kalska, H., Ylikoski, R., Madureira, S., Verdelho, A., Gouw, A., et al. (2009). MRI-defined subcortical ischemic vascular disease: Baseline clinical and neuropsychological findings. The LADIS Study. *Cerebrovascular Disorders, 27*(4), 336–344.

Kanaya, A. M., Barrett-Connor, E., Gildengorin, G., & Yaffe, K. (2004). Change in cognitive function by glucose tolerance status in older adults: A 4-year prospective study of the Rancho Bernardo study cohort. *Archives of Internal Medicine, 164*(12), 1327–1333.

Kaplan, E., Goodglass, H., & Weintraub, S. (1983). *The Boston Naming Test*. Philadelphia: Lea & Febiger.

Kempler, D., Teng, E. L., Dick, M., Taussig, I. M., & Davis, D. S. (1998). The effects of age, education, and ethnicity on verbal fluency. *Journal of the International Neuropsychological Society, 4*, 531–538.

Kennedy, K. M., & Raz, N. (2005). Age, sex and regional brain volumes predict perceptual-motor skill acquisition. *Cortex, 41*(4), 560–569.

Kertesz, A., & McMonagle, P. (2009). Behavior and cognition in corticobasal degeneration and progressive supranuclear palsy. *Journal of Neurological Science, 289*(1–2), 138–143.

Kirsch, I. S., Jungeblut, A., Jenkins, L., & Kolstad, A. (1993). *Adult literacy in America: The National Adult Literacy Survey. National Center for Education Statistics, US Department of Education*. Washington DC: US Government Printing Office.

Kral, V. A. (1958). Neuro-psychiatric observation in an old peoples' home. Studies of memory dysfunction in senescence. *Journals of Gerontology, 13*, 169–176.

Landrine, H., & Klonoff, E. A. (1994). The African American Acculturation Scale: Development, reliability, and validity. *Journal of Black Psychology, 20*, 104–127.

Langa, K., Llewellyn, D., Lang, I., Weir, D., Wallace, R., Kabeto, M., et al. (2009). Cognitive health among older adults in the United States and in England. *BMC Geriatrics, 9*(1), 23.

Lemstra, A. W., Eikelenboom, P., & van Gool, W. A. (2003). The cholinergic deficiency syndrome and its therapeutic implications. *Gerontology, 49*(1), 55–60.

Lezak, M. D., Howieson, D. B., Loring, D. W., Hannay, H. J., & Fischer, J. S. (2004). *Neuropsychological Assessment* (4th ed.). Oxford, UK: Oxford University Press.

Listerud, J., Powers, C., Moore, P., Libon, D. J., & Grossman, M. (2009). Neuropsychological patterns in magnetic resonance imaging-defined subgroups of patients with degenerative dementia. *Journal of the International Neuropsychological Society, 15*(3), 459–470.

Lopez, O. L., Hamilton, R. L., Becker, J. T., Wisniewski, S., Kaufer, D. I., & DeKosky, S. T. (2000). Severity of cognitive impairment and the clinical diagnosis of AD with Lewy bodies. *Neurology, 54*(9), 1780–1787.

Luchsinger, J. A., Brickman, A. M., Reitz, C., Cho, S. J., Schupf, N., Manly, J. J., et al. (2009). Subclinical cerebrovascular disease in mild cognitive impairment. *Neurology, 73*(6), 450–456.

Luria, A. R. (Ed.), (1980). *Higher Cortical Functions*. New York: Basic Books.

Malmstrom, T. K. P., Miller, D. K. M. D., Coats, M. A. R. N. M. S. N., Jackson, P. M. A. B. S. N., Miller, J. P. A. B., & Morris, J. C. M. D. (2009). Informant-based dementia screening in a population-based sample of African Americans. *Alzheimer Disease & Associated Disorders April/June, 23*(2), 117–123.

Manly, J. J., Byrd, D., Touradji, P., & Stern, Y. (2004). Acculturation, reading level, and neuropsychological test performance among African American elders. *Applied Neuropsychology, 11*, 37–46.

Manly, J. J., Jacobs, D. M., Sano, M., Bell, K., Merchant, C. A., Small, S. A., et al. (1998). Cognitive test performance among nondemented elderly African Americans and Whites. *Neurology, 50*, 1238–1245.

Manly, J. J., Jacobs, D. M., Sano, M., Bell, K., Merchant, C. A., Small, S. A., et al. (1999). Effect of literacy on neuropsychological test performance in nondemented, education-matched elders. *Journal of the International Neuropsychological Society, 5*, 191–202.

Manly, J. J., Jacobs, D. M., Touradji, P., Small, S. A., & Stern, Y. (2002). Reading level attenuates differences in neuropsychological test performance between African American and White elders. *Journal of the International Neuropsychological Society, 8*, 341–348.

Manly, J. J., & Mayeux, R. (2004). Ethnic differences in dementia and Alzheimer's disease. In N. A. Anderson, R. A. Bulatao, & B. Cohen (Eds.), *Critical perspectives on racial and ethnic differentials in health in late life* (pp. 95–141). Washington, DC: National Academies Press.

Manly, J. J., Touradji, P., Tang, M. X., & Stern, Y. (2003). Literacy and memory decline among ethnically diverse elders. *Journal of Clinical and Experimental Neuropsychology, 5*, 680–690.

McArdle, J. J., Smith, J. P., & Willis, R. (2009). Cognition and Economic Outcomes in the Health and Retirement Survey. *National*

Bureau of Economic Research Working Paper Series, No. 15266.

Metzler-Baddeley, C. (2007). A review of cognitive impairments in dementia with Lewy bodies relative to Alzheimer's disease and Parkinson's disease with dementia. *Cortex, 43*(5), 583–600.

Meyers, J., & Meyers, K. (1995). *Rey Complex Figure Test and Recognition Trial (RCFT)*. Odessa, FL: Psychological Assessment Resources, Inc.

Miller, S. W., Heaton, R. K., Kirson, D., & Grant, I. (1997). Neuropsychological (NP) Assessment of African Americans. *Journal of the International Neuropsychological Society, 3*, 49.

Mitrushina, M., Boone, K. B., Razani, J., & D'Elia, L. F. (2005). *Handbook of normative data for neuropsychological assessment*. Oxford, UK: Oxford University Press.

Morris, J. C. (1993). The Clinical Dementia Rating (CDR): Current version and scoring rules. *Neurology, 43*(11), 2412–2414.

Mortimer, J. A., Henderson, A. S., & Henderson, J. H. (1988). Do psychosocial risk factors contribute to Alzheimer's disease. In *Etiology of dementia of Alzheimer's type* (pp. 39–52). Chichester, UK: John Wiley and Sons.

Mungas, D., Yeo, G., & Gallagher-Thompson, D. (1996). The process of development of valid and reliable neuropsychological assessment measures for English- and Spanish-speaking elderly persons. In *Ethnicity and the dementias* (pp. 33–46). Washington DC: Taylor & Francis.

Murray, R., Neumann, M., Forman, M. S., Farmer, J., Massimo, L., Rice, A., et al. (2007). Cognitive and motor assessment in autopsy-proven corticobasal degeneration. *Neurology, 68*(16), 1274–1283.

National Research Council & Committee on Future Directions for Cognitive Research on Aging. (2000). *The Aging Mind: Opportunities in Cognitive Research*. Washington, DC: National Academies Press.

Negy, C., & Woods, D. J. (1992). The importance of acculturation in understanding research with Hispanic-Americans. *Hispanic Journal of Behavioral Sciences, 14*, 224–247.

Padilla, A. M. (1980). *Acculturation: theory, models, and some new findings*. Boulder, CO: Westview Press for the American Association for the Advancement of Science.

Piquard, A., Lacomblez, L., Derouesne, C., & Sieroff, E. (2009). Problems inhibiting attentional capture by irrelevant stimuli in patients with frontotemporal dementia. *Brain and Cognition, 70*(1), 62–66.

Plassman, B. L., Langa, K. M., Fisher, G. G., Heeringa, S. G., Weir, D. R., Ofstedal, M. B., et al. (2007). Prevalence of dementia in the United States: The aging, demographics, and memory study. *Neuroepidemiology, 29*(1–2), 125–132.

Potter, G. G., & Attix, D. K. (2005). An Integrated model for geriatric neuropsychological assessment. In D. K. Attix & K. A. Welsh-Bohmer (Eds.), *Geriatric Neuropsychology* (pp. 5–26). New York: The Guilford Press.

Rascovsky, K., Salmon, D. P., Ho, G. J., Galasko, D., Peavy, G. M., Hansen, L. A., et al. (2002). Cognitive profiles differ in autopsy-confirmed frontotemporal dementia and AD. *Neurology, 58*(12), 1801–1808.

Reitan, R. (1958). Validity of the Trail Making Test as an indicator of organic brain damage. *Perceptual Motor Skills, 8*, 271–276.

Reitan, R. M., & Wolfson, D. (1987). *The Halstead-Reitan Neuropsychological Test Battery.* Tucson, AZ: Neuropsychological Press.

Richards, M., & Sacker, A. (2003). Lifetime antecedents of cognitive reserve. *Journal of Clinical and Experimental Neuropsychology, 25*, 614–624.

Rivera-Mindt, M., Arentoft, A., Kubo-Germano, K., D'Aquila, E., Scheiner, D., Pizzirusso, M., et al. (2008). Neuropsychological, cognitive, and theoretical considerations for evaluation of bilingual individuals. *Neuropsychology Review, 18*(3), 255–268.

Rosen, W., Mohs, R., & Davis, K. (1984). A new rating scale for Alzheimer's disease. *American Journal of Psychiatry, 141*, 1356–1364.

Sano, M., Ernesto, C., Thomas, R. G., et al. (1997). A controlled trial of Selegiline, alpha-tocopherol, or both as treatment for Alzheimer's disease. *New England Journal of Medicine, 336*, 1216–1222.

Satz, P. (1993). Brain reserve capacity on symptom onset after brain injury: A formulation and review of evidence for threshold theory. *Neuropsychology, 7*, 273–295.

Sawamoto, N., Honda, M., Hanakawa, T., Aso, T., Inoue, M., Toyoda, H., et al. (2007). Cognitive slowing in Parkinson disease is accompanied by hypofunctioning of the striatum. *Neurology, 68*(13), 1062–1068.

Sawamoto, N., Honda, M., Hanakawa, T., Fukuyama, H., & Shibasaki, H. (2002). Cognitive slowing in Parkinson's disease: A behavioral evaluation independent of motor slowing. *Journal of Neuroscience, 22*(12), 5198–5203.

Simmons, W. K., & Martin, A. (2009). The anterior temporal lobes and the functional architecture of semantic memory. *Journal of the International Neuropsychological Society, 15*(5), 645–649.

Spencer, S. J., Steele, C. M., & Quinn, D. M. (1999). Stereotype threat and women's math performance. *Journal of Experimental and Social Psychology, 35*, 4–28.

Stern, Y. (2002). What is cognitive reserve? Theory and research application of the reserve concept. *Journal of the International Neuropsychological Society, 8*, 448–460.

Stern, Y. (2009). Cognitive reserve. *Neuropsychologia, 47*(10), 2015–2028.

Stern, Y., Albert, S., Tang, M. X., & Tsai, W. Y. (1999). Rate of memory decline in AD is related to education and occupation: Cognitive reserve? *Neurology, 53*, 1942–1947.

Stern, Y., Alexander, G. E., Prohovnik, I., & Mayeux, R. (1992). Inverse relationship between education and parietotemporal perfusion deficit in Alzheimer's disease. *Annals of Neurology, 32*(3), 371–375.

Stern, Y., Tang, M. X., Denaro, J., & Mayeux, R. (1995). Increased risk of mortality in Alzheimer's disease patients with more advanced educational and occupational attainment. *Annals of Neurology, 37*, 590–595.

Storandt, M., Botwinick, J., Danziger, W. L., Berg, L., & Hughes, C. P. (1984). Psychometric differentiation of mild senile dementia of the Alzheimer type. *Archives of Neurology, 41*(5), 497–499.

Story, T. J., & Attix, D. K. (2010). Models of developmental neuropsychology: Adult and geriatric. In J. Donders & S. J. Hunter (Eds.), *Principles and Practice of Lifespan Developmental Neuropsychology*. Cambridge, UK: Cambridge University Press.

Strauss, E., Sherman, E. M. S., & Spreen, O. (2006). *A compendium of neuropsychological tests: administration, norms, and commentary* (3rd ed.). New York: Oxford University Press.

Sullivan, E. V., & Pfefferbaum, A. (2006). Diffusion tensor imaging and aging. *Neuroscience and Biobehavioral Reviews, 30*(6), 749–761.

Teng, E. L., Yeo, G., & Gallagher-Thompson, D. (1996). Cross-cultural testing and the Cognitive Abilities Screening Instrument. In *Ethnicity and the dementias* (pp. 77–85). Washington DC: Taylor & Francis.

Teri, L., McCurry, S. M., Edland, S. D., Kukull, W. A., & Larson, E. B. (1995). Cognitive decline in Alzheimer's disease: A longitudinal investigation of risk factors for accelerated decline. *Journals of Gerontology: Biological and Medical Sciences, 50A*, M49–M55.

Tiraboschi, P., Salmon, D. P., Hansen, L. A., Hofstetter, R. C., Thal, L. J., & Corey-Bloom, J. (2006). What best differentiates Lewy body from Alzheimer's disease in early-stage dementia? *Brain, 129*(Pt 3), 729–735.

Unverzagt, F. W., Hui, S. L., Farlow, M. R., Hall, K. S., & Hendrie, H. C. (1998). Cognitive decline and education in mild dementia. *Neurology, 50*, 181–185.

Wang, L., Zhang, Z., McArdle, J. J., & Salthouse, T. A. (2008). Investigating ceiling effects in longitudinal data analysis. *Multivariate Behavioral Research, 43*(3), 476–496.

Wechsler, D. (2008a). *Wechsler Adult Intelligence Scale — Fourth Edition: Technical and interpretive manual.* San Antonio, TX: Pearson.

Wechsler, D. (2008b). *Wechsler Memory Scale — Fourth Edition.* San Antonio, TX: Pearson.

Weiss, B. D., Reed, R., Kligman, E. W., & Abyad, A. (1995). Literacy and performance on the Mini-Mental State Examination. *Journal of the American Geriatric Society, 43*, 807–810.

West, R. (2000). In defense of the frontal lobe hypothesis of cognitive aging. *Journal of the International Neuropsychological Society, 6*(6), 727–729, discussion 730.

Wilson, R. S., Li, Y., Bienias, L., & Bennett, D. A. (2006). Cognitive decline in old age: Separating retest effects from the effects of growing older. *Psychology and Aging, 21*(4), 774–789.

Woodward, M., Jacova, C., Black, S. E., Kertesz, A., Mackenzie, I. R., & Feldman, H. (2009). Differentiating the frontal variant of Alzheimer's disease. *International Journal of Geriatric Psychiatry*.

Chapter | 23 |

Family Caregiving for Cognitively or Physically Frail Older Adults: Theory, Research, and Practice

Bob G. Knight,[1] Andres Losada[2]

[1]School of Gerontology, University of Southern California, Los Angeles, California, USA; [2]Department of Psychology, Universidad Reg Juan Carlos, Madrid, Spain

CHAPTER CONTENTS

Introduction 353
Stress and Coping Models for Caregiving 354
Mental Health Outcomes 354
Physical Health Outcomes 354
Potential Influences on Outcomes of Caregiving 355
Caregiving Stressors 355
Potential Diathesis 355
Appraisal of Caregiving as Stressful 355
Coping Styles 355
Social Support 355
Efficacy of Interventions 356
Clinical Significance 356
Treatment Implementation 356
Cross-Cultural Issues and Caregiving 357
Ethnic Differences in Mental Health Outcomes 357
Ethnic Differences in Physical Health Outcomes 357
Coping Styles 357
Social Support 358
Cultural Values 358
Ethnic Group Differences in Treatment Responsiveness 358
Abuse Within the Caregiving Dyad 359
Aggression from the Care-Recipient to the Caregiver 359
Predictors of Aggression from the Caregiver to the Care-Recipient 359
Stages of Caregiving 359
Becoming a Caregiver 359
Institutionalization and Caregiving Effects 360
Grief After Caregiving 361
Conclusions 361
References 362

INTRODUCTION

Research and practice concerning stress and coping processes among family caregivers of frail older adults have grown exponentially in the last 30 years. The interest in this area has been enhanced by the effects on society of population aging which increases the number of frail elders needing care, as well as the decrease in the birth rate and the incorporation of women to the work force, which potentially decrease the pool of family caregivers.

In this chapter, we review the literature on family caregiving to assess the current status of stress and coping models of the effects of caregiving on physical and mental health and the efficacy of interventions to assist stressed family caregivers. As caregivers become more culturally diverse within nations and caregiving research becomes more transnational, there has been increased attention to the role of culture in stress and coping process among family caregivers, so we next turn our attention to cultural and individual

DOI: 10.1016/B978-0-12-380882-0.00023-1

diversity issues as they influence the caregiving process. Finally, we discuss less commonly explored issues including research on whether abuse within caregiving dyads is related to caregiving stress and to whether the stress processes cease when in-home caregiving ends by institutional placement or by the death of the care recipient. Throughout the review, we give priority to longitudinal studies of caregiving and to meta-analyses.

STRESS AND COPING MODELS FOR CAREGIVING

Research on caregiving has mainly been guided by theoretical frameworks such as the stress and coping model (Haley et al., 1987; Knight et al., 2000; Lazarus & Folkman, 1984), the stress process model (Pearlin et al., 1990), and the diathesis-stress model (Gatz et al., 1996; Russo et al., 1995; Schulz & Beach, 1999). These models share much in common, having a focus on potential individual differences in responses to caregiving, identifying objective caregiving stressors; and attending to coping styles and/or social support as important mediators between stressors and health outcomes. Diathesis-stress models emphasize the preexisting vulnerabilities of some caregivers. The stress and coping models emphasize the appraisal of caregiving as burdensome. Stress process models emphasize conflicts among the caregiver's social roles (e.g., work and family). In the remainder of this section, we discuss the health consequences of caregiving and then explore the influences on those outcomes.

Mental Health Outcomes

Meta-analyses have found strong evidence that caregivers have higher distress (depression, stress, less subjective well-being, etc.) than non-caregivers, more so for older caregivers, women, and for spouses (e.g., Pinquart & Sörensen, 2003). While gender and familial relationships are generally discussed as independent factors, they are partly confounded in that the three major categories of caregivers within non-Hispanic White caregivers are husbands, wives, and daughters. Risk emotional distress is higher for dementia caregivers than for samples of caregivers of the physically frail and for mixed samples. The adverse mental health effects of caregiving are smaller when studies use stronger research designs, such as representative samples versus samples recruited from memory clinics and/or support groups. Longitudinal data with Alzheimer caregivers suggest that distress remains relatively stable for caregivers as a whole over several years at a time (e.g., Clay et al., 2008; Schulz & Williamson, 1991). This stability is especially consistent for female caregivers (Li et al., 1999; Schulz & Williamson, 1991). Thus, there is little evidence for natural adjustment to the stresses of caregiving over time.

Physical Health Outcomes

In contrast to mental health outcomes, differences in physical health outcomes between caregivers and non-caregivers have been found to be significant, but smaller (Pinquart & Sörensen, 2003; Vitaliano et al., 2003). For example, Pinquart and Sörensen (2003) reported that caregiving status alone explained 7.8% of variance in mental health but only 0.8% of physical health outcomes. However, as noted by Vitaliano et al. (2003), this finding should not understate the clinical relevance of such difference, considering the millions of people who are caregivers: the number of persons affected and the implications (economic, personal, and social costs) are significant. Caregiving strain also contributes to all-cause mortality. Schulz and Beach (1999) found that 56% of their sample of spousal caregivers of elderly with disabilities reported caregiver strain. Caregivers who experienced strain had a mortality risk 63% higher than those who were not caring for a disabled spouse and was higher than for those caregivers not reporting strain.

Most studies of caregivers' health have used global self-report measures of health (Pinquart & Sörensen, 2007). Those studies suggest that caregiver depression is a stronger correlate of health status than caregiving stressors. Among stressors, behavior problems are more strongly associated with health status than recipient functional status or caregiving workload. The associations between caregiving stressors and health were stronger among older caregivers, dementia caregivers, and men (Pinquart & Sörensen, 2007).

The Vitaliano et al. (2003) meta-analysis noted that caregiving has significant health effects as measured by stress hormones, antibodies, and self-reported health measures. They also suggested a model for understanding the impact of caregiving on health that links emotional distress to physiological stress responses and poorer health care behaviors, which then lead to illness and increased risk of mortality. They also noted that the type of health measure influenced gender differences in health of caregivers versus non-caregivers: female caregivers reported worse health on subjective health but not on biomarkers (hormone, cardiovascular, or metabolic measures), which showed worse health for male caregivers compared to non-caregivers.

In summary, there is consistent evidence for strong effects of caregiving on mental health of caregivers, especially for dementia caregivers in convenience samples. Psychological distress is in turn related to poor physical health outcomes, including lower antibody counts, higher stress hormones, and all may cause mortality in caregivers reporting strain. Dementia caregivers and male caregivers appear to be more likely to experience physical health consequences of caregiving stressors than are women.

Potential Influences on Outcomes of Caregiving

While negative physical and mental outcomes have been consistently reported in the caregiving literature, caregiver status seems to explain less than 8% of the variance of the physical and mental health outcomes (Pinquart & Sörensen, 2003). In this section, we explore potential influences on caregiving health outcomes that are suggested by the stress and coping models.

Caregiving Stressors

Data from meta-analyese and from longitudinal studies suggest that patient problem behaviors and patients' poor physical health contribute to caregivers' distress and physical health outcomes and that caregiving workload affects physical health (Pinquart & Sörensen, 2005, 2007). Facing severe early problem behaviors seems to predict increases in distress and probability of institutionalization three years later (Gaugler et al., 2005). Care-recipient level of depression seems to be an independent factor that contributes longitudinally to lower mental health of caregivers (McCusker et al., 2007).

Potential Diathesis

Several studies have analyzed variables that may make caregivers vulnerable or predisposed to the effects of stressors. First of all, as it has been commented that being a caregiver is an independent risk factor for mortality in strained caregivers (Schulz & Beach, 1999). As Russo et al. (1995) showed, caregivers with a history of mental health problems prior to caregiving are more likely to experience psychiatric disorders after the onset of their relative's illness as compared with controls. Also, Hooker et al. (1998) found that the personality traits of neuroticism and pessimism influence caregivers' mental and physical health both directly and indirectly through stress and social support. Neuroticism and pessimism may influence stress proliferation and caregivers scoring in these variables "may have impoverished social supports in part because they are not the type of people with whom one would choose to spend time" (Hooker et al., 2008, p. 81).

Appraisal of Caregiving as Stressful

Sörensen and Pinquart (2005) suggested a common core model for caregiver distress that considers behavior problems in the person with dementia as stressors for family caregivers, includes the caregivers' appraisal of burden as a key mediator of those stressors, and finds higher levels of burden appraisal associated with worse mental and physical health outcomes. It is likely that a similar model with functional disability substituting for behavioral problems would be the corresponding model for caregivers of the physically frail (cf. Pinquart & Sörensen, 2005, 2007). Perhaps the strongest evidence for the role of appraisal was reported by Schulz and Beach (1999) who found a higher risk of mortality for caregivers who appraised caregiving as stressful as compared to both non-caregivers and to caregivers who did not view caregiving as stressful.

Coping Styles

In a one-year follow-up study, Cooper et al. (2008) analyzed how coping strategies mediated the relationship between burden and anxiety. The use of dysfunctional coping strategies (e.g., behavioral disengagement or denial) was related with anxiety both at baseline and one year later. Using positive emotion-coping strategies at Time 1 baseline (e.g., acceptance, positive reframing, humor) protected caregivers from developing higher anxiety levels a year later, while problem-focused strategies (e.g., active coping, instrumental support, planning) did not protect against the impact of greater burden on anxiety. In general, the use of avoidant emotion-focused coping strategies has been linked with increases in depressive symptoms, while the use of problem-focused strategies has been linked with decreases in depressive symptoms (Li et al., 1999).

Social Support

In their modeling of influences on outcomes of caregiving across ethnic groups using the REACH data set, Sörensen and Pinquart (2005) found that informal, but not formal, social support was associated with better outcomes for both depression and for physical health across all ethnic groups in the sample. In a five-year longitudinal study, Clay et al. (2008) found that satisfaction with social support partially explained depressive symptoms and life satisfaction. These authors suggested that low quality of social support could be viewed as a precursor of poor psychological outcomes (e.g., higher depression and lower life satisfaction). In contrast, Ducharme et al. (2007), in a longitudinal study with husband caregivers, found that greater use of instrumental support at the initial assessment predicted greater psychological distress one year later. They interpreted the finding as meaning that men wait until they are overwhelmed to ask for help.

In short, caregivers who report high levels of emotional distress appear to continue to stay distressed for long periods of time, a finding that raises the possibility of a diathesis that predisposes some caregivers to high levels of distress, which may well be present before caregiving begins. Behavior problems in persons with dementia, physical disability in the physically frail, and care recipient depression all act as key stressors in the stress and coping process. Appraisal of caregiving as stressful appears to be a key and consistent element in producing poor outcomes. Among resource variables, avoidant coping consistently leads to poor outcomes, whereas positive emotion focused coping and perceived positive support are protective. These findings, and especially the key role of appraisal, lend support to the stress and coping models descended from Lazarus and Folkman (1984), although the suggestion of a potential diathesis (e.g., the affects of personality variables such as neuroticism or optimism on the adaptation to caregiving; Hooker et al., 1998) suggests a need for further research into diathesis-stress models and more generally into understanding the influences of pre-caregiving factors on caregivers' reactions to caregiving stressors.

EFFICACY OF INTERVENTIONS

Attention to developing and evaluating interventions to reduce caregiver distress have increased over the last 20 years. On the whole, the evidence shows that the effects of interventions for caregivers are small to moderate in size (e.g., see meta-analyses by Knight et al., 1993; Pinquart & Sörensen, 2006), and the effects are smaller on younger caregivers, spouses, and caregivers of relatives with dementia (Sörensen et al., 2002). The nationwide collaborative REACH studies (e.g., Belle et al., 2006; Gitlin et al., 2003) also showed small effect sizes with some variations by site.

Theory-based development of the intervention has been suggested as a way to increase effectiveness, by establishing the mechanism of expected improvements, and which outcomes will be modified through the intervention. Knight et al. (2006) suggested that family systems theory, which frames distress as a family issue and takes the family as the unit of analysis for theory and the focus of intervention for treatment, is a logical choice and one that has shown promise in applications by Mittelman's group (e.g., Mittelman et al., 2006) and by the Miami site of REACH I (Eisdorfer et al., 2003).

Pinquart and Sörensen's (2006) meta-analysis provided evidence for outcomes of caregiving interventions varying by both treatment type and by the targeted outcome (see Table 2, pp. 586–587 of their paper). For example, cognitive behavior therapy had significant and large effects on depression and on knowledge about caregiving; whereas, respite care and structured multicomponent interventions had significant and large effects on institutionalization.

Clinical Significance

According to Jacobson et al. (1999), a change will be clinically significant if (a) the magnitude of the change is statistically reliable and (b) participants' symptoms or problems are comparable to those of well-functioning people. Schulz et al. (2002) reviewed interventions for caregivers and analyzed their effects in terms of the clinical significance of their results. They considered four domains that could reflect important outcomes for individuals or society: reduced symptomatology, improved quality of life, importance of the outcomes for society, and social validity (experts or participants find treatment goals, procedures, and outcomes acceptable). According to Schulz et al. (2002), social validity is well-established in that caregivers are consistently positive about the interventions. They also found that there is "...promise of achieving clinically significant outcomes in improving depressive symptoms, and, to a lesser degree, in reducing anxiety, anger, and hostility" (p. 598). They found that the success of efforts to improve the overall quality of life for caregivers has been "limited," but that there are socially important outcomes for delay of institutionalization of the care recipient. While using a different framework, the findings of greater clinical significance with regard to depressive symptoms and delay of institutionalization are similar to those reported by Pinquart and Sörensen (2006).

Treatment Implementation

The effectiveness of caregiver interventions might also be improved by greater attention to fidelity of treatment implementation. Treatment implementation in caregiving interventions may be assessed by three components (Burgio et al., 2001): treatment delivery (Have the interventionists performed the intervention as planned?), treatment receipt (Is the caregiver able to put in practice the knowledge and skills that have been trained?), and treatment enactment (Does the caregiver use the skills and mastery acquired in the actual caregiving context?).

Bourgeois et al. (2002) provide examples of the monitoring of treatment, including tracking participant attendance, testing knowledge gained from the workshop, and tracking percentage of caregivers who implemented the intervention programs for an average of 24 weeks. Teri et al. (2005) also assessed consultants' adherence to the treatment delivery as intended. This assessment of treatment implementation can provide important information for improving the interventions and their effects. For example, Márquez-González et al. (2007) tested the efficacy of a cognitive-behavioral intervention aimed at modifying dysfunctional thoughts about caregiving. Although they found positive results for this intervention (e.g., reduction of depressive symptomatology, appraisals of behavioural problems and dysfunctional thoughts), the analysis of the quantity of homework done by participants suggested that more attention to increasing homework completion could produce greater change in future studies.

In summary, available evidence suggest that significant, although moderate or low, effects on caregivers' distress reduction can be obtained through interventions such as cognitive-behavior therapy. However, as Pinquart and Sörensen (2006) stated, "there is room for further improvements in interventions" (p. 577). Guiding assessment through theoretically valid models, developing interventions targeted to specific outcome goals, and paying greater attention to treatment fidelity are strategies for improving the effects of interventions for caregivers (Zarit & Femia, 2008).

CROSS-CULTURAL ISSUES AND CAREGIVING

In recent years, the literature on cultural issues in caregiving has increased significantly (see, for example, reviews by Aranda & Knight, 1997; Dilworth-Anderson et al., 2002; Janevic & Connell, 2001; Pinquart & Sörensen, 2005, and Sörensen & Pinquart, 2005) in response to the growing population of minority groups in many nations and to increasing internationalization of research in caregiving. Introducing cultural values and other cultural variables enriches the available knowledge about caregiving and the related theoretical models. For example, the sociocultural stress and coping model (Aranda & Knight, 1997; Knight & Sayegh, 2010) added cultural values to the stress and coping model previously discussed. In the updated model, Knight and Sayegh (2010) proposed that there is a common core that was shared by different cultural groups (e.g., the patient's disruptive behaviors lead to burden, and burden leads to depression and anxiety), but differences exist between cultures as to whether and how social support and coping styles impact emotional distress outcomes. Similar results have been reported by Hilgeman et al. (2009), who provided support for the Pearlin et al. (1990) stress process model as a whole, but found significant differences in individual components by race. So, although caregiving seems to have similar negative consequences for cultural groups, several differences between cultural groups have been found for dimensions usually included in the stress and coping models.

Ethnic Differences in Mental Health Outcomes

Pinquart & Sörensen (2005), in their meta-analysis, found lower scores in burden and depression for African American caregivers, when compared with White caregivers. Roth et al. (2001) found, in a two-year follow-up of White and African American caregivers, that African American caregivers showed better adaptation over time than White caregivers. Specifically, they found that White caregivers showed more deterioration over time in life satisfaction. Also, White caregivers showed increased depression levels while African American caregivers did not show changes through the study period. In Pinquart and Sörensen's (2005) meta-analysis, higher scores on depression were found for Hispanic and Asian American caregivers when compared with Whites. African American and Hispanic caregivers also reported greater number of perceived uplifts (i.e., positive experiences related to caregiving).

Ethnic Differences in Physical Health Outcomes

Regarding physical health outcomes, ethnic minority caregivers show worse health than White caregivers (Pinquart & Sörensen, 2005). Kim et al. (2007) found that ethnicity had a direct effect on physical health outcomes. Specifically, being African American (as compared with White caregivers) was directly associated with poorer health indicators (self-reported physical health and blood pressure). Similar predictors have been found for physical health for different cultural groups (Sörensen & Pinquart, 2005). More memory and behavioral problems, lower mental status, and lower income are associated with poorer health. An important unresolved issue is whether the physical health effects found for minority caregivers are specific to caregiving or reflect the health disparities for their populations as a whole. Knight et al. (2007) and Kim and Knight (2008) point out that these comparisons are further complicated by evidence that some minority caregivers show increased stress in biomarkers without associated differences in self-reported physical health, the measure used in most caregiving studies.

Coping Styles

Regarding differences in use of coping styles, Pinquart and Sörensen's (2005) meta-analysis reported that caregivers from ethnic minorities use more cognitive and emotion-focused coping strategies than Whites, while no differences were found for instrumental coping. Sörensen and Pinquart (2005) reported that all ethnic groups in the REACH dataset benefited from religious coping with regard to depressive symptoms, but not for physical health outcomes. Knight and Sayegh (2010) noted that there may be different coping styles in different cultural groups: while the factor structure of the COPE and Brief COPE were invariant across African American and White caregivers, Korean heritage caregivers showed a different factor structure, with an active coping factor that included elements of acceptance and positive cognitive coping, no avoidant coping factor, and a social support coping factor.

Social Support

Regarding social support, Dilworth-Anderson et al. (2002) noted in their review that most research has reported that ethnic minorities rely more on informal support as compared with formal support. African American caregivers report more unmet needs for caregiving than Whites (Navaie-Waliser et al., 2001). In Pinquart and Sörensen's (2005) meta-analysis, ethnic minority caregivers reported greater levels of informal support than White caregivers. In contrast, Asian American caregivers used fewer formal resources when compared with Whites, African Americans, and Hispanics. Clay et al. (2008) followed African American and White caregivers for a five-year period and found that African American caregivers reported higher satisfaction with social support and had significantly lower depressive symptoms than White caregivers.

Cultural Values

The influence of cultural values on the stress and coping model has also been studied, and data have been obtained that suggest the commonly assumed positive influences of familism values or of East Asian cultural values such as filial piety on caregiving should be considered with caution. A review of the literature and revision of the sociocultural stress and coping model by Knight and Sayegh (2010) argued that the effects of cultural values are complex, multidirectional, and operate through coping styles and social support rather than through lower burden appraisals as has been commonly assumed. Familism values are composed of values centering on obligation rather than those facilitating a view of caregiving as a natural part of family life as hypothesized in the early years of cross-cultural caregiving theory and research. For example, studies, done with different cultural groups (Knight et al., 2002, 2007; Rozario & DeRienzis, 2008), have either found no effects or negative effects of familism on distress; it now appears that familism largely measures values related to obligation rather than to family solidarity and support (Knight & Sayegh, 2010).

Ethnic Group Differences in Treatment Responsiveness

Taking into account the cultural aspects that define each group and how they affect caregiving may be important for designing and implementing interventions adapted to these cultural differences. Significant efforts have already been made regarding these issues. For example, Gallagher-Thompson and colleagues (2003b) reviewed culturally significant values from different ethnic groups and suggested ways to develop interventions culturally appropriate for these groups. Therapists should develop cultural competence (knowledge, culturally sensitive skills, etc.) regarding the population they serve. However, in agreement with Gallagher-Thompson et al. (2003b), individual variability in the assumption of values and norms should be considered, and generalizations must be avoided to prevent stereotypes influencing the interventions.

A few evaluations of interventions with comparisons across cultural groups have suggested differences in outcomes. For example, in the study by Burgio et al. (2003), African American caregivers that participated in the skills training condition showed greater improvements in behavioral bother when compared with White caregivers and African Americans who participated in minimal support control condition. Caregivers in both interventions experienced reduced levels of problem behaviors, burden, and higher satisfaction with leisure activities, but no change in depressive or anxiety symptoms. Burgio et al. (2003) suggested that African Americans were more responsive to the therapeutic relationship in the skills training condition.

Eisdorfer and colleagues (2003), from the REACH team, assessed a family-based therapy intervention, family therapy augmented by technology, and a minimal support control condition in Whites and Cuban American caregivers. The family therapy intervention was aimed to restructure interactions within the family, and between the family and other systems that could be related to the caregiver's burden. Family therapy alone reduced depressive symptoms in Cuban American caregivers at the 18-month follow-up whereas Whites showed increases in depressive symptoms. Belle et al. (2006), from the REACH II initiative, found that Hispanic and Caucasian caregivers who participated in a multicomponent intervention showed significant improvements in quality of life when compared with caregivers from a control group. Among African American caregivers, this intervention only yielded improvement for spouses.

In the study by Burgio et al. (2003), Whites showed a greater improvement in subjective burden and African Americans in positive aspects of caregiving, a self-report measure of ways that caregiving has a positive impact on the caregiver's life. However, no ethnicity effects have been found for other interventions, such as the one developed by Gallagher-Thompson et al. (2003a), who found no significant ethnicity by treatment effects on their study that included Latino and Anglo female caregivers.

Thus, both the theoretical perspectives on stress and coping and the small body of existing intervention research offer mixed perspectives on the effects of cultural differences on stress outcomes and on psychosocial interventions, with both commonalities and differences receiving support in the literature. When differential effects have been found, they seem plausible with regard to what we think we know about ethnic differences. African Americans were more responsive to an intervention that involved greater personal contact with the interventionist. Cuban Americans were more responsive to a family intervention. Our confidence in these differences would be greater if the contrasts had been planned and if the underlying cultural differences had been explicitly measured. As with the literature on White caregivers, greater attention to theory and a more specific focus on the experience and needs of specific cultural groups could advance the field in the future.

ABUSE WITHIN THE CAREGIVING DYAD

There is a widespread assumption that abuse within the caregiver-care receiver dyad is often the result of excessive stress. If this is true, then findings about stress and coping processes and results of caregiving interventions could be helpful in responding to this problem. As Pillemer and Finkelhor (1988) stated, elder abuse or mistreatment is a serious public policy issue, and a very difficult area to study, as reflected in the wide range of differences in prevalence rates between studies and types of abuse or neglect (e.g., economic, physical, or psychological).

Aggression from the Care-Recipient to the Caregiver

Lyketsos et al. (1999) found that a minority (15%) of care-recipients with dementia exhibit physically aggressive behavior toward the family caregiver. Those with moderate to severe depression scores were more likely to act aggressively. Being male and having greater activities of daily living (ADL) impairments were also characteristics associated with aggressive behaviors. Hamel et al. (1990) found that a troubled pre-morbid relationship between the caregiver and the care-recipient, higher levels of pre-morbid care-recipient aggression, and greater number of care-recipient problems predicted care-recipient aggression.

Predictors of Aggression from the Caregiver to the Care-Recipient

Pillemer and Suitor (1992) differentiated between violent feelings (fear of becoming violent or potential for violence) and violent behaviors. They found small differences in the predictors for each phenomenon: differences between potential for and actual violence were found in only three of the ten risk factors assessed: Being older, being a spouse caregiver, and having experienced violence from the care-recipient were associated with caregivers who committed violence. Fear of becoming violent and becoming violent were both associated with caring for a relative showing behavioral problems, low scores on self-esteem, and living with the relative. Sasaki et al. (2008), in a two-year longitudinal study, found that the only caregiver factor related to institutionalization at Time 2 was potentially harmful behaviors toward the care-recipient.

Beach et al. (2005) studied potentially harmful behaviors (e.g., psychological, such as threatening with nursing home placement, or physical, such as handling roughly) in caregiving dyads, and found the following independent risk factors for the presence of potentially harmful caregiver behavior: higher levels of ADL/IADL (instrumental activities of daily living) needs for care, spouse caregivers, higher levels of caregiver cognitive impairment, more caregiver physical symptoms in the previous week, and caregivers at risk for clinical depression. Depression and anxiety have also been reported as determinants of abusive behaviors in a study done by Cooper et al. (2009). However, in this case, the influence of depression and anxiety on abuse was mediated by dysfunctional coping styles and burden. Considering that elder abuse is a priority for many developed countries' social and health policies, the lack of interventions aimed at reducing abuse risks is surprising. Many of the risk factors for abuse within the caregiving dyad are key elements of the stress and coping models of caregiving and could be the focus of caregiving interventions. Thus, interventions and prevention could be targeted to caregivers at risk (e.g., with depression or other distress indicators) or caregivers of relatives showing behavioral problems.

STAGES OF CAREGIVING

It is well known that caregiving usually lasts for years, and researchers have used the term "career" as a metaphor for describing the different transitions that caregivers face during this period (e.g., Pearlin et al., 1990).

Becoming a Caregiver

According to Gaugler et al. (2003), "how long caregivers remain in their role is not as important as determining how caregivers actually acquire their roles during the onset of dementia care" (p. 177). Caregiving onset is unexpected (Pearlin & Aneshensel,

1994) and not "entered into by choice" (Seltzer & Li, 2000; p. 165). Even the moment of the onset may not be easily identified by the caregivers (Seltzer & Li, 2000). In addition to the personal reaction to their relatives' physical or cognitive decline, the caregiver may experience changes in family relations or a reduction in participation in leisure activities or work (Berecki-Gisolf et al., 2008; Seltzer & Li, 2000). Gaugler et al. (2003) found that those caregivers who experienced the less abrupt entry into caregiving were less likely to institutionalize their relative or experience poor adaptation over time. Also, the likelihood of experiencing social or psychological effects when entering the caregiving role seems to be lower for daughter caregivers than for wives (Seltzer & Li, 2000). Although overall negative effects on psychological well-being are usually associated with caregiving, Marks et al. (2002) found in a prospective study that benefits such as more positive relations with others, personal growth, purpose in life or self-acceptance, were also reported by caregivers.

Institutionalization and Caregiving Effects

Mixed results have been found so far with regard to changes in the caregiver's felt distress following the transition to institutional care. Skaff et al. (1996) found that mastery declined while continuing home care but, when the relative was placed in an institution, mastery levels remained stable until the relative died, after which mastery increased. Grant et al. (2002) found reductions in caregivers' depressive symptoms immediately following long-term care placement, with continued reductions over time. These authors found also that caregivers reported fewer serious medical symptoms immediately after placement, and this improved health was sustained over time. These results point in the same direction as those found by Gräsel (2002), who compared caregivers who remained in the community caregiving role with a group of former caregivers, composed of caregivers who ceased to care for at least six months due to institutionalization or death of their relative. The self-reported physical health of former caregivers improved even though a small but significant increase in illnesses was found, and the number of visits to physicians by this group increased. The increase in illnesses was considered a consequence of the increase in number of doctor visits and was interpreted as resulting from an increase in time for considering self-care needs.

However, the findings do not all favor reduction in caregiver distress with institutionalization of the recipient. Schulz et al. (2004) found that anxiety, but not depression, declined over time for caregivers who institutionalized their relatives. Following placement, a significant proportion of caregivers (48.3%) showed depression scores suggesting risk for clinical depression. Lieberman and Fisher (2001), when comparing caregivers who institutionalized their relative with caregivers who did not institutionalize them in a two-year longitudinal study, found no differences between these two groups in terms of changes in physical and mental outcomes. So, no relief was found due to institutionalization, and female caregivers and spouses showed poorer health and well-being scores.

Gaugler et al. (2007) found that, although significant decreases in role overload and anxiety following institutionalization were reported by caregivers, significant variations in caregivers' adaptation to placement were found for longer post-placement panels. Gaugler et al. (2009) found that burden and depression were lower at 6-month post-placement, with burden also reduced at 12-month follow-up. However, in their study, those caregivers who experienced increased burden scores at post-placement were found to differ on contextual characteristics including being a spouse, the availability of affordable home care services, use of overnight hospital stay during transition to home care, and pre-placement depressive symptoms. Several issues may explain the mixed findings that have been found regarding caregivers well-being after institutionalization. Although institutionalizing the relative may have benefits such as not facing the round-the-clock care of the relative, other sources of burden may appear, such as financial strains (Skaff et al., 1996). Caregiver characteristics such as gender may also contribute to the mixed findings. The finding that wife caregivers are more vulnerable to negative consequences of institutionalization (e.g., Lieberman & Fisher, 2001; Schulz et al., 2004) is highlighted in some of the reviewed studies. On the contrary, daughter caregivers may show decline in caregiving burden and increases in social participation (e.g., Seltzer & Li, 2000). Feelings of guilt, being dissatisfied with help received from others, frequent visits and trips to the long-term care facility, and so on are also factors that may contribute to the maintenance of distress feelings after placement. Programs similar to the one developed by Pillemer and colleagues (2003) that assist families and staff in ways to increase the opportunities for adaptive processes during institutionalization (e.g., successful family-staff communication and understanding differences in values) are needed. Participating in intervention programs prior to institutionalization, such as the one developed by Mittelman and colleagues (2003), that includes family and individual ad hoc counselling, may also be helpful for caregivers. A recent study by Gaugler et al. (2008) has shown that caregivers that received guidance and support during nursing home admission showed lower levels of depression and burden than those caregivers who received usual care.

Grief After Caregiving

Caregivers also experience anticipatory grief about the death of their loved one and, finally, the death of the relative. Although conventional wisdom might argue that older adults in general, and caregivers for a family member with a chronic illness in particular, might find the death of a loved one more expected and therefore have an easier bereavement, Hebert et al. (2006) reported that a significant percentage of caregivers (23%) reported that the death of their relative was "extremely" unexpected. Hebert et al. (2006) further showed that being unprepared for the death of the relative was associated with negative outcomes such as depression or complicated grief. Pre-bereavement depression and other variables such as lower educational level or income and ethnicity (African American caregivers were less prepared than White caregivers) were variables associated with less preparedness for the death of the loved one and, so, may show those caregivers at greater risk for mental health problems (Hebert et al., 2006).

A review of studies that have been conducted regarding caregivers' psychological and physical health after the death of their relative shows a mixed picture. Robinson-Whelen et al. (2001) compared active caregivers with former caregivers and non-caregivers. While decreases in perceived stress and negative affect were found, reaching similar levels to non-caregivers, these changes were not observed for other variables such as depression, positive affect, and loneliness. In these variables, former caregivers were similar to active caregivers. The authors suggested that caregiving can have long-lasting psychological consequences on caregivers that last well past the death of the care-recipient. During a three-year follow-up of former caregivers, depressive symptoms did not return to levels comparable to those of non-caregivers. On the contrary, they had similar depression levels to those of current caregivers. This finding is similar to the one reported by Bodnar and Kiecolt-Glaser (1994).

Among bereaved caregivers, no difference in serious medical symptoms were found immediately following patient death, but by one-year post-death there was a 30% reduction in symptoms (Grant et al., 2002). Mausbach et al. (2007) followed bereaved caregivers for 18 months and caregivers that placed their relative for 30 months. They found a long-term normalization of caregivers' physical outcomes that began to occur at six months following the transitions, suggesting a reduction of cardiovascular risk.

Interventions to reduce psychological distress during active caregiving may also have long-term effects after the loss of the care-recipient. A recent study by Holland et al. (2009), done with the REACH I study sample, shows that caregivers who participated in active interventions aimed at teaching caregivers skills to enhance emotional well-being reported fewer normal grief symptoms than those in a control condition, and a trend to fewer complicated grief symptoms. Although nonsignificant effects were found for depressive symptoms in the Holland et al. (2009) study, significant effects for depressive symptoms have been found by Haley et al. (2008) in bereaved caregivers that participated in the New York University Caregiver Intervention.

CONCLUSIONS

It seems clear that caring for dependent elderly relatives, especially if they have dementia, increases the risk of suffering negative consequences for mental and physical health. The negative effects of caregiving last for years, and in some caregivers continue after the frail older relative is placed in 24-hour care and even past the death of the care-recipient. There are gender differences in effects of caregiving stress, with female caregivers reporting worse mental and subjective physical health while male caregivers show worse physical health on biomarkers.

Stress and coping models of various types have guided most of the research on caregiving, and our understanding of psychosocial influences on caregivers' health outcomes has increased over time. At this point in time, the stress and coping models that include a major role for appraisal of caregiving as stressful appear to have garnered the most support, with some indication of a need for future research to attend more to the possibility of pre-caregiving diatheses for stress vulnerability. This understanding includes a greater attention to cultural differences in the operation of stress and coping processes. Greater methodological sophistication, including the more frequent use of longitudinal studies and of meta-analytic reviews, has also contributed to the advancement of knowledge about the caregiving career.

The increase in the evaluation of interventions aimed at helping caregivers lead first to the finding that the effect sizes of most interventions were small to moderate at best. However, attention to matching interventions to the goals for which they have the largest effects is promising (cf. Pinquart & Sörensen, 2006) as is the success of interventions focused on the family system as a unit. Researchers have also analyzed ways to improve the effects of these interventions, and several methodological suggestions have been proposed for improving their effects (e.g., Zarit & Femia, 2008), including greater attention to treatment fidelity. We would add our voices to those who have called for interventions that are more clearly rooted in theory and research on caregiving outcomes as a way to identify the points in the stress and coping process most likely to result in changes in outcomes, as opposed to the use of "off-the-shelf" treatments.

As we look to the future of caregiving research and development of evidenced-based interventions, we would expect to see greater attention to the whole career of caregiving, beginning with the ways in which caregivers choose (or are chosen) for this career and extending to the health consequences that continue for some caregivers after caregiving ends. Greater attention to the specifics of caregiving careers in research (e.g., differences by gender, spouse/child relationship, ethnicity, and between dementia and physical frailty) will hopefully be matched by similar trends in targeting interventions. Emerging attention to abuse within the caregiving dyad and to the nature of grief after extended caregiving in research could lead to the development of appropriate intervention and prevention programs as well.

REFERENCES

Aranda, M. P., & Knight, B. G. (1997). The influence of ethnicity and culture on the caregiver stress and coping process: A sociocultural review and analysis. *The Gerontologist, 37*, 342–354.

Beach, S. R., Schulz, R., Williamson, G. M., Miller, L. S., Weiner, M. F., & Lance, C. E. (2005). Risk factors for potentially harmful informal caregiver behavior. *Journal of the American Geriatrics Society, 53*, 255–261.

Belle, S. H., Burgio, L., Burns, R., Coon, D., Czaja, S . J., Gallagher-Thompson, D., et al. (2006). Resources for enhancing Alzheimer's caregiver health (REACH) ii investigators. Enhancing the quality of life of dementia caregivers from different ethnic or racial groups: A randomized, controlled trial. *Annals of Internal Medicine, 145*, 727–738.

Berecki-Gisolf, J., Lucke, J., Hockey, R., & Dobson, A. (2008). Transitions into informal caregiving and out of paid employment of women in their 50s. *Social Science and Medicine, 67*, 122–127.

Bodnar, J. C., & Kiecolt-Glaser, J. K. (1994). Caregiver depression after bereavement: Chronic stress isn't over when it's over. *Psychology and Aging, 9*, 372–380.

Bourgeois, M., Schulz, R., Burgio, L. D., & Beach, S. (2002). Skills training for spouses of patients with Alzheimer´s disease: Outcomes of an intervention study. *Journal of Clinical Geropsychology, 8*, 53–73.

Burgio, L., Corcoran, M., Lichstein, K. L., Nichols, L., Czaja, S., Gallagher-Thompson, D., et al. (2001). Judging outcomes in psychological interventions for dementia caregivers: The problem of treatment implementation. *The Gerontologist, 41*, 481–489.

Burgio, L., Stevens, A., Guy, D., Roth, D. L., & Haley, W. E. (2003). Impact of two psychosocial interventions on White and African American family caregivers of individuals with dementia. *The Gerontologist, 43*, 568–579.

Clay, O. J., Roth, D. L., Wadley, V. G., & Haley, W. E. (2008). Changes in social support and their impact on psychosocial outcome over a 5-year period for African American and White dementia caregivers. *International Journal of Geriatric Psychiatry, 23*, 857–862.

Cooper, C., Katona, C., Orrell, M., & Livingston, G. (2008). Coping strategies, anxiety and depression in caregivers of people with Alzheimer's disease. *International Journal of Geriatric Psychiatry, 23*, 929–936.

Cooper, C., Selwood, A., Blanchard, M., Walker, Z., Blizard, R., & Livingston, G. (2010). The determinants of family carers' abusive behaviour to people with dementia: Results of the CARD study. *Journal of Affective Disorders*, 121, 136–142.

Dilworth-Anderson, P., Williams, I. C., & Gibson, B. E. (2002). Issues of race, ethnicity, and culture in caregiving research: A 20-year review (1980–2000). *The Gerontologist, 42*, 237–272.

Ducharme, F., Lévesque, L., Zarit, S. H., Lachance, L., & Giroux, F. (2007). Changes in health outcomes among older husband caregivers: A one-year longitudinal study. *International Journal of Aging and Human Development, 65*, 73–96.

Eisdorfer, C., Czaja, S. J., Loewenstein, D. A., Rubert, M. P., Argüelles, S., Mitrani, V. B., et al. (2003). The effect of a family therapy and technology-based intervention on caregiver depression. *The Gerontologist, 43*, 521–531.

Gallagher-Thompson, D., Coon, D. W., Solano, N., Ambler, C., Rabinowitz, Y., & Thompson, L. W. (2003a). Change in indices of distress among Latina and Caucasian female caregivers of elderly relatives with dementia: Site-specific results from the REACH National Collaborative Study. *The Gerontologist, 43*, 580–591.

Gallagher-Thompson, D., Haley, W., Guy, D., Rupert, M., Arguelles, S., Zeiss, L. M., et al. (2003b). Tailoring psychological interventions for ethnically diverse dementia caregivers. *Clinical Psychology: Science and Practice, 10*, 423–438.

Gatz, M., Kasl-Godley, J. E., & Karel, M. J. (1996). Aging and mental disorders. In J. E. Birren & K. W. Schaie (Eds.), *Handbook of the psychology of aging* (4th ed.) (pp. 365–382). San Diego: Academic Press.

Gaugler, J. E., Kane, R. L., Kane, R. A., & Newcomer, R. (2005). The longitudinal effects of early behavior problems in the dementia caregiving career. *Psychology and Aging, 20*, 100–116.

Gaugler, J . E., Mittelman, M. S., Hepburn, K., & Newcomer, R. (2009). Predictors of change in caregiver burden and depressive symptoms following nursing home admission. *Psychology and Aging, 24*, 385–396.

Gaugler, J. E., Pot, A. M., & Zarit, S. H. (2007). Long-term adaptation to institutionalization in dementia caregivers. *The Gerontologist, 47*, 730–740.

Gaugler, J. E., Roth, D. L., Haley, W. E., & Mittelman, M. S. (2008). Can counseling and support reduce burden and depressive symptoms in caregivers of people with Alzheimer's disease during the transition to institutionalization? Results from the New York University caregiver intervention study. *Journal of the American Geriatrics Society, 56*, 421–428.

Gaugler, J. E., Zarit, S. H., & Pearlin, L. I. (2003). The onset of dementia caregiving and its longitudinal implications. *Psychology and Aging, 18*, 171–180.

Gitlin, L. N., Belle, S. H., Burgio, L. D., Czaja, S. J., Mahoney, D., Gallagher-Thompson, D., et al. (2003). Effect of multicomponent interventions on caregiver burden and depression: The REACH Multisite Initiative at 6-month follow-up. *Psychology and Aging, 18*, 361–374.

Grant, I., Adler, K. A., Patterson, T. L., Dimsdale, J. E., Ziegler, M. G., & Irwin, M. R. (2002). Health consequences of Alzheimer's caregiving transitions: Effects of placement and bereavement. *Psychosomatic Medicine, 64*, 477–486.

Gräsel, E. (2002). When home care ends — changes in the physical health of informal caregivers caring for dementia patients: A longitudinal study. *Journal of the American Geriatrics Society, 50*, 843–849.

Haley, W. E., Bergman, E. J., Roth, D. L., McVie, T., Gaugler, J. E., & Mittelman, M. S. (2008). Long-term effects of bereavement and caregiver intervention on dementia caregiver depressive symptoms. *The Gerontologist, 48*, 732–740.

Haley, W. E., Levine, E. G., Brown, L., & Bartolucci, A . A. (1987). Stress, appraisal, coping, and social support as predictors of adaptational outcome among dementia caregivers. *Psychology and Aging, 2*, 323–330.

Hamel, M., Pushkar, D., Andres, D., Reis, M., Dastoor, D., Grauer, H., et al. (1990). Predictors and consequences of aggressive behavior by community-based dementia patients. *The Gerontologist, 30*, 206–211.

Hebert, R. S., Dang, Q., & Schulz, R. (2006). Preparedness for the death of a loved one and mental health in bereaved caregivers of patients with dementia: Findings from the REACH study. *Journal of Palliative Medicine, 9*, 683–693.

Hilgeman, M. M., Durkin, D. W., Sun, F., DeCoster, J., Allen, R. S., Gallagher-Thompson, D., et al. (2009). Testing a theoretical model of the stress process in Alzheimer's caregivers with race as a moderator. *The Gerontologist, 49*, 248–261.

Holland, J. M., Currier, J. M., & Gallagher-Thompson, D. (2009). Outcomes from the Resources for Enhancing Alzheimer's Caregiver Health (REACH) program for bereaved caregivers. *Psychology and Aging, 24*, 190–202.

Hooker, K., Monahan, D. J., Bowman, S. R., Frazier, L. D., & Shifren, K. (1998). Personality counts for a lot: Predictors of mental and physical health of spouse caregivers in two disease groups. *Journals of Gerontology: Psychological Sciences, 53*, 73–85.

Jacobson, N. S., Roberts, L . J., Berns, S . B., & McGlinchey, J . B. (1999). Methods for defining and determining the clinical significance of treatment effects: Description, application, and alternatives. *Journal of Consulting and Clinical Psychology, 67*, 300–307.

Janevic, M. R., & Connell, C. M. (2001). Racial, ethnic, and cultural differences in dementia caregiving: Recent findings. *The Gerontologist, 41*, 334–347.

Kim, J. H., & Knight, B. G. (2008). Effects of caregiver status, coping styles, and social support on the physical health of Korean American caregivers. *The Gerontologist, 48*, 287–299.

Kim, J. H., Knight, B. G., & Longmire, C. V. (2007). The role of familism in stress and coping processes among African American and White dementia caregivers: Effects on mental and physical health. *Health Psychology, 26*, 564–576.

Knight, B. G., Kaskie, B., Shurgot, G. R., & Dave, J. (2006). Improving the mental health of older adults. In J. E. Birren & K. W. Schaie (Eds.), *Handbook of the psychology of aging* (6th ed.) (pp. 407–424). San Diego, CA: Elsevier.

Knight, B. G., Longmire, C. V., Dave, J., Kim, J. H., & David, S. (2007). Mental health and physical health of family caregivers for persons with dementia: A comparison of African American and white caregivers. *Aging & Mental Health, 11*, 538–546.

Knight, B. G., Lutzky, S. M., & Macofsky-Urban, F. (1993). A meta-analytic review of interventions for caregiver distress: Recommendations for future research. *The Gerontologist, 33*, 240–248.

Knight, B. G., Robinson, G. S., Longmire, C. V. F., Chun, M., Nakao, K., & Kim, J. H. (2002). Cross cultural issues in caregiving for persons with dementia: Do familism values reduce burden and distress? *Ageing International, 27*, 70–94.

Knight, B. G., & Sayegh, P. (2010) Cultural values and caregiving: Updated sociocultural stress and coping model. *Journals of Gerontology: Psychological Sciences,* 65, 5–13.

Knight, B. G., Silverstein, M., McCallum, T. J., & Fox, L. S. (2000). A Sociocultural Stress and Coping Model for mental health outcomes among African American caregivers in Southern California. *Journals of Gerontology: Psychological Sciences, 55*, 142–150.

Lazarus, R. S., & Folkman, S. (1984). *Stress, appraisal, and coping.* New York: Springer.

Li, L. W., Seltzer, M. M., & Greenberg, J. S. (1999). Change in depressive symptoms among daughter caregivers: An 18-month longitudinal study. *Psychology and Aging, 14*, 206–219.

Lieberman, M. A., & Fisher, L. (2001). The effects of nursing home placement on family caregivers of patients with Alzheimer's disease. *The Gerontologist, 41*, 819–826.

Lyketsos, C. G., Steele, C., Galik, E., Rosenblatt, A., Steinberg, M., Warren, A., et al. (1999). Physical aggression in dementia patients and its relationship to depression. *American Journal of Psychiatry, 156*, 66–71.

Marks, N. F., Lambert, J. D., & Choi, H. (2002). Transitions to caregiving, gender, and psychological well-being: A prospective U.S. National Study. *Journal of Marriage and Family, 64*, 657–667.

Márquez-González, M., Losada, A., Izal, M., Pérez-Rojo, G., & Montorio, I. (2007). Modification of dysfunctional thoughts about caregiving in dementia family caregivers: Description and outcomes of an intervention program. *Aging & Mental Health, 11*, 616–625.

Mausbach, B. T., Aschbacher, K., Patterson, T. L., von Känel, R., Dimsdale, J. E., Mills, P. J., et al. (2007). Effects of placement and bereavement on psychological well-being and cardiovascular risk in Alzheimer's caregivers: A longitudinal analysis. *Journal of Psychosomatic Research, 62*, 439–455.

McCusker, J., Latimer, E., Cole, M., Ciampi, A., & Sewitch, M. (2007). Major depression among medically ill elders contributes to sustained poor mental health in their informal caregivers. *Age and Ageing, 36*, 400–406.

Mittelman, M. S., Haley, W. E., Clay, O. J., & Roth, D. L. (2006). Improving caregiver well-being delays nursing home placement of patients with Alzheimer disease. *Neurology, 67*, 1592–1599.

Navaie-Waliser, M., Feldman, P. H., Gould, D. A., Levine, C., Kuerbis, A. N., & Donelan, K. (2001). The experiences and challenges of informal caregivers: Common themes and differences among whites, blacks, and Hispanics. *The Gerontologist, 41*, 733–741.

Pearlin, L. I., & Aneshensel, C. S. (1994). Caregiving: The unexpected career. *Social Justice Research, 7*, 373–390.

Pearlin, L. I., Mullan, J. T., Semple, S. J., & Skaff, M. M. (1990). Caregiving and the stress process: An overview of concepts and their measures. *The Gerontologist, 30*, 583–591.

Pillemer, K., & Finkelhor, D. (1988). The prevalence of elder abuse: A random sample survey. *The Gerontologist, 28*, 51–57.

Pillemer, K., & Suitor, J. J. (1992). Violence and violent feelings: What causes them among family caregivers? *Journals of Gerontology, 47*, 165–172.

Pillemer, K., Suitor, J. J., Henderson, C. R., Meador, R., Schultz, L., Robison, J., et al. (2003). A cooperative communication intervention for nursing home staff and family members of residents. *The Gerontologist, 43*, 96–106.

Pinquart, M., & Sörensen, S. (2003). Differences between caregivers and noncaregivers in psychological health and physical health: A meta-analysis. *Psychology and Aging, 18*, 250–267.

Pinquart, M., & Sörensen, S. (2005). Ethnic differences in stressors, resources, and psychological outcomes of family caregiving: A meta-analysis. *The Gerontologist, 45*, 90–106.

Pinquart, M., & Sörensen, S. (2006). Helping caregivers of persons with dementia: Which interventions work and how large are their effects? *International Psychogeriatrics*, 18, 577–595.

Pinquart, M., & Sörensen, S. (2007). Correlates of physical health of informal caregivers: A meta-analysis. *Journals of Gerontology: Psychological Sciences, 62*, 126–137.

Robinson-Whelen, S., Tada, Y., MacCallum, R. C., McGuire, L., & Kiecolt-Glaser, J. K. (2001). Long-term caregiving: What happens when it ends? *Journal of Abnormal Psychology, 110*, 573–584.

Roth, D. L., Haley, W. E., Owen, J. E., Clay, O. J., & Goode, K. T. (2001). Latent growth models of the longitudinal effects of dementia caregiving: A comparison of African American and White family caregivers. *Psychology and Aging, 16*, 427–436.

Rozario, P. A., & DeRienzis, D. (2008). Familism beliefs and psychological distress among African American women caregivers. *The Gerontologist, 48*, 772–780.

Russo, J., Vitaliano, P. P., Brewer, D. D., Katon, W., & Becker, J. (1995). Psychiatric disorders in spouse caregivers of care recipients with Alzheimer's disease and matched controls: A diathesis-stress model of psychopathology. *Journal of Abnormal Psychology, 104*, 197–204.

Sasaki, M., Arai, A., & Arai, Y. (2008). Factors related to institutionalization among disabled older people; A two-year longitudinal study. *International Journals of Geriatric Psychiatry, 23*, 113–115.

Schulz, R., & Beach, S. R. (1999). Caregiving as a risk factor for mortality: The caregiver health effects study. *JAMA, 282*, 2215–2219.

Schulz, R., Belle, S. H., Czaja, S. J., McGinnis, K. A., Stevens, A., & Zhang, S. (2004). Long-term care placement of dementia patients and caregiver health and well-being. *JAMA, 25*, 961–967.

Schulz, R., O'Brien, A., Czaja, S., Ory, M., Norris, R., Martire, L. M., et al. (2002). Dementia Caregiver Intervention Research: In search of clinical significance. *The Gerontologist, 42*, 589–602.

Schulz, R., & Williamson, G. M. (1991). A 2-year longitudinal study of depression among Alzheimer's caregivers. *Psychology and Aging, 6*, 569–578.

Seltzer, M. M., & Li, L. W. (2000). The dynamics of caregiving: Transitions during a three-year prospective study. *The Gerontologist, 40*, 165–178.

Skaff, M. M., Pearlin, L. I., & Mullan, J. T. (1996). Transitions in the caregiving career: Effects on sense of mastery. *Psychology & Aging, 11*, 247–257.

Sörensen, S., Pinquart, M., & Duberstein, P. (2002). How effective are interventions with caregivers? An updated meta-analysis. *The Gerontologist, 42*, 356–372.

Sörensen, S., & Pinquart, M. (2005). Racial and ethnic differences in the relationship of caregiving stressors, resources, and sociodemographic variables to caregiver depression and perceived physical health. *Aging & Mental Health, 9*, 482–495.

Teri, L., McCurry, S. M., Logsdon, R., & Gibbons, L. E. (2005). Training community consultants to help family members improve dementia care: A randomized controlled trial. *The Gerontologist, 45*, 802–811.

Vitaliano, P. P., Zhang, J., & Scanlan, J. M. (2003). Is caregiving hazardous to one's physical health? A meta-analysis. *Psychological Bulletin, 129*, 946–972.

Zarit, S. H., & Femia, E. E. (2008). A future for family care and dementia intervention research? Challenges and strategies. *Aging & Mental Health, 12*, 5–13.

Chapter | 24 |

Decision Making Capacity

Jennifer Moye,[1] Daniel Marson,[2] Barry Edelstein,[3] Stacey Wood,[4] Aida Saldivar[5]

[1]Director, Geriatric Mental Health, VA Boston Healthcare System, Massachusetts, USA; [2]Department of Neurology, University of Alabama-Birmingham, Birmingham, Alabama, USA; [3]Department of Psychology, West Virginia University, Morgantown, West Virginia, USA; [4]Department of Psychology, Scripps College, Claremont, California, USA; [5]Boston VA Medical Center, Boston, Massachusetts, USA

CHAPTER CONTENTS

Introduction **367**
What is Meant by the Term Capacity? 368
Where are Matters of Capacity Resolved? 368
Evolution of Capacity as a Prominent Concern in Society, Practice, and Research 368
A Conceptual Framework for Capacity Assessment **369**
Legal Standards for Capacity 369
Capacity as Defined in Guardianship Law 369
Capacity as Defined in Health Care Consent Law 370
The Relationship of Law to the Science of Decision Making 370
Consent Capacities **371**
Capacity to Consent to Medical Treatment 371
Studies of Medical Conditions Associated with Medical Consent Capacity 371
Studies of Cognitive Abilities Needed for Medical Consent Capacity 371
Capacity to Consent to Research 372
Studies of Medical Conditions Associated with Research Consent Capacity 372
Capacity to Consent to Sexual Relations 372
Everyday Skill-Based Capacities **372**
Capacity to Manage Finances 372
Studies of Medical Conditions Associated with Financial Capacity 373
Studies of Cognitive Abilities Needed for Financial Capacity 373
Capacity to Live Independently 373
Studies of Medical Conditions Associated with Independent Living Capacity 373
Studies of Cognitive Abilities Needed for Independent Living Capacity 374
Capacity to Drive 374
Studies of Medical Conditions Associated with Driving Capacity 374
Studies of Cognitive Abilities Needed for Driving Capacity 374
Planning for Future Incapacity: Capacities to Designate and Direct Surrogates and Executors **374**
Capacity to Appoint an Agent Under a Durable Power of Attorney or Healthcare Proxy 375
Capacity to Execute a Will 375
Assessment of Capacity **375**
Future Directions **376**
Acknowledgments **376**
References **377**

INTRODUCTION

This chapter reviews the conceptual and empirical basis for the assessment of legal capacities in older adults. Legal capacities (formerly called competencies) are distinguished from the important conceptual, empirical, and clinical work to date in defining, measuring, and maintaining functional everyday competence (e.g., Willis et al., 1997). This chapter summarizes a framework

DOI: 10.1016/B978-0-12-380882-0.00024-3

for clinical assessment but is not a "how to" guide to clinical assessment. This chapter draws upon material developed by the authors for *Assessment of Older Adults with Diminished Capacity: A Handbook for Psychologists* (*ABA–APA Handbook*) under the auspices of a joint working group of the American Bar Association (ABA) and American Psychological Association (APA; American Bar Association and American Psychological Association Assessment of Capacity in Older Adults Project Working Group, 2008). For more in-depth direction regarding clinical assessment, readers may refer to the *ABA–APA Handbook* as well as other sources on clinical assessment (Grisso, 2003; Lichtenberg, 1999).

What is Meant by the Term Capacity?

"Decision making capacity," "decisional capacity," "capacity," and "competency" are terms used in clinical and legal settings – often used differently or incorrectly (Ganzini et al., 2003) – that can be confusing. Therefore, it is important to be quite precise in their use. In this chapter, the term clinical "capacity" will refer to a professional clinical judgment as to whether a specific individual has the requisite cognitive, decisional, affective, and practical abilities to adequately complete a specific task (e.g., drive a car) or make a specific decision (e.g., refuse a medical treatment). The term is frequently used when an individual who has a neuropsychiatric condition makes a decision that puts his or her health, assets, property, or self at significant risk – typically a risk that is new for the person and incongruent with past behavior. Clinicians or family members may raise the question, "Does this individual have decision making capacity?" and seek the authority to make, or appoint, or enact a surrogate to make decisions for the older adult. The term capacity is favored in clinical settings and legal settings, as less pejorative and more precise, although the term competency is still encountered in both settings.

Where are Matters of Capacity Resolved?

In health care settings, questions of capacity are often encountered in regard to medical consent, sexual consent, financial management, independent living, and driving. In contrast, a host of specific financial capacities that are less likely to arise in health care settings may arise in court settings and be referred to clinicians in forensic private practice, including testamentary capacity, donative capacity, capacity to contract, and capacity to convey real property (Marson et al., 2000). These "civil" capacities are distinguished from "criminal" capacities that arise when an individual has been charged with a crime (e.g., capacity to stand trial, capacity for criminal responsibility, etc.).

Decisions about capacity are ultimately legal judgments enforced by the power of the state. However, in practice, most clinical judgments of capacity are made without court involvement, by clinicians, attorneys, adult protective service workers, and other professional groups working with the elderly. In cases where there exists a previously appointed surrogate (such as a health care proxy), the authority of the surrogate springs into effect on the basis of a clinical finding of diminished capacity without judicial review. Further, in practice, many situations of diminished capacity are managed without appointment of a surrogate. For example, a caregiver of an adult with dementia may simply assume responsibility for bill paying and investments, or strategically disallow driving. The variable roles of the family, clinician, and judicial system in managing diminished capacities in older adults can create considerable confusion but are important to recognize (Ganzini et al., 2003).

Evolution of Capacity as a Prominent Concern in Society, Practice, and Research

A number of sociodemographic forces have made capacity assessment an emerging concern. The U.S. population is aging rapidly. While age itself does not infer loss of cognitive functioning or incapacity, cognitive and physical losses accompanying diseases such as dementia are intimately linked with declines in everyday functioning (Karlawish & Schmitt, 2000). Attention to capacity issues is also increasing due to large-scale financial and cultural changes, and associated risks of elder abuse and undue influence. The current older generation has amassed wealth, and consequently our society is undergoing a massive transfer of wealth from the World War II to the Baby Boomer generation (Havens & Schervish, 2003) within families that are increasingly blended and living at geographical distance. As a result, probate courts are seeing a marked rise in contested guardianships and wills. There is a high prevalence of elder abuse, exploitation, and undue influence by strangers, friends, and family members (National Center for Elder Abuse, 2005) who seek to take financial advantage of vulnerable seniors and their assets, resulting in an increased need for experts in these areas.

In response to these rapid societal shifts, capacity assessment has emerged as a distinct field of research (Marson et al., 1996). The origins of the field lie in a series of important articles reviewing legal standards and ethical issues in the capacity to consent to treatment (Appelbaum & Grisso, 1988; Berg et al., 1996; President's Commission, 1982; Roth et al., 1977), followed by later efforts to integrate and summarize the field of capacity (Smyer et al., 1996). The emergence of assessment frameworks and forensic assessment tools, growing out of this early work, has enabled empirical study of the assessment of capacity in older adults, although many important areas remain virtually without study.

A CONCEPTUAL FRAMEWORK FOR CAPACITY ASSESSMENT

In this chapter we will use the capacity assessment framework developed in the ABA–APA Handbook (2008). This framework will guide our summary of assessment as well as our review of the empirical literature in this chapter. The ABA–APA framework expands upon Grisso's seminal conceptual work on capacity (Grisso, 1986, 2003) by setting out nine components necessary for clinical capacity assessment of older adults: (1) Legal Standard, (2) Functional Elements, (3) Diagnosis, (4) Cognitive Underpinnings, (5) Psychiatric or Emotional Factors, (6) Values, (7) Risk Considerations, (8) Steps to Enhance Capacity, and (9) Clinical Judgment of Capacity, as shown in Figure 24.1.

In this framework, a key element in coming to a professional judgment regarding capacity is measuring and defining the relationships of the medical diagnoses, cognitive abilities, and psychiatric symptoms to the functional abilities. These relationships that have been the main focus of empirical efforts will be summarized in each capacity section later.

Legal Standards for Capacity

All adults are presumed to have capacity in the eyes of the law unless otherwise determined in a court of law. Capacity, when used as a legal term, refers to a judicial finding regarding an individual, as raised in the context of a legal hearing or dispute, and in consideration of the legal standard. A legal standard (sometimes called a legal test), refers to how capacity is defined in statute and case law. The components of the legal capacity found in the law define the constituent functional elements around which clinicians will want to organize their evidence collection and opinion formation.

Capacity as Defined in Guardianship Law

Questions of civil capacity of older adults come to the court often in guardianship proceedings. States use the term guardianship differently. Some states use the term conservatorship for all guardianship, while other states use the term guardianship to refer to guardianship of the person, and conservatorship to refer to guardianship of the estate. The legal process for guardianship begins when a family member or other interested party files a petition for guardianship of another individual, followed by a hearing to determine the legal capacity of the alleged incapacitated person. If incapacity is found by the judge, a guardian is appointed. In many states there is a distinction

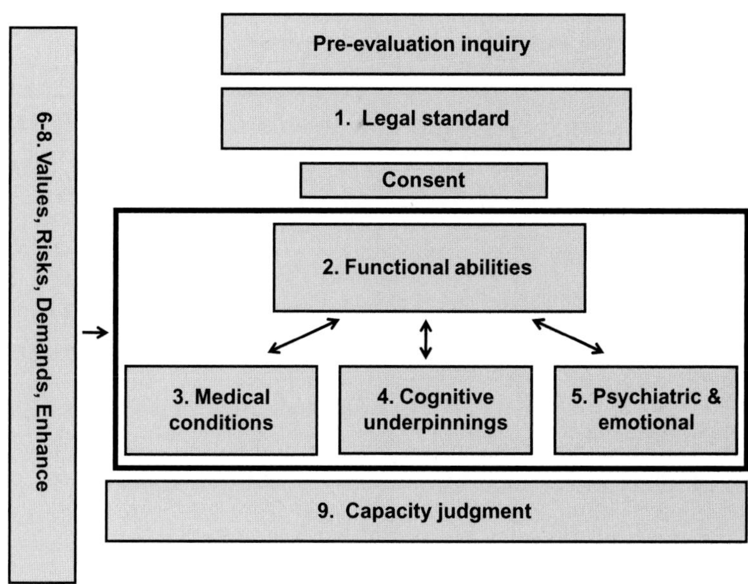

Figure 24.1 Capacity assessment framework.

between a guardian of the person (e.g., responsible for day-to-day issues of care, residence, activities) versus guardian of estate (e.g., responsible for managing assets; Quinn, 2004).

In determining capacity in guardianship hearings, judges rely upon "medical evidence," usually in the form of a clinical report or certificate completed by a physician, psychologist, or other qualified health care provider. Clinical evaluations for the purposes of guardianship have historically, and for the most part remain to this date, very brief and conclusory (meaning the clinician offers a conclusion but does not describe the data that supports the conclusion; Bulcroft et al.,1991; Dudley & Goins, 2003; Moye et al., 2007a,b).

In response to these problems, state statutes for guardianship have undergone massive reform over the past twenty years to enhance due process protections. Legal definitions of incapacity under guardianship have shifted away from diagnosis-based definitions to "functional" definitions. In most states, a diagnosis is considered relevant but not dispositive for finding incapacity. Courts are interested in diagnoses but often more in how the disorders or symptoms of the disorder impact functioning (e.g., decision making, judgment, behavior, etc.; Parry, 1988), allowing them for "limited guardianships" that provide the guardians with limited authority to make decisions in only those areas where the individuals requires assistance, and preserves rights in other domains.

Capacity as Defined in Health Care Consent Law

Capacity to consent to medical treatment is rooted in the concept of informed consent as voluntary (the person must not be coerced), knowledgeable (the person must be informed about the condition, treatments, and alternatives), and the person must have the capacity to make the decision (Berg et al., 2001). The Uniform Health Decisions Act defines medical consent capacity as an individual's "ability to understand the significant benefits, risks, and alternatives to proposed health care and to make and communicate a health care decision" (National Conference of Commissioners on Uniform State Laws, 1993). State-specific definitions regarding medical consent capacity are often located in advance directive statutes, durable power of attorney statutes, and in the body of case law. The capacity to consent to medical treatment is perhaps the most well studied and articulated civil capacity.

In reviewing consent capacity law within the United States, various scholars have identified four discrete abilities that are often present in legal standards for medical consent capacity: the ability to understand diagnostic and treatment information, appreciate the significance of this information, reason about the risks and benefits of treatment alternatives, and evidence a choice (Grisso & Appelbaum, 1998a). A problem in one or more of these areas, in concert with other factors, may lead to legal determinations of incapacity to make a medical decision. "Understanding" refers to the ability to comprehend diagnostic and treatment-related information. This concept includes not only the ability to remember newly presented words and phrases but also the ability to comprehend the meaning of these words and phrases, and to exhibit that comprehension to the physician or evaluator. "Appreciation" refers to the ability to determine the significance of the treatment information relative to the individual's situation, focusing on the nature of the diagnosis and the possibility that treatment would be beneficial, and involves both cognitive and emotional appreciation. Thus, "understanding" refers to whether the individual can comprehend basic information about a condition and treatment, while "appreciation" refers to whether the individual believes that the information is accurate and applies to him or her. "Reasoning" is the process of deciding on treatment by comparing alternatives in light of consequences, and through integrating, analyzing, and manipulating information. Reasoning involves including drawing inferences about the impact of alternatives on everyday life considering one's own personal values and preferences. Although it is not usually explicitly stated, the verb "to make" in some health care capacity statutes may refer to the process of reasoning. "Expressing a choice" concerns the basic ability to communicate a decision about treatment, and applies to individuals who cannot or will not express a choice, or who are ambivalent (Grisso & Appelbaum, 1995a).

The Relationship of Law to the Science of Decision Making

Because fundamental ethical issues of autonomy and legal issues of rights are at stake, it is critical that clinical assessments of capacity be reliable and valid. Clinical assessments must be reliable, that is, reasonably consistent across evaluators and time (assuming no clinical changes), rather than being subjective, or overly influenced or biased by the subjective opinion of one person. Clinical assessments must also be valid, that is, comprehensively assess the cognitive, emotional, and functional abilities that are relevant to the capacity, based on the body of scientific evidence supporting practice. One considerable challenge in exercising evidence-based practice in capacity assessment is the fact that capacity assessments must be grounded in the law. Legal conceptualizations of capacity are developed in a framework of justice, not science, based on what lawmakers have thought to define as rational or sound decision making (Moye, 1996).

These legal definitions of capacity, however, are not consistent with what we know about how humans approach and arrive at decisions. For example, in decision science there have been challenges to the rational models of decision making that appear to dominate the legal constructs and assessments of capacity (Kahneman, 2003). At present, capacity assessments measure explicit, conscious, analytic processes through the evaluation of discrete neuropsychological domains. However, it is now accepted that decision making occurs through a dual-process model incorporating a recognition of unconscious, affective heuristic processes important for decision making (Loewenstein et al., 2001). Although this may be an oversimplification, it points to the role of non-rational, less conscious factors in decision making. For example, Damasio's Somatic Marker Hypotheses emphasizes the importance of affective cues in the assessment of risk using the Iowa Gambling Task (Bechara & Damasio, 1997). Other tasks used to assess risk and "hot" (emotional) versus "cold" (calm) decision making are being used in experimental work, but have not yet been incorporated into capacity assessments (Figner et al., 2009). Finally, there is work in decision science on the importance of health literacy and financial literacy on decision making, but these constructs are not always assessed in the field (Peters et al., 2007). As capacity research evolves, it will hopefully incorporate decision science, and together these will inform clinical practice and the law. Until then, the individual clinician expert must be guided in the assessment approach and clinical judgment through a skillful integration of the law and science.

CONSENT CAPACITIES

Perhaps the most commonly evaluated capacity in the health care setting is the capacity to consent to treatment, which relies upon the modern doctrine of informed consent previously described. Informed consent to medical treatment is similar to other consent situations, such as consent to research and consent to sexual relations, in that it involves cognitive and affective skills and judgment, rather than performance or procedural skills such as are needed for driving, managing finances, or day-to-day living.

Capacity to Consent to Medical Treatment

The capacity to consent to treatment is considered to involve four decision-making abilities that match legal standards for medical consent previously reviewed: understanding, appreciation, reasoning, and expressing a choice. There are numerous standardized instruments including The Capacity Competency to Consent to Treatment Instrument (Marson et al., 1995a); Hopemont Capacity Assessment Interview (Edelstein et al., 1993); MacArthur Competence Assessment Tool–Treatment (Grisso & Appelbaum, 1998b); and Assessment of the Capacity to Consent to Treatment (Moye et al., 2008). Some of these instruments use a standardized vignette; others provide semi-structured interview questions. Across these instruments, the inter-rater reliability is fair to good, however, test-retest and internal consistency reliability have rarely been studied, and normative data are scant. Validity has been studied by comparing scores obtained on these capacity instruments with ratings by clinicians, experts, and scores on neuropsychological tests. Most validity studies, however, are based in relatively small samples with limited replication.

Studies of Medical Conditions Associated with Medical Consent Capacity

Consent capacity of individuals with dementia is reduced compared to healthy controls (Kim & Caine, 2002; Marson et al., 1996; Moye et al., 2004) specifically due to impairments in understanding and reasoning. In these same studies, the capacity to personally appreciate the diagnosis and the risks and benefits of treatment was inconsistently impaired in older adults with dementia. In control-comparison studies with younger individuals with schizophrenia, results are mixed, with some studies showing impairment relative to controls and others not (Grisso & Appelbaum, 1995b; Wong et al., 2000). In general, the pattern of decisional impairment associated with schizophrenia is quite variable, possibly related to the vast heterogeneity found within the disorder.

Studies of Cognitive Abilities Needed for Medical Consent Capacity

Diminished consent capacity has been associated with impairments in memory, executive functions, and comprehension. Specifically, difficulties understanding diagnostic and treatment information have been strongly related to impaired memory, as well as impaired conceptualization, and comprehension (Gurrera et al., 2006; Marson et al., 1995a, 1996). In these same studies, appreciation has been weakly associated with executive functions and conceptualization. Reasoning, involving contrasting risks and benefits, and relating them to personal preferences, has been associated with executive abilities, such as attention, mental flexibility, and additional to the ability to recall information after a delay. Expressing a choice is a basic consent ability, and has been empirically associated with auditory comprehension and confrontation naming.

Capacity to Consent to Research

Capacity to provide informed consent for research participation has some commonalities with capacity to consent to medical treatment; both require a person's consent, often involving a medical treatment, and the ability to consent is influenced by cognitive and affective factors. Capacity to consent to research participation differs from medical consent in two critical ways. First, the purpose of participation is to advance knowledge, and unlike medical treatment, participation may provide no direct benefit to the patient. Second, the principal investigator and research staff have a research relationship with the patient, not a treatment relationship (Kim et al., 2001). These differences may be difficult for some patients to grasp, but they must be distinguished and understood by the patient for true informed consent (ABA–APA Handbook, 2008). In addition, federal and local regulations will stipulate what must be disclosed in the informed consent form (Dukoff & Sunderland, 1997). While these stipulations are intended to inform and protect the research participant, they can be detailed and esoteric — involving the maintenance of research records and the audit of research studies by regulatory authorities. All these factors, as well as the inherent complexity of the research study itself, make the task of disclosure, understanding, appreciation, and reasoning, potentially much more difficult and wrought with conflicts of interest than informed consent for medical treatment. Instruments to assess the capacity to consent to research are now being developed, such as the MacArthur Competence Assessment Tool - Clinical Research (Dunn, 2006; Dunn et al., 2006; Sturman, 2005).

Studies of Medical Conditions Associated with Research Consent Capacity

Adults with Alzheimer's disease have a reduced ability to provide informed consent for participating in research (Karlawish et al., 2002; Kim et al., 2001). Among patients with schizophrenia, psychiatric symptoms are generally not predictive of decisional capacity (Palmer & Salva, 2007). In bipolar disorder, manic symptoms may decrease the capacity to consent to research (Misra et al., 2008; Palmer et al., 2007). Other research, such as on the cognitive abilities needed for research consent capacity, is needed.

Capacity to Consent to Sexual Relations

For older adults, questions of sexual consent capacity arise infrequently and occur most often in long-term care facilities where individuals with varying degrees of cognitive deficit are engaging in sexual activities, and staff are concerned that one or both partners may be so impaired as to not have the capacity to consent to the activity (Lichtenberg & Strzepek, 1990). Long-term care facilities that are licensed by their states have a legal obligation to protect their residents from unreasonable harm (Lyden, 2007), while also promoting autonomy and individual rights. Under American law, all individuals who have reached the age of consent have the right, and are assumed to have the capacity, to consent to sexual relations.

Like informed consent for medical treatment, informed consent to sexual relations requires some degree of being "informed" (i.e., having knowledge about the sexual activities, associated risks and responsibilities). Capacity to consent to sexual activity is thought to include the ability to understand the options related to the sexual behavior, appreciate the consequences of various courses of action, and express a choice that is based on a rational or logical consideration of relevant knowledge, including the personal benefits and risks of the sexual activity, and is consistent with the individual's values and preferences. Unique aspects of sexual consent capacity - including its physical, relational, and affective nature — differentiate it from other forms of consent capacity (Kennedy, 1999). There are no instruments to assess sexual consent capacity, although frameworks exist (see ABA–APA Handbook, 2008).

EVERYDAY SKILL-BASED CAPACITIES

In contrast to consent capacities that are chiefly cognitive and affective, other types of capacity that may come into question for older adults with neurological or psychiatric illness, are those capacities of everyday living, such as the capacity to manage finances, the capacity to manage independent living, and the capacity to drive. These capacities have in common their reliance on having content related knowledge and judgment as well as the application of skills to practice.

Capacity to Manage Finances

Financial capacity is a medical-legal construct that represents the ability to independently manage one's financial affairs in a manner consistent with personal self-interest and values (Marson & Hebert, 2008a). Financial capacity, thus, involves not only performance skills (e.g., counting coins/currency accurately, completing a check register accurately, paying bills), but also judgment skills that optimize financial self-interest and promote independence, and values that guide personal financial choices. Due to differences in background and experience, financial experience and skills can vary widely among cognitively normal individuals and are associated with factors of education and socioeconomic status.

From a legal standpoint, financial capacity represents the financial skills sufficient for handling one's estate and financial affairs, and is the basis for determinations of conservatorship of the estate (or guardianship of the estate, depending on the state legal jurisdiction). Broadly construed, financial capacity also conceptually encompasses more specific legal capacities, such as contractual capacity, donative capacity, and testamentary capacity. Thus, financial capacity is an important area of assessment in the civil legal system (Marson & Hebert, 2008a). Marson and colleagues (2000) have proposed a clinical model of financial capacity that represents an initial effort at identifying functional elements constituent to this capacity (Griffith et al., 2003), including basic monetary skills, conceptual knowledge, cash transactions, checkbook management, bank statement management, financial judgment, bill payment, knowledge of assets, and investment decision making. The model focuses on both performance and judgment skills and conceptualizes financial capacity at these three increasingly complex levels.

Functional assessment instruments for the evaluation of the capacity to manage finances include: the Financial Capacity Instrument (FCI), a comprehensive assessment of nine financial domains (Marson et al., 2000); Decision-making Interview for Guardianship (DIG), four vignettes assessing social judgment in financial situations (Anderer, 1997); Hopemont Capacity Assessment Interview (HCAI), three vignettes assessing social judgment in financial situations (Edelstein, et al., 1993); and the Independent Living Scales (ILS), one subscale with questions assessing financial knowledge and skills (Loeb, 1996). In addition there are a number of tools for the assessment of instrumental activities of daily living (IADLs) that include direct assessment of financial skills such as the Direct Assessment of Functional Status (DAFS; Loewenstein et al., 1989).

Studies of Medical Conditions Associated with Financial Capacity

Existing empirical research in this area has focused on changes in financial capacity occurring in the context of Alzheimer's disease and related disorders. Patients with amnestic mild cognitive impairment, the prodrome or transitional stage to Alzheimer's disease, already show emerging deficits in higher order financial skills, such as conceptual knowledge, bank statement management and bill payment, and also in overall financial capacity (Griffith et al., 2003). Patients with mild Alzheimer's disease have emerging global impairment across almost all financial tasks and most domains, while patients with moderate Alzheimer's disease have advanced global impairment in all financial areas (Marson et al., 2000). While financial capacity is already impaired in patients with mild Alzheimer's disease, a longitudinal study has also shown that there is rapid decline, in both simple and complex financial tasks, in mild Alzheimer's disease patients over a one-year period (Martin et al., 2008). In mild cognitive impairment (MCI) patients demonstrate detectable declines in complex financial skills such as using a checkbook and register in the year prior to conversion to Alzheimer's disease, (Triebel et al., 2009).

Studies of Cognitive Abilities Needed for Financial Capacity

Due to the functional complexity of the financial capacity construct, it is not surprising that there are a wide variety of cognitive abilities that inform financial capacity. Global financial capacity is associated primarily with written arithmetic abilities, and to a lesser extent with memory and executive function skills, across cognitively normal older adults, patients with amnestic MCI, and patients with mild Alzheimer's disease (Sherod et al., 2009).

Capacity to Live Independently

An older adult's capacity to live independently may be questioned when he or she develops a medical or neurological condition making it increasingly difficult to manage health and safety in the community, even when provided with environmental supports. A question may arise as to whether an older adult needs to move to a more supportive living setting such as assisted living or skilled nursing facility, and/or whether the person would benefit from the appointment of a guardian of the person. In most states, there is unlikely to be a specific legal standard for "the capacity to live independently." Instead, the most relevant legal standards for the capacity to live independently are those that are defined in guardianship law.

A number of instruments exist for assessing the capacity to live independently, such as the ILS; (Loeb, 1996) and the Texas Functional Living Scale (TFLS; Cullum et al., 2001). Clinical approaches to assessing such a broad capacity will likely utilize a wide array of traditional cognitive measures, as well as behavioral, psychiatric, and functional measures. Incorporating both subjective (i.e., what patient self-reports he or she can do) and objective (i.e., performance-based or direct observation) assessments of functional abilities is recommended because they can significantly vary from each other (Glass, 1997).

Studies of Medical Conditions Associated with Independent Living Capacity

In older adults, the most common disorder likely to affect the capacity to live independently is dementia. Innumerable studies have documented the relationship between the severity of dementia and the performance of functional abilities key to independent living (Hill et al., 1995; Tatemichi et al., 1994). Additionally, psychotic disorders are often associated with difficulties with independent living, associated with negative symptoms (Meeks & Walker, 1990). Furthermore, alcohol dependence and even moderate alcohol use is related to increased risk of functional impairment (Stuck et al., 1999).

Studies of Cognitive Abilities Needed for Independent Living Capacity

Specific cognitive predictors of independent living capacity are varied. Visuospatial and memory deficits are associated with a person's ability to manage medications (Richardson et al., 1995), while visuospatial problem solving and memory have been found to affect money management skills, as well as overall safety (Richardson et al., 1995). Attention deficits have been correlated with balance, falls, and activities of daily living (ADL) function (Hyndman & Ashburn, 2003). However, cognitive impairments are not the sole predictor of functional decline. A literature review of longitudinal studies published between 1985 and 1997 (Stuck et al., 1999) found that in addition to cognitive impairments, other factors associated with decline in functional status in older adults who live in the community included: depression, disease burden, increased or decreased body mass index, lower extremity functional limitation, low frequency of social contacts, poor self-perceived health, smoking, vision impairments, and low level of physical activity.

Capacity to Drive

Although there is variability across states in older driver re-licensing laws, the license to drive is generally dependent on a person's mental and/or physical condition and ability to follow traffic laws and rules, regardless of age (ABA–APA Handbook, 2008). The tremendous variety of physical, mental, and emotional problems that can result in an inability to operate a motor vehicle safely results in substantial assessment variability, but regardless of the nature or source of impairment, the legal standard considers the impact of a medical condition on the individual's ability to operate a motor vehicle with reasonable and ordinary control (National Committee on Uniform Traffic Laws and Ordinances, 2000).

A comprehensive assessment of driving capacity relies on a medical exam, neuropsychological evaluation, and driving evaluation. Important considerations are visual acuity, mental flexibility, and reaction time, as well as knowledge of road rules, judgment about driving, and appreciation of functional limits (ABA–APA Handbook, 2008).

Studies of Medical Conditions Associated with Driving Capacity

Medical conditions that are associated with abrupt changes in cognition, such as epilepsy, diabetes, or heart disease, can place an individual at higher risk for a motor vehicle accident, as do neurodegenerative diseases such as dementia. A close review of medications associated with these medical conditions is critical, as many prescription drugs can be sedating and impair driving ability. Medications known to impair driving include: opioids, benzodiazepines, antidepressants, hypnotics, antipsychotics, antihistamines, glaucoma agents, nonsteroidal anti-inflammatory drugs, and muscle relaxants (Carr, 2000).

Studies of Cognitive Abilities Needed for Driving Capacity

Consistent evidence has supported the notion that driving performance in older adults is related to visual attention and processing speed (Lee et al. 2003; Roenker et al., 2003). Changes in functional visual field, that area from which a person can attain visual information in a quick glance, has received particular interest. The useful-field-of-view (UFOV) test is a measure commonly used to assess functional visual field by testing visual processing speed and visual attention during higher order processing tasks. Studies have found a relation between performance on UFOV tests and future at-fault motor vehicle accidents (Ball et al., 2006; Owsley et al., 1998). The size of the functional visual field has been found to be affected by visual sensory function, delays in processing ability, difficulties with divided attention, and inability to ignore distracters (Ball et al., 1990; Owsley et al., 1995). Other important cognitive mechanisms associated with driving difficulties include impaired memory, impaired visual acuity, decline in peripheral vision, and decreased ability to perform two tasks simultaneously (Bravo & Nakayama, 1992; McGwin et al., 2000).

PLANNING FOR FUTURE INCAPACITY: CAPACITIES TO DESIGNATE AND DIRECT SURROGATES AND EXECUTORS

In recognition of the potential for future incapacities, individuals of all ages are encouraged to complete legal documents that direct others as to the person's plans and preferences in the event of one's incapacity or death. Legal documents that direct actions and appoint others in the event of one's incapacity are called durable powers of attorney for health care or finances, advance directives, living wills, or health care proxies. The legal document that directs the disposition of assets upon one's death is a will. Although quite different in scope, all of these documents require that the individual has capacity during execution of the document and is free of coercion.

Capacity to Appoint an Agent Under a Durable Power of Attorney or Healthcare Proxy

An individual's capacity to execute an advance directive for health care is different than the capacity to make specific medical decisions. The legal standard for capacity to execute a health care power of attorney is generally parallel to that of capacity to contract, focusing on understanding the nature and extent of the act. Similarly, the legal standard for creating a power of attorney has traditionally been based on the capacity to contract (ABA–APA Handbook, 2008). Some courts have held that the standard is similar to that for making a will (Regan & Gilfix, 2003), however, as litigation of this matter is nonexisting, specific guidance is lacking.

Although degree of cognitive impairment is associated with the capacity to appoint a power of attorney (Gregory et al., 2007), there is little research available on the topic and is an area in which clinicians are seeking more guidance. At times an individual is recognized to not have the capacity to make health care or financial decisions. A question then arises whether the individual can still appoint someone else to make decisions, typically considered a lower standard of capacity, and therefore avoiding the need for a guardian or conservator. Of note, some states have default surrogate laws that allow next of kin to make medical decisions in the absence of previously appointed health care agents (Karp & Wood, 2003).

Capacity to Execute a Will

Testamentary capacity is a legal construct that represents the level of mental capacity necessary to execute a valid will. If testamentary capacity is absent, then the will is void and fails. For reasons of public policy supporting the orderly probating of wills and distribution of assets to heirs, courts have traditionally applied a low legal threshold for finding testamentary capacity (Marson & Hebert, 2008b). Although requirements for testamentary capacity vary across states, four criteria have generally been identified. A testator must have (1) knowledge of what a will is, (2) knowledge of that class of individuals that represents the testator's potential heirs ("natural objects of one's bounty"), (3) knowledge of the nature and extent of one's assets, and (4) a general plan of distribution of assets to heirs (ABA–APA Handbook, 2008). The absence of one or more of these elements can serve as grounds for a court to invalidate a will due to lack of testamentary capacity. The way that courts weigh legal elements of testamentary capacity in determining the validity of a will varies across states. State laws may also specify unique psycho-legal standards for a will's validity or lack of validity, such as an "insane delusion" or "lucid interval." There is very little empirical research to date in the area of testamentary capacity and none specific to the effects of different diagnostic conditions or neurocognitive abilities on testamentary capacity. This remains an area where considerable valuable research can be done.

ASSESSMENT OF CAPACITY

Capacity assessments, grounded in the relevant legal standard, consider functional, cognitive, and emotional abilities in the context of values, risks, and the means to enhance capacity. Age, race, ethnicity, culture, gender, sexual orientation, and religion may affect a person's values and preferences for health care, where or how he or she lives, how money is spent, with whom time is spent, and the level of risk or comfort that is desirable to make life good or meaningful, among other factors (Blackhall et al., 1995; Hornung et al., 1998). Such values lay the personal foundation for decisions. Consideration of values is one of the key areas where issues of diversity and individual differences enter into a capacity assessment. The extent to which an individual's current decisions are consistent with long-standing values may be an indicator of capacity (American Bar Association, 2003), although it should be noted that values may change with experience, so a change in values does not in itself indicate a change in capacity. Capacity assessments often involve understanding the process by which a person came to a decision. The evaluator's job is to evaluate the decision-making *process*, but not the outcome. Thus, it is important to remember that an individual has the right to make a decision that the examiner may personally think is unwise for the individual, especially when those decisions are consistent with long held values, preferences.

Risk assessment plays a key role in capacity evaluation (Ruchinskas, 2005), which considers the seriousness of the risk and the likelihood of risk in the context of the supports available (or that could be made available) to minimize the risk. Although some degree of risk is present in making any decision or doing any task, the evaluator examines whether the risk facing the individual is significant, and more than his or her peers face in similar situations.

At times, an older adult may be thought to lack capacity, but would not if appropriate accommodations were made, such as those to enhance hearing or vision or comprehension. Like any geriatric assessment, capacity evaluation can provide an opportunity to outline interventions and to determine whether capacity needs to be reconsidered after interventions have been given time to work. Familiarity with common interventions to help older adults compensate for sensory, cognitive, and physical deficits is therefore useful for those doing capacity evaluation.

One thing that distinguishes capacity assessment from general geriatric assessments is the extent of work that typically occurs prior to the actual assessment. The evaluator must first be an investigator to clarify the referral; namely what capacities are in question, the background to the referral, why the question is being raised, and where the outcome of the assessment may lead. Once the specific capacity in question is understood, the evaluator can define the relevant legal standard and functional elements to consider. A review of the record, interviews with collaterals, and preparing for accommodations to maximize functioning during the standardized assessment often pre-date testing with the individual.

Informed consent must be obtained prior to completing a capacity assessment. Such consent should involve disclosure of the procedure, the associated risks and benefits, and assess the individual's understanding of these. The final report should describe in detail what was disclosed and how the person conveyed his or her consent or assent. The individual may lack the capacity to consent to the evaluation, but still assent (i.e., agreement to participate without fully demonstrating an understanding of the risks and benefits), which should then be distinguished and detailed in the written report.

The standardized assessment likely considers the functional elements relevant to the capacity, and includes a cognitive battery using neuropsychological tests, and a psychiatric evaluation. One of the most critical ways in which a capacity evaluation is distinguished from a neuropsychological evaluation is the inclusion of the functional assessment, ideally through the inclusion of standardized capacity instruments geared to assess the core functional elements, and/or a home visit, and/or observation of sample demonstrations of the task, and/or collaboration with other professionals (e.g., Occupational Therapists).

As a general rule it is useful to evaluate the cognitive functioning of the individual, focusing on those neuropsychological tasks most relevant to the capacity in question. Neuropsychological findings are relevant evidence, but like diagnosis, a level of evidence secondary to that of the core functional abilities. For example, if the capacity evaluation request is for an individual who is mildly delirious after one week of refusing dialysis, and the question surrounds the individuals' capacity to continue to refuse dialysis, it will be critical to evaluate mental status and determine the extent to which delirium is impacting the person's consent capacity. At the same time, the degree of delirium may make completion of extensive neuropsychological testing impossible and invalid. Therefore clinical judgment is always necessary in the selection of the neuropsychological battery. For a higher functioning person who is medically stable, and for whom the capacity issue is complex and high risk, a thorough neuropsychological assessment can be invaluable. The assessment of values and risks is typically completed through a clinical interview with the older adult, as well as through interviews with collaterals and review of history.

After all assessment data have been gathered, the clinician arrives at a clinical judgment of capacity. A professional clinical judgment is just that: it is the evaluator's opinion, bringing together all the data and weighing it in light of the person's values, risks, and interventions to maximize capacity. Like a neuropsychological report, a capacity report may well elucidate the diagnosis and describe the cognitive and psychiatric strengths and weaknesses. The capacity report, however, goes beyond these general clinical findings to offer an opinion about the capacity or capacities in question.

A professional finding of capacity involves weighing the obligation to promote autonomy versus protection from harm — a task that can be onerous but more clear in light of a careful and comprehensive standardized assessment. Clinical supervision and consultation are important in gaining clarity and confidence in offering clinical judgments about capacity, especially as the evaluator becomes familiar with the process, and when results of tests or procedures are inconsistent.

FUTURE DIRECTIONS

As the population continues to age and the need for assessment of capacities increases, it will be important to expand attention to capacity assessment in clinical training and in research. To optimize the understanding of capacity and its application in clinical practice and law, vigorous collaboration between clinical and legal professionals (e.g., attorneys, judges, courts, etc.) should continue to be encouraged. Additionally, enhancing knowledge about capacity in the general population will be useful to assist individuals in planning for future incapacities, recognizing diminished capacity in their loved ones, and to protect vulnerable adults from elder abuse and exploitation. Many areas of civil capacity as relevant to the aging society remain ripe for study, including all the specific capacity domains, as well as issues of undue influence.

ACKNOWLEDGMENTS

This chapter draws from material developed by the authors for the *Assessment of Older Adults with*

Diminished Capacity: A Handbook for Psychologists, a work product of the American Bar Association (ABA) and American Psychological Association (APA) Assessment of Capacity in Older Adults Project Working Group, established in 2003 under the auspices of the interdisciplinary Task Force on Facilitating APA/ABA Relations. The goal of the working group was to develop resources for members of the ABA and APA who were confronting challenges assessing civil capacities of older adults. The members of the ABA/APA Working Group for the *Handbook for Psychologists* were Barry Edelstein, PhD; Peter Lichtenberg, PhD, ABPP; Daniel Marson, JD, PhD; Jennifer Moye, PhD (co-editor); David Powers, PhD; Charles Sabatino, JD; Aida Saldivar, PhD, ABPP; Erica Wood, JD; Stacey Wood, PhD (co-editor). Deborah DiGilio, MPH, Director of the APA Office on Aging provided major staff support for the ABA-APA Handbook series. The handbooks are available online at www.apa.org/pi/aging.

REFERENCES

American Bar Association. (2003). *Model rules of professional conduction.* Washington DC: American Bar Association.

American Bar Association and American Psychological Association Assessment of Capacity in Older Adults Project Working Group. (2008). *Assessment of older adults with diminished capacity: A handbook for psychologists.* Washington DC: American Bar Association and American Psychological Association.

Anderer, S. J. (1997). Development of an instrument to evaluate the capacity of elderly persons to make personal care and financial decisions. Unpublished Dissertation, Allegheny University of the Health Sciences.

Appelbaum, P. S., & Grisso, T. (1988). Assessing patients' capacities to consent to treatment. *New England Journal of Medicine, 319,* 1635–1638.

Ball, K. K., Roenker, D. L., & Bruni, J. R. (1990). Developmental changes in attention and visual search throughout adulthood. In J. Enns (Ed.), *Advances in Psychology* (pp. 489–508). Amsterdam: North-Holland-Elsevier Science Publishers.

Ball, K. K., Roenker, D. L., Wadley, V. G., Edwards, J. B., Roth, D. L., McGwin, G., et al. (2006). Can high-risk older drivers be identified through performance-based measures in a department of motor vehicles setting? *Journal of the American Geriatrics Society, 54,* 77–84.

Bechara, A., & Damasio, H. (1997). Deciding advantageously before knowing the advantageous strategy. *Science, 275,* 1293.

Berg, J. W., Appelbaum, P. S., & Grisso, T. (1996). Constructing competence: Formulating standards of legal competence to make medical decisions. *Rutgers Law Review, 48,* 345–396.

Berg, J. W., Appelbaum, P. S., Lidz, C. W., & Parker, L. S. (2001). *Informed consent: Legal theory and clinical practice.* New York: Oxford.

Blackhall, L. J., Murphy, S. T., Frank, G., Michel, V., & Azen, S. (1995). Ethnicity and attitudes toward patient autonomy. *Journal of the American Medical Association, 274,* 820–825.

Bravo, M., & Nakayama, K. (1992). The role of attention in visual search tasks. *Perceptual Psychophysiology, 51,* 465–472.

Bulcroft, K. A., Kielkopf, M. R., & Tripp, K. (1991). Elderly wards and their legal guardians: Analysis of country probate records in Ohio and Washington. *Gerontologist, 31*(2), 156–164.

Carr, D. B. (2000). The older adult driver. *American Family Physician, 61,* 141–148.

Cullum, C. M., Saine, K., Chan, L. D., Martin-Cook, K., Gray, K. F., & Weiner, M. F. (2001). Performance-based instrument to assess functional capacity in dementia: The Texas Functional Living Scale. *Neuropsychiatry, Neuropsychology, and Behavioral Neurology, 14,* 103–108.

Dudley, K. C., & Goins, R. T. (2003). Guardianship capacity evaluations of older adults: Comparing current practice to legal standards in two states. *Journal of Aging and Social Policy, 15,* 97–115.

Dukoff, R., & Sunderland, T. (1997). Durable power of attorney and informed consent with Alzheimer's disease patients: A clinical study. *American Journal of Psychiatry, 154,* 1070–1075.

Dunn, L. B. (2006). Capacity to consent to research in schizophrenia: The expanding evidence base. *Behavioral Sciences & the Law, 24*(4), 431.

Dunn, L. B., Nowrangi, M. A., Palmer, B. W., Jeste, D. V., & Saks, E. R. (2006). Assessing decisional capacity for clinical research or treatment: A review of instruments. *American Journal of Psychiatry, 163*(8), 1323–1334.

Edelstein, B., Nygren, M., Northrop, L., Staats, N., & Pool, D. (1993, August). *Assessment of capacity to make financial and medical decisions.* Paper presented at the annual meeting of the American Psychological Association, Toronto.

Figner, B., Mackinlay, R., Wilkening, F., & Weber, E. (2009). Affective and deliberative processes in risky choice: Age differences in risk taking in the Columbia Card Task. *Journal of Experimental Psychology: Learning, Memory, and Cognition,* 709–730.

Ganzini, L., Volicer, L., Nelson, W., & Derse, A. (2003). Pitfalls in the assessment of decision-making capacity. *Psychosomatics, 44*(3), 237–243.

Glass, K. C. (1997). Refining definitions and devising

instruments: Two decades of assessing mental competence. *International Journal of Law and Psychiatry, 20*, 5–33.

Gregory, R., Roked, F., Jones, L., & Patel, A. (2007). Is the degree of cognitive impairment in patients with Alzheimer's disease related to their capacity to appoint an enduring power of attorney. *Age and Ageing, 36*, 527–531.

Griffith, H. R., Belue, K., Sicola, A., Krzywanski, S., Zamrini, E., Harrell, L., et al. (2003). Impaired financial abilities in mild cognitive impairment: A direct assessment approach. *Neurology, 60*, 449–457.

Grisso, T. (1986). *Evaluating Competencies*. NY: Plenum.

Grisso, T. (2003). *Evaluating competences* (2nd ed.). New York: Plenum.

Grisso, T., & Appelbaum, P. S. (1995a). Comparison of standards for assessing patient's capacities to make treatment decisions. *American Journal of Psychiatry, 152*, 1033–1037.

Grisso, T., & Appelbaum, P. S. (1995b). The MacArthur treatment competency study III: Abilities of patients to consent to psychiatric and medical treatment. *Law and Human Behavior, 19*, 149–174.

Grisso, T., & Appelbaum, P. S. (1998a). *Assessing competence to consent to treatment*. New York: Oxford.

Grisso, T., & Appelbaum, P. S. (1998b). *MacArthur competency assessment tool for treatment (MacCAT-T)*. Sarasota, FL: Professional Resource Press.

Gurrera, R. J., Moye, J., Karel, M. J., Azar, A. R., & Armesto, J. C. (2006). Cognitive performance predicts treatment decisional abilities in mild to moderate dementia. *Neurology, 66*, 1367–1372.

Havens, J. J., & Schervish, P. G. (2003). Why the $41 trillion wealth transfer estimate is still valid: A review of challenges and questions. *The Journal of Gift Planning, 7*, 11–15.

Hill, R. D., Backman, L., & Fratiglioni, L. (1995). Determinants of functional abilities in dementia. *Journal of the American Geriatrics Society, 43*, 1092–1097.

Hornung, C. A., Eleazer, G. P., Strothers, H. S., Wieland, G. D., Eng, C., McCann, R., et al. (1998). Ethnicity and decision-makers in a group of frail older people. *Journal of the American Geriatrics Society, 46*, 280–286.

Hyndman, D., & Ashburn, A. (2003). People with stroke living in the community: Attention deficits, balance, ADL ability and falls. *Disability and Rehabilitation, 25*, 817–822.

Kahneman, D. (2003). A perspective on judgment and choice: Mapping bounded rationality. *American Psychologist, 58*, 697–720.

Karlawish, J. H., Casarett, D. J., & James, B. D. (2002). Alzheimer's disease patients' and caregivers' capacity, competency, and reasons to enroll in an early-phase Alzheimer's disease clinical trial. *Journal of the American Geriatrics Society, 50*(12), 2019–2024.

Karlawish, J. H. T., & Schmitt, F. A. (2000). Why physicians need to become more proficient in assessing their patients' competency and how they can achieve this. *Journal of the American Geriatric Society, 48*, 1014–1016.

Karp, N., & Wood, E. (2003). *Incapacitated and alone: Health care decision-making for the unbefriended elderly*. Washington DC: American Bar Association.

Kennedy, C. (1999). Assessing competency to consent to sexual activity in the cognitively impaired population. *Journal of Forensic Neuropsychology, 1*, 17–33.

Kim, S. Y. H., & Caine, E. D. (2002). Utility and limits of the mini mental state examination in evaluating consent capacity in Alzheimer's disease. *Psychiatric Services, 53*(10), 1322–1324.

Lee, H. C., Lee, A. H., & Cameron, D. (2003). Validation of a driving stimulator by measuring the visual attention skill of older adult drivers. *The American Journal of Occupational Therapy, 57*, 324–328.

Lichtenberg, P. A., & Strzepek, D. M. (1990). Assessments of institutionalized dementia patients' competencies to participate in intimate relationships. *The Gerontologist, 30*, 117–120.

Lichtenberg, P. A. E. (1999). *Handbook of assessment in clinical gerontology*. New York: Wiley.

Loeb, P. (1996). *Independent Living Scales*. San Antonio: Psychological Corporation.

Loewenstein, D. A., Amigo, E., Duara, R., Guterman, A., Hurwitz, D., Berkowitz, N., et al. (1989). A new scale for the assessment of functional status in Alzheimer's disease and related disorders. *Journals of Gerontology Psychological Sciences, 44*, 114–121.

Loewenstein, G., Weber, E., Hsee, C., & Welch, N. (2001). Risk as feelings. *Psychological Bulletin, 127*, 267–286.

Lyden, M. (2007). Assessment of sexual consent capacity. *Sexual Disabilities, 25*, 3–20.

Marson, D. C., Chatterjee, A., Ingram, K. K., & Harrell, L. E. (1996). Toward a neurologic model of competency: Cognitive predictors of capacity to consent in Alzheimer's disease using three different legal standards. *Neurology, 46*, 666–672.

Marson, D. C., & Hebert, T. (2008a). Financial capacity. In B. L. Cutler (Ed.), *Encyclopedia of psychology and the law* (pp. 313-316). New York: Sage.

Marson, D. C., & Hebert, T. (2008b). Testamentary capacity. In B. L. Cutler (Ed.), *Encyclopedia of Psychology and the Law*. New York: Sage.

Marson, D. C., Sawrie, S., McInturff, B., Snyder, S., Chatterjee, A., Stalvey, T., et al. (2000). Assessing financial capacity in patients with Alzheimer's disease: A conceptual model and prototype instrument. *Archives of Neurology, 57*, 877–884.

Martin, R., Griffith, R., Belue, K., Harrell, L., Zamrini, E., Anderson, B., et al. (2008). Declining financial capacity in patients with mild Alzheimer's disease: A one-year longitudinal study. *American Journal of Geriatric Psychiatry, 16*, 209–219.

McGwin, G., Chapman, V., & Owsley, C. (2000). Visual risk factors for driving difficulty among older drivers. *Accident Analysis and Prevention., 32*, 735–744.

Meeks, S., & Walker, J. (1990). Blunted affect, blunted lives? Negative symptoms, ADL functioning, and mental health among older adults. *International Journal of Geriatric Psychiatry, 5*, 233–238.

Misra, S., Socherman, R., Park, B. S., Hauser, P., & Ganzini, L. (2008). Influence of mood state on capacity to consent to research in patients with bipolar disorder. *Bipolar Disorder, 10*, 303–309.

Moye, J. (1996). Theoretical frameworks for competency in cognitively impaired elderly adults. *Journal of Aging Studies, 10*(1), 27.

Moye, J., Butz, S. W., Marson, D. C., Wood, E., & ABA–APA Capacity Assessment of Older Adults Working Group. (2007a). A conceptual model and assessment template for capacity evaluation in adult guardianship. *The Gerontologist, 47*, 591–603.

Moye, J., Karel, M. J., Azar, A. R., & Gurrera, R. J. (2004). Capacity to consent to treatment: Empirical comparison of three instruments in older adults with and without dementia. *Gerontologist, 44*(2), 166.

Moye, J., Karel, M. J., Edelstein, B., Hicken, B., Armesto, J. C., & Gurrera, R. J. (2008). Assessment of capacity to consent to treatment: Current research, the "ACCT" approach, future directions. *Clinical Gerontologist, 31*, 37–66.

Moye, J., Wood, S., Edelstein, B., Armesto, J. C., Bower, E. H., Harrison, J. A., et al. (2007b). Clinical evidence for guardianship of older adults is inadequate: Findings from a tri-state study. *The Gerontologist, 47*, 604–612.

National Center for Elder Abuse. (2005). Fifteen questions and answers about elder abuse.

National Committee on Uniform Traffic Laws and Ordinances. (2000). *Uniform Vehicle Code*. Retrieved October 2, 2009, from www.ncutlo.org/modellaws.htm.

Uniform Health Decisions Act (1993).

Owsley, C., Ball, K., & Keeton, D. M. (1995). Relationship between visual sensitivity and target localization in older adults. *Vision Search*, 579–587.

Owsley, C., Ball, K., McGwin, G., Sloane, M. E., Roenker, D. L., & White, M. F. (1998). Visual processing impairment and risk of motor vehicle crash among older adults. *Journal of American Medical Association, 279*, 1083–1088.

Palmer, B. W., Dunn, L. B., Depp, C. A., Eyler, L. T., & Jeste, D. V. (2007). Decisional capacity to consent to research among patients with bipolar disorder: Comparison with schizophrenia patients and healthy subjects. *Journal of Clinical Psychiatry, 68*, 689–696.

Palmer, B. W., & Salva, G. N. (2007). The association of specific neuropsychological deficits with capacity to consent to research or treatment. *Journal of the International Neuropsychological Society, 13*, 1047–1059.

Parry, J. (1988). Mental and Physical Disability Law Reporter. Selected recommendations from the national guardianship symposium at Wingspread, *12*, 398–406.

Peters, E., Hibbard, J., Slovic, P., & Dieckmann, N. (2007). Numeracy skill and the communication, comprehension, and use of risk-benefit information. *Health Affairs, 26*, 741–748.

President's Commission for the study of ethical problems in medicine and biomedical and behavioral research: Making health care decisions. *Vol. 1*. (1982). Washington DC: Author.

Quinn, M. J. (2004). *Guardianships of adults: Achieving justice, autonomy, and safety*. New York: Springer.

Regan, J. J., & Gilfix, M. (2003). Tax, estate, and financial planning for the elderly: Forms and practice.

Richardson, E. D., Nadler, J. D., & Malloy, P. F. (1995). Neuropsychologic prediction of performance measures of daily living skills in geriatric patients. *Neuropsychology, 9*, 565–572.

Roenker, D. L., Cissell, G. M., Ball., K. K., Wadley, V. G., & Edwards, J. D. (2003). Speed-of-processing and driving stimulator training result in improved driving performance. *Human Factors, 45*, 218–233.

Roth, L. H., Meisel, C. A., & Lidz, C. A. (1977). Tests of competency to consent to treatment. *Canadian Journal of Psychiatry, 134*, 279–284.

Ruchinskas, R. A. (2005). Risk assessment as an integral aspect of capacity evaluations. *Rehabilitation Psychology, 50*, 197–200.

Sherod, M. G., Griffith, H. R., Copeland, J., Belue, K., Krzywanski, S., Zamrini, E. Y., et al. (2009). Neurocognitive predictors of financial capacity across the dementia spectrum: Normal aging, mild cognitive impairment, and Alzheimer's disease. *Journal of the International Neuropsychologcal Society, 15*(2), 258–267.

Stuck, A. E., Walthert, J. M., Nikolaus, T., Bula, C. J., Hohmann, C., & Beck, J. C. (1999). Risk factors for functional status decline in community-living elderly people: A systemic literature review. *Social Science & Medicine, 48*, 445–469.

Sturman, E. D. (2005). The capacity to consent to treatment and research: A review of standardized assessment tools. *Clinical Psychology Review, 25*, 954–974.

Tatemichi, T. K., Desmond, D. W., Stern, Y., Paik, M., & Bagiella, E. (1994). Cognitive impairment after stroke: Frequency, patterns, and relationship to functional abilities. *Journal of Neurology, Neurosurgery, and Psychiatry, 57*, 202–207.

Triebel, K., Martin, R., Griffith, H. R., Marceaux, M. A., Okonkwo, O. C., Harrell, L., et al. (2009). Declining financial capacity in patients with mild cognitive impairment: A one-year longitudinal study. *Neurology, 73*, 928–934.

Willis, S. L., Schaie, K. W., & Hayward, M. (Eds.), (1997). *Societal mechanisms for maintaining competence in old age*. New York: Springer Publishing Co.

Wong, J. G., Clare, I. C. H., Holland, A. J., Watson, P. C., & Gunn, M. (2000). The capacity of people with a "mental disability" to make a health care decision. *Psychological Medicine, 30*, 295–306.

Author Index

Page numbers in *italic* denote references. Page numbers in roman denote citations.

A

ABA-APA Capacity Assessment of Older Adults Working Group, 368, *377*, *379*
Abakoumkin, G., 319, *323*
Abe, O., 80, *85*
Abeles, N., 318, *320*, 343, *349*
Abeles, R., 177, *186*
Abeles, R. A., 42, *54*
Abelskov, K., 328, *335*
Aber, M. S., 144, *146*
Abraham, W. T., 266, *276*
Abrams, D., 257, *259*
Abrams, L., 241, *246*
Abrams, R., 314, *323*, 326, *337*
Abrams, R. C., 328, 330, *334*
Abramson, J. H., 209, *214*
Abreu, B. C., 154, *167*
Abyad, A., 346, *352*
Achenbaum, A., 5, 10, *20*
Achenbaum, A. W., 281, 282, *288*
Achenbaum, W. A., 42, 49, *50*, *51*, *54*, 282, *290*
Achten, E., 77, 78, *86*, 340, *349*
Acker, J. D., 66, *71*, 75, 76, 77, 78, 79, 84, *88*, *90*, 99, *107*
Ackerman, M., 47, *50*
Ackerman, P. L., 163, *165*, 267, *274*
Acosta, O., 83, *87*
Adalsteinsson, E., 80, 81, *89*
Adamec, R. E., 193, *200*
Adams, K. M., 346, *349*
Adams, M. M., 209, *215*
Adams, R. G., 228, *229*
Adey, M., 327, *337*
Adler, K. A., 360, 361, *363*
Adler, N., 209, *214*
Adler, N. E., 179, 183, *186*, 209, 212, *214*
Adolfsson, R., 101, 102, *105*
Afshin-Pour, B., 112, *118*
Agartz, I., 103, *107*
Aggen, S. H., 33, 34, *38*
Agrigoroaei, S., 181, *186*
Agronin, M. E., 330, 333, *334*, *337*
Aguilar-Navarro, S., 315, *321*
Ahern, F., 95, *106*
Ahsaduddin, O. N., 158, 159, *168*
Aizenstein, H. J., 83, *85*
Akbudak, E., 60, *71*, 80, *88*, 110, *118*, 125, *130*
Akincigil, A., 314, *320*
Akiskal, H. S., 326, *334*
Albert, M., 125, *129*, 181, *189*
Albert, M. S., 46, 49, *50*, 160, *165*, 198, *204*, 345, *349*
Albert, S., 346, 347, *350*, *351*
Aldwin, C. M., 47, *50*, 192, *200*, 281, 284, 287, *290*, 302, *306*
Alea, N., 326, *333*
Aleksandrowicz, P., 271, *272*
Alexander, D. M., 101, *104*
Alexander, G. E., 343, 347, *348*, *351*
Alexander, M., 159, *171*
Alexander, M. P., 159, *170*
Alexopoulos, G. S., 82, *87*, 111, *118*, 315, 316, *320*, *322*, 328, *334*
Alhakami, A. S., 136, *146*, *147*
Ali, S., 208, *214*
Allain, A. N., Jr., 198, *205*
Allain, P., 154, *165*
Allaire, J. C., 208, 209, *215*
Allali, G., 154, *165*
Allen, J. K., 208, 211, 213, *218*
Allen, J. L., 303, *308*
Allen, N. B., 327, *335*
Allen, R. S., 357, *363*
Alley, D., 196, *202*
Allik, J., 297, *309*
Allison, P. D., 27, *36*
Allman, J. M., 137, 138, *148*
Allore, H. G., 226, *229*
All Politics, 249, *259*
Allport, G. W., 286, *298*
Almeida, D. M., 26, *39*, 184, *189*, 192, 193, 194, 195, 196, 197, 198, 199, 200, *200*, *202*, *204*, *205*, *206*, 295, 297, 298, 299, 300, 301, 302, 304, 305, *306*, *307*, *309*, *310*
Alpérovitch, A., 78, 79, *86*, *87*, *91*
Altemus, M., 197, *201*, *203*, *205*
Altendorf, A., 315, *320*
Altieri, P. A., 155, *168*
Alvarez, W., 199, *202*
Alves de Moraes, S., 345, *348*
Alwin, D. F., 44, 45, 46, *50*, *53*
Amato, P. R., 219, 221, *229*
Ambler, C., 358, *362*
American Academy of Clinical Neuropsychology, 339, *348*
American Bar Association, 375, *377*
American Psychiatric Association, 313, *320*, 329, *334*, 342, *348*
Ames, D., 328, *334*
Amico, J. A., 197, *203*
Amieva, H., 141, *146*
Amigo, E., 373, *378*
Amlien, I., 77, *87*
Anas, A. P., 236, 237, 242, *244*, *246*, 251, *261*
Ancelin, L., 315, *322*
Andel, R., 95, *107*, 265, *272*, *273*, *274*
Anderberg, U. M., 197, *201*
Anderer, S. J., 373, *377*
Anderson, B., 197, *205*, 373, *378*
Anderson, E., 4, *21*
Anderson, N., 207, *217*
Anderson, N. B., 195, *201*, 214, *218*
Anderson, N. D., 6, 11, 16, *19*, 111, *117*, 122, *130*
Anderson, T. M., 314, 316, *323*
Anderson-Hanley, C., 185, *186*
Andersson, M., 77, *85*, 125, 127, *131*
Andersson, R., 99, *104*
Andreasen, N., 111, *117*
Andreassen, O. A., 103, *105*
Andreoletti, C., 170, 180, 182, *186*, *188*, 257, *259*
Andres, D., 241, *246*, 359, *363*

Andrés, P., 69, *69*, *71*
Andresen, E. M., 327, *334*
Andreski, P. M., 211, *217*
Andrews, G., 314, 316, *323*
Andrews-Hanna, J. R., 83, *86*, 112, *117*
Aneshensel, C., 220, *229*
Aneshensel, C. S., 268, *277*, 359, *364*
Angleitner, A., 266, *275*, 304, *309*
Annerbrink, K., 101, 102, *105*
Annweiler, C., 154, *165*
Anstey, K. J., 6, 8, 14, 16, 17, *19*, 46, 49, *50*, 63, 68, *69*, 78, *86*, 102, *105*, 180, *190*, 304, *308*, 314, *320*
Anthony, J. C., 46, *53*, 66, *72*, 76, *90*, 327, *335*
Antonucci, T. C., 43, *52*, 179, 181, *186*, *187*, 223, 224, 225, 226, *229*, *232*
Anzai, Y., 78, *88*
Aoki, S., 80, *85*
Appelbaum, P. S., 368, 370, 371, *377*, *378*
Appelman, J., 158, 159, *168*
Aquilino, W., 219, 221, 222, *229*
Arai, A., 359, *364*
Arai, Y., 359, *364*
Aranda, M. P., 357, *362*
Arbuckle, T. Y., 241, *246*
Ardelt, M., 281, 282, 283, 284, 285, 286, 287, *288*
Arentoft, A., 347, *351*
Argüelles, S., 356, 358, *362*
Arias, E., 209, *217*
Arigita, E. J., 112, *117*
Armeli, S., 194, *202*
Armesto, J. C., 370, 371, *378*, *379*
Armstead, C., 207, *217*
Armstrong, C. L., 82, *85*
Arnau, R. C., 327, *336*
Arndt, S., 345, *349*
Arnold, B. R., 346, *348*
Arnold, E., 328, 329, *336*
Arnold, S. E., 68, *72*, 198, 199, *205*, *206*, 304, *310*, 347, *348*
Aronson, J., 256, *262*, 346, *348*
Arthur, A., 317, *321*
Artiola i Fortuny, L., 346, 347, *348*
Artola, A., 164, *165*
Arvey, R. D., 253, 258, *260*, 269, *274*
Aschbacher, K., 196, *201*, 361, *364*
Ashburn, A., 374, 375, *378*
Ashburner, J. A., 74, *85*, 113, *118*, 141, *147*, 162, *168*, 340, *349*
Ashe, M. C., 161, *168*
Ashman, O., 179, *186*
Ashmore, R. D., 249, 253, *259*
Aso, T., 342, *351*
Assmann, A., 283, 285, *288*
Assmann, S. F., 185, *187*
Astin, A. W., 46, *50*
Astone, N. M., 212, *215*
Atiya, M., 126, 127, *130*
Atkinson, M. P., 220, *229*
Atkinson, R. C., 60, *69*
Atkinson, T. M., 61, 62, 63, 64, 69, *72*
Attias-Donfut, C., 222, *229*
Attix, D. K., 340, 347, *351*, *352*
Augustine, A. M., 66, *72*, 76, *90*
Auman, C., 256, 257, 259, *259*, *260*, 301, *308*
Avia, M. D., 304, *309*
Avila-Funes, J. A., 315, *321*
Avolio, B. J., 48, *50*
Aycock, J., 145, *151*, 304, *310*
Aylward, E. H., 66, *72*, 76, *90*
Aysan, F., 192, *202*
Aytac, I. A., 222, *230*
Ayutyanont, N., 129, *130*
Azar, A. R., 371, *378*, *379*
Azen, S., 375, *377*
Azjen, I., 253, *260*

B

Babb, J. S., 85, *87*
Babiloni, C., 111, *119*
Bach, J., 30, *39*
Bachar, J. R., 327, *334*
Bachmann, M. O., 211, *215*
Bach-Peterson, J., 220, *232*
Bachrach, D. G., 268, *275*
Bäckman, L., 7, 11, 12, 14, 16, 18, *19*, *20*, *21*, 34, *38*, 101, *104*, 114, 115, 116, *117*, 121, 122, 123, 124, 125, 127, 128, *129*, *130*, *131*, 155, 158, 163, 164, *166*, *170*, 181, *187*, 267, *272*
Baden, L., 270, *273*
Bagby, R. M., 328, 332, *334*
Bagiella, E., 374, *379*
Bagne, A. G., 303, *308*
Bagwell, D. K., 155, 156, *165*, *170*, 183, *186*
Bailey, A., 287, *288*
Bajuscak, L., 75, 79, *91*
Baker, C. I., 113, *117*
Baker, D., 145, *149*
Baker, D. P., 47, *50*
Baker, D. W., 210, *218*
Baker, S., 127, *130*
Baker, S. L., 83, *89*
Baker, S. R., 183, *186*
Bakermans-Kranenburg, M. J., 228, *229*
Balaban, R. S., 82, *91*
Balcerak, L. J., 155, *169*
Baldo, J. V., 344, *348*
Ball, K., 6, *19*, 49, *55*, 156, 157, 159, *165*, *167*, *171*, 268, *272*, 374, *379*
Ball, K. K., 374, *377*, *379*
Ballmaier, M., 75, *87*
Balluerka, N., 29, 30, 32, *36*
Balsis, S., 329, 330, 331, 333, *334*
Balsters, J. H., 129, *129*
Baltes, B. B., 269, *275*
Baltes, M. M., 5, 6, 10, 11, *19*, 154, *165*, 177, 178, 181, *186*, 194, *201*, 228, *229*, 242, *243*, 300, *306*
Baltes, P. B., 4, 5, 6, 7, 8, 9, 10, 11, 12, 14, 15, 18, *19*, *20*, *21*, 25, 26, *38*, 43, 45, *50*, 111, 114, *118*, 154, 155, 158, *165*, *168*, *169*, *171*, 191, 194, *201*, 242, *243*, 250, *260*, 263, 267, 272, *272*, *274*, *276*, 280, 281, 283, 284, 285, 286, 287, *288*, *289*, *290*, *291*, 300, *306*
Balzarini, E., 319, *321*
Banaji, M. R., 253, 254, *260*
Bandeen-Roche, K., 157, *168*
Bandura, A., 155, *165*, 177, 181, 183, 184, 185, *186*
Bandura, M., 184, *188*
Bandy, D., 129, *130*
Bangert, A., 111, *118*
Bangert, M., 113, *117*
Banich, M. T., 67, *71*
Baradell, J. G., 198, *201*
Barbeite, F. G., 259, *262*, 269, *274*
Barber, C., 280, 281, *290*
Barceló, F., 68, *69*
Bardell, L., 164, *168*
Barden, N., 213, *215*
Barker, G. J., 82, *89*, *90*
Barker, M., 236, *245*
Barker, V., 233, 238, 240, 243, *243*
Barkhof, F., 112, *117*
Barko, J. J., 46, *51*
Barlow, D., 326, *334*
Barnes, D., 160, *171*, 198, *203*
Barnes, L. L., 30, *39*, 159, *171*, 304, *310*
Barnes, R. F., 196, *201*
Barnes-Farrell, J. L., 270, *272*
Barnetson, L., 48, *51*
Barnett, S. M., 159, *165*
Baron, J. C., 67, *71*, 284, *289*
Barrett-Connor, E., 345, *350*
Barrick, T. R., 76, 80, 81, 82, *86*, *87*, *90*
Barry-Walsh, J., 317, *322*
Barsalou, L. W., 162, *165*
Bartels, S. J., 316, *320*
Bartolucci, A. A., 354, *363*
Bartolucci, G., 233, 235, 238, *246*, 254, *262*
Bartzokis, G., 74, 80, *85*, *88*, 340, *348*
Basak, C., 160, 163, *165*, *167*

Author Index

Basevitz, P., 298, *306*
Basser, P. J., 79, *89*
Bastin, M. E., 80, 81, 82, *85*, *86*, *90*
Batalova, J., 49, *55*
Bates, J. F., 126, 127, *130*
Bauer, I., 303, *306*
Baum, A., 198, *201*
Bauman, K. J., 346, *348*
Bavelier, D., 160, *167*
Baxendale, S., 197, *201*
Baxter, J. D., 313, *320*
Bayan, U., 94, *107*
Bayley, P. J., 342, *348*
Baynes, K., 61, 66, *71*
Beach, S. R., 354, 355, 356, 359, *362*, *364*
Beason-Held, L. L., 123, *129*
Beattie, L., 161, *168*
Bechara, A., 16, *19*, 137, 138, *146*, 371, *377*
Becic, E., 158, *166*
Beck, A. T., 327, 328, 329, *334*, *337*
Beck, C. J., 78, *88*
Beck, J. C., 374, *379*
Beck, J. G., 329, *337*
Becker, G., 221, 223, *229*
Becker, J., 354, 355, *364*
Becker, J. T., 344, *350*
Beckett, L. A., 30, *39*
Beckmann, C. F., 112, *117*
Beckson, M., 74, *85*, 340, *348*
Beehr, T. A., 269, 270, *272*, *274*
Beekman, A. T., 315, *323*, 327, 328, *334*
Beekman, A. T. F., 313, 314, 315, *320*, *321*, *333*
Beglinger, L. J., 313, *323*, 345, *349*
Beier, M. E., 62, 63, *71*, 163, *165*
Bell, C. B., 210, *215*
Bell, K., 346, *350*
Bell, R. Q., 26, *36*
Belle, S. H., 356, 358, 360, *362*, *363*, *364*
Belue, K., 373, *378*, *379*
Benedetti, B., 82, *85*
Bengtson, V. L., 5, 7, 10, 11, *19*, 220, 223, 224, 227, *229*, *230*, *231*
Benjamin, L. S., 332, 333, *335*, *337*
Benjamins, M., 212, *216*
Bennett, C. A., 137, *146*
Bennett, D. A., 68, *72*, 195, 199, *205*, *206*, 345, 347, *348*, *352*
Bennett, E. L., 113, *119*
Benounissa, Z., 265, *274*
Ben-Porath, Y. S., 194, *201*
Berch, D. B., 6, *19*, 156, 159, *165*, 268, *272*
Berecki-Gisolf, J., 356, 358, *362*
Bereket, Y., 155, 158, 160, 161, *167*
Berg, C. A., 297, 301, 302, 303, *310*
Berg, J. W., 368, 370, *377*
Berg, L., 342, *352*
Berg, S., 14, 16, 18, *21*, 48, *52*, 95, 96, 97, 99, *106*, *107*
Bergeman, C. S., 181, 183, 184, *186*, *189*, 299, *309*
Berger, A. K., 254, *261*
Berger, K., 79, *91*
Berger, U., 271, *273*
Bergman, E. J., 361, *363*
Berish, D. E., 61, 62, 63, 64, 69, *72*
Berkman, L., 46, 49, *50*, 160, *165*, 345, 346, *349*
Berkowitz, N., 373, *378*
Berman, K. F., 127, *131*
Berman, W. H., 331, *336*
Bernard, B. A., 344, *348*
Bernieri, F., 97, *106*
Berns, S. B., 356, *363*
Bernstein, L., 196, *203*
Berntson, G. G., 16, *19*
Berry, J. D., 295, 305, *308*
Berry, J. M., 159, 164, *165*, 182, 183, *186*
Berryhill, J. S., 327, *335*
Bersick, M., 61, 62, 68, 69, *70*
Best, D. L., 155, *165*
Bettman, J. R., 134, *149*
Beveridge, R., 301, 302, *310*
Beyenburg, S., 100, *104*
Beyene, Y., 221, 223, *229*
Bhakta, M., 129, *130*
Bhattacharyya, S., 257, *259*
Bherer, L., 115, *117*, 154, 158, 164, *166*, *167*, 264, *274*
Bialystok, E., 7, 14, *20*
Bianchi, E. C., 285, 286, *288*
Bianchi, S. M., 222, *229*
Bickel, J.-F., 6, *20*, 264, *274*
Bidlingmaier, F., 100, *104*
Bielak, A. A. M., 265, *273*
Bieman-Copland, S., 242, *246*
Bienias, J. L., 68, *72*, 159, *171*, 195, 199, *206*
Bienias, L., 345, *352*
Bierman, A., 226, *231*
Bigler, E. D., 78, *88*
Bilder, R. M., 101, *104*
Binns, M. A., 159, *166*, *168*, *171*
Birditt, K. S., 219, 220, 221, 222, 223, 224, 225, 226, 227, 228, *229*, *230*, *232*, 298, 301, *306*
Birmingham, W., 297, *310*
Birren, B. A., 4, 7, 14, *19*
Birren, J. E., 4, 5, 6, 7, 8, 9, 14, 16, *19*, *22*, 279, 280, 281, 282, 287, *288*, *289*
Bisconti, T. L., 181, 183, 184, *186*, *189*, 299, *309*
Bjork, R., 163, *169*
Black, F. W., 344, *348*
Black, M. C., 197, *203*
Black, S., 159, *170*
Black, S. E., 75, 83, *91*, 343, *352*
Blackhall, L. J., 375, *377*
Blackwell, D. L., 212, *215*
Blair, C., 47, *50*
Blais, A.-R., 138, 140, *151*
Blanchard-Fields, F., 16, *19*, 135, 137, 142, *146*, 256, *262*, 281, 282, 284, *288*, 297, 301, *306*, *310*
Blankenship, L., 327, *336*
Blatt-Eisengart, I., 182, *186*
Blatter, C. W., 195, *201*
Blau, P. M., 48, *50*
Blauw, G. J., 82, *91*
Blazer, D., 46, 49, *50*, 160, *165*, 326, 327, *334*, *335*
Blazer, D. G., 214, *216*, 314, *322*, 326, 327, *334*, *335*
Bleszner, R., 26, *36*, 242, *244*
Block, J., 282, 285, *288*
Bloor, L., 225, *232*
Bloor, L. E., 295, 303, *310*
Bloss, C. S., 101, *104*, *105*
Bluck, S., 280, 284, *288*, *289*, 326, *334*
Blum, N., 333, *336*
Blumcke, I., 100, *104*
Blumenthal, J. A., 161, *166*
Boals, A., 198, 199, *203*
Bockmühl, Y., 214, *217*
Bodammer, N., 83, *87*
Bodke, A., 129, *129*
Bodnar, J. C., 361, *362*
Boduroglu, A., 251, *259*
Boeninger, D. K., 302, *306*
Bogdahn, U., 114, *117*, 162, *166*
Bogg, T., 266, *276*
Bogner, H. R., 315, *320*
Böhmig-Krumhaar, S. A., 285, 287, *288*
Boich, L. H., 234, 235, 236, 238, 242, *246*
Boker, S. M., 35, *36*, 181, *186*
Boland, L. L., 48, *52*
Boland, S. M., 250, 251, *262*
Bolea, N., 115, *117*
Bolger, N., 192, 193, 194, *201*, 318, *320*
Bollen, E. L., 82, *91*
Bollen, K., 32, *36*
Bollini, A. M., 183, *187*
Bolstad, C. A., 139, 142, *147*
Bonanno, G. A., 318, 319, *320*, *322*
Bonatti, E., 138, *151*
Bondi, M. W., 101, *104*, 342, *348*
Bongers, G., 101, *107*
Bonneson, J. L., 234, 238, 240, *244*, *245*, 254, *261*
Bonneville, L. P., 283, *290*
Bontempo, D., 29, *36*
Bookheimer, S. Y., 77, *86*

Boomsma, D. I., 96, 99, *105*, *107*
Boone, K. B., 339, 347, *351*
Boot, W. R., 160, 163, *165*, *167*
Booth, A., 49, *54*
Booth, H., 68, *69*
Bordia, P., 281, *291*
Borenstein, A. R., 198, *204*
Borkovec, T. D., 329, *336*
Borman, W. C., 270, *274*
Börsch-Supan, A., 267, *273*
Bos, I. M., 42, 50, *52*
Bos, M. W., 138, *147*
Bosma, H., 156, *170*, 265, *273*
Bossé, R., 270, *273*
Bosworth, H. B., 154, *166*, 259, *259*
Bottiroli, S., 156, *166*
Botwinick, J., 342, *352*
Bouchard, G., 192, *201*
Bouchard, T. J., Jr., 96, 102, 103, *104*
Bound, J., 212, 213, *215*
Bourgeat, P., 83, *87*, 111, *119*
Bourgeois, M., 356, *362*
Bourhis, R. Y., 235, 236, *246*
Bowen, C. E., 266, 267, 269, *273*, *276*
Bowen, J. D., 49, *52*
Bowen, K. R., 163, *165*
Bowen, M. E., 211, *215*
Bowen-Reid, T., 210, 211, *216*
Bower, E. H., 329, *335*, 370, *379*
Bower, J. H., 304, *307*
Bowles, R. P., 30, *37*
Bowman, S. R., 355, 356, *363*
Boyce, T., 209, *214*
Boyce, W. T., 179, 183, *186*
Boyd, J. H., 328, *336*
Boyd, R., 45, *50*
Boyke, J., 114, *117*
Bozoki, A., 343, *349*
Braam, A. W., 327, 328, *334*
Bradley, C. J., 208, *215*
Bradley, E. H., 270, *273*
Bradley, G. W., 282, *288*
Bradway, K. P., 33, *38*
Brady, C. B., 6, 8, 14, 16, *22*
Brailey, K., 198, *205*
Bramson, R., 327, *336*
Brandon, D. T., 208, 211, 213, *218*
Brandtstädter, J., 177, 178, *187*, 255, *262*, 300, *310*
Brandt, J., 156, *169*, *189*, 342, *348*
Branscombe, N. R., 259, *260*
Braskie, M. N., 77, 83, *86*
Brassen, S., 125, 126, *129*
Braus, D. F., 125, 126, *129*
Braveman, P., 208, 209, 210, 211, *215*
Bravo, M., 374, *377*
Breen, G., 100, *105*, *106*
Brehmer, Y., 125, 127, 128, *129*, *130*, 154, *166*
Breil, F., 157, 158, *166*
Bremmer, M. A., 328, *334*
Bremner, J. D., 198, *201*
Brenes, M., 240, 241, 242, 243, *244*
Brennan, P. L., 316, *321*
Brenner, H. G., 284, *289*
Breteler, M. M., 75, 78, 79, *87*, *91*, 160, *170*
Brett, M., 197, *201*
Brewer, D. D., 354, 355, *364*
Brewer, M., 251, 253, *259*
Brewin, C. R., 192, *201*
Brickman, A. M., 75, 82, *87*, 111, *118*, 340, *348*, *350*
Bridenbaugh, S., 154, *165*
Bridges, K., 159, *166*
Brierley, B., 137, *148*
Briggs, S. D., 74, 76, *90*
Brim, O. G., 177, 181, *187*, 235, *245*
Brink, T. L., 327, *337*
Britt, M., 328, *336*
Broad, K. D., 228, *229*
Broadhead, W. W., 326, *334*
Brodaty, H., 314, 315, 316, *320*, *323*
Brodersen, A. M., 328, *335*
Brodscholl, J. C., 143, *151*
Broese Van Groenou, M. I., 319, *322*
Bromberger, J. T., 195, *202*
Bronfenbrenner, U., 43, *50*
Brooks, J. O., 155, *166*
Brose, A., 27, *36*
Brosschot, J. F., 198, *201*
Brown, A. A., 103, *107*
Brown, C. H., 313, *321*
Brown, D., 33, *39*
Brown, E. E., 179, *187*
Brown, G., 329, *334*
Brown, G. K., 327, *334*
Brown, G. W., 192, 195, *201*
Brown, J., 346, *348*
Brown, J. L., 314, *321*
Brown, L., 354, *363*
Brown, S., 197, *202*, 314, *320*
Brown, S. C., 141, *146*, 287, *289*
Brown, T., 326, *334*
Browne, M. W., 32, 33, *36*
Brownley, K. A., 197, *203*
Bruce, M. A., 180, *187*
Bruce, M. L., 226, *229*, 315, 316, 318, *320*, *323*
Bruder, C. E., 99, *104*
Brugman, G. M., 281, 284, 285, 286, *289*
Bruine de Bruin, W., 134, 135, 142, *146*
Bruni, J. R., 374, *377*
Bryan, J., 59, 61, 62, 63, 65, 67, *69*, *70*, *71*
Bryant, C., 328, *334*
Bryant, J., 257, *259*
Bryk, A. S., 32, *36*
Buchel, C., 114, *117*, 125, 126, *129*
Buchler, N. G., 80, *86*
Buchmann, C., 209, *215*
Buchsbaum, M. S., 340, *348*
Buckner, R. L., 60, 66, *70*, *71*, 77, 80, 83, *86*, *88*, *90*, 110, 113, *118*, 121, 124, 125, 129, *129*, *130*
Bucur, A., 213, *217*
Bucur, B., 80, 81, 82, *86*, *88*
Budde, M., 112, *117*
Budge, M. M., 48, *51*
Buhler, M., 101, *107*
Bui, B. K., 342, *348*
Bukov, A., 271, *273*
Bukowski, W. M., 5, *22*
Bula, C. J., 374, *379*
Bulcroft, K. A., 370, *377*
Bumpass, L. L., 195, *203*
Bunce, D., 78, *86*
Bunzeck, N., 83, *86*, *87*
Burane, G. J., 328, 329, *336*
Burdette, J. H., 80, *88*
Burdorf, A., 265, *273*
Bureau of Labor Statistics, 196, *201*
Burell, G., 200, *202*
Burgess, N., 162, *168*
Burgess, P., 317, *322*
Burgess, P. W., 63, 69, *70*
Burgio, L., 356, 358, *362*
Burgio, L. D., 356, *362*, *363*
Burgmans, S., 75, *86*
Burianova, H., 297, *308*
Burke, C. T., 318, *320*
Burke, H. M., 197, *202*
Burke, J. D., 328, *336*
Burleson, M. H., 305, *306*
Burmeister, M., 94, *106*
Burnett, D. L., 78, *88*
Burnight, K. P., 122, *131*
Burns, A. S., 109, *119*
Burns, R., 356, 358, *362*
Burns, W., 332, *337*
Burton, L. M., *215*
Busa, E., 77, *90*
Busch, J. C., 266, *274*
Busch, V., 114, *117*, 162, *166*
Buschke, H., 31, *39*, 74, 75, *91*
Buschkuehl, M., 157, 158, *166*, *167*
Busemeyer, J. R., 138, 140, *151*
Bushke, H., 342, *348*
Butterfield, B., 344, *348*
Butterworth, P., 102, *105*
Buttini, M., 101, *107*
Butz, S. W., 370, *379*
Byers, A. L., 226, *229*
Byles, J. E., 68, *69*
Bylsma, F. W., 156, *169*
Byrd, D., 346, *350*
Byrd, M., 11, *20*
Byrne, D. G., 209, *215*
Byrne, E. J., 314, *323*

Author Index

C

Cabeza, R., 6, 7, 9, 11, 14, 16, *19*, *22*, 66, 67, 68, *70*, *71*, 75, 80, 81, 82, *86*, *88*, *89*, 111, 112, *117*, 121, 122, *130*, *131*, 297, *310*
Cacioppo, J. T., 16, *19*, 184, *187*, 193, *201*, 226, *229*, 295, 304, 305, *306*, *307*, *308*
Cahill, B. S., 328, *336*
Cai, D., 236, 237, *244*, 251, *260*
Caine, E. D., 326, 327, *334*, *336*, 371, *378*
Cajko, L., 160, *167*
Callahan, H., 83, *88*
Callan, M. J., 184, *187*
Callon, V. J., 236, *245*
Camerer, C. F., 137, 138, *148*
Cameron, D., 374, *378*
Camp, C., 135, *146*
Camp, C. J., 154, *168*
Campbell, D. T., 30, *36*, 325, *334*
Campbell, D. W., 180, *187*
Campbell, R. T., 220, *229*
Campbell, W., 129, *129*
Campion, M. A., 259, *262*, 269, *275*
Campo, R. A., 295, 297, 303, *310*
Campos, J. J., 94, *105*
Canavan, M., 228, *230*
Canli, T., 295, 297, 302, *309*
Cannon, W. B., 191, *201*
Capadano, H. L., 253, *262*
Capaldi, D., 161, *167*
Caplan, L. J., 48, *54*, 180, *187*
Caporael, L. R., 234, *244*
Cappa, S. F., 111, *119*
Cappell, K., 16, *22*, 112, *119*
Caracciolo, E. A., 258, 259, *261*
Carbonare, L. D., 313, *320*
Cardenas, V. A., 75, *86*
Cardillo, V., 319, *321*
Carlin, B. P., 34, *37*
Carlin, N. C., 42, *51*
Carlson, M. C., 61, *70*, 115, *117*, 157, 161, 163, 164, *166*, *167*, *168*, *169*, 284, 287, *290*
Carmelli, D., 48, *54*, 78, 80, *86*, *89*
Carmody, J., 199, *201*
Carnelley, K. B., 318, *320*
Caro, F. G., 271, *273*
Carr, D. B., 374, *377*
Carstensen, L. L., 5, 6, 7, 8, 11, 12, 14, *19*, *20*, *22*, 60, 61, *70*, 136, 137, 138, 139, 140, *146*, *147*, *148*, *149*, 163, *166*, 181, *187*, 193, *201*, *203*, 284, *289*, 295, 296, 297, 298, 299, 300, 301, 302, 303, 304, *306*, *307*, *308*, *309*, *310*
Carter, C. S., 197, *201*
Carter, W. B., 327, *334*
Caruso, M. J., 156, *168*
Carver, C. S., 302, *310*
Cary, M. S., 315, *320*
Casanova, R., 80, *88*
Casarett, D. J., 372, *378*
Caselli, R. J., 129, *130*
Casillas, A., 332, *335*
Casper, L. M., 222, *229*
Caspi, A., 135, *146*, 266, *275*, 283, 284, *289*
Cassidy, E., 234, *246*
Castaneda, I., 346, *348*
Caswell, L. W., 198, *201*
Cattell, A. K. S., 33, *36*
Cattell, R. B., 30, 33, *36*
Cavallini, E., 156, *166*
Cavalli-Sforza, L. L., 45, *51*
Cavanaugh, J. C., 5, 10, *20*, 159, 164, *165*
Ceballos, R. M., 197, *203*
Ceci, S. J., 159, *165*
Cella, D., 345, *349*
Cercignani, M., 82, *90*
Cerella, J., 64, *72*
Cezayirli, E., 76, *87*
Chaddock, L., 115, *117*
Chaikelson, J., 298, *306*
Chan, A. C. M., 242, *244*
Chan, C. C., 139, *148*
Chan, L. D., 373, *377*
Chan, W., 221, 222, 223, *230*
Chandler, M. J., 280, 282, *289*
Chang, B. H., 184, *190*
Chang, H., 143, *151*
Chao, L. L., 75, *86*
Chapman, C. N., 266, *275*
Chapman, D., 298, *308*
Chapman, V., 374, *378*
Charil, A., 82, *85*
Charles, S. T., 11, *20*, 184, *189*, 193, 194, 195, *201*, 228, *230*, 284, *289*, 295, 296, 297, 298, 299, 300, 301, 302, 304, 305, *307*, *309*
Charlton, R. A., 80, 81, 82, *86*, *90*
Charness, N., 155, *167*, 180, *187*, 267, 268, *273*
Chasteen, A. L., 253, 255, 257, 259, *259*, *261*
Chatterjee, A., 368, 373, *378*
Chatters, L., 304, *310*
Chatters, L. M., 221, 226, *229*
Chavez, G., 209, *215*
Chee, M. W., 111, *117*
Chelune, G. J., 339, *349*
Chen, H., 316, *320*
Chen, J., 209, *216*, 345, *349*
Chen, K. W., 129, *130*
Chen, L. S., 46, *53*
Chen, P. C., 221, 225, 226, 227, *230*
Chen, S. P., 100, *107*
Chen, W. J., 103, *104*
Chen, Y., 137, 142, 144, *146*
Cheng, J. C., 82, *87*, 111, *118*
Cheng, S.-T., 242, *244*
Chernew, M. E., 304, *308*
Chesla, C. A., 180, 183, *190*
Chesney, M. A., 179, 183, *186*, 209, *214*
Cheung, H., 234, *245*
Chicherio, C., 101, 102, *106*, 122, 125, 127, 129, *130*, *131*
Chideya, S., 208, 209, 210, *215*
Chiew, K., 297, *308*
Chiou, J. Y., 75, 83, *91*
Chipperfield, J. G., 180, *187*, 296, *307*
Chiriboga, D. A., 192, 195, 199, *201*, *203*
Chisum, H. J., 74, *86*
Chiu, W. T., 328, *335*
Cho, I. H., 82, *88*
Cho, S. J., 340, *350*
Choca, J. P., 332, *335*
Choi, H., 227, *229*, *231*, 360, *364*
Chou, L. N., 103, *104*
Chou, P., 318, *321*
Chow, S.-M., 295, *307*
Chow, T. W., 137, *146*
Christensen, B. C., 99, *104*
Christensen, H., 16, *19*, 46, 49, *50*, 78, *86*, 102, *105*, 304, *308*, 327, *334*
Christensen, K., 95, 96, 97, *104*, *106*, *107*, 153, *166*
Christie, B. R., 164, *167*
Chrousos, G. P., 191, 197, *201*, *205*
Chulef, A. S., 143, *147*
Chun, M., 358, *363*
Chun, W. Y., 136, *148*
Chung, P., 228, *230*
Ciampi, A., 355, *364*
Cichy, K. E., 220, 221, 222, 223, 225, 226, 227, *230*
Ciliberti, C., 327, 328, 329, *335*
Cissell, G. M., 374, *379*
Clapp, W. C., 68, *72*
Clare, I. C. H., 371, *379*
Clark, A. E., 305, *309*
Clark, C. A., 80, 81, *86*
Clark, C. R., 80, 81, *87*
Clark, J. E., 160, *166*
Clark, L. A., 316, *322*, 331, 332, *334*, *335*
Clark, L. W., 326, *337*
Clark, M. H., 35, *39*
Clark, R., 214, *218*, 313, *320*
Claudio, L., 212, *217*
Clausen, J. A., 266, *273*
Clay, O. J., 354, 355, 356, 357, 358, *362*, *364*
Clayden, J. D., 80, 81, 82, *85*, *86*

Clayton, V. P., 280, 281, 282, 285, 286, *289*
Cleary, P. D., 195, *203*
Clemence, M., 82, *89*
Clément, R., 237, *244*
Clore, G. L., 139, *150*
Clusmann, H., 100, *104*
Coakley, E., 316, *320*
Coats, M. A. R. N. M. S. N., 345, *350*
Cohen, A.-L., 6, 16, 17, *21*
Cohen, C. I., 317, *321, 322*
Cohen, G., 141, *146*, 234, *244*
Cohen, H. J., 326, *335*
Cohen, J. D., 60, 61, *70*
Cohen, L. H., 194, *202*
Cohen, N. J., 114, 116, *117*, 161, *166*
Cohen, P., 315, *323*
Cohen, S., 209, *215*, 220, 226, *229*
Cohn, L. D., 283, *289, 290*
Colby, A., 283, *289*
Colcombe, S., 49, *51, 260, 274*
Colcombe, S. J., 6, *21*, 74, 75, 80, 84, *87, 88*, 115, 116, *117, 118*, 129, *130*, 141, *148*, 154, 158, 161, 164, *166, 167, 168*, 256, 257, *260*, 264, *274*
Cole, C. A., 134, *151*
Cole, M., 355, *364*
Cole, R., 236, *246*
Cole, T., 42, *51*
Cole, T. R., 42, *51*
Coleman, L. M., 234, *244*
Coleman, M., 223, *230*
Collie, A., 343, 345, *348, 349*
Colligan, R. C., 304, *307*
Collins, A., 226, *229*
Collins, C., 208, 210, *218*
Collins, C. L., 240, *244*
Collins, J., 145, *149*
Collins, K. S., 207, *215*
Colliver, J. D., 318, *320*
Comi, G., 82, *89*
Committee on Understanding and Eliminating Racial and Ethnic Disparities in Health Care, 211, *215*
Compton, W. M., 318, *320*
Condon, T., 318, *320*
Conger, R. D., 226, *232*
Conlee, E. W., 78, 79, *86*
Connell, C., 304, *310*
Connell, C. M., 357, *363*
Connell, F. A., 208, *217*
Connidis, I. A., 225, *229*
Connor, B. B., 158, 159, *168*
Connor, L. T., 156, *166*
Connors, L., 327, *334*
Conroy, S., 223, *231*
Consedine, N. S., 296, 299, 301, 304, *307, 309*
Constans, J. I., 198, *205*
Constantion, G., 316, *320*
Contugna, N., 211, *216*
Conturo, T. E., 60, *71*, 80, *88*, 110, *118*, 125, *130*
Convit, A., 75, *87*, 198, *203*
Conway, M., 298, *306*
Conwell, Y., 316, *320, 323*, 326, *336*
Cook, I. A., 78, 79, *86, 88*
Coolidge, F. L., 328, 329, 330, 331, 332, *335, 336*
Coon, D. W., 356, 358, *362*
Cooper, B. P., 154, *167*, 197, *205*
Cooper, R. S., 211, *216*
Copeland, J., 373, *379*
Corbitt, E. M., 333, *337*
Corcoran, C., 101, *105*
Corcoran, M., 356, *362*
Corder, L., 99, *104*
Cordner, S. M., 317, *322*
Corey-Bloom, J., 344, *352*
Corkin, S., 137, *148*
Corley, R. P., 61, 62, 68, 69, *70*
Cornelius, S. W., 135, *146*
Cortina, K. S., 179, *187*
Corwin, E. J., 188, 197, *203*
Cosentino, S., 344, *348*
Costa, P. T., Jr., 11, *21*, 194, *202*, 265, 266, *273, 275*, 283, *290*, 298, 299, 304, *307, 309*
Costello, M. C., 80, *89*
Costigan, M., 194, *206*
Cotman, C. W., 83, *88, 350*
Coupland, J., 233, 234, 235, 240, 241, *244*
Coupland, N., 233, 234, 235, 240, 241, *244*
Courchesne, E., 74, *86*
Courtet, P., 315, *322*
Covington, J., 74, *86*
Covinsky, K., 160, *171*
Cowan, D. N., 313, *323*
Cowles, A., 74, *86*
Cox, C., 316, *320*, 326, *336*
Cox, C. R., 138, 140, *151*
Cox, H., 196, *202*
Coyle, N., 193, *202*
Coyle, T., 80, *88*
Craik, F. I. M., 7, 11, 14, 18, *20*, 121, *130*, 159, 163, *166, 168, 171*
Crawford, J. D., 142, *146*
Crawford, J. R., 62, 67, *70*, 96, *105*
Crawford, L. E., 305, *306*
Crimmins, E., 196, *202*, 213, *217*, 265, *272*
Crimmins, E. M., 209, 210, 212, *215, 216*
Crockett, W. H., 250, 253, *259*
Crook, T. J., 326, 327, *335*
Crouter, A., 43, *50*
Crowe, M., 265, *272*
Croyle, K. L., 198, *201*
Cruts, M., 129, *130*
Crystal, S., 210, *215*, 314, *320*
Csikszentmihalyi, M., 282, 283, 285, *289*
Cubbin, C., 208, 209, 210, *215*
Cuddy, A. J. C., 251, 252, 253, 254, *260*
Cudeck, R., 32, 35, *36*
Cuijpers, P., 318, *322*
Culgin, S., 234, *246*
Cullum, C. M., 373, *377*
Cully, M., 268, *277*
Cummings, J., 143, 145, *147*
Cummings, J. L., 137, *146*
Cummings, J. R., 143, *146*
Cummings, S. R., 49, *53*
Cumsille, P. E., 29, *37, 38*
Cunningham, J., 236, *244*
Cunningham, W. R., 5, 6, 7, 8, 14, *19*
Cupples, L. A., 100, *105*
Curham, K. B., 49, *53*
Curley, J. P., 228, *229*
Curran, P. J., 32, *36*
Currier, J. M., 361, *363*
Curtain, R., 268, *277*
Cushman, M., 345, *350*
Czaja, S. J., 180, *187*, 268, *273*, 356, 358, 360, *362, 363, 364*
Czienskowski, U., 135, *149*
Czobor, P., 101, *104*

D

Daatland, S. O., 221, 223, *231*
D'Agostino, R. B., 48, *51*
Dahle, C. L., 84, *90*
Dahlin, E., 114, 115, 116, *117*, 125, 127, *131*, 158, 163, 164, *166*
Dailey, R. M., 233, 241, *244, 245*
Dajani, S., 109, *119*
Dale, A. M., 77, *87, 91*, 103, *105*
D'Alessio, A. C., 99, *106*
Dalton, C., 298, *306*
Daly, J., 242, *245*
Damasio, A. R., 136, 138, *146*
Damasio, H., 371, *377*
Damoiseaux, J. S., 112, *117*
Damos, D. L., 158, *166*
Daneman, M., 158, *166*
Dang, Q., 361, *363*
Daniels, K., 60, 61, 62, 64, 65, 68, *70*
Dannefer, D., 26, *38*, 212, *215*, 264, 268, *273, 275*
Danner, D., 242, *244*
Danziger, W. L., 342, *352*
Däpp, C., 157, 158, *166*
D'Aquila, E., 347, *351*
Darby, D. G., 343, 345, *348, 349*
Dark-Freudeman, A., 155, 156, *170*, 183, *190*

Author Index

Darmopil, S., 164, *168*
Darowski, E. S., 9, *20*, 62, *70*
Daruwala, A., 198, *201*
Darwin, C., 296, *307*
Das, S., 127, *131*
Daselaar, S. M., 67, *70*, 112, *117*
Dastoor, D., 359, *363*
Daumit, G. L., 313, *321*
Davatsikos, C., 141, *150*
Dave, J., 356, 357, 358, *363*
Davey, A., 221, *229*, 298, *307*
Davey Smith, G., 211, *215*
David, J. P., 194, *202*
David, S., 78, 79, *86*, 357, 358, *363*
Davidson, N. S., 110, *119*
Davidson, P. S., 75, 79, *91*
Davidson, R. J., 94, *105*, 199, *202*
Davidsson, P., 111, *117*
Davis, A., 76, *90*, 192, *201*
Davis, A. A., 184, *189*
Davis, D. S., 347, *350*
Davis, H., 138, 140, *151*
Davis, K., 345, *351*
Davis, M., 299, *309*
Davis, R., 332, *336*
Davis, S. W., 66, *72*, 80, *86*, 112, *117*, 155, *165*
Davison, M. L., 284, *289*
Dawkins, R., 45, *51*
Dawson, 318, *321*
Dear, K., 16, *19*, 78, *86*
Dear, K. B. G., 304, *308*
Dearden, L., 268, *273*
Deary, I. J., 17, *20*, 48, *54*, 80, 81, 82, *85*, *86*, *90*, 96, 99, 100, *105*, 345, *349*
Debanne, S. M., 265, *273*
De Beurs, E., 328, *334*
deBeurs, E., 315, *320*
Debner, J. A., 65, *71*
DeCarli, C., 78, 79, *86*, *89*, *91*, 99, *105*, 125, 126, *131*, 340, *349*
DeCoster, J., 357, *363*
de Craen, A. J., 82, *91*
Deeg, D. J., 315, *323*, 327, 328, *334*
Deeg, D. J. H., 315, 328, *320*, *334*
de Frias, C. M., 6, *23*, 62, 63, 64, 69, *70*, 101, 102, *105*, 181, *187*
DeFries, J. C., 61, 62, 68, 69, *70*, 94, 97, 103, *105*, *107*
De Fruyt, F., 283, *290*
de Geus, E. J., 96, 97, *105*, *107*
de Groot, J. C., 77, 78, *86*, 340, *349*
Dehaene, S., 134, *146*
Deibler, A. R., 80, *88*
DeJong, G. F., 49, *51*
Dekngger, N., 316, *321*
DeKosky, S. T., 344, *350*
Delano-Wood, L., 343, *349*
Delazer, M., 138, *151*
Del Boca, F. K., 249, 253, *259*
de Leeuw, F. E., 77, 78, *86*, 340, *349*
de Leon, M. J., 75, *87*, 198, *203*, 340, *349*
D'Elia, L. F., 339, 347, *351*
Delis, D. C., 101, 102, *104*, *105*, 342, 343, 344, *348*, *349*
Della Sala, S., 137, 138, 141, *146*, *149*
Deller, J., 270, *273*
DeLong, M. R., 343, *348*
DeLongis, A., 192, *201*
DelVecchio, W. F., 331, *336*
Demler, O., 328, *335*
Demoulin, S., 252, *260*
Denaro, J., 347, *352*
Denburg, N. L., 138, 140, 145, *146*, *151*
den Heijer, T., 75, *87*
Denney, N. W., 264, *273*
Dennis, M. S., 314, *323*
Dennis, N. A., 67, *70*, 80, *86*, 112, *117*
Department of Health and Human Services, 318, *321*
DePaulo, B. M., 234, *244*
Depp, C. A., 242, *244*, *245*, 314, 315, 316, 317, *321*, *322*, 372, *379*
Der, G., 271, *273*
Derby, C., 113, *118*
Derby, C. A., 153, 163, *170*
DeRienzis, D., 358, *364*
Derksen, J. J. L., 333, *337*
Derouesne, C., 343, *351*
Derse, A., 368, *377*
Desai, A. K., 317, *321*
de Santi, S., 198, *203*
Desgranges, B., 67, *71*
Desikan, R. S., 77, *86*, *90*
Desmond, D. W., 374, *379*
D'Esposito, M., 111, *119*, 121, 122, 123, 125, 129, *130*, *131*
Desrichard, O., 183, *187*
Desson, J. F., 67, *71*
de Stahl, T. D., 99, *104*
De Stefano, N., 82, *90*
Devoe, M., 193, *203*
Devos, T., 254, 255, *262*
De Vries, M. Z., 327, 328, *334*
DeWaal, F. B. M., 94, *105*
DeYoung, C. G., 17, *20*
Dhar, R., 137, *147*
Dibbs, E., 270, *273*
Dick, M., 347, *350*
Dickens, W. T., 42, *51*
Dickerson, B., 16, *23*
Dickerson, B. C., 77, *86*, 126, 127, *130*
Dickerson, F. B., 313, *321*
Dickerson, S. S., 182, *187*, 197, *202*
Dieckmann, N., 134, 143, 145, *149*, 371, *379*
Dieckmann, N. F., 143, 146, *150*
Diederichs, Y., 270, *273*
Diefenbach, M. A., 134, 136, *149*
Diehl, M., 193, *202*
Diener, E., 266, *276*, 298, 305, *307*, *309*, 325, *335*
Diez Roux, A. V., 211, *217*
Diggle, P. J., 30, 31, 32, 34, *37*, *38*
DiGiorgio, A., 316, *320*
Dijksterhuis, A., 138, *147*
Dillon, M., 285, 286, *291*
Dilworth-Anderson, P., 357, 358, *362*
Dimsdale, J. E., 360, 361, *363*, *364*
Diniz, B. S., 111, *117*
DiPrete, T., 209, *215*
Dixon, A., 234, *245*
Dixon, R. A., 4, 5, 6, 7, 8, 9, 10, 11, 12, 14, 16, 17, 18, *20*, *21*, *23*, 121, *131*, 161, *167*, 178, 180, 181, 183, *187*, 250, *260*, 263, 265, 267, *272*, *273*
Dixon, R. F., 62, 63, 64, 69, *70*
Djurovic, S., 103, *107*
Dobie, D. J., 197, *204*
Doblhammer, G., 153, *166*
Dobson, A., 34, *37*, 356, 358, *362*
Dobson-Stone, C., 101, *104*
Dohrenwend, B. S., 192, 195, *202*
Doi, S., 95, *105*
Dolan, C. V., 35, *37*
Dolcos, F., 16, *22*, 112, *117*, 297, *310*
Donahue, C., 329, 330, 331, 333, *334*
Donchin, E., 160, *166*
Donelan, K., 358, *364*
Dong, W., 154, *168*, 264, *274*
Donlan, C., 9, *22*
Donlon, M. M., 242, *244*
Donnellan, M. B., 265, *273*
Dooneief, G., 346, *350*
Dorfman, K., 330, 332, *336*
Dorjee, T., 242, *244*
Dornan, B., 159, *169*
Dörner, J., 266, 267, *276*, 285, 287, *291*
Doubal, S., 6, 17, *21*
Draganski, B., 114, *117*, 162, *166*
Drevets, W. C., 103, *105*
Driemeyer, J., 114, *117*
Dronkers, N. F., 344, *348*
Drozdick, L., 327, 328, 329, *335*
Drummer, O. H., 317, *322*
Drungle, S. C., 143, 144, *148*
Du, A., 75, *86*
Duara, R., 373, *378*
Duarte, A., 75, *86*
Duberstein, P. R., 316, *320*, 326, *336*, *364*
Dubois, B., 343, *349*
Ducharme, F., 355, *362*

Ducimetière, P., 78, *91*
Dudley, K. C., 370, *377*
Duff, K., 345, *349*
Dufouil, C., 78, 79, *86*, *87*, *91*
Dufour, M., 318, *321*
Duke, L. M., 198, *205*
Dukoff, R., 372, *377*
Duley, A. R., 303, *310*
Dull, V., 251, *259*
Dumke, H. A., 135, *151*
Duncan, D. J., 50, *51*
Duncan, G., 209, *215*
Duncan, G. J., 209, *217*
Duncan, J., 66, 69, *70*
Duncan, O. D., 48, *50*
Dunham, N. C., 326, *336*
Dunham, W. H., 45, *51*
Dunkin, J. J., 78, *88*
Dunlosky, J., 156, *166*, 181, *187*
Dunn, D. S., 136, *151*
Dunn, L. B., 372, *377*, *379*
Dupont, P., 84, *89*
Dupuis, J. H., 74, 75, 76, *90*
Dupuy, A., 315, *322*
Durkin, D. W., 357, *363*
Dustman, R. E., 160, *167*
Dustman, T. J., 160, *167*
Du Toit, S. H. C., 32, *36*
Dutta, R., 94, *107*
Düzel, S., 83, *86*, *87*
Dweck, C. S., 155, *168*
Dykstra, P. A., 305, *307*, 319, *322*
Dymov, S., 99, *106*
Dzung, L. P., 141, *150*

E

Eachus, J., 211, *215*
Easteal, S., 102, *105*
Eaton, W. W., 266, *274*
Eaves, L. J., 96, 97, *106*
Eberling, J. L., 79, *89*
Eckenrode, J., 192, 200, *202*
Eckerdt, D. J., 50, *51*
Edelstein, B., 327, 328, 329, *335*, 370, 371, 373, *377*, *379*
Edelstein, P. H., 211, *215*
Edge, N., 297, 298, *310*
Edland, S. D., 347, *352*
Edman, J. S., 154, *167*
Edwards, C. L., 95, *107*
Edwards, D., 161, *169*
Edwards, H., 234, 235, 236, *244*
Edwards, J. B., 374, *377*
Edwards, J. D., 374, *379*
Edwards, M., 159, *166*
Edwards, N., 74, *85*, 340, *348*
Eefsting, J. A., 313, *323*
Egaas, B., 74, *86*
Egerter, S., 208, 209, 210, *215*
Eggebeen, D. J., 220, 222, *229*, *232*
Eichele, T., 125, *130*
Eid, M., 325, *335*
Eikelenboom, P., 342, *350*
Eimicke, J., 314, *323*, 327, *337*
Einstein, G. O., 6, *20*
Eisdorfer, C., 356, 358, *362*
Eisen, S. A., 95, 103, *106*
Eisses, A. M. H., 314, *321*
Eizenman, D., 26, *36*
Eizenman, D. R., 177, 178, 184, *187*
Ekerdt, D. J., 270, *273*
Ekman, P., 94, *105*
Elbert, T., 113, *119*
Elder, G. H., Jr., 42, 43, *51*, *54*, 220, 225, 226, *232*, 266, *273*, *276*, *277*
Elderkin-Thompson, V., 75, *87*
Eleazer, G. P., 375, *378*
Elger, C. E., 100, *104*
Elias, J., 49, *55*, 156, 159, *171*
Elias, M. F., 48, *51*, *55*
Elias, P. K., 48, *51*
Eller, A., 257, *259*
Eller, T. J., 210, *215*
Elliott, E., 184, *188*
Elliott, J. C., 197, *203*
Ellis, C. G., 333, *337*
Ellis, C. H., 242, *246*
Ellis, K. A., 111, *119*
Emerson, M. J., 60, 62, 63, 64, *71*, 114, *118*, 161, *168*
Emery, C. F., 161, *166*
Emery, L., 257, 259, *260*
Emirbayer, M., 47, *51*
Emmerson, R. Y., 160, *167*
Endres, T. E., 161, *167*
Eng, C., 375, *378*
Engdahl, R. A., 300, *310*
Engelen, G. J., 333, *337*
Engle, R. W., 158, *167*
English, T., 295, 297, 302, *309*
Engstler, H., 270, *277*
Ennis, G. E., 184, *189*
Enos, T., 197, *205*
Ensminger, M., 212, *215*
Enzinger, C., 78, 82, *87*
Enzmann, D. R., 82, *89*
Epel, E. S., 197, *202*, *205*
Epstein, D. B., 32, *37*
Epstein, N., 329, *334*
Epstein, R. M., 134, *147*
Epstein, S., 135, 136, *147*
Era, P., 14, 16, 18, *21*
Erb, H.-P., 136, *148*
Erber, J. T., 253, *260*
Ercoli, L. M., 161, *169*
Erickson, K. I., 6, *21*, 67, *71*, 74, 75, 80, 84, *87*, *88*, 115, 116, *117*, 129, *130*, 141, *148*, 158, 160, 161, 164, *165*, *166*, *167*
Erickson, S., 99, *104*
Ericsson, K. A., 5, *20*, 155, *166*
Eriksen, H., 268, *275*
Erikson, E. H., 282, 285, *289*
Erikson, E. K., 227, *230*
Erikson, J. M., 282, *289*
Eriksson, E., 101, 102, *105*
Eriksson, J. G., 315, *322*
Eriksson, P. S., 113, *118*
Erlinghagen, M., 271, *273*, *274*
Ernesto, C., 347, *351*
Ernfors, P., 164, *168*
Ernst, J. M., 305, *306*
Esiri, M. M., 48, *51*
Esler, M., 196, *202*
Esopenko, C., 183, *190*
Espeseth, T., 75, 77, *87*, *91*
Essex, M. J., 265, *275*
Ettner, S., 195, *202*
Evans, A. C., 75, *91*
Evans, D. A., 30, *39*, 68, *72*, 159, *171*, 195, 347, *348*
Evans, J. D., 317, *322*
Evans, M. K., 211, *216*
Ewing, F. M. E., 48, *54*
Eyer, J., 212, *218*
Eyler, L. T., 103, *106*, 372, *379*

F

Fabel, K., 84, *87*
Fabiani, M., 160, *165*, *166*
Fabsitz, R. R., 48, *54*
Fahy, L., 159, *168*
Falba, T. A., 270, *273*
Falk, S. B., 332, *336*
Fan, J., 17, *20*
Fang, C. Y., 195, *202*
Fang, S. A., 266, *276*
Fannes, K., 84, *89*
Farberow, N., 319, *321*
Farde, L., 16, *19*, *129*
Farlow, M. R., 347, *352*
Farmer, J., 164, *167*, 344, *351*
Farmer, M. E., 46, *51*
Farr, A. L., 48, *51*
Farrer, L. A., 100, *105*
Farvolden, P., 332, *334*
Fasang, A., 271, *272*
Fast, J., 300, *307*
Faulkner, D., 234, *244*
Fazekas, F., 78, 82, *87*
Featherman, D. L., 26, *36*, 44, 46, *52*, 177, 178, 184, *187*
Feczko, E., 16, *23*
Fedorikhin, A., 136, *150*
Feher, E. P., 326, 327, *335*
Fein, G., 138, *147*
Feinberg, F., 257, *262*
Feldman, D. C., 267, 268, 270, 271, 272, *273*, *274*, *275*
Feldman, H., 343, *352*

Feldman, J. J., 196, *202*
Feldman, M. W., 45, *51*
Feldman, P. H., 358, *364*
Felsten, G., 192, *202*
Feng, D., 224, *230*
Fennema-Notestine, C., 103, *106*
Fenstermacher, E., 77, *86*
Fera, F., 127, *131*
Ferguson, J. N., 197, *202*
Fermia, E. E., 357, 361, *365*
Fermont, P. C. J., 164, *165*
Fernandez, M. E., 270, *275*
Ferrari, E., 100, *105*
Ferrari, M., 287, *289*
Ferrario, S. R., 319, *321*
Ferraro, F. R., 139, *147*
Ferraro, K., 227, *230*
Ferrer, E., 29, 30, 31, 32, 33, 34, 35, *36*, *37*
Ferrer-Caja, E., 32, *37*
Ferris, S. H., 75, *87*, 340, *349*
Ferrucci, L., 175, 180, *188*, 256, 257, 258, 259, *261*
Field, N. P., 318, *321*
Figner, B., 371, *377*
Filippi, M., 82, *89*
Finch, C. E., 46, *51*
Fine, E. M., 342, *349*
Fingerman, K. L., 219, 220, 221, 222, 223, 224, 225, 226, 227, 228, *229*, *230*, *231*, 298, 299, 300, 301, *306*, *307*, *309*
Fink, A., 158, *169*
Finkel, D., 95, 96, 99, *105*, *107*, 265, *273*
Finkelhor, D., 359, *364*
Finn, P., 138, *147*
Finucane, M. L., 134, 136, 143, 145, *147*, *148*
Fiorri, K. L., 179, *187*
First, M., 326, 333, *335*
Firth, K. M., 177, 180, 183, *188*
Fiscella, K., 209, *215*
Fischer, D., 214, *217*
Fischer, H., 125, 127, 128, 129, *129*, *130*
Fischer, J. S., 339, *350*
Fischhoff, B., 134, 135, 142, *146*
Fischl, B., 75, 77, *87*, *91*
Fishbein, M., 253, *260*
Fisher, C. L., 242, *246*
Fisher, G. G., 345, *351*
Fisher, L., 180, 183, *190*, 270, *275*, 360, *363*
Fisher, P. J., 100, *107*
Fishman, N. O., 211, *215*
Fisk, A. D., 135, 138, *147*, *149*, 154, *167*, 180, *187*, 268, *273*, *334*
Fisk, J. E., 138, *147*
Fiske, A., 297, 305, *307*, 316, *321*, 327, *335*
Fiske, D. W., 26, 33, *36*, 325, *334*
Fiske, S. T., 16, *23*, 249, 251, 252, 253, 254, *260*, *262*
Fitzsimmons, C., 155, *168*
Fjell, A. M., 75, 77, *87*, *91*
Flatt, T., 94, *105*
Fleck, M. S., 112, *117*
Flegal, K. E., 159, 164, *168*
Fleming, S., 319, *321*
Fletcher, E., 78, 79, *89*, *91*, 125, 126, *131*
Flinders, J. B., 196, *205*, 303, *310*
Flint, A. J., 316, *321*
Floderus-Myrhed, B., 95, *106*
Flory, J. H., 211, *215*
Flynn, J. R., 42, 45, 46, 47, *51*
Foch, T., 93, *106*
Folkman, S., 179, 183, *186*, 192, *202*, *203*, *214*, 354, 356, *363*
Folsom, A. R., 48, *52*
Folstein, M. F., 342, 345, *349*
Folstein, S. E., 342, *349*
Foner, A., 41, 43, *53*
Fong, T. G., 343, *349*
Ford, G. A., 77, *87*
Forgas, J. P., 139, *147*
Forkstam, C., 122, *131*
Forlenza, O. V., 111, *117*
Forman, M. S., 344, *351*
Forsen, T., 315, *322*
Forsgren, L., 125, 127, *131*
Fortmann, S. P., 209, *218*
Fossella, J. A., 17, *20*
Foster, M., 192, *201*
Fotenos, A. F., 83, *86*, 113, *118*
Fowler, F., 240, *244*
Fox, L. S., 354, *363*
Fox, N. A., 296, *307*, 345, *349*
Fox, P. T., 67, *72*, 139, *148*
Fox, S., 235, 236, 237, 238, *244*, *245*
Frackowiak, R. S., 111, 113, *118*, 141, *147*, 162, *168*, 340, *349*
Frank, E., 197, *205*, 209, *218*
Frank, G., 375, *377*
Frankenburg, F. R., 333, *337*
Franklin, S. S., 196, *202*
Franks, M. M., 221, 222, 223, 227, *230*
Franz, C. E., 96, 97, 103, *106*
Fratiglioni, L., 34, *38*, 100, *107*, 124, *130*, 374, *378*
Frazier, L. D., 355, 356, *363*
Frederickson, J. R., 160, *167*
Fredrickson, B. L., 296, 298, 299, *307*
Freedman, M., 161, *167*, 344, *349*
Freedman, V. A., 211, *217*
Freud, S., 227, *230*
Freund, A. M., 8, *19*, 45, *53*
Friberg, L., 95, *106*
Frick, K. D., 161, *167*, 208, 211, 213, *218*
Fried, L. P., 161, *167*, 208, 211, 213, *218*, 284, 287, *290*
Friedland, R. P., 265, *273*
Friedman, D., 61, 62, 68, 69, *70*
Friedman, L., 155, *166*
Friedman, N. P., 60, 61, 62, 63, 64, 68, 69, *70*, *71*, 114, *118*, 161, *168*
Frier, B. M., 48, *54*
Fries, J. F., 154, *167*
Friesen, W., 242, *244*
Friesinger, G. C., 17, 18, *20*
Fripp, J., 83, *87*
Friston, K. J., 74, *85*, 141, *147*, 340, *349*
Fritsch, T., 265, *273*
Fry, C. L., 50, *51*
Fuhrer, R., 78, 79, *87*, *91*
Fukuyama, H., 343, *351*
Fuligni, A. I., 49, *51*
Fultz, N. H., 315, *321*
Fung, H. H., 137, *147*, 242, *244*
Furnham, A., 192, *201*
Furstenberg, F., 222, *230*
Fuster, J. M., 69, *70*
Futterman, A., 319, *321*

G

Gabrieli, J. D. E., 9, 16, *20*, 121, 122, 123, *130*
Gächter, S., 137, *148*
Gadian, D. G., 113, *118*, 162, *168*
Gaeth, G. J., 138, *148*
Gage, F. H., 113, *118*, 164, *167*, *170*, 264, *276*
Gagne, D. D., 181, *188*
Gairrusso, R., 223, *231*
Gajewski, B., 235, *247*
Galasko, D., 342, 344, *349*, *351*
Galik, E., 359, *363*
Galinsky, A. D., 184, *190*
Gallagher-Thompson, D., 319, *321*, 328, *336*, 347, *351*, *352*, 356, 357, 358, 361, *362*, *363*
Gallo, J. J., 327, *335*
Gallo, W. T., 270, *273*
Gallois, C., 234, 236, *244*, *245*, 249, *258*
Gamaldo, A., 95, *107*
Gamboz, N., 138, *151*
Gamson, D. A., 47, *50*
Ganong, L. H., 223, *230*
Gans, D., 220, *231*
Ganslandt, O., 80, *91*
Ganzini, L., 368, 372, *377*, *378*, *379*
Gao, F. Q., 75, 83, *91*
Gao, J. H., 139, *148*
Gao, S. J., 49, *52*
Garavan, H., 67, *71*
Garcia-Fabela, L., 315, *321*
Garcia-Lara, J. M., 315, *321*

Garde, E., 79, *87*
Gardiner, P., 179, *190*
Gardner, C. O., 194, 195, *203*, 316, *322*
Garner, J., 99, *105*
Garrett, D. D., 12, 16, *20*
Garris, J. M., 300, *310*
Garstka, T. A., 234, 238, *245*, 250, 251, 252, 253, 254, 255, 257, 258, 259, *260*, *261*, *262*
Gary, T., 210, 211, *216*
Gaser, C., 114, *117*, 162, *166*
Gaskin, D., 210, 211, *216*
Gass, K. A., 319, *321*
Gatt, J. M., 101, *104*
Gatz, M., 99, *107*, 178, *187*, *201*, 265, *273*, 297, 298, 299, 301, 304, 305, *307*, 311, 316, *321*, *322*, 327, 329, *335*, *337*, 354, *362*
Gaucher, D., 184, *187*
Gaudreau, S., 182, *188*
Gaugler, J. E., 355, 359, 360, 361, *362*, *363*
Gauvain, M., 45, *51*
Gazmararian, J. A., 209, *215*
Gazzaley, A., 68, *72*, 129, *130*
Ge, Y., 85, *87*
Geda, Y. E., 304, *307*
Gee, S., 251, *261*
Geeraedts, T., 82, *91*
Geerlings, S. W., 315, *320*
Geiss, S., 271, *273*
Gelfand, M., 179, *190*
Gensicke, T., 271, *273*
George, A. E., 340, *349*
George, L. K., 161, *166*, 212, *215*, 326, *334*
Georgellis, Y., 305, *309*
Gerevini, S., 82, *90*
Gergen, K. J., 319, *323*
Gergen, M., 319, *323*
Gerin, W., 198, *201*
Germain, C. M., 61, 66, 67, *70*, *71*, 144, *147*
Geronimus, A. T., 212, 213, *215*
Gerrish, I. F., 82, *85*
Gershon, R. C., 345, *349*
Gerstel, N., 221, *231*
Gerstorf, D., 30, *38*
Gfroerer, J. C., 318, *320*
Gharapetian, L., 80, *89*
Ghisletta, P., 6, 16, 17, *20*, *21*, 28, 31, 32, 33, 34, *36*, *37*, 74, 76, 84, *87*, *90*, 264, *274*
Giannini, S., 313, *320*
Giarrusso, R., 224, *229*, *230*
Gibbens, C., 142, *149*
Gibbon, M., 333, *335*
Gibbons, L. E., 356, *365*
Gibbs, J., 283, *289*
Gibson, B. E., 357, 358, *362*
Gibson, C. J., 49, *51*
Gierveld, J., 305, *307*
Gierz, M., 313, *321*
Gijsbers, A. A., 99, *104*
Gilbert, D. T., 253, *260*
Gildengorin, G., 345, *350*
Gilens, M., 266, *273*
Giles, H., 233, 234, 235, 236, 237, 238, 239, 240, 241, 242, 243, *243*, *244*, *245*, *246*, *247*, 251, 254, *260*, *262*
Gilfix, M., 375, *379*
Gillette, J. A., 78, *86*, 340, *349*
Gilliland, G., 319, *321*
Gillum, R. F., 196, *202*
Ginn, J., 300, *307*
Giorgetti, M. M., 185, *187*
Giroux, F., 355, *362*
Girton, L. E., 60, *71*, 80, *88*, 110, *118*
Giskes, K., 271, *276*
Gispen, W. H., 164, *165*
Gitlin, L. N., 356, *363*
Given, C. W., 208, *215*
Gladsjo, J. A., 317, *322*
Glascher, J., 101, *107*
Glaser, R., 191, *202*, *203*, 305, *308*
Glass, K. C., 373, *377*
Glass, T. A., 61, *70*, 161, 163, 164, *166*, *167*
Gleason, M. E. J., 329, *334*
Glenn, N. D., 46, *52*
Glick, P., 251, 252, 254, *260*
Glisky, E. L., 75, 79, *91*
Glück, J., 280, 284, *288*, *289*
Glymour, M., 345, 346, *349*
Go, R. C., 345, *350*
Gobeski, K. T., 270, *274*
Godde, B., 116, *119*
Goedert, K. M., 142, *149*
Goesling, B., 208, *216*
Goetestam Skorpen, C., 139, *147*
Goffaux, J., 17, 18, *20*
Gofin, J., 209, *214*
Gofin, R., 209, *214*
Goh, J. O., 111, 115, *117*, *118*
Goins, R. T., 370, *377*
Gold, B. T., 80, *87*
Gold, P. W., 197, *201*
Goldberg, R. W., 313, *321*
Goldberg, T. E., 100, 102, *105*, *106*
Golden, C. J., 343, *349*
Goldman, N., 213, *218*
Goldman-Rakic, P. S., 101, *107*
Goldstein, D., 137, 141, 143, *148*, *151*
Goldstein, J., 160, *167*
Golomb, J., 75, *87*, 340, *349*
Golshan, S., 242, *245*, 317, *322*
Gomez, C. R., 345, *350*
Gomez-Pinilla, F., 164, *170*
Gong, Q. Y., 76, *87*
Gonzaga, G. C., 197, *205*
Good, C. D., 111, 113, *118*, 141, *147*, 162, *168*, 340, 346, *348*, *349*
Goode, K. T., 357, *364*
Goodglass, H., 343, 344, *349*, *350*
Goodman, E., 249, *260*
Goossens, L., 155, 156, *170*
Gootjes, L., 78, *87*
Gopher, D., 155, 158, 160, 161, *167*
Gorani, F., 78, 82, *87*
Gordon, E., 80, 81, *87*
Gordon, N. P., 318, *322*
Gordon, R. A., 253, 258, *260*, 269, *274*
Gordon, T. L., 328, *337*
Gordon-Larsen, P., 211, *215*
Goren, D., 301, 302, *308*
Gorlick, M. A., 303, *309*
Gorzelle, G. J., 154, *168*
Gottesman, I. I., 103, *105*
Gottfredson, L. S., 345, *349*
Gottman, J. M., 301, 302, *306*
Gould, D. A., 358, *364*
Gould, O. N., 183, *188*, 234, 240, *244*, *245*
Gould, T. D., 103, *105*
Gouw, A., 78, 79, *89*, 342, *350*
Gove, W. R., 46, *55*
Grace, A. A., 101, *104*
Grady, C. L., 60, 66, 67, *70*, *72*, 78, *86*, 112, *118*, 122, *130*, 137, *147*, 297, *308*
Graf, N. L., 346, *348*
Graf, P., 161, *168*
Graham, C., 317, *321*
Graham, J. W., 27, 28, 29, *37*, *38*
Grahn, J. A., 109, *119*
Grainger, K., 241, *245*
Grant, B. S., 318, *321*
Grant, I., 346, *349*, *351*, 360, 361, *363*
Grant, M. D., 96, 97, 103, *106*
Gräsel, E., 360, *363*
Gratton, B., 49, *52*
Gratton, G., 160, *166*
Grauer, H., 359, *363*
Gravenstein, S., 191, *203*
Gravina, S., 99, *105*
Gray, J. R., 17, *20*
Gray, K. F., 373, *377*
Green, A. E., 17, *20*
Green, C. S., 160, *167*
Green, J., 347, *349*
Greenberg, J. S., 222, *230*, 354, 355, *363*
Greendale, G. A., 197, *205*
Greene, J. C., 162, *169*, *170*
Greenlee, I., 253, *260*
Greenough, W. T., 154, *168*, 264, *274*
Greenwald, A. G., 253, 254, 255, 257, 258, *260*, *261*

Greenwood, P. M., 59, 66, *70*, 340, *349*
Gregory, R., 134, 137, *147*, *150*, 375, *378*
Greicius, M. D., 112, *118*
Greiner, L. H., 48, *54*
Greiner, P. A., 48, *54*
Greist, J. H., 332, *335*
Gretarsdottir, E. S., 316, *321*
Grether, D. M., 137, 138, *148*
Greve, D. N., 77, 80, *90*, 126, 127, *130*
Grieve, S. M., 75, 78, 80, 81, *87*, *89*
Griffin, L. J., 44, *53*
Griffin, P. W., 193, 194, *204*
Griffith, H. R., 373, *378*, *379*
Griffith, R., 373, *378*
Grimm, K. J., 30, 35, *37*, *38*
Grisso, T., 368, 369, 370, 371, *377*, *378*
Grodstein, F., 160, *170*, 198, *203*, 345, *349*
Gronenschild, E. H. B. M., 75, 84, *86*
Gross, J. J., 139, *147*, 301, 302, *307*
Grossardt, B. R., 304, *307*
Grossberg, G. T., 317, *321*
Grossman, M., 342, *350*
Grossman, R. I., 85, *87*
Grover, D. R., 178, *187*
Growdon, J. H., 137, *148*
Gruber-Baldini, A., 94, *107*
Gruenewald, T. L., 191, *205*, 213, *217*
Grühn, D., 297, 299, *308*
Grundy, E., 221, 222, 223, *230*
Gruneir, A. J. S., 242, *246*
Grzywacz, J. G., 195, *202*
Gubarchuk, J., 234, *245*
Guerra, M., 211, *217*
Gulmann, N., 328, *335*
Gum, A. M., 314, 316, 317, *321*, *322*
Gumbrecht, G., 196, *201*
Gunn, M., 371, *379*
Gunning, F. M., 74, *90*
Gunning-Dixon, F., 66, *70*, *71*, 76, *88*, 111, *118*
Gunning-Dixon, F. M., 75, 76, 78, 82, *87*, 75, 76, *90*, 315, *320*
Gunstad, J., 75, 78, *89*
Günther, A., 182, *189*
Gunthert, K. C., 194, *202*
Guo, X., 34, *37*
Gurrera, R. J., 371, *378*, *379*
Gurtman, M. B., 254, 255, *262*
Gurucharri, C., 283, *289*
Gurung, R. A. R., 191, *205*
Gusnard, D. A., 112, *119*
Gutchess, A., 67, *71*, 111, *117*, *118*, 121, 122, *131*
Guterman, A., 373, *378*
Gutierrez, P. R., 49, *53*
Gutierrez-Robledo, L. M., 315, *321*
Gutzmann, H., 154, *165*
Guy, D., 358, *362*
Guyll, M., 195, *202*

H

Ha, J. H., 219, 221, 222, 225, *230*
Haan, N., 285, *289*
Habeck, C., 340, *348*
Habel, I., 182, *189*
Haber, C., 49, *52*
Habib, J., 209, *214*
Habib, R., 122, *130*
Hackert, V. H., 75, *87*
Haddy, C., 332, *335*
Hagestad, G. O., 50, *52*, 219, *230*
Hagler, D. J., Jr., 80, *89*
Haines, J. L., 100, *105*
Hajek, C., 234, *245*
Haley, W. E., 354, 355, 356, 357, 358, 360, 361, *362*, *363*, *364*
Hall, A., 207, *215*
Hall, B., 253, *260*
Hall, C., 31, *39*, 178, *190*
Hall, C. B., 9, *22*, 113, *118*, 153, 163, *170*
Hall, G. S., 42, *52*
Hall, K. S., 49, *52*, 347, *352*
Halligan, E. M., 78, 79, *89*
Hallman, T., 200, *202*
Halter, J. B., 196, *201*
Halverson, C. F. J., 298, *307*
Halverson, K., 326, *336*
Hamagami, F., 28, 29, 30, 32, 33, *36*, *37*, *38*, 295, *307*
Hamaker, E. L., 35, *37*
Hamann, S., 183, *187*
Hamarat, E., 192, *202*
Hambrick, D. Z., 9, 16, *20*, *22*, 62, *70*, 141, *150*, 158, *167*
Hamel, M., 359, *363*
Hamer, D., 213, *215*
Hamil-Luker, J., 210, *216*
Hamilton, A. C., 62, 63, *71*
Hamilton, J. M., 342, 344, *349*
Hamilton, M., 328, *335*
Hamilton, R. L., 344, *350*
Hamlett, K. W., 155, *165*
Hammen, C., 197, *202*
Hammen, T., 80, *91*
Hammond, K. R., 136, *147*
Hampes, W. P., 237, *246*
Hampshire, A., 109, *119*
Han, P., 143, *150*
Hanakawa, T., 342, 343, *351*
Hancock, G. R., 29, *37*
Hancock, H. E., 65, *72*
Handen, B., 328, 329, *337*
Handy, T. C., 161, *168*
Hank, K., 271, *273*, *274*
Hannah, M. K., 271, *273*
Hannan, A., 164, *169*
Hannay, H. J., 339, *350*
Hanoch, Y., 143, 144, 145, *146*, *147*, *150*
Hansen, J. J., 254, 255, *262*
Hansen, L. A., 342, 344, *349*, *352*
Hanson, N. R., 4, *20*
Hansson, P., 142, *147*
Hanusa, B. H., 177, 184, 185, *189*
Haque, O., 78, *89*
Harden, T., 234, *245*
Harding, C. M., 317, *321*
Hardy, J. L., 158, 159, *168*
Hardy, S., 30, *38*
Hareven, T. K., 220, *230*
Harford, T. C., 318, *321*
Haring, M., 318, 319, *320*
Hariri, A. R., 127, *131*
Harley, E., 328, 329, *336*
Harlowe, D., 326, *336*
Harper, S., 269, *274*
Harrell, L., 373, *378*, *379*
Harrell, L. E., 368, 371, *378*
Harrington, F., 77, *87*
Harris, B. A., 175, 183, 185, *187*, *188*
Harris, M., 97, *106*
Harris, M. J., 317, *322*
Harris, S., 180, 183, *189*
Harris, S. E., 17, *20*, 99, *105*
Harris, T. O., 192, 195, *201*
Harrison, J. A., 370, *379*
Hart, A. D., 314, *323*
Hart, S., 197, *204*
Hartel, C. R., 181, *187*
Hartley, A., 111, *119*
Hartley, T., 162, *168*
Harwood, J., 233, 234, 236, 237, 238, 239, 240, 241, 243, *243*, *244*, *245*, *246*, 251, *260*
Haselgrove, J. C., 82, *85*
Hasher, L., 9, 11, *20*, *21*, *23*, 60, 62, 65, *70*, 135, 137, 141, 142, 143, *147*, *148*, *151*, 257, *259*, *262*
Hasler, G., 103, *105*
Hassing, L. B., 48, *52*
Hastings, E., 155, 156, 159, 164, *165*, *167*
Häubl, G., 143, *148*
Hauger, R. L., 198, *203*
Hausdorff, J. M., 180, 181, *188*, 258, *259*, *261*
Hauser, P., 372, *379*
Hauser, R. M., 44, 46, *52*, 153, *167*
Hausmann, E., 270, *273*
Havens, J. J., 368, *378*
Havighurst, R. J., 270, *274*
Havlik, R. J., 345, *349*
Hawkins, H. L., 161, *167*
Hawkley, L. C., 16, *20*, 226, *229*, 295, 304, 305, *306*, *307*, *308*

Haworth, C. M., 96, 97, *105*
Haxby, J. V., 78, *86*, 340, *349*
Hay, E. L., 219, 220, 221, 222, 223, 224, 225, 226, 227, *230*
Hay, J. F., 65, *71*
Hayakawa, K., 95, *105*
Hayasaka, S., 75, *86*, 115, *118*
Hayashi, K. M., 83, *86*
Hayashi, N., 80, *85*
Hayden, K. M., 101, *105*
Hayes, S. M., 67, 68, *70*
Haynes, S. N., 325, *335*
Hayward, M. D., 50, *52*, 209, 210, 212, *215*, *216*, 367, *379*
Hazlitt, J. E., 6, 16, 17, *21*
He, W., 153, *168*
Head, D., 16, *22*, 59, 60, 61, 63, 65, 66, 69, *71*, 74, 75, 76, 77, 80, 83, *88*, *90*, 110, 112, *117*, *118*, 123, 124, 125, *130*, *131*, 141, *150*
Head, E., 75, 83, *91*, 343, *350*
Healey, M. K., 141, 142, *147*, *148*
Heatherton, T. F., 297, *308*
Heaton, R. K., 66, *71*, 317, *322*, 339, 343, 346, 347, *348*, *349*, *351*
Hebert, R. S., 361, *363*
Hebert, T., 372, 373, 375, *378*
Hebrank, A. C., 67, *71*, 112, *119*
Heckhausen, J., 177, 179, 181, *187*, *189*, *190*, 235, *245*, 250, *260*, 300, *308*
Hedden, T., 5, 9, 14, 16, *20*, *22*, 62, 63, 65, *71*, 83, *86*, 110, 111, *118*, *119*, 122, *130*, 143, *147*
Hedehus, M., 80, 81, *89*
Hedge, J. W., 270, *274*
Heekeren, H. R., 101, 102, *106*, 125, 127, 129, *130*, 138, *149*
Heeringa, S. G., 345, *351*
Heffner, K. L., 305, *308*
Heijboer, R., 77, 78, *86*, 340, *349*
Heijmans, B. T., 99, *105*
Heiman, N., 97, *105*
Heinonen, K., 315, *322*
Heinze, H. J., 83, *86*, *87*, 303, *308*
Heisel, M. J., 329, *335*
Helder, E., 9, *20*, 62, *70*
Helenius, H., 111, *118*
Hellemann, G., 75, *87*
Hellhammer, D. H., 182, *187*
Helmers, K. F., 6, *19*, 156, 159, *165*, 268, *272*
Helms, J. E., 346, *349*
Helms, M. J., 265, *275*
Helson, R., 43, *52*, 266, *274*, 284, 285, 286, 287, *289*, *291*
Hemingway, H., 270, *275*
Hencke, R., 180, 181, *188*, 258, 259, *261*
Henderson, A. S., 327, *334*, 347, *351*
Henderson, C. R., 360, *364*
Henderson, J. H., 347, *351*
Henderson, R., 34, *37*
Hendricks, J., 5, 10, *20*
Hendricks, T., 163, *168*
Hendrie, H. C., 49, *52*, 345, 347, *349*, *352*
Henning, K., 68, *72*
Henretta, J. C., 221, 222, 223, *230*
Henry, C., 234, *245*, 253, 254, *261*
Henry, J. D., 59, 60, 61, 62, 66, 67, 68, *70*, *71*, *72*, 297, 298, *309*, *310*
Henry, N. J. M., 301, 302, *310*
Henson, J. W., 46, *50*
Henson, R. N., 340, *349*
Henson, R. N. A., 141, *147*
Henwood, K., 233, 234, 235, 238, 240, 241, *244*, *246*, 254, *262*
Hepburn, K., 360, *362*
Hepworth, J. T., 208, *217*
Herd, P., 208, *216*
Herman, R., 235, *247*
Hermosillo, D., 346, 347, *348*
Hernandez, L. M., 214, *216*
Herrmann, A., 137, *148*
Hersen, M., 329, 332, *335*, *336*
Hershey, D. A., 143, *147*
Hertzog, C., 5, 6, 10, 12, 18, *20*, 29, 32, *37*, 110, 113, *118*, 154, 156, 161, *166*, *167*, 178, 180, 181, 183, *187*, *190*, 254, 256, *261*, *262*, 265, 268, *273*, *274*
Herzog, A. R., 208, 209, 210, *216*, 271, *274*, 304, *308*, 345, *349*
Hess, T. M., 61, 66, 67, *70*, *71*, 138, 139, 142, 144, *147*, *150*, 175, 181, *187*, 250, 253, 256, 257, 259, *259*, *260*, 301, *308*
Hetherington, H. P., 75, *91*
Hevelone, N. D., 80, *90*
Hewitt, J. K., 97, *105*
Heyn, P., 154, *167*
Hibbard, J. H., 134, 143, 145, 146, *147*, *148*, *149*, 371, *379*
Hicken, B., 371, *379*
Hicken, M., 212, 213, *215*
Hietala, J., 111, *118*
Higdon, R., 49, *52*
Hilgeman, M. M., 357, *363*
Hill, J., 161, *167*
Hill, R. D., 156, 161, *167*, *170*, 374, *378*
Hillemeier, M. M., 212, *215*
Hillman, C. H., 84, *88*, 303, *310*
Hinson, J. T., 256, 257, 259, *260*
Hinterlong, J., 271, 272, *275*
Hirschberger, G., 301, 302, *310*
Hirschman, C., 49, *52*
Hirstein, W., 113, *119*
Hixon, J. G., 253, *260*
Hjerling-Leffler, J., 164, *168*
Ho, D. Y. F., 251, *260*
Ho, G. J., 344, *351*
Hockey, R., 356, 358, *362*
Hodges, E. A., 144, *147*, 257, 259, *260*
Hofer, S. M., 6, 9, 11, 14, 16, 17, 18, *21*, *22*, 26, 29, 31, *36*, *37*, *39*, 48, *52*, 63, *69*, 94, 97, *105*, *107*, 178, *188*, *190*, 194, *205*
Hoffman, C., 211, *216*
Hofheimer, J. A., 197, *203*
Hofman, A., 75, *87*
Hofman, P., 84, *86*
Hofstetter, R. C., 344, *352*
Hogan, M. J., 60, 61, 68, *71*
Hogan, R., 265, *274*
Hogervorst, E., 101, *105*
Hogg, M. A., 241, *246*
Hohmann, C., 374, *379*
Hoijtink, H. J. A., 333, *337*
Holahan, C. J., 316, *321*
Holahan, C. K., 316, *321*
Holen, A., 318, *321*
Holland, A. J., 371, *379*
Holland, F., 30, 31, 32, *38*
Holland, J. M., 361, *363*
Holliday, S. G., 138, 140, *148*, 280, 282, *289*
Hollon, N. G., 137, *148*
Holm, N. V., 95, 99, *104*, *107*
Holmes, D., 327, *337*
Holmes, T. H., 192, *202*
Holt-Lundstad, J., 196, *205*, 225, *232*, 295, 297, 303, *310*
Homans, G. F., 220, *230*
Homes, D., 314, *323*
Honda, M., 342, 343, *351*
Hong, C. J., 100, *107*
Hong, J., 222, *230*
Hong, S., 196, *201*
Hongwanishkul, D., 112, *118*, 297, *308*
Hooijer, C., 327, 328, *334*
Hook, J. N., 332, *336*
Hooker, K., 34, *39*, 176, 177, 185, *187*, 225, *231*, 355, 356, *363*
Hooper, H. E., 344, *350*
Hopkins, R. O., 78, *88*
Hopper, C. D., 211, *215*
Horan, M., 9, *22*, 66, 67, 68, *72*
Horhota, M., 257, *259*
Horn, J. L., 29, 30, *37*, *38*
Horn, M. C., 192, 193, *200*, 302, *306*
Horne, N. R., 343, *349*
Hornung, C. A., 375, *378*
Horowitz, M., 199, *202*
Horowitz, M. J., 318, *321*
Horowitz, S. V., 330, *334*
Hosie, J. A., 297, 298, *309*
Hosterman, S., 220, 222, 223, 225, 227, *230*

Hotchkiss, L., 211, *216*
Hoth, K., 78, *89*
Houck, P. R., 326, *336*
House, J. S., 208, 209, 210, 212, *216*, *217*, *218*
Houseman, E. A., 95, *104*
Housen, P., 157, 158, 159, *169*
Houx, P. J., 265, *273*
Howard, G., 48, *52*
Howard, R., 317, *321*
Howard, V. J., 345, *350*
Howe, F. A., 80, 81, *86*
Howerter, A., 60, 62, 63, 64, *71*, 114, *118*, 161, *168*
Howieson, D. B., 339, *350*
Howland, J., 175, 183, 184, 185, *188*, *190*
Hrebickova, M., 304, *309*
Hsee, C. K., 135, *149*, 371, *378*
Hsu, A. Y. C., 139, *147*
Hu, J., 100, *106*
Hu, L., 115, *117*
Hu, P., 197, *205*
Hu, X., 81, 82, *88*
Hu, X. Z., 101, *107*
Huan, Z. D., 129, *130*
Huang, M. H., 213, *217*
Huang, V., 327, *337*
Hubler, D., 100, *106*
Hudson, P., 212, *216*
Huettel, S. A., 81, *88*
Hugdahl, K., 125, *130*
Hugenschmidt, C. E., 80, *88*
Hughes, C. P., 342, *352*
Hughes, D. C., 327, *334*
Hughes, H. B., 17, *23*
Hughes, M. E., 222, *230*
Hughes, M. H., 50, *52*
Hughes, T. F., 265, *273*
Hui, S. L., 49, *52*, 347, *352*
Hulbert, A., 226, *230*
Hull, R., 62, 63, *71*
Hultsch, D. F., 4, 5, 9, 11, 17, *20*, *21*, 26, 33, *37*, *167*, 178, 180, 183, *187*
Hummer, R., 212, *216*
Hummer, R. A., 208, 210, *217*
Hummert, M. L., 233, 234, 235, 236, 238, 239, 240, 241, 242, *244*, *245*, *246*, 247, *247*, 249, 250, 251, 252, 253, 254, 255, 257, 258, 259, *259*, *260*, *261*, *262*
Hunt, C., 114, *117*
Hunter, J. V., 82, *85*
Hunter, M. A., 26, 33, *37*
Hurd, M. D., 210, *216*
Hurley, M. M., 253, *262*
Hurt, S. W., 331, *336*
Hurwitz, D., 373, *378*
Husted, J., 332, *335*
Huston, A. C., 42, 50, *52*
Hutchison, S., 157, 158, *166*
Hutson, M. A., 211, *217*
Huyck, M. H., 266, *274*
Hybels, C., 326, 327, *335*
Hyer, L., 332, *335*
Hyler, S. E., 332, *335*
Hyman, B., 100, *105*
Hyndman, D., 374, *378*

I

Iannucci, G., 82, *90*
Ikels, C., 50, *52*
Imfeld, A., 113, *118*
Ingersoll-Dayton, B., 225, *230*, 304, *310*
Ingram, K. K., 368, 371, *378*
Ingvar, M., 16, *22*, 81, 82, *89*, 114, *118*, *119*, 122, 123, 124, 125, 129, *130*, *131*, 156, *169*
Inoue, M., 342, *351*
Inouye, S. K., 343, *349*
Insel, T. R., 197, *202*
Institute of Medicine, 154, *167*
Irving, S., 227, *230*
Irwin, M. R., 360, 361, *363*
Isaacowitz, D. M., 193, *201*, 300, 301, 302, *307*, *308*
Isaacs, S. L., 208, *216*
Iso-Ahola, S. E., 184, *189*
Ivnik, I., 339, *349*
Izal, M., 360, *364*
Izard, C. E., 296, *308*

J

Jack, C. R., 83, *88*, 111, *118*
Jack, C. R., Jr., 83, *88*
Jack, L. M., 78, *86*, *91*
Jackey, L. M. H., 224, 225, 226, *229*
Jacko, J. A., 113, *119*
Jackson, E. S., 313, *321*
Jackson, H., 328, *334*
Jackson, J., 210, 211, *217*
Jackson, J. H., 60, *71*
Jackson, J. S., 49, *52*, 213, *216*
Jackson, P. M. A. B. S. N., 345, *350*
Jackson, S. H. D., 16, *21*
Jacobs, D. M., 346, *350*
Jacobs, H. I., 75, *86*
Jacobs, S., 197, *202*, 281, 282, 283, *288*, 318, *320*
Jacobsen, J. J., 195, *201*
Jacobson, K. C., 96, 97, *106*
Jacobson, M. W., 342, *349*
Jacobson, N. S., 356, *363*
Jacoby, L., 60, 61, 62, 64, 65, 68, *70*, *71*
Jacomb, P. A., 327, *334*
Jacova, C., 343, *352*
Jaeggi, S. M., 157, 158, *166*, *167*
Jäger, T., 299, *308*
Jagust, W., 83, *88*, 121, 123, 125, 129, *130*
Jagust, W. J., 79, *89*, 125, 126, 127, *130*, *131*
Jahng, G. H., 75, *86*
Jahnke, H., 135, *146*
Jain, E., 303, *308*
Jakobsson-Mo, S., 125, 127, *131*
James, B. D., 372, *378*
James, J. B., 42, *52*, 270, *274*
Jancke, L., 113, *118*
Janevic, M. R., 357, *363*
Janicki-Deverts, D., 220, 226, *229*
Janke, M., 221, *229*
Janowsky, J. S., 75, 76, *90*
Jatulis, D. E., 209, *218*
Jaussent, I., 315, *322*
Jax, C., 287, *289*
Jencks, C. S., 345, 346, *349*
Jenkins, K. R., 315, *321*
Jenkins, L. J., 111, 112, *119*, 346, *350*
Jennings, G., 196, *202*
Jennings, J. M., 159, *166*
Jennings, P. A., 281, 284, 287, *290*
Jernigan, T. L., 103, *106*
Jeste, D. V., 242, *244*, 282, *289*, 313, 314, 315, 316, *321*, 326, *335*, 372, *377*, *379*
Jette, A., 183, 184, 185, *188*, *190*
Jette, A. M., 185, *187*, 211, *218*
Jicha, G. A., 80, *87*
Jin, Y.-S., 251, *261*
Jobe, J. B., 6, *19*, 156, 159, *165*, *167*, 268, *272*
Jobin, J., 303, *306*
Joffe, M., 211, *215*
Johansson, B., 95, *106*, 265, *272*
Johansson, L., 223, *231*
Johansson, U., 113, *118*
Johns, J. M., 197, *203*
Johnson, B. N., 67, 68, *72*
Johnson, B. T., 250, 253, 258, *261*
Johnson, E. J., 137, 143, *148*, *151*
Johnson, J. K., 343, *350*
Johnson, K., 157, *170*
Johnson, M. J., 41, 43, *53*
Johnson, M. K., 141, *149*
Johnson, M. L., 5, 11, *19*
Johnson, M. M., 143, 144, *148*, *150*
Johnson, N. J., 209, *217*
Johnson, R. E., 162, *167*
Johnson, R., Jr., 61, 62, 68, 69, *70*
Johnson, S. M., 136, *147*
Johnson, W., 97, *105*
Johnsrude, I. S., 113, *118*, 141, *147*, 162, *168*, 340, *349*
Jokinen, H., 342, *350*
Jolles, J., 66, *72*, 75, *86*, *91*, 156, *170*, 265, *273*

Jones, C. J., 33, *37*, 313, *321*
Jones, D. K., 80, *89*
Jones, E., 236, *245*
Jones, G., 111, *119*
Jones, K., 46, 49, *50*, 160, *165*, 303, *309*
Jones, L., 375, *378*
Jones, M., 31, *37*
Jones, M. P., 316, *323*
Jones, R., 157, *171*
Jones, S., 114, *118*, *119*, 156, *169*
Jongenelis, K., 314, *321*, *322*
Jongenelis, L., 313, *323*
Jonides, J., 111, *119*, 158, *167*
Jordan, J., 281, 282, 283, *289*
Jorm, A. F., 16, *19*, 102, *105*, 304, *308*, 327, *334*
Joyner, A. H., 103, *105*
Ju, C., 80, 81, *91*
Juardo, M. B., 60, *71*
Judd, L. L., 314, *321*, 326, *335*
Judica, E., 82, *85*
Jukema, J. W., 271, *276*
June, A., 329, *336*
Jungeblut, A., 346, *350*
Juon, H. S., 212, *215*
Juslin, P., 142, *147*
Juslin, P. N., 297, *308*

K

Kaasinen, V., 111, *118*
Kabacoff, R. I., 329, 332, *335*, *336*
Kabani, N. J., 84, *89*
Kabat-Zinn, J., 199, *202*
Kabeto, M., 345, *350*
Kabeto, M. U., 304, *308*, 315, *321*
Kadish, I., 17, *21*, 99, *106*
Kahana, E., 181, *188*
Kähler, A. K., 103, *107*
Kahn, A. S., 286, *290*
Kahn, R. L., 43, *52*, 175, 180, *189*, 194, *204*, 209, *217*
Kahn, S. A., 196, *202*
Kahneman, D., 133, 135, 136, 137, *148*, *151*, 198, *202*, 371, *378*
Kail, R. V., 35, *37*
Kajantie, E., 197, *202*, 315, *322*
Kalisch, R., 101, *107*
Kalska, H., 342, *350*
Kamal, A., 164, *165*
Kamo, Y., 221, *230*
Kamp Dush, C. M., 220, 222, 223, 225, 227, *229*, *230*
Kamphuis, C. B. M., 271, *276*
Kanamori, M., 95, *105*
Kanaya, A. M., 345, *350*
Kane, M. J., 158, *167*
Kane, R. A., 355, *362*
Kane, R. L., 355, *362*
Kanellopoulos, D., 315, *320*
Kanfer, R., 163, *165*, 267, *274*
Kang, J. H., 160, *170*
Kang, S. K., 257, 259, *261*
Kannel, W. B., 196, *202*
Kanwisher, N. G., 113, *117*
Kaplan, D., 343, *349*
Kaplan, E., 102, *105*, 342, 343, 344, *349*, *350*
Kaplan, G. A., 209, *217*
Kaplan, K., 344, *349*
Kaplan, R. M., 317, *322*
Kaprio, J., 98, *107*
Karel, M., 311, *321*
Karel, M. J., 178, *187*, 354, *362*, 371, *378*, *379*
Karlamangla, A. S., 213, *216*
Karlawish, J. H., 368, 372, *378*
Karlsson, E., 138, *150*
Karlsson, P., 125, 127, 128, 129, *129*, *130*
Karlsson, S., 125, 127, 128, 129, *129*, *130*
Karp, N., 372, *378*
Kasen, S., 315, *323*
Kaskie, B., 356, *363*
Kasl, S. V., 226, *229*, 250, 257, 258, 259, *261*, 263, 270, *273*
Kasl-Godley, J. E., 311, *321*, 327, *335*, 354, *362*
Kasper, J. D., 208, 211, 213, *218*, 219, 223, *232*
Kasten, L., 157, *170*, 184, 185, *190*
Katlin, E. S., 197, *204*
Kato, K., 95, 97, *105*, *106*, *201*, 304, *307*
Katon, W., 354, 355, *364*
Katona, C., 355, *362*
Katz, I., 327, *336*
Katz, I. R., 313, 316, *320*, *322*
Katz, M., 9, *22*
Katz, M. J., 75, *91*, 113, *118*, 153, 163, *170*
Kaufer, D. I., 344, *350*
Kaufman, J. S., 211, *216*
Kaufmann, J., 83, *86*, *87*
Kaup, A. R., 138, 145, *146*
Kausler, D. H., 141, *148*
Kawachi, I., 198, *203*, 345, 346, *349*
Kay, A. C., 184, *187*, *188*
Kaye, D., 196, *202*
Kaye, J. A., 75, 76, *90*, 124, *130*
Keene, D., 212, 213, *215*
Keeton, D. M., 374, *379*
Keightley, M., 297, *308*
Keinan, A., 143, *148*
Keith, S. J., 317, *321*
Kekes, J., 280, 281, 282, 283, 285, 286, *289*
Keller, S., 76, *87*
Keller-Cohen, D., 241, *246*
Kelly, J. F., 198, 199, *205*
Kemeny, M. E., 182, *187*, 197, *202*
Kemp, B. J., 83, *88*, 111, *118*, 314, *321*
Kemper, H. C. G., 200, *205*
Kemper, S., 69, *71*, 234, 238, *245*, 247, *247*
Kemper, T. L., 74, *88*
Kempermann, G., 84, *87*, 113, *118*, 164, *167*, 264, *276*
Kempler, D., 347, *350*
Kendler, K. S., 98, *106*, 194, 195, *203*, 316, *322*
Kennaley, D. E., 237, *246*
Kennedy, C., 162, *168*, 372, *378*
Kennedy, J. L., 101, *104*
Kennedy, K. M., 16, *22*, 59, 60, 61, 63, 65, 66, 69, *71*, 74, 75, 76, 77, 78, 79, 80, 81, 83, 84, *87*, *88*, *89*, *90*, 110, 111, *118*, *119*, 123, 124, 125, 129, *131*, 141, *148*, *150*, 340, *350*
Kennedy, Q., 301, 303, *308*
Kennison, R. F., 43, *55*, 157, 158, 159, *169*
Kenntner-Mabiala, R., 297, *310*
Kensinger, E. A., 137, *148*, 297, 298, *308*
Keough, K., 346, *348*
Kepe, V., 83, *86*
Kerkhof, A. J., 315, *323*
Kern, S., 270, *273*
Kertesz, A., 343, *350*, *352*
Kessler, E.-M., 264, 266, 267, 268, *274*, *276*
Kessler, R. C., 192, 195, *201*, *203*, 208, 209, 210, *216*, 314, *322*, 328, *335*
Kestler, L., 183, *187*
Keverne, E. B., 228, *229*
Khan, H. T. A., 269, *274*
Kiddoe, J., 95, *107*
Kiecolt-Glaser, J. K., 191, *203*, 305, *308*, 361, *362*, *364*
Kieffer, K. M., 327, *335*
Kielkopf, M. R., 370, *377*
Killiany, R. J., 125, 126, 127, *129*, *130*
Kim, J. E., 195, *203*
Kim, J. H., 357, 358, *363*
Kim, J. K., 196, *202*
Kim, J. S., 116, *117*, 129, *130*, 161, *166*
Kim, K., 318, *320*
Kim, R., 343, *350*
Kim, S., 135, 137, 141, *148*, 270, 271, *274*
Kim, S. Y. H., 371, *378*
Kim, T. K., 82, *88*
King, B., 139, *147*
King, D. A., 326, 327, *334*, *336*
King, H., 200, *200*

King, L., 298, *309*
King, P. M., 284, *289*
King-Kallimanis, B., 314, 316, 317, *321*, *322*
Kington, R. S., 209, *216*
Kinney, A. M., 208, 209, 210, *216*
Kinsella, K., 153, *168*
Kinzel, E. N., 113, *119*
Kirkwood, T. B., 46, *51*
Kirsch, I. S., 346, *350*
Kirschbaum, C., 182, *187*
Kirson, D., 346, *351*
Kisley, M. A., 302, *310*
Kitayama, S., 179, *188*
Kitchener, K. S., 284, *289*
Kite, M. E., 250, 253, 258, *261*
Kittner, S. J., 46, *51*
Kivela, S., 304, *308*
Kivett, V. R., 220, *229*, 266, *274*
Kivimaki, M., 304, *308*
Kivnick, H. Q., 282, *289*
Klebe, K. J., 32, 35, *36*
Kleemeier, R. W., 34, *37*
Klein, D. M., 313, *323*, 326, *337*
Klein, K., 191, 197, 198, 199, *201*, *203*
Klein, L. C., 191, 197, *203*, *205*
Klein, M. H., 332, *335*, *337*
Klein, S., 101, *107*
Klemera, P., 6, 17, *21*
Kliegel, M., 299, *308*
Kliegl, R., 114, *118*, 154, *165*, *168*, 234, *245*, 267, *274*
Kligman, E. W., 346, *352*
Klimstra, S., 315, *320*
Klonoff, E. A., 346, *350*
Kluger, A., 75, *87*, 340, *349*
Kluiter, H., 314, *321*
Klunder, A. D., 83, *86*
Kluth, J. T., 76, *89*
Knight, B. G., 139, *148*, 354, 356, 357, 358, *362*, *363*
Knight, K. M., 49, *52*, 213, *216*
Knight, M., 16, *21*, 139, 141, *149*
Knight, M. R., 140, *149*, 298, *309*
Knopman, D. S., 48, *52*, 83, *88*, 345, *348*
Knops, U., 235, 236, *246*
Knouf, N., 113, *117*
Knowlton, B., 122, *131*
Knutson, B., 137, *148*
Ko, S., 82, *88*
Kobau, R., 298, *308*
Koch, H. E., 145, *151*, 304, *310*
Kocha, J., 264, *276*
Kochunov, P., 80, *88*
Koenig, C. S., 286, *288*
Koenig, H. G., 326, 327, *335*, *336*
Koepke, K. M., 49, *55*, 156, 157, 159, *171*
Koepsell, T. D., 208, *217*
Kogan, J., 328, 329, *335*
Kohlberg, L., 283, *289*
Kohli, M., 221, *230*
Kohn, M. L., 44, 48, *52*, 266, *274*
Kohn, R., 314, 316, 317, *321*, *322*
Kolarz, C. M., 298, 299, *309*
Koling, A., 138, 140, *151*
Koloski, N., 328, 329, *336*
Kolson, D. L., 85, *87*
Kolstad, A., 346, *350*
Kompus, K., 125, *130*
Köpetz, C., 183, *187*
Korkeila, J., 304, *308*
Korkeila, K., 304, *308*
Korner, A., 328, *335*
Korol, D. L., 84, *87*
Korten, A. E., 327, *334*
Koskenvuo, M., 98, *107*
Kosten, T., 197, *202*
Kotz, S. A., 297, *309*
Koudstaal, P. J., 75, *87*
Koutstall, W., 162, *170*
Kovacevic, N., 67, *70*, 112, *118*
Kovacs, D., 100, *106*
Kovalchik, S., 137, 138, *148*
Kowalewski, R. B., 305, *306*
Koyama, A. K., 80, *89*
Kozma, A., 159, *169*
Krabbe, K., 79, *87*
Kraft, D., 136, *151*
Kraft, R. A., 80, *88*
Kral, V. A., 340, *350*
Kramer, A. F., 6, *21*, 49, *51*, 67, *71*, 74, 75, 80, 84, *88*, 110, 113, 115, *117*, *118*, 129, *130*, 141, *148*, 154, 157, 158, 160, 161, 163, 164, *165*, *166*, *167*, *168*, 264, 265, *274*
Kramer, D. A., 282, 283, 285, 286, 287, *289*
Kramer, J., 75, *86*, 102, *105*
Kramer, J. H., 342, 343, *349*
Kramer, M., 328, *336*
Krampe, R. T., 154, 159, *171*
Krasnow, B., 112, *118*
Krause, N., 49, *52*, *54*, 178, 180, *187*, *190*, 301, 304, *309*, *310*
Kraut, M., 78, 79, *91*
Kraut, M. A., 123, *129*, 141, *150*
Kray, J., 64, *71*
Kremen, W. S., 95, 103, *106*
Kremer, D., 99, *105*
Krendl, A. C., 297, *308*
Kressig, R. W., 154, *165*
Krey, L. C., 197, 198, *204*
Krienen, F. M., 83, *86*
Krings, F., 255, *261*
Kristeller, J., 199, *201*
Kritchevsky, S. B., 210, *217*
Krivoshekova, Y. S., 296, 299, 301, *309*
Kröger, E., 265, *274*
Krueger, K. R., 97, *105*, 304, *310*
Kruglanski, A. W., 136, *148*
Krumholz, H. M., 270, *273*
Kruse, A., 264, 268, *274*
Krzywanski, S., 373, *378*, *379*
Kua, E. H., 125, *131*
Kuan, S. A., 101, *104*
Kubat-Silman, A. K., 156, *166*
Kubo-Germano, K., 347, *351*
Kuczmarski, M. F., 211, *216*
Kudadjie-Gyamfi, E., 296, 299, 301, *309*
Kuerbis, A. N., 358, *364*
Kühl, K.-P., 154, *165*
Kuhlen, R. G., 41, *52*
Kuhn, H. G., 113, *118*
Kuhn, T. S., 4, *21*
Kuin, Y., 333, *337*
Kukull, W. A., 48, 49, *52*, *53*, 100, *105*, 347, *352*
Kumar, A., 75, *87*, 327, *335*
Kumka, D., 44, *53*
Kunik, M. E., 317, *322*
Kunimatsu, A., 80, *85*
Kunkel, S. R., 257, *261*
Kunzmann, U., 180, *187*, 266, *276*, 283, 285, 286, 287, *289*, *291*, 297, 298, 299, *308*
Kuo, P. H., 103, *104*
Kuo, T. Y., 75, 79, *91*
Kuo, W., 29, *37*
Kuperman, J. M., 80, *89*
Kupfer, D. J., 197, *205*
Kupperbusch, C. S., 299, *308*
Kupperman, J. J., 285, 287, *290*
Kurbanyan, K., 327, *335*
Kuslansky, G., 153, 163, *170*
Kwan, V. S. Y., 252, *260*
Kwong See, S. T., 233, 242, *246*, 254, *262*
Kyvik, K., 95, *107*

L

Labonte, B., 99, *106*
Labouvie-Vief, G., 5, *21*, 137, 139, 145, *148*, *151*, 193, *202*, *203*, 303, 304, *308*, *310*
Labuda, M. C., 97, *105*
Lachance, L., 355, *362*
Lachin, J. M., 164, *168*
Lachman, H. M., 102, *104*
Lachman, M. E., 176, 177, 178, 179, 180, 181, 182, 183, 184, 185, 186, *186*, *187*, *188*, *189*, *190*, 251, 257, *259*, *262*
LaClere, F., 212, *216*
Lacomblez, L., 343, *351*
Laggnäs, E., 138, *150*
Lal, R., 127, *130*

LaLoggia, A., 138, 145, *146*
Lambert, J. D., 227, *231*, 360, *364*
Lambert, W., 17, 18, *20*
Lamme, S., 319, *322*
Lammlein, S. E., 270, *274*
Lampert, T., 271, *273*
Lancaster, J. L., 80, *88*
Lance, C. E., 359, *362*
Land, S., 84, *90*
Land, S. J., 80, 84, *88*
Landau, S., 80, 81, *86*
Landau, S. M., 127, *130*
Landeau, B., 67, *71*
Landrigan, P. J., 212, *217*
Landrine, H., 346, *350*
Lane, A., 60, 61, 62, 63, 65, 66, 67, 68, *71*
Lane, D., 62, 63, *71*
Lane, R. D., 298, 299, *308*
Lang, F. R., 138, *148*, 193, *203*, 300, 301, *308*
Lang, I., 345, *350*
Langa, K. M., 304, *308*, 315, *321*, 345, *350*, *351*
Langbaum, B. S., 155, 156, 157, 161, 164, *168*, *169*
Langenecker, S. A., 67, *71*
Langer, E., 184, *188*, 251, 257, *261*
Langer, E. J., 177, 178, *189*, 258, *262*
Langeslag, S. J. E., 302, *308*
Langley, L. K., 303, *308*
Languay, R., 67, 68, *72*
Lanphear, A. K., 160, *166*
Lantz, P. M., 209, 212, *216*
Lapage, M., 198, *203*
LaPierre, T. A., 222, *230*
Larish, J. F., 158, *168*
Larish, J. L., 164, *168*
Larkin, G. R., 137, *149*
Larkin, K., 328, *335*
LaRossa, G., 83, *86*
Larrabee, G. J., 326, 327, *335*
Larson, E. B., 347, *352*
Larson, M. D., 196, *202*
Larsson, A., 16, *22*, 81, 82, *89*, 101, *104*, 112, 114, 115, 116, *117*, *119*, 122, 123, 124, 125, 127, 129, *130*, *131*, 158, 163, 164, *166*
Larsson, H. B., 79, *87*
Larsson, L., 138, *150*
LaRue, A., 48, *54*
Latimer, E., 355, *364*
LaTourette, T., 234, 236, *245*
Latoussakis, V., 315, *320*
Lau, A., 328, *335*
Laub, J. H., 42, 46, *52*, *53*
Laukka, P., 297, *308*
Launer, L. J., 125, *131*
Laurienti, P. J., 115, *118*
Laurin, D., 265, *274*
Laurin, K., 184, *187*, *188*
Lauriola, M., 138, 140, *148*
Lauritzen, L., 328, *335*
Lautenschlager, G., 110, *119*
LaVeist, T. A., 208, 209, 210, 211, 213, *215*, *216*, *217*, *218*
Laviolette, P. S., 83, *91*
Lavretsky, H., 161, *169*, 327, *335*
Lawrence, F. R., 29, *37*
Lawton, M. P., 139, *148*, 193, *203*, 313, *322*, 327, *336*
Lazarus, R. S., 192, 193, 200, *202*, *203*, 302, *308*, 354, 356, *363*
Le, T. N., 286, 287, *290*
Leach, L., 344, *349*
Leaf, P. J., 318, *320*
Leaper, S., 100, *105*
Leclerc, C. M., 144, *147*, 297, 298, *308*
Lecours, A. R., 198, *203*
Ledakis, G. E., 82, *85*
Lee, A. H., 374, *378*
Lee, C., 159, 164, *165*
Lee, H. C., 374, *378*
Lee, J. A., 99, *106*
Lee, K. Y., 82, *88*
Lee, M. P., 134, *151*
Lee, S., 198, *203*
Lee, T. M., 139, *148*
Lee, Y. J., 222, *230*
Leeson, G., 269, *274*
Lefcourt, H. M., 177, *188*
LeFevour, A., 101, *107*
Lefkowitz, E. S., 220, 221, 222, 225, 226, 227, 228, *229*, *230*
Legro, R. S., 196, *203*
Lehman, D. R., 318, 319, *320*
Lehmann, D. J., 101, *105*
Lehmbeck, J. T., 125, 126, *129*
Leifheit-Limson, E., 256, 257, 258, 259, *261*
Leinsinger, G., 78, *87*
Leip, E. P., 196, *202*
Leirer, V. O., 155, *168*
Leland, J., 179, *188*
Lemmon, H., 96, 100, *105*
Lemstra, A. W., 342, *350*
Lennartsson, C., 159, *168*
Lennon, E., 49, *51*
Leon, J., 145, *149*
Lepkowski, J. M., 208, 209, 210, 212, *216*
Leproult, R., 197, *205*
Lerner, J. S., 137, *148*
Lerner, R. M., 4, 5, *20*
Le Roux, H., 326, 328, *337*
Lesher, E. L., 327, *335*
Leshikar, E. D., 67, *71*
Leuchter, A. F., 78, 79, *86*, *88*
Leuenberger, B., 101, *107*
Leung, A. W., 139, *148*
Leung, C. C., 137, *150*
Leung, Y. J., 103, *106*
LeValley, A., 113, *118*
Leveck, M. D., 6, *19*, 156, 159, *165*, 268, *272*
Levenson, C., 185, *187*
Levenson, M. R., 47, *50*, 281, 284, 287, *290*
Levenson, R. W., 296, 297, 299, 301, 302, 303, *306*, *308*, *310*
Leventhal, E. A., 42, 48, 49, *52*
Leventhal, H., 42, 48, 49, *52*, *54*
Leverenz, J., 48, *53*
Lévesque, L., 355, *362*
Levin, I., 137, *150*
Levin, I. P., 138, 140, *148*, *151*
Levine, B., 159, *168*, *171*
Levine, C., 358, *364*
Levine, E. G., 354, *363*
Levitt, H. M., 282, *290*
Levitzki, N., 222, *230*
Levy, B. R., 175, 179, 180, 181, *186*, *188*, 226, 228, *229*, *230*, 241, 242, *244*, *245*, 250, 251, 256, 257, 258, 259, *261*
Lévy, C., 78, *91*
Levy, G., 159, *169*
Lewinsohn, P. M., 313, *323*, 327, *335*
Lewis, B. P., 191, *205*
Lewis, G., 197, *205*
Lewis, K. L., 43, *55*
Lewkowicz, C. J., 184, *188*
Leyens, J.-P., 250, 252, 253, *260*, *261*, *262*
Lezak, M. D., 339, *350*
Li, K. Z. H., 11, *23*, 64, *71*
Li, L. W., 354, 355, 360, *363*, *364*
Li, M. D., 94, *106*
Li, S., 295, *310*
Li, S.-C., 5, 6, 8, 9, 14, 16, *19*, *21*, 45, *52*, *53*, 101, 102, *106*, 123, 124, 125, 127, 129, *129*, *130*, *131*, 154, 163, *166*, *169*, 178, *189*
Li, Y., 68, *72*, 199, *206*, 345, *352*
Li, Z., 81, 82, *88*
Libon, D. J., 342, *350*
Lichstein, K. L., 356, *362*
Lichtenberg, P. A., 368, 372, *378*
Lichtenstein, P., 94, 96, 97, 103, *106*, *107*
Lichtenstein, S., 133, 134, *147*, *148*
Lidz, C. A., 368, *379*
Lidz, C. W., 370, *377*
Lieberman, M., 283, *289*
Lieberman, M. A., 192, 199, 200, *204*, 360, *363*
Liedtke, P. M., 270, *273*
Light, K. C., 197, *203*
Light, L. L., 11, *21*
Lighthall, N. R., 303, *309*

LiJuan, F., 313, *321*
Lillie-Blanton, M., 208, *217*
Lim, A., 48, *53*
Lim, K. O., 80, 81, 82, *89*, *91*
Lima, M. P., 266, *275*
Lin, C. C., 103, *104*, 209, *217*
Lin, C. H., 100, *107*
Lin, M., 239, 240, *245*, *247*
Lin, M.-C., 239, 241, *245*
Lin, Y. H., 213, *218*
Lincoln, K. D., 221, *229*
Lind, J., 16, *22*, 81, 82, *89*, 112, *119*, 122, 123, 124, 125, 129, *130*, *131*
Lindenberger, U., 5, 8, 9, 11, 12, 14, 16, 17, *19*, *21*, *22*, 27, 29, 31, 32, *36*, *37*, 64, *71*, 74, 76, 77, 83, 84, *87*, *90*, 101, 102, *106*, 110, 111, 113, *118*, *119*, 123, 124, 125, 127, 129, *129*, *130*, *131*, 141, *150*, 154, 158, 163, *167*, *168*, *169*, 178, *186*, 191, *201*, 265, 267, *274*
Lindenthal, J. J., 195, *204*
Lindheim, S. R., 196, *203*
Lindner, N. M., 254, 255, *262*
Lindsay, J., 265, *274*
Lindström, T., 138, *150*
Lindstrom, T. C., 318, *322*
Lineweaver, T. T., 181, *187*, 254, *261*
Link, B. G., 208, *217*
Linville, P. W., 250, *261*
Lipkus, I. M., 134, 136, *149*
Lippstreu, M., 259, *262*
Lipsitt, L. P., 272, *272*
Lipton, R., 9, *23*
Lipton, R. B., 31, *39*, 113, *118*, 153, 163, *170*
Lisle, D. J., 136, *151*
Lisspers, J., 200, *202*
Listerud, J., 342, *350*
Little, R. T. A., 27, 28, *37*
Little, T. D., 29, *37*, 180, *187*, 298, *308*
Litvan, I., 343, *349*
Liu, H., 49, *53*, 83, *86*, 208, 210, *217*
Liu, J. H., 251, *261*
Liu, L., 17, *21*, 99, *106*
Liu, L. L., 111, *118*
Liu, S., 270, *276*
Liu, X., 100, *106*
Liu-Ambrose, T., 161, *168*
Livesley, W. J., 326, *337*
Livingstone, V., 297, *310*
Llaneras, R. E., 164, *170*
Llewellyn, D., 345, *350*
Locantore, J. K., 6, 11, 16, *19*, 111, *117*, 122, *130*
Lo Cascio, V., 313, *320*
Löckenhoff, C. E., 140, *148*, 298, 299, *308*
LoConto, D. G., 318, *322*
Loeb, P., 373, *378*
Loenneker, T., 113, *118*
Loevinger, J., 266, *274*, 283, *290*
Loewenstein, D. A., 356, 358, *362*, 371, 373, *378*
Loewenstein, G., 135, 137, *148*, *149*, *378*
Logan, J. M., 129, *130*
Logan, J. R., 220, *230*
Logsdon, R., 356, *365*
Longmire, C. V., 357, 358, *363*
Longoria, R., 346, *348*
Looman, C., 271, *276*
Loong, C., 251, *261*
Lopatto, D. E., 142, *149*
Lopez, D. F., 285, 286, *291*
Lopez, O. L., 344, *350*
Lopez-Aqueres, W., 314, *321*
Loranger, A. W., 333, *336*
Lorenze, F. O., 226, *232*, 266, *276*
Loring, D. W., 339, *350*
Losada, A., 360, *364*
Losada, M. F., 296, 298, 299, *307*
Lovasi, G. S., 211, *217*
Lövdén, M., 6, 12, 16, *20*, *21*, 27, 31, *36*, *37*, 110, *119*, 264, *274*
Love, G., 299, *307*
Loving, T. J., 305, *308*
Lowe, C., 30, *37*, 66, 67, 68, *72*
Lowe, V. J., 83, *88*, 111, *118*
Lowenstein, A., 220, 221, 223, 225, 226, 227, 228, *230*, *231*
Lowenthal, M. F., 195, *203*
Lowery, A. J., 329, *335*
Lozano, P., 208, *217*
Lu, P. H., 74, *85*, 340, *348*
Lubin, D. A., 197, *203*
Lucas, R. E., 265, *273*, 305, *309*
Luce, M. F., 134, *149*
Luchsinger, J. A., 340, *350*
Luciano, M., 96, 97, *105*
Lucke, J., 356, 358, *362*
Lueger, R. J., 318, *322*
Luescher, K., 225, *231*
Lufkin, R. B., 78, 79, *86*, *88*
Lui, L., 251, 253, *259*
Lui, L. Y., 160, *171*
Lum, O., 327, *337*
Lumley, M. A., 303, *308*
Lundervold, A., 75, 77, *85*, *87*, *91*
Lundervold, A. J., 75, 77, *85*, *91*
Luo, L., 163, *168*
Luo, T., 251, *259*
Luo, Y., 222, *230*
Luoh, M.-C., 271, *274*
Luong, G., 295, 299, 301, *307*
Lupien, S. J., 122, *130*, 182, *188*, 198, *203*
Lupski, J. R., 99, *106*
Luria, A. R., 343, *350*
Lussier, I., 198, *203*
Lustig, C., 9, 11, 16, *21*, *22*, 110, 111, 112, *117*, *118*, *119*, 129, *130*, 154, 158, 159, 164, *168*
Lustina, M. J., 346, *348*
Luszcz, M. A., 59, 60, 61, 62, 63, 65, 66, 67, 68, *69*, *70*, *71*, 314, *320*
Lutzky, S. M., 356, *363*
Lyden, M., 372, *378*
Lyketsos, C. G., 46, *53*, 359, *363*
Lynch, J. W., 209, 212, *216*, *217*
Lyness, J. M., 316, *320*, 326, 327, *334*, *336*
Lyons, M. J., 95, 96, 97, *106*
Lyubomirsky, S., 298, *309*

M

Maas, I., 265, 271, *273*, *274*
Mabry, J. B., 224, *229*
MacCallum, R. C., 361, *364*
MacCarthy, B., 192, *201*
Macdonald, S., 127, 129, *130*
MacDonald, S. W. S., 6, 9, 11, 16, 17, *21*, *23*, 26, 33, *37*, 178, *187*
Macera, C., 207, *217*
MacFall, J. R., 81, *88*
Macgillivray, T. J., 81, *90*
MacGregor, D. G., 134, *147*
Maciejewski, P. K., 197, *203*
Maciel, A. G., 281, 287, *291*
Mackenbach, J. P., 209, *218*
Mackenzie, I. R., 343, *352*
MacKenzie, S. B, 268, *275*
Mackinlay, R., 371, *377*
Mackinnon, A. J., 327, *334*
Maclean, M., 235, 236, *246*
MacLeod, A. M., 112, *119*
MacManus, D. G., 82, *90*
Macofsky-Urban, F., 356, *363*
MacPherson, S. E., 137, 138, *149*
Madden, D. J., 80, 81, 82, *86*, *88*, *89*, 161, *166*
Madison, C., 75, 76, *86*, *89*
Madureira, S., 342, *350*
Magai, C., 296, 299, 301, 304, *307*, *309*
Maggi, S., 313, *320*
Magri, F., 100, *105*
Maguire, E. A., 113, *118*, 162, *168*
Maguire, R. P., 77, *86*
Mahan, T. L., 301, *309*
Maher, B. S., 17, *23*
Maheu, F., 182, *188*
Mahncke, H. W., 157, 158, 159, *168*, *169*
Mahon, M. J., 184, *189*
Mahoney, D., 356, *363*
Main, K. L., 113, *119*
Maines, M. L., 139, *148*
Maitland, S. B., 11, *21*, 49, *53*, 121, *131*

Makoni, S., 233, 241, *244*
Makris, N., 77, *91*
Makuc, D. M., 196, *202*
Malarkey, W. B., 191, *202*, *203*, 305, *308*
Maletta, G., 333, *334*
Malhotra, A. K., 101, *104*
Malley, M., 161, *167*
Malloy, P. F., 374, *379*
Malmberg, B., 223, *231*
Malmgren, J. A., 327, *334*
Malmstrom, T. K. P., 345, *350*
Malone, M. L., 154, *168*
Mance, G. A., 210, *217*
Mancini, A. D., 318, *322*
Mandic, M., 159, *168*
Mandler, G., 198, *203*
Mangine, S., 333, *337*
Mangione, C. M., 49, *53*
Manji, H. K., 103, *105*
Manley, A., 253, *260*
Manly, J., 159, *169*, 339, 345, 346, *349*
Manly, J. J., 340, 346, 347, *350*
Mannetti, L., 136, *148*
Mannheim, K., 42, *53*
Mannon, L. J., 85, *87*
Manson, J. E., 160, *170*
Manuck, S. B., 77, *91*
Marceaux, M. A., 373, *379*
Marchi, K., 209, *215*
Marchi, K. S., 208, 209, 210, *215*
Marcoen, A., 155, 156, *170*
Margrett, J. A., 163, *168*
Marin, J., 77, *89*
Marinkovic, K., 318, *322*
Marino, F., 209, *218*
Markesbery, W. R., 48, *54*
Marks, N. F., 195, *203*, 227, *229*, *231*, 360, *364*
Marks, W., 76, *90*
Markus, H. R., 49, *53*, *89*, 179, *188*
Markus, H. S., 80, 81, *86*, *90*
Marmar, C. R., 197, *204*
Marmot, M., 195, *203*, 209, *217*, 270, *275*
Marmot, M. G., 180, *188*
Marques, J. M., 253, *262*
Márquez-González, M., 360, *364*
Marschner, A., 138, *149*
Marsh, M. A., 185, *186*
Marshall, M. B., 328, *334*
Marshuetz, C., 121, 122, *131*
Marsiske, M., 6, *19*, 49, *55*, 156, 157, 159, *165*, *167*, *170*, *171*, 268, *272*
Marsit, C. J., 95, *104*
Marson, D. C., 368, 370, 371, 372, 373, 375, *378*, *379*
Martikainen, P., 270, *275*
Martin, A., 344, *351*
Martin, L. G., 211, *217*
Martin, M., 48, *55*, 178, *188*
Martin, N. G., 96, 97, *105*, *106*
Martin, R., 157, *171*, 373, *378*, *379*
Martin, R. C., 62, 63, *71*
Martin-Cook, K., 373, *377*
Martinez, R. M., 208, *217*
Martire, L. M., 223, 227, *231*, 356, *364*
Maruff, P., 83, *89*, 343, 345, *348*, *349*
Masi, C. M., 295, 305, *308*
Masliah, E., 342, 344, *349*
Mason, J., 197, *202*
Massimo, L., 344, *351*
Mata, R., 135, *149*
Matheny, K. B., 192, *202*
Mather, K. A., 102, *105*
Mather, M., 6, 11, 12, 16, *20*, *21*, 60, 61, *70*, 136, 139, 140, 141, *149*, 163, *166*, 295, 296, 297, 298, 301, 302, 303, *307*, *308*, *309*
Mathis, C. A., 83, *85*
Mattay, V. S., 100, *106*, 127, *131*
Matthews, C. G., 346, *349*
Matthews, K. A., 195, *202*
Maurer, T. J., 259, *262*
Maurer, T. M., 269, *274*
Mausbach, B. T., 196, *201*, 361, *364*
Mausner-Dorsch, H., 266, *274*
Mavandadi, S., 301, *310*
Maxin, L. M., 270, *273*
May, A., 114, *117*, *166*
May, C., 135, *151*
May, J., 258, 259, *261*
May, M., 182, *187*
Mayen, N., 221, 223, *229*
Mayes, A., 76, *87*
Mayeux, R., 100, *105*, 347, *350*, *351*, *352*
Mayhorn, C. B., 138, *149*
Mayr, U., 297, 298, 299, *307*
Mazloff, D., 234, *245*
Mazloff, D. C., 253, *259*
Mazure, C. M., 197, *203*
McAdams, D. P., 176, 177, 185, *187*, 284, *289*
McAlpine, D. D., 317, *322*
McArdle, J. J., 4, *21*, 28, 29, 30, 31, 32, 33, 34, *36*, *37*, *38*, 99, *107*, 144, *146*, 157, *168*, 345, *350*, *352*
McAuley, E., 6, *21*, 116, *117*, 129, *130*, 161, *166*
McAvay, G., 181, *189*
McBroom, J., 101, *105*
McCallum, T. J., 354, *363*
McCammon, R. J., 46, *50*
McCann, R., 233, *245*, *245*, 251, *260*, 375, *378*
McCarthy, M., 17, 18, *20*
McCarthy, M. M., 197, *203*
McCartney, K., 97, *106*
McClearn, G. E., 17, *21*, 48, *52*, 93, 94, 95, 96, 97, 103, *105*, *106*, *107*, 213, 214, *218*
McCormick, W. C., 48, 49, *52*, *53*
McCrae, R. R., 11, *21*, 194, *202*, 265, 266, *273*, *275*, 283, *290*, 304, *309*
McCurry, S. M., 347, *352*, 356, *365*
McCusker, J., 355, *364*
McDaniel, M., 163, *169*
McDaniel, M. A., 6, *20*
McDonald, C. R., 80, *89*
McDonald-Miszczak, L., 183, *188*
McDonough, P., 209, *217*
McDowd, J., 69, *71*
McDowd, J. M., 121, *130*
McEvoy, C. L., 198, *204*
McEwen, B. S., 182, *188*, 191, 193, 196, 197, 198, *203*, *204*, 212, 213, *216*, *217*, *218*
McFadden, S. H., 286, *290*
McFall, J. P., 135, *150*
McFall, R. M., 298, 299, 301, 304, *307*
McGarry, K., 221, *231*
McGee, D. L., 211, *216*
McGee, K. A., 138, 142, *147*
McGhee, D. E., 254, *260*
McGill, S., 61, *70*, 161, 163, 164, *166*
McGillivray, S., 138, *147*
McGinnis, K. A., 360, *364*
McGlinchey, J. B., 356, *363*
McGonagle, K., 200, *200*
McGovern, P. G., 48, *52*
McGowan, P. O., 99, *106*
McGue, M., 95, 96, 97, 99, 102, 103, *104*, *105*, *106*
McGuffin, P., 94, 97, 103, *106*
McGuiness, T., 197, *205*
McGuire, C. L., 156, *166*, 181, *187*
McGuire, L., 191, *203*, 361, *364*
McGuthry, K. E., 16, *22*, 141, *150*
McGwin, G., 374, *377*, *378*, *379*
McHugh, P. R., 342, *349*
McInnes, L., 9, *22*, 30, 31, 32, *38*
McIntosh, A. R., 6, 11, 16, *19*, 111, 112, *117*, *118*, *130*
McInturff, B., 368, 373, *378*
McIntyre, D. J., 80, 81, *86*
McKee, J., 239, *245*
McKee, P., 280, 281, *290*
McKeith, I. G., 77, *87*
McLaughlin, D., 209, 210, *216*
McMonagle, P., 343, *350*
McMullin, J. A., 225, *229*
McPherson, R., 296, 299, 301, *309*
McQuain, J. M., 74, *90*
McStephen, M., 343, 345, *348*, *349*
McVie, T., 361, *363*
Meacham, J. A., 281, 283, *290*
Meador, K. G., 326, *335*

Meador, R., 360, *364*
Meagher, M. W., 327, *336*
Meagher, S. E., 332, *336*
Meaney, M. J., 198, *203*
Mecum, L., 326, *336*
Medford, N., 137, *148*
Meeks, S., 234, 236, *245*, 313, 314, 315, 316, 317, *321*, *322*, 374, *379*
Mehta, C. M., 135, *150*
Mehta, K. M., 210, *217*
Mehta, R. C., 82, *89*
Mein, G., 270, *275*
Meisel, C. A., 368, *379*
Melano-Carranza, E., 315, *321*
Mell, T., 138, *149*
Mellott, D. S., 254, 255, 257, 258, *261*
Meltzer, C. C., 78, 79, *89*
Menaghan, E. G., 192, *204*
Mendes de Leon, C. F., 159, *171*, 195, 199, *206*, 304, *310*, 347, *348*
Meneer, W. B., 233, *246*
Menon, V., 112, *118*
Merchant, C. A., 346, *350*
Meredith, M. W., 29, 30, *38*
Meredith, S. D., 236, *246*
Meredith, W., 29, 30, 32, 33, *37*, *38*, 313, *321*
Merikangas, K. R., 328, *335*
Merikle, P. M., 158, *166*
Mero, R. P., 208, 209, 210, 212, *216*
Merriam, P., 199, *201*
Merrill, S., 181, *189*
Mertz, C. K., 134, 143, *147*, *149*
Meshberg, S. R., 185, *186*
Mestre, J. P., 163, *168*
Metcalfe, J., 344, *348*
Metlay, J. P., 211, *215*
Metzger, R. L., 329, *336*
Metzler, M., 208, 209, 210, *215*
Metzler-Baddeley, C., 343, *351*
Meyer, B. J. F., 135, 144, *149*
Meyer, M., 113, *118*
Meyer, T. J., 329, *336*
Meyers, B. S., 315, *323*
Meyers, J., 342, 344, *351*
Meyers, J. M., 33, 34, *38*
Meyers, K., 342, 344, *351*
Mezzacappa, E. S., 197, *204*
Mezzapesa, D. M., 82, *89*
Micale, V., 214, *217*
Michel, V., 375, *377*
Michielsen, M., 160, *167*
Mickler, C., 266, 267, *275*, *276*, 285, 287, *291*
Midlarsky, E., 181, *188*
Mielke, M., 115, *117*
Mienaltowski, A., 135, *146*, 301, *306*
Mikels, J. A., 6, 11, 12, *20*, 60, 61, *70*, 121, 122, *131*, 137, 138, 140, 143, *149*, *150*, 163, *166*, 295, 302, *307*
Mikkelsen, A., 268, *275*
Milch, K. F., 143, *151*
Miles, J. R., 156, *168*, *170*
Miles, T. P., 209, 210, *216*, *217*
Milgram, N. W., 83, *88*
Milham, M. P., 67, *71*
Milkie, M. A., 226, *231*
Mill, A., 297, *309*
Miller, A., 111, *119*, 193, *204*
Miller, B. L., 75, 76, 78, *86*, *89*, *91*, 99, *105*
Miller, D. H., 82, *90*
Miller, D. K. M. D., 345, *350*
Miller, G. E., 177, *190*, 196, 200, *204*
Miller, J. P. A. B., 345, *350*
Miller, K. J., 83, *86*, 161, *169*
Miller, L. M., 221, 222, 223, *229*, *230*, 299, *309*
Miller, L. M. S., 177, 181, 182, *188*
Miller, L. S., 359, *362*
Miller, M. L., 329, *336*
Miller, S. W., 346, *351*
Millikan, A. M., 313, *323*
Millon, C., 332, *336*
Millon, T., 332, *336*
Mills, C. J., 283, *290*
Mills, P. J., 196, *201*, 361, *364*
Mills, W. L., 332, *335*
Milne, A. B., 297, 298, *309*
Minear, M., 111, *118*, *119*
Mineka, S., 316, *322*
Miniussi, C., 111, *119*
Minthon, L., 111, *117*
Mintun, M. A., 113, *118*
Mintz, J., 74, *85*, 340, *348*
Mirowsky, J., 177, 179, *188*, *189*, 208, 209, *217*
Misra, S., 372, *379*
Mistry, R. S., 42, 50, *52*
Mitchell, P., 68, *69*
Mitchell, R. L. C., 297, *309*
Mitrani, V. B., 356, 358, *362*
Mitrushina, M., 339, 347, *351*
Mittelman, M. S., 75, *87*, 354, 360, 361, *362*, *363*, *364*
Miwa, Y., 78, *89*
Miyake, A., 60, 61, 62, 63, 64, 68, 69, *70*, *71*, 114, *118*, 161, *168*
Miyao, K., 6, 17, *21*
Moane, G., 43, *52*
Moayer, M., 101, *107*
Mock, S. E., 226, *231*
Modat, M., 83, *87*
Moen, P., 195, 196, *203*, *204*
Moffat, S. D., 76, 84, *89*
Moffitt, T. E., 266, *276*
Mogapi, O., 66, 67, 68, *72*
Mohammed, A. H., 164, *168*
Mohr, D. C., 197, *204*
Mohs, R., 345, *351*
Molden, D. C., 155, *168*
Molenaar, P. C. M., 27, 33, 34, 35, *36*, *37*, *38*
Molinari, V., 330, 331, 332, 333, *336*
Mollenkopf, H., 49, *54*
Moloney, K. P., 113, *119*
Monahan, D. J., 355, 356, *363*
Montenegro, X., 270, *275*
Montepare, J. M., 253, *262*
Montgomery, G. T., 346, *348*
Monti, D. A., 154, *167*
Montorio, I., 360, *364*
Montrose, L. P., 242, *245*
Moody, H. R., 282, 287, *290*
Moore, A. B., 81, 82, *88*
Moore, D., 242, *245*
Moore, J. H., 99, *106*
Moore, L. V., 211, *217*
Moore, P., 208, *217*, 342, *350*
Moos, R. H., 316, *321*
Morales, K., 315, *320*
Morcom, A. M., 111, *118*
Morgan, M. L., 78, 79, *86*
Morgan, W. R., 44, *53*
Mori, H., 80, *85*
Moriarty, D. G., 298, *308*
Moritz, T. E., 17, 18, *20*
Mormino, E. C., 83, *89*
Morris, J., 157, *170*
Morris, J. C., 83, *90*, 113, *118*, 129, *130*, 157, 345, *351*
Morris, J. C. M. D., 345, *350*
Morris, K. S., 115, *117*
Morris, R. G., 80, 82, *89*, *90*
Morrow, D. G., 155, 162, 163, *168*, *169*, *170*
Morrow-Howell, N., 271, *272*, *275*
Morse, C. K., 328, 329, *337*
Mortensen, E. L., 79, *87*
Mortimer, J. A., 48, *54*, 198, 265, *272*, 347, *351*
Mortimer, J. T., 44, *53*
Moscona, S., 317, *322*
Moscovitch, D. A., 184, *188*
Moscovitch, M., 137, *149*
Moseley, M., 80, 81, *89*
Moser, D. J., 345, *349*
Mosing, M. A., 97, *106*
Mosley, T. H., 48, *52*
Moss, S. A., 83, *89*
Mottershead, J. P., 82, *89*
Moye, J., 370, 371, *378*, *379*
Mozolic, J. L., 115, *118*
Mroczek, D. K., 184, *189*, 193, 194, 198, *204*, 220, 225, 226, 228, *230*, 265, *275*, 298, 299, 304, *309*, 331, *336*
Mucke, L., 101, *107*
Muggenburg, B. A., 83, *88*
Mühlberger, A., 297, *310*
Mühlig-Verson, A., 272, *275*

Mulatu, M. S., 48, *54*, *169*, 209, *217*, *276*
Muldoon, M. F., 77, *91*
Mullan, J. T., 180, *190*, 192, 199, 200, *204*, 220, *229*, 354, 357, 359, 360, *364*
Mullaney, H., 347, *348*
Mullen, P. E., 317, *322*
Muller, D., 199, *202*
Müller, M. M., 182, *189*
Müller, V., 154, *166*
Mulsant, B. H., 315, 316, *320*, 326, *336*
Munafo, M. R., 17, *20*
Mungas, D., 79, *89*, 347, *351*
Münte, T. F., 83, *87*
Muraskin, J., 340, *348*
Murgatroyd, C., 214, *217*
Murphy, C. F., 315, *320*
Murphy, D. G., 78, *86*, 340, *349*
Murphy, M. D., 156, *168*
Murphy, M. P., 100, *106*
Murphy, S. T., 139, *149*, 375, *377*
Murray, R., 344, *351*
Murrell, S. A., 313, 314, 317, *322*
Musen, G., 122, *131*
Musick, M. A., 212, *216*
Musumeci, T. J., 42, 48, 49, *52*
Muthén, B. O., 32, 34, *38*, 327, *335*
Muthén, L. K., 32, 34, *38*
Mutran, E. J., 270, *275*
Mutrie, N., 271, *273*
Mutter, S. A., 142, *149*
Myers, H. F., 195, *202*
Myers, J. K., 195, *204*, 328, *336*
Myers, L. M., 261, *263*

N

Nadler, J. D., 374, *379*
Nagamatsu, L. S., 161, *168*
Nagel, I. E., 101, 102, *106*, 122, 125, 127, 129, *130*, *131*
Nagourney, A., 249, *262*
Nägren, K., 111, *118*
Nagy, Z., 48, *51*
Nair, N. P. V., 182, *188*, 198, *203*
Nair, S. N., 180, *187*, 268, *273*
Nakamura, E., 6, 17, *21*
Nakamura, J., 283, 285, *289*
Nakao, K., 358, *363*
Nakayama, K., 374, *377*
Nam, C. B., 46, 47, *53*
Napier, J. L., 184, *187*
Nash, C., 114, *117*
National Association of Chronic Disease Directors, 208, *217*
National Center for Elder Abuse, 368, *379*
National Committee on Uniform Traffic Laws and Ordinances, 374, *379*
National Guardianship Network Members, *379*
National Institute on Aging, 14, 15, 16, 17, *21*
National Research Council & Committee on Future Directions for Cognitive Research on Aging, 345, *351*
Navaie-Waliser, M., 358, *364*
Navarro, V., 210, *217*
Nduaguba, M., 331, *336*
Neale, M. C., 103, *106*
Nebes, R. D., 78, 79, 83, *85*, *89*
Neckerman, K. M., 211, *217*
Neely, A. S., 114, 115, 116, *117*, *118*, *119*, 158, 163, 164, *166*
Negy, C., 346, *351*
Neider, M. R., 160, *165*, *166*, *167*
Neighbors, H. W., 226, *229*, *231*
Neill, C. M., 286, *290*
Nelissen, N., 84, *89*
Nelson, A. R., 208, *218*
Nelson, E. A., 26, *38*, 264, *275*
Nelson, J. K., 111, *119*
Nelson, K. L., 301, 302, *310*
Nelson, M. C., 211, *215*
Nelson, T. D., 250, *262*
Nelson, W., 143, *150*, 368, *377*
Nesse, R. M., 319, *320*
Nesselroade, C. S., 155, *170*
Nesselroade, J. R., 6, 14, 18, *20*, *21*, *22*, 25, 26, 29, 30, 32, 33, 34, *36*, *37*, *38*, *39*, 154, *167*, 177, 178, 184, *187*, *189*, 295, 297, 298, 299, *307*
Nessler, D., 61, 62, 68, 69, *70*
Neubauer, A. C., 158, *169*
Neuchterlein, K. H., 74, 340, *348*
Neugarten, B. L., 270, *274*
Neuhaus, C., 207, *215*
Neumann, M., 344, *351*
Neundorfer, M., 154, *168*
Neupert, S. D., 183, 184, *189*, 193, 194, 195, 198, 199, *202*, *204*, *274*, 277, 297, 300, *309*
Nevitt, M., 160, *171*
Newall, N. E., 296, *307*
Newcomer, R., 355, 360, *362*
Newman, A. B., 210, *217*
Newman, K., 209, 212, *214*
Newmann, J. P., 314, *322*
Newsom, E., 221, 223, *229*
Newsom, J. T., 301, *309*
Newton, T. E., 78, *88*
Neylan, T. C., 197, *204*
Ng, R., 192, *201*
Ng, S., 83, *89*
Ng, S. H., 236, *246*, 251, *260*
Ng, T. W. H., 267, 268, 272, *275*
Nguyen, H. T., 327, *336*
Nguyen, T. V., 100, *106*
Ni, X., 101, *104*
Nichols, C., 318, *321*
Nichols, L., 356, *362*
Niebuhr, D. W., 313, *323*
Nielson, K. A., 67, *71*
NIH State-of-the-Science Conference Preventing Alzheimer's Disease and Cognitive Decline, 109, *118*
Nikolaus, T., 374, *379*
Nilsson, G.-G., 6, *23*
Nilsson, L.-G., 7, 14, 16, 18, *20*, *22*, 78, 79, 81, 82, *89*, *91*, 101, 102, *105*, 112, *119*, 122, 123, 124, 125, 127, *130*, *131*, 142, *147*
Nilsson, M., 113, *118*
Nilsson, S. E., 48, *52*
Nisbett, R. E., 5, 14, *22*
Nithianantharajah, J., 164, *169*
Niti, M., 125, *131*
Noack, C. M. G., 269, *275*
Noack, H., 110, *119*
Noale, M., 313, *320*
Nochlin, D., 48, *53*
Noels, K., 236, 237, *244*, *246*
Noh, S. R., 156, *170*
Noice, H., 162, *169*
Noice, T., 162, *169*
Noller, P., 234, 235, 236, *244*
Nordahl, C. W., 79, *89*, 125, 126, *131*
Nordberg, A., 129, *131*
Nordgren, L. F., 138, *147*
Norris, L., 137, *146*, 281, 282, *288*
Norris, M. P., 327, *336*
Norris, R., 356, *364*
Northrop, L., 371, 373, *377*
Norton, M. C., 101, *105*, 314, *323*
Norton, M. I., 252, *260*
Nosek, B. A., 254, 255, *260*, *262*
Novacek, J., 192, *202*
Novak, D. L., 136, *149*
Nowrangi, M. A., 372, *377*
Nuechterlein, K. H., 74, *85*
Nussbaum, J. F., 233, 241, 242, *244*, *246*
Nyberg, L., 7, 9, 11, 14, 16, *19*, *21*, *22*, 67, *71*, 81, 82, *89*, 112, 114, 115, 116, *117*, *118*, *119*, 121, 122, 123, 124, 125, 127, 128, 129, *129*, *130*, *131*, 156, 158, 163, 164, *166*, *169*
Nygren, M., 371, 373, *377*

O

Oakes, P. J., 241, *246*
Oates, G., 48, *54*, *276*
Ober, B., 102, *105*
Ober, B. A., 342, *349*
O'Brien, A., 356, *364*
O'Brien, J., 83, *91*

O'Brien, L. T., 254, 255, 257, 258, 259, *261*, *262*
O'Brien, W. H., 325, *335*
Ochsner, K., 295, 297, 302, *309*
O'Connell, R. G., 129, *129*
Odato, C. V., 241, *246*
Oden, A., 200, *202*
Oechslin, M. S., 113, *118*
Oettel, M., 100, *106*
Ofstedal, M. B., 304, *308*, 345, *351*
Ogay, T., 234, *244*
Ogier, S., 142, *149*
Ohashi, M. M., 179, *190*
Ohayon, M. M., 314, *322*
Ohmine, T., 78, *89*
Okamoto, K., 258, *262*
O'Keefe, K., 83, *91*
Okonkwo, O. C., 373, *379*
Olchowski, A. E., 29, *37*
Olichney, J., 342, *348*
Olsson, H., 111, *118*
Oltmanns, T. F., 326, 329, *334*, *337*
Omenn, G. S., 93, *106*
O'Neil, J. P., 127, *130*
Ong, A. D., 183, 184, *189*, 299, *309*
Onoi, M., 95, *105*
Onrust, S. A., 318, *322*
Oosterbroek, M., 160, *167*
Oosterman, J. M., 78, 79, *89*
Operario, D., 249, 253, *262*
Orange, J. B., 235, 236, *246*
Organisation for Economic Cooperation and Development, 268, 269, 270, *275*
O'Riley, A. A., 316, *321*, 327, 328, *335*, *336*
Orrell, M., 355, *362*
Orwar, O., 113, *118*
Orwoll, L., 281, 282, *290*, *298*
Ory, M., 356, *364*
Orzechowski, S., 210, *217*
Osbeck, L. M., 279, 282, *290*
Osberg, J. S., 208, *214*
Oscar-Berman, M, 318, *322*
Osgood, C. E., 136, *149*
Osherson, D. N., 134, 135, *150*, *151*
Oslin, D., 316, *320*
Osowski, N. L., 61, 66, *71*
Östberg, M., 68, *72*
Ostbye, T., 315, *321*
Ostendorf, F., 266, *275*, 304, *309*
Ostfeld, A., 197, *202*
Ostrander, D. R., 195, *204*
O'Sullivan, M., 80, 81, *86*, *89*
Oswald, F., 49, *54*
Ota, H., 233, 237, *245*, *246*, 251, *260*
Ott, C. H., 318, *322*
Otte, C., 197, *204*
Ottenbacher, K. J., 154, *167*
Oudkerk, M., 75, 77, 78, *86*, *87*, 340, *349*
Overton, W. F., 4, 11, *21*, *22*, 281, 282, 284, 286, 287, *291*
Owen, A. M., 109, *119*
Owen, J. E., 357, *364*
Owen, M. J., 100, *107*
Owens, W. A., 48, *53*
Owsley, C., 374, *378*
Oxman, T. E., 316, *320*

P

Pacak, K., 212, *217*
Pachana, N. A., 328, 329, *336*
Pachur, T., 135, *149*
Padilla, A. M., 346, *351*
Pagani, E., 82, *89*
Page, P., 211, *215*
Paik, M., 374, *379*
Paillard-Borg, S., 124, *130*
Paine, J. B., 268, *275*
Palkovits, M., 212, *217*
Palmer, B. W., 317, *322*, 372, *377*, *379*
Palmer, H., 159, *166*
Palmersheim, K. A., 49, *53*
Pamuk, E. R., 209, *215*
Pan, J. W., 75, *91*
Panizzon, M. S., 103, *106*
Panksepp, J., 193, *204*
Papenberg, G., 125, 127, 129, *130*
Pardo, T. B., 226, *231*
Parisi, J. M., 162, 163, *169*, *170*, 284, 287, *290*
Park, B. S., 372, *379*
Park, D., 121, *130*, 143, *147*
Park, D. C., 5, 6, 7, 9, 11, 14, 16, *19*, *21*, *22*, 59, 60, 66, 67, *71*, 75, 83, 84, *89*, *90*, 110, 111, 112, 115, *118*, *119*, 121, 122, *131*, 141, 142, *146*, *150*, 162, 163, *170*, 251, 255, *259*, 264, 265, *275*
Park, M., 82, *88*
Park, N., 287, *290*
Park, R., 111, *119*
Parker, A. M., 134, 135, 142, *146*
Parker, L. S., 370, *377*
Parker, W. D., 283, *290*
Parmalee, P. A., 327, *336*
Parmelee, P. A., 313, *322*
Parry, J., 370, *379*
Parsons, T., 220, *231*
Partridge, T., 76, *88*
Pascualy, M., 197, *204*
Pashler, H., 163, *169*
Pasqualetti, P., 111, *119*
Pasupathi, M., 139, *147*, 283, *290*, 297, 298, 299, *307*
Patchev, A. V., 214, *217*
Patchev, V., 100, *106*
Patel, A., 375, *378*
Patrick, D. L., 327, *334*
Patterson, D., 197, *205*
Patterson, T. L., 317, *322*, 360, 361, *363*, *364*
Pattie, A., 80, 81, 82, *85*, *86*
Paul, R. H., 75, 78, 80, 81, *87*, *89*
Pauli, P., 297, *310*
Paulmann, S., 297, *309*
Paulos, J. A., 134, *149*
Paulsen, J. S., 345, *349*
Paulus, M. P., 314, *321*
Paus, T., 67, *72*
Payne, J. W., 134, *149*
Payne, M., 329, *336*
Payne, T. W., 158, *167*
Pearce, G., 301, 302, 303, *310*
Pearl, J., 35, *38*
Pearlin, L. I., 176, 177, *189*, 192, 199, 200, *204*, 220, *229*, 354, 357, 359, 360, *363*, *364*
Pearlson, G. D., 66, *72*, 76, 78, 79, *90*, *91*
Pearson, J. L., 316, *323*
Pearson, N. J., 211, *215*
Peavy, G., 342, *349*
Peavy, G. M., 344, *351*
Pecchioni, L. L., 241, *246*
Pedersen, N. L., 48, *52*, 93, 94, 95, 96, 97, 99, 103, *105*, *106*, *107*, *201*, 265, *272*, *273*, 304, *307*, 316, *321*
Peeters, R., 84, *89*
Peiffer, A. M., 80, *88*
Peiris, L., 226, *232*
Pekarski, K., 139, *147*
Peli, E., 113, *117*
Pell, M. D., 297, *309*
Pendleton, N., 9, *22*
Penley, J. A., 192, *204*
Pennak, S., 42, 43, 46, *54*, 110, *119*
Penner, R. G., 269, *275*
Pepper, M. P., 195, *204*
Pepper, S. C., 4, *22*
Perdue, C. W., 254, 255, *262*
Pérez-Rojo, G., 360, *364*
Perfilieva, E., 113, *118*
Perrig, W., 158, 162, *167*, *169*
Perrig, W. J., 157, 158, *166*
Perrig-Chiello, P., 162, *169*
Perry, M. E., 80, *89*
Perry, R. P., 180, *187*, 296, *307*
Persson, J., 16, *22*, 81, 82, *89*, 111, 112, *119*, 122, 124, 125, 126, 129, *130*, *131*, 159, *169*
Perun, P., 269, *275*
Peskind, E. R., 197, *204*
Pesonen, A., 315, *322*
Peters, C. L., 225, *231*
Peters, E., 134, 136, 137, 138, 143, 145, 146, *147*, *148*, *149*, *150*, 371, *379*
Peters, K., 212, *216*

Peterson, C., 287, *290*
Peterson, E., 175, 183, *188*
Peterson, E. W., 184, 185, *190*
Peterson, J., 319, *321*
Peterson, J. S., 158, *166*
Peterson, M. S., 116, *118*, 158, 164, *167*
Petersson, K. M., 114, *118*, *119*, 122, *131*, 156, *169*
Petit Taboué, M. C., 67, *71*
Petkov, C. I., 79, *89*
Petot, G., 265, *273*
Petrill, S. A., 95, *106*
Petrovic, K., 78, 82, *87*
Petty, R. E., 256, 257, *262*
Pew Internet Survey, 228, *231*
Pfefferbaum, A., 80, 81, *89*, *91*, 340, *352*
Pfohl, B., 333, *336*
Pham, D., 75, *87*
Phelan, J., 208, *217*
Phillips, C., 316, *323*
Phillips, D. I. W., 197, *202*
Phillips, L. H., 59, 60, 61, 66, 68, *71*, *72*, 137, 138, 141, *146*, *149*, 297, 298, 299, *308*, *309*, *310*
Piaget, J., 283, *290*
Piasecki, M., 143, *150*
Piazza, J. R., 194, 197, 199, *200*, *201*, 296, 299, 301, 305, *307*, *309*
Piccinin, A. M., 26, *37*
Pickering, R., 318, *321*
Picot, S., 271, *273*
Pienta, A., 209, 210, *216*
Pieper, C., 326, 327, *335*
Pierpaoli, C., 79, *89*
Pierro, A., 136, *148*
Pierson, H., 237, *244*
Pierson, H. D., 251, *260*
Pietrucha, M., 49, *54*
Pihlajamaki, M., 83, *91*
Pike, C. J., 100, *106*
Pike, G. B., 82, *89*
Pike, K. E., 83, *87*, *89*, 111, *119*
Pilcher, J., 42, *53*
Pillemer, K., 220, 221, 222, 223, 225, 226, *231*, 359, 360, *364*
Pillon, B., 343, *349*
Pillow, D. R., 192, *204*
Pilver, C. E., 258, 259, *261*
Pimley, S., 192, *202*
Pinquart, M., 50, *54*, 223, 227, *231*, 271, *275*, 354, 355, 356, 357, 358, 361, *364*
Pinto, J. A., 111, *117*
Pioli, M. F., 176, 177, *189*
Piotrowski, A., 99, *104*
Piquard, A. M., 343, *351*
Pitzer, L., 220, 221, 222, 223, 225, 226, 227, 228, *230*, *231*
Pizzirusso, M., 347, *351*
Plakans, A., 49, *53*
Plante, E., 75, 79, *91*
Plassman, B. L., 265, *275*, 314, *323*, 345, *351*
Plemons, J. K., 155, *169*
Pliske, R. M., 142, *149*
Plomin, R., 93, 94, 95, 97, 100, 103, *105*, *106*, *107*
Plott, C. R., 137, 138, *148*
Podsakoff, P. M., 268, *275*
Pogash, R., 143, *150*
Poggesi, A., 78, 79, *89*
Pointer, S., 59, 61, 62, 63, *70*
Polk, T. A., 111, 112, *119*, 121, 122, *131*
Pollard, C. A., 135, *149*
Pollen, D. A., 345, *349*
Ponds, R. W. H. M., 265, *273*
Pool, D., 371, 373, *377*
Pope, S. K., 210, *217*
Popkin, B. M., 211, *215*
Porges, S. W., 212, *217*
Posluszny, D. M., 198, *201*
Post, G. M., 143, *150*
Posthuma, D., 96, *107*
Posthuma, R. A., 259, *262*, 269, *275*
Pot, A. M., 313, 314, *321*, *323*, 360, *363*
Potter, G. G., 265, *275*, 347, *351*
Potworowski, G., 287, *289*
Powell, D. K., 80, *87*
Powell, F. C., 237, *246*, 284, *291*
Powers, C., 342, *350*
Powers, W. J., 112, *119*
Prager, I. G., 253, *260*
Prakash, R., 116, *117*, 129, *130*, 161, *166*
Prakash, R. S., 116, *117*, 160, *167*
Pratt, M. W., 237, *246*
Prelec, D., 137, *148*
Prentice, D., 16, *23*
President's Commission, 368, *379*
Pressor, S. C., 196, *203*
Preuschhof, C., 122, 127, 129, *131*
Price, J. C., 83, *85*
Pridan, H., 209, *214*
Prigerson, H. G., 197, *203*
Primo, S. A., 113, *119*
Prince, S. E., 112, *117*
Prindle, J. J., 157, *168*
Prineas, R. J., 345, *350*
Prohovnik, I., 347, *351*
Prom-Wormley, E., 103, *106*
Propper, C., 211, *215*
Protas, H., 83, *86*
Protzner, A. B., 67, *70*, 112, *118*
Provenzale, J. M., 80, 81, 82, *86*, *88*
Pruessner, J. C., 75, *91*
Pudrovska, T., 220, 226, *231*
Puka, B., 283, *289*
Pullen, S. M., 138, *147*
Pulley, L., 345, *350*
Pushkar, D., 5, *22*, 298, *306*, 359, *363*
Pushkar, D. P., 241, *246*

Q

Quadagno, J., 49, *54*
Queen, T. L., 138, *150*, 257, 259, *260*
Quinn, B. T., 75, 77, *87*, *91*
Quinn, D. M., 346, *351*
Quinn, M. J., 370, *379*

R

Rabbitt, P., 9, *22*, 30, 31, 32, *37*, *38*, 60, 61, 62, 66, 67, 68, *72*
Raber, J., 100, 101, *107*
Rabin, M. L., 85, *87*
Rabinovici, G. D., 76, *89*
Rabinowitz, Y., 358, *362*
Radloff, L. S., 327, *336*
Radvansky, G., 143, *151*
Rae, D. S., 46, *51*, 317, *321*, 328, *336*
Rafaeli, E., 192, *201*
Rafferty, J. A., 213, *216*
Rahe, R. H., 192, *202*
Rahhal, T. A., 256, 257, *260*, *262*
Raichle, M. E., 83, *90*, 112, *117*, *119*
Raikkonen, K., 315, *322*
Rajah, M. N., 67, 68, *72*
Rakic, P., 103, *107*
Ram, N., 14, *22*, 30, 35, *38*
Ramachandran, V. S., 113, *119*
Ramirez, M., 314, *323*, 327, *337*
Ramos, L. M., 77, 78, *86*, 340, *349*
Ramos, M. A., 340, *348*
Ramsden, M., 100, *106*
Ranganath, C., 79, *89*, 125, 126, *131*
Ranganath, K. A., 254, 255, *262*
Raniga, P., 83, *87*
Ransom, R. L., 49, *53*
Rapaport, M. H., 314, *321*
Rapp, S. R., 328, *336*
Rascovsky, K., 344, *351*
Raskind, M. A., 196, 197, *201*, *204*
Rasmusson, D. X., 156, *169*, 180, *189*
Rathunde, K., 282, *289*
Rau, R., 153, *166*
Raudenbush, S. W., 32, *36*
Raue, P. J., 315, 316, *322*, *323*
Rauh, V. A., 212, *217*
Raynor, J. O., 283, *290*
Raz, N., 16, *22*, 59, 60, 61, 63, 65, 66, 69, *70*, *71*, *72*, 74, 75, 76, 77, 78, 79, 80, 81, 84, *87*, *88*, *89*, *90*, 99, *107*, 110, 111, 116, *117*, *118*, *119*, 123, 124, 125, 129, *131*, 141, *150*, 340, *350*
Razani, J., 339, 347, *351*

Read, D., 139, *150*
Read, N. L., 139, *150*
Read, S. J., 143, *147*
Ready, R. E., 303, *309*
Realo, A., 297, *309*
Rebok, G. W., 61, *70*, 155, 156, 157, 161, 163, 164, *166*, *168*, *169*, *170*, 180, *189*, 284, 287, *290*
Rebucal, K. A., 145, *151*, 304, *310*
Redmore, C. D., 283, *290*
Reeb, B. C., 296, *307*
Reed, A. E., 138, 140, 143, *149*, *150*
Reed, G., 199, *201*
Reed, H., 268, *273*
Reed, M., 154, *171*
Reed, R., 346, *352*
Reed, T., 78, *86*, *91*, 99, *105*
Reed, T. E., 48, *54*
Reese, H. W., 4, 11, *21*, *22*, 272, *272*
Reese, R. J., 327, *335*
Reever, K. E., 220, *232*
Regan, J. J., 375, *379*
Regier, D. A., 46, *51*, 314, 317, *321*, *322*, 328, *336*
Reich, J., 331, *336*
Reich, J. W., 185, *189*, 299, *309*
Reicher, S. D., 241, *246*
Reichstadt, J., 242, *245*
Reid, S. A., 242, *244*
Reiman, E. M., 129, *130*
Reinvang, I., 75, 77, *87*, *91*
Reis, M., 359, *363*
Reischies, F. M., 138, *149*
Reise, S. P., 29, *39*
Reiss, A. L., 112, *118*
Reitan, R., 343, *351*
Reitan, R. M., 342, *351*
Reitz, C., 340, *350*
Reitzes, D. C., 270, *275*
Reitzle, M., 50, *54*
Remez, S., 270, *275*
Renner, G., 177, *187*
Rentz, D. M., 83, *91*
Repetti, R. L., 304, *310*
Resnick, S. M., 84, *89*, 123, *129*, 141, *150*
Reus, V. I., 100, *107*
Reuter-Lorenz, P. A., 6, 8, 9, 15, 16, *19*, *22*, 59, 60, 66, 67, *71*, 75, 84, *89*, 110, 111, 112, *118*, *119*, 121, 122, *131*, 137, *149*, 154, 158, 159, 164, *168*, *169*, 264, 265, *275*
Reyna, V. F., 135, 140, 143, *150*
Reynolds, C. A., 96, 97, *106*, *107*, 298, 299, 301, 304, *307*
Reynolds, C. F. III, 197, *205*, 315, 316, *320*, 326, *336*
Reznitskaya, A., 287, *290*
Rhymer, R. M., 33, *36*
Ribbe, M. W., 313, 314, *321*, *323*
Rice, A., 344, *351*
Rice, C. J., 5, 11, *19*
Rice, K., 234, *245*
Rice, L., 26, 33, *36*
Rice, T., 143, 144, 145, *146*, *147*, *150*
Richards, M., 164, *169*, 347, *351*
Richardson, E. D., 374, *379*
Richardson, M. J., 283, *290*
Richerson, P. J., 45, *50*
Rick, S., 137, *148*
Ridderinkhof, K. R., 64, *72*
Riddick, C. C., 160, *166*
Rieckmann, A., 127, 128, *129*, *130*
Riediger, M., 163, *169*
Rieskamp, J., 135, *149*
Riggle, E. D. B., 143, *150*
Rikli, R., 161, *169*
Riley, J. W., Jr., 41, *53*, 162, 164, 165, *169*
Riley, K. P., 48, *54*
Riley, M. W., 41, 43, *53*, 162, 164, 165, *169*
Rimajova, M., 111, *119*
Rimol, L. M., 103, *107*
Risam, J., 139, *147*
Rissmiller, D. J., 328, *337*
Ritchie, K., 315, *322*
Ritter, W., 61, 62, 68, 69, *70*
Rivera-Mindt, M., 347, *351*
Rivers, C. S., 81, *90*
Robbins, M. A., 48, *51*
Robbins, R. J., 182, *189*
Robert, S., 210, *217*
Roberts, B. W., 11, *22*, 265, 266, *274*, *275*, 283, 284, *289*, 331, *336*
Roberts, C., 208, *215*
Roberts, L. J., 356, *363*
Roberts, M. L., 178, *189*
Roberts, R. C., 18, *22*
Roberts, R. E., 327, *335*
Robertson, I. H., 129, *129*, 159, *171*
Robins, L. R., 314, *322*
Robins, R. W., 266, *275*
Robinson, A. E., 181, *187*
Robinson, D. N., 279, 282, 290, *290*
Robinson, G. S., 139, *148*, 358, 360, *363*
Robinson, J. D., 233, *246*
Robinson-Whelen, S., 361, *364*
Robison, J., 359, *364*
Robles, T. F., 191, *203*
Rocca, M. A., 82, *89*
Rocca, W. A., 304, *307*
Röcke, C., 178, 180, 181, *188*, *189*, 295, *310*
Rockstroh, B., 182, *189*
Roddey, C., 103, *105*
Roddey, J. C., 103, *107*
Rodgers, B., 304, *308*
Rodin, J., 176, 177, 178, 180, 181, 183, 184, *188*, *189*, 258, *262*
Rodrigue, K. M., 16, *22*, 59, 60, 61, 63, 65, 66, 69, *71*, 74, 75, 76, 77, 78, 79, 80, 83, 84, *87*, *88*, *89*, *90*, 99, *107*, 110, 111, *119*, 123, 124, *131*, 141, *148*, *150*
Rodriguez-Martinez, M. A., 77, *89*
Roenker, D. L., 374, *377*, *379*
Roepke, S. K., 196, *201*
Rogers, R., 212, *216*
Rogers, W. A., 135, *147*, 180, *187*, 268, *273*
Rogot, E., 209, *217*
Rohde, P., 313, *323*
Roher, D., 163, *169*
Rohlfing, T., 81, *91*
Rojas, V. A., 184, *189*
Roked, F., 375, *378*
Rokke, P. D., 303, *308*
Rolfhus, E. L., 163, *165*
Rollman, B. L., 326, *336*
Romine, L., 114, *117*
Ronning, B., 139, *147*
Rönnlund, M., 11, *21*, 121, 122, 123, 124, *131*, 138, 142, *147*, *150*
Rook, K. S., 221, 227, *231*, 301, *309*, *310*
Rooks, R., 210, *217*
Rooks, R. N., 210, *217*
Rootwelt, H., 75, *91*
Roozendaal, B., 198, *204*
Ropele, S., 78, 82, *87*
Rosario, E. R., 100, *106*
Rosch, E. H., 251, *262*
Rose, R. J., 98, *107*
Rose, T. L., 327, *337*
Roselli, M., 60, *71*
Rosen, W., 345, *351*
Rosenberg, D. C., 144, *147*
Rosenblatt, A., 359, *363*
Rosenfeld, R., 332, *335*
Rosenkoetter, M. M., 300, *310*
Rosenkranz, M., 199, *202*
Rosenmayr, L., 270, *275*
Rosenzweig, M. R., 113, *119*
Rosler, F., 8, 9, 15, *19*
Roßnagel, C., 269, 270, *276*
Rosnick, C. B., 100, *107*, 178, 180, 181, *188*, 198, *204*
Rosowsky, E., 329, 330, 331, *336*
Ross, C., 179, *188*
Ross, C. E., 177, 179, *189*, 208, 209, *217*
Ross, C. W., 209, *217*
Ross, J. M., 286, *288*
Ross, K. E., 222, *231*
Rossi, A. S., 220, 224, 226, *231*
Rossi, P. H., 220, 224, 226, *231*
Rossi, S., 111, *119*
Rossini, P. M., 111, *119*
Rostrup, E., 79, *87*

Roth, D. L., 354, 355, 356, 357, 358, 360, 361, *362*, *363*, *364*, 374, *377*
Roth, H., 156, *166*
Roth, L., 332, *337*
Roth, L. H., 368, *379*
Rothermund, K., 178, *187*, 301, *310*
Rott, L., 224, 225, 226, *229*
Rotter, J. B., 176, 177, *189*
Rovaris, M., 82, *85*, *90*
Rowe, C. C., 111, *119*
Rowe, J., 26, *36*
Rowe, J. W., 175, 177, 178, 180, 184, *187*, *189*, 193, 198, *204*, 209, 213, *216*, *217*, *218*
Rozario, P. A., 271, 272, *275*, 358, *364*
Rozzini, R., 313, *320*
Rubert, M. P., 356, 358, *362*
Rubin, D. B., 27, 28, *37*, *38*, *217*
Rubin, S. M., 210, *217*
Ruchinskas, R. A., 375, *379*
Ruff, R., 157, 158, 159, *169*
Ruffman, T., 297, 298, *310*
Rugg, M. D., 111, *118*
Rumbaut, R. G., 42, 49, *53*
Rupert, M., 358, *362*
Ruschena, D., 317, *322*
Ruscher, J. B., 253, *262*
Russell, K. C., 287, *288*
Russell, S., 226, *229*
Russo, C., 135, 144, *149*
Russo, F. A., 154, *171*
Russo, J., 354, 355, *364*
Ryall, A. L., 258, 259, *261*
Ryan, C. M., 77, *91*
Ryan, E. B., 233, 234, 235, 236, 237, 238, 239, 242, *244*, *245*, *246*, 251, 253, 254, *261*, *262*
Ryan, J., 114, *117*
Ryder, A. G., 328, *334*
Ryder, N. B., 42, *53*
Ryff, C. D., 49, *53*, 180, 181, *188*, 195, *203*, 265, *275*, 285, *290*, 299, *307*
Ryff, C. R., 195, *201*
Rypma, B., 111, *119*, 122, *131*

S

Sabir, M., 226, *231*
Sacco, J. M., 343, *349*
Sachdev, P., 78, *86*
Sachdev, P. S., 314, 315, 316, *320*, *323*
Sachs, R., 83, *86*
Sachweh, S., 236, *246*
Sacker, A., 347, *351*
Sacker, M., 164, *169*
Saczynski, J. S., 61, *70*, 161, 163, 164, *166*
Safran, M. A., 298, *308*
Sager, M. A., 326, *336*
Saine, K., 373, *377*
Saks, E. R., 372, *377*
Saksvik, P. Ö., 268, *275*
Salari, S. M., 234, *246*
Salat, D. H., 75, 76, 77, 80, *86*, *87*, *90*, 126, 127, *130*
Salganicoff, A., 208, *217*
Salmon, D. P., 101, *104*, 342, 344, *348*, *349*, *351*, *352*
Salomonowitz, E., 80, *91*
Salovey, P., 197, *205*
Salthouse, T. A., 5, 9, 10, 11, 12, 14, 16, 17, 18, *20*, *22*, 31, *36*, 61, 62, 63, 64, 65, 69, *72*, 122, *131*, 141, *150*, 153, 154, 158, 159, 164, *169*, 178, *189*, 264, 267, *276*, 345, *352*
Salva, G. N., 372, *379*
Salvedera, F., 160, *167*
Sambamoorthi, U., 314, *320*
Sambataro, F., 100, *106*
Samnaliev, M., 313, *320*
Sampson, R. J., 42, 46, *52*, *53*
Sandblom, J., 114, *118*, *119*, 156, *169*
Sander, N., 62, *72*
Sander, T., 101, 102, *106*, 122, *131*
Sanders, A. L., 129, *130*
Sanders, R. E., 156, *168*
Sandler, I., 192, *204*
Sanford, N., 26, *36*, 242, *244*
Sangree, W. H., 50, *53*
Sano, M., 346, 347, *350*, *351*
Santorelli, S. F., 199, *202*
Sanz, A., 183, *189*
Sanz Arigita, E. J., 75, *91*
Sapolsky, R. M., 182, *188*, 197, 198, *204*
Sargent, M., 283, *290*
Sargent-Cox, K., 314, *320*
Sarkar, J. M., 233, *244*
Sarkisian, C. A., 49, *53*
Sarkisian, N., 221, *231*
Sarmany-Schuller, I., 237, *246*
Sasaki, A., 99, *106*
Sasaki, M., 359, *364*
Sastry, J., 179, *189*
Sato, R., 345, *348*
Satre, D. D., 318, *322*
Satz, P., 347, *351*
Saudino, K. J., 94, *107*
Savage, A., 111, *119*
Savage, C. R., 46, 49, *50*, 160, *165*
Savage, G., 83, *89*
Saville, A. L., 303, *308*
Savla, J., 221, *229*
Sawamoto, N., 342, 343, *351*
Sawrie, S., 368, 373, *378*
Saxby, B. K., 77, *87*
Saxena, A., 269, *274*
Saxton, J. A., 78, 79, 83, *85*, *89*
Sayegh, P., 357, 358, *363*
Sayer, A. G., 29, *38*
Scalf, P., 6, *21*, 84, *87*
Scalf, P. E., 116, *118*, 129, *130*, 158, 161, 164, *166*, *167*
Scanlan, J. M., 198, *201*, 354, *365*
Scanlon, J. M., 78, 79, *89*
Scaravilli, F., 82, *89*
Scarmeas, N., 159, *169*, 340, *348*
Schacter, D. L., 83, *86*, 122, *131*
Schadron, G., 250, 253, *261*
Schaefer, S., 12, 16, *21*
Schafer, J. L., 27, 28, *38*
Schaie, K. W., 4, 5, 6, 7, 8, 9, 10, 11, 14, 18, *19*, *22*, 26, 30, 31, 34, *38*, *39*, 41, 42, 43, 45, 46, 48, 49, *52*, *53*, *54*, *55*, 94, 96, *107*, 110, *119*, 122, 123, *131*, 143, *150*, 180, *190*, 367, *379*
Schapiro, M. B., 340, *349*
Scheier, M. F., 302, *310*
Schein, R. L., 327, *336*
Scheiner, D., 347, *351*
Schellenberg, G. C., 49, *52*
Scheltens, P., 78, 79, *87*, *89*, 112, *117*
Scherder, E. J., 78, *89*
Schervish, P. G., 368, *378*
Schettler, P. J., 326, *335*
Schiavone, F., 80, 81, 82, *86*, *90*
Schieman, S., 226, *231*, *310*
Schilling, E. A., 192, 194, *201*
Schindler, I., 271, *275*
Schkade, D. A., 134, *149*
Schlaug, G., 113, *117*
Schmidt, D. F., 250, 251, *262*
Schmidt, P. S., 94, *105*
Schmiedek, F., 12, 16, *21*, 27, *36*, 110, *119*
Schmierer, K., 82, *89*
Schmitt, F. A., 156, *168*, 368, *378*
Schmitt, M., 259, *260*
Schneider, J. A., 30, *39*, 68, *72*, 159, *171*, *205*, 347, *348*
Schneider, J. S., 199, *206*
Schneider, S. L., 138, *148*
Schneider, W., 60, 65, *72*
Schniebolk, S., 161, *166*
Schoeni, R., 211, *217*, 222, *231*
Schoevers, R. S., 315, *320*
Schofield, P., 346, *350*
Schömann, K., 258, 270, 271, *272*
Schooler, C., 42, 44, 48, *52*, *54*, 159, 162, *169*, 180, *187*, 209, *217*, 265, 266, *274*, *276*
Schooler, L. J., 135, *149*
Schork, N. J., 103, *105*
Schott, A.-M., 154, *165*
Schrama, L. H., 164, *165*
Schretlen, D., 66, *72*, 76, *90*
Schretlen, D. J., 78, 79, *91*

Schroeder, K., 101, *107*
Schroeder, S. A., 208, *216*
Schroepfer, T., 221, *229*
Schroots, J. J. F., 4, 6, 7, *19*, *22*
Schuff, N., 75, *86*
Schuierer, G., 114, *117*, 162, *166*
Schulberg, H. C., 316, *320*, 326, *336*
Schuller, K. L., 135, *150*
Schuller, M. D., 328, *334*
Schultz, L., 360, *364*
Schultz, N. R., 48, *51*
Schultz, S. K., 313, *323*, 345, *349*
Schulz, R., 177, 179, 184, 185, *187*, *189*, *190*, 210, *217*, 223, *231*, 300, *308*, 326, *336*, 354, 355, 356, 359, 360, 361, *362*, *363*, *364*
Schumacher, E. H., 113, *119*
Schumacher, J., 199, *202*
Schumann, G., 101, *107*
Schupf, N., 340, *350*
Schut, H., 319, *323*
Schutte, K. K., 316, *321*
Schütze, H., 83, *86*, *87*
Schwall, A. R., 48, *51*
Schwantes, A., 326, *336*
Schwarb, H., 67, 68, *72*
Schwartz, B. S., 31, *36*
Schwartz, G., 198, *203*
Schwartz, J. L. K., 254, *260*
Schwartz, K., 211, *216*
Schwartz, S., 344, *348*
Schwartzman, A. E., 5, *22*
Schwarz, N., 139, 142, *150*, 255, *259*, 326, *336*
Schwarz, R., 78, *87*
Scollon, C. N., 266, *276*
Scott, M., 66, 67, 68, *72*
Sdrolias, H. A., 184, *189*
Searle, M. S., 184, *189*
Seay, R. B., 135, *146*, 301, *306*
Sechrist, J., 220, 221, 222, 223, 226, *231*
Seeley, D. G., 49, *53*
Seeley, J. R., 313, *323*, 327, *335*
Seeman, T., 46, 49, *50*, 61, *70*, 160, 161, 163, 164, *165*, *166*, *189*
Seeman, T. E., 181, 182, 184, 193, 197, 198, *204*, *205*, 213, *216*, *217*, *218*, 268, *277*, 284, 287, *290*, 304, *310*
Sees, A. C., 211, *216*
Seewann, A., 78, 82, *87*
Segal, D. L., 328, 329, 330, 331, 332, 333, *334*, *335*, *336*, *337*
Segal, D. R., 46, *54*
Segerstrom, S. C., 196, 200, *204*
Seider, B. H., 301, 302, *310*
Seidler, R., 110, *118*, 154, 158, 164, *168*
Seidlitz, L., 316, *320*
Seignourel, P. J., 317, *322*
Selman, R. L., 283, *289*
Seltzer, M. M., 222, *230*, 354, 355, 360, *363*, *364*
Selye, H., 191, *204*, 218, *218*
Semegon, A. B., 326, *334*
Semple, S. J., 317, *322*, 354, 357, 359, *364*
Senjem, M. L., 83, *88*, 111, *118*
Sepielli, P., 210, *217*
Seplaki, C. L., 208, 211, 213, *218*
Sepulcre, J., 83, *86*
Sergeant, J. A., 78, *89*
Serido, J., 192, 200, *204*
Setterlind, S., 200, *202*
Sewitch, M., 355, *364*
Seymour, R. M., 139, *150*
Shadish, W. R., 35, *39*
Shafir, E., 134, *150*
Shafir, S., 138, 140, *151*
Shah, P., 110, *118*, 154, 158, 164, *168*
Shake, M. C., 156, *170*
Shallice, T., 69, *70*
Shamoian, C. A., 328, *334*
Shanahan, M. J., 17, *22*, 94, *107*
Shaner, J. L., 234, 238, *245*, 250, 251, 252, 253, 254, *261*
Shankman, S., 326, *337*
Shannon, B. J., 83, *86*
Shantz, G. D., 236, *246*
Shapiro, A., 224, *231*
Sharma, S., 182, *188*, 198, *203*
Shaw, B., 304, *310*
Shaw, B. A., 180, *190*
Shaw, W., 317, *322*
Shea, D., 210, *215*
Shearer, D. E., 160, *167*
Shekar, S. N., 97, *106*
Sheline, Y. I., 83, *90*
Shema, S. J., 209, *217*
Shen, Y., 80, 81, *86*
Shenkin, S. D., 81, *90*
Sheridan, J. F., 191, *202*, *203*
Sheridan, P. L., 258, 259, *261*
Sherman, E. M. S., 347, *352*
Sherod, M. G., 373, *379*
Sherrill, J. T., 197, *205*
Sherwood, G. G., 282, *290*
Shibasaki, H., 343, *351*
Shiffrin, R. M., 60, 65, *69*, *72*
Shifren, K., 34, *39*, 355, 356, *363*
Shim, M. S., 42, 50, *52*
Shimony, J. S., 60, *71*, 80, *88*, 110, *118*, 125, *130*
Shiner, R. L., 283, 284, *289*
Shiomura, K., 179, *186*
Shipley, M., 195, *203*
Shiraishi, R. W., 281, 284, 287, *290*, 302, *306*
Shiung, M. M., 83, *88*, 111, *118*
Shiv, B., 136, *150*
Shivapour, D. M., 138, 145, *146*
Short, J.-A. C., 283, *290*
Shroyer, L. W., 17, 18, *20*
Shubert, T., 164, *170*
Shuey, K. M., 220, 225, 226, *232*
Shulman, G. L., 112, *119*
Shulman, K. I., 344, *349*
Shultz, K. S., 270, *276*, *276*
Shumovich, M. A., 237, *246*
Shupe, D. R., 179, *190*
Shurgot, G. R., 356, *363*
Sickel, A. E., 333, *327*
Sicola, A., 373, *378*
Siddarth, P., 161, *169*
Siddle, H., 328, 329, *336*
Siegel, D., 155, 158, 160, 161, *167*
Sieroff, E., 343, *351*
Silbereisen, R. K., 50, *54*
Silberman, C. S., 332, *337*
Silbershatz, H., 48, *51*
Sillanmaki, L., 304, *308*
Silver, N. C., 82, *90*
Silverman, D. H. S., 161, *169*
Silverstein, M., 159, *168*, 220, 223, 224, 227, *229*, *231*, 242, *246*, 354, *363*
Simmons, W. K., 344, *351*
Simms, L. J., 332, *335*
Simoes, A., 266, *275*
Simon, K. I., 143, *150*
Simoni-Wastila, L., 318, *322*
Simons, D. J., 160, *165*, *166*
Simonsick, E. M., 208, 210, 211, 213, *217*, *218*, 316, *323*
Singer, B. H., 193, 198, *204*, 213, *216*, *217*, *218*
Singer, J. D., 32, 34, *39*
Sinz, H., 138, *151*
Sirey, M. P., 316, *322*
Siwak, C. T., 75, 83, *91*
Skaff, M. M., 179, 180, 181, *190*, 192, *204*, 354, 357, 359, 360, *364*
Skill, T., 233, *246*
Skinner, E. A., 177, *190*
Skinner, M., 303, *310*
Skirbekk, V., 267, *276*
Skoog, I., 314, *323*
Skrajner, M. J., 154, *168*
Skurnik, I., 142, *150*
Skytthe, A., 95, *107*
Slachevsky, A., 343, *349*
Slade, M. D., 175, 180, *188*, 250, 256, 257, 258, 259, *261*
Slagboom, P. E., 99, *105*
Slingerland, A. S., 271, *276*
Sliwinski, M. J., 9, 11, *21*, *22*, 26, 31, *39*, 74, *91*, 178, 188, *190*, 193, 194, 199, 201, *205*, 300, *310*
Sloane, M. E., 374, *379*

Sloggett, A., 197, *205*
Sloman, S. A., 135, *150*
Slovic, P., 133, 134, 136, 137, 138, 143, 145, 146, *146*, *147*, *148*, *149*, *150*, 371, *379*
Sluming, V., 76, *87*
Smalbrugge, M., 313, *323*
Small, B. J., 34, *38*, 100, 101, *104*, *107*, 121, *129*, 161, *167*, 180, 183, *187*, 198, *204*, 265, *273*
Small, D. A., 137, *148*
Small, G. W., 77, *86*, 161, *169*
Small, S. A., 346, *350*
Smedley, B. D., 208, *218*
Smit, J. H., 315, 327, 328, *320*, *334*
Smith, A., 142, *149*
Smith, A. D., 48, *51*, 101, *105*, 110, *119*
Smith, A. P., 209, *215*
Smith, C. D., 80, *87*
Smith, D., 30, 31, 32, *38*, 156, 157, *167*, *170*, *171*
Smith, D. P., 303, *310*
Smith, E., 235, 236, *244*
Smith, E. E., 111, *119*, 134, *150*
Smith, G. E., 157, 159, *169*
Smith, G. T., 326, *337*
Smith, J., 5, 8, 9, 14, *19*, *20*, 114, *118*, 154, *168*, 178, 180, *187*, *189*, 198, *205*, 267, *276*, 280, 281, 283, 286, 287, *288*, *290*, *291*, 295, 298, *308*, *310*
Smith, J. L., 265, *275*
Smith, J. P., 209, *216*, 345, *350*
Smith, M. R., 111, *119*
Smith, M. Z., 48, *51*
Smith, P. K., 110, *119*
Smith, S., 80, *88*
Smith, S. M., 137, *150*
Smith, S. S., 328, *336*
Smith, T. E., 197, *203*
Smith, T. L., 332, *337*
Smith, T. S., 303, *310*
Smith, T. W., 225, *232*, 301, 302, *310*
Smolka, M. N., 101, *107*
Smyth, F. L., 254, 255, *262*
Smyth, J., 26, *39*
Smyth, J. M., 193, 194, 198, 199, *205*, 300, *310*
Smyth, K. A., 265, *273*
Smyth, R., 50, *54*
Sneed, J. R., 315, *323*
Snel, J., 200, *205*
Snow, L., 317, *322*
Snowdon, D., 242, *244*
Snowdon, D. A., 48, *54*
Snow-Turek, A. L., 327, *336*
Snyder, A. Z., 77, 83, *86*, *90*, 112, 113, *117*, *118*, *119*, 129, *130*
Snyder, S., 368, 373, *378*
Socherman, R., 372, *379*
Söderlund, H., 78, 79, *91*, 125, *131*
Solano, N., 358, *362*
Solano, N. H., 317, *323*
Soliz, J., 234, 240, *244*, *246*
Somera, L. P., 237, *246*, 251, *260*
Somerfield, M. R., 194, *202*
Sommer, T., 101, *107*, 125, 126, *129*
Song, I. C., 82, *88*
Sonnega, J., 318, 319, *320*
Sorensen, S., 223, 227, *231*
Sörensen, S., 354, 355, 356, 357, 358, 361, *364*
Sorenson, A. M., 192, 199, *205*
Sorkin, D. H., 301, *310*
Sorlie, P. D., 209, *217*
Sormani, M. P., 82, *85*, *90*
Sorrentino, R. M., 283, *290*
Sowarka, D., 154, *165*
Sozou, P. D., 139, *150*
Spaniol, J., 80, 81, 82, *86*, *88*, *89*
Spencer, S. J., 256, *262*, 346, *351*
Sperling, R. A., 83, *91*
Spiegel, D., 136, *148*
Spielberger, C. D., 329, *337*
Spiers, H. J., 162, *168*
Spilt, A., 82, *91*
Spiro, A. III, 6, 8, 14, 16, *22*, 181, 184, *188*, *189*, 191, 194, 195, 198, *204*, *205*, 270, *274*, 298, 302, 304, *306*, *309*
Spitze, G. D., 220, *230*
Spitzer, R. L., 333, *335*
Spreen, O., 347, *352*
Spreng, R. N., 60, 66, 67, *72*
Springer, M. V., 112, *118*
Squire, L. R., 122, *131*
Srivastava, S., 287, *289*
St. Clair, D., 100, *105*
St. Jacques, P., 16, *22*, 297, *310*
Staats, N., 371, 373, *377*
Stack, D. M., 5, *22*
Stadlbauer, A., 80, *91*
Stallforth, S., 83, *86*, *87*
Stallings, M. C., 97, *105*
Stalvey, T., 368, 373, *378*
Stanczyk, F. Z., 196, *203*
Stankov, L., 142, *146*
Stanley, J. C., 30, *36*
Stanley, J. T., 297, *310*
Stanley, M., 329, *337*
Stanley, M. A., 317, *322*
Stanovich, K. E., 135, *150*
Stansfeld, S., 270, *275*
Staples, F., 314, *321*
Stark, A. C., 303, *308*
Starr, A., 343, *350*
Starr, J. M., 17, *20*, 80, 81, 82, *86*, *90*, 96, 99, *105*
Statham, J. A., 256, 257, *260*
Staudinger, U. M., 5, 8, 9, 11, 12, 14, 18, *19*, 116, *119*, 178, *186*, 191, 193, *201*, *203*, 263, 264, 265, 266, 267, 268, 269, 270, 271, 272, *272*, *273*, *274*, *275*, *276*, 281, 283, 284, 285, 286, 287, *288*, *290*, *291*
Stawski, R. S., 9, *22*, 26, *39*, 188, 193, 194, 197, 199, *200*, 201, *204*, *205*, 300, *310*
Steel, D., 68, *69*
Steele, C. M., 256, *262*, 346, *348*, *351*, *352*, 359, *363*
Steele, D., 192, *202*
Steer, R., 329, *334*
Steer, R. A., 327, *337*
Steffens, D. C., 314, *323*
Stein, M. B., 297, 305, *310*
Stein, R., 256, *262*
Steinberg, M., 359, *363*
Steiner, P. M., 35, *39*
Steinhaus, L. A., 160, *167*
Stellar, E., 191, 196, 197, *203*, 212, *217*
Stenton, R., 109, *119*
Stephens, E. C., 144, *150*
Stephens, M. A. P., 227, *231*
Stephenson, D., 183, *186*
Sterling, P., 212, *218*
Stern, P. C., 6, 7, 11, 14, *22*
Stern, Y., 11, 14, 16, *22*, 59, 66, *72*, 75, *91*, 113, *119*, 122, *131*, 153, 159, 165, *169*, 340, 344, 346, 347, *348*, *350*, *351*, *352*, 374, *379*
Sternäng, O., 122, *131*
Sternberg, R. J., 265, *276*, 280, 281, 282, 283, 284, 285, 287, *290*, *291*
Steuerle, E., 269, *275*
Steunenberg, B., 315, *323*
Stevens, A., 358, 360, *362*, *364*
Stevenson, M. L., 228, *229*
Stewart, A. J., 43, *54*
Stewart, R., 315, *322*
Stewart, W. F., 31, *36*
Stigsdotter-Neely, A. S., 125, 127, *131*, 155, 156, *169*, *170*
Stine-Morrow, E. A. L., 156, 159, 162, *168*, *169*, *170*
Stith, A. Y., 208, *218*
Stockdale, G. D., 250, 253, 258, *261*
Stokes, D. E., 164, *170*
Stones, M. J., 159, *170*
Storandt, M., 161, *167*, 342, *352*
Story, T. J., 340, *352*
Story, T. N., 301, 302, *310*
Strachan, M. W. J., 48, *54*
Strack, S., 332, *335*
Strahm, S., 238, *245*, 250, 251, 252, 253, 254, *261*
Strange, J. J., 137, *150*
Stratakis, C. A., 191, *205*

Strauss, E., 26, 33, *37*, 62, 63, 64, 69, *70*, 347, *352*
Strayer, D. L., 158, *168*
Street, D., 49, *54*
Streeten, D. H., 48, *51*
Streich, D. D., 283, *290*
Streufert, S., 143, *150*
Strick, P. L., 343, *348*
Stroebe, M., 319, *323*
Stroebe, M. S., 319, *323*
Stroebe, W., 319, *323*
Stronks, K., 209, *218*
Stroop, J. R., 109, *119*
Strother, S. C., 67, *70*, 112, *118*
Strothers, H. S., 375, *378*
Stroud, L. R., 197, *205*
Strough, J., 135, *150*
Strunk, G., 80, *91*
Stryker, S., 178, 183, *187*
Strzepek, D. M., 372, *378*
Stuck, A. E., 374, *379*
Stuck, S., 271, *274*
Studholme, C., 75, *86*
Stump, T. E., 179, *190*
Sturm, M., 299, *307*
Sturman, E. D., 372, *379*
Stuss, D. T., 159, *168*, *170*
Sub, H. M., 62, *72*
Subramaniam, H., 314, *323*
Substance Abuse and Mental Health Services Administration, 318, *323*
Suci, G. J., 136, *149*
Sudano, J. J., 210, *218*
Suh, E. M., 298, *307*
Suitor, J. J., 220, 221, 225, 226, *231*, 359, 360, *364*
Sullivan, E. V., 80, 81, *89*, *91*, 340, *352*
Sullivan, L., 142, *149*
Sullivan, S., 297, 298, *310*
Suls, J., 194, *202*, *205*
Summers, P. E., 80, *89*
Sun, F., 357, *363*
Sun, X., 100, *106*
Sunderland, T., 372, *377*
Sundstrom, G., 223, *231*
Sung, K. T., 220, *231*
Sunstein, C. R., 145, *150*
Surjadi, F. F., 266, *277*
Sutch, R., 49, *53*
Sutker, P. B., 198, *205*
Sutton, B., 111, *117*
Sutton, B. P., 67, *71*
Suzuki, A., 111, 115, *118*
Svedberg, P., 96, *106*
Svensson, C. M., 279, 287, *288*
Swaim, E. L., 61, 66, *71*
Swan, G. E., 48, *54*, 78, *86*, *91*, 99, *105*
Swartz, M., 314, *322*
Swartz, T. T., 223, *231*
Swezy, R. W., 164, *170*
Syme, S. L., 179, 183, *186*, *214*
Szanton, S. L., 208, 211, 213, *218*
Szekely, C. A., 84, *89*
Szklo, M., 345, *348*
Szuchman, L., 253, *260*
Szyf, M., 99, *106*

T

Tada, Y., 361, *364*
Tadorov, A., 16, *23*
Takahashi, M., 281, 282, 284, 286, 287, *291*
Takashima, Y., 78, *89*
Talbot, A., 135, 144, *149*
Tallent, E. M., 82, *85*
Talukdar, T., 83, *86*
Tam, R., 257, *259*
Tan, E. J., 284, 287, *290*
Tan, J. C., 111, *117*
Tanaka, Y., 258, *262*
Tang, F., 271, 272, *275*
Tang, M. X., 159, *169*, 346, 347, *350*, *351*, *352*
Tang, Y., 198, 199, *205*
Tanius, B. E., 144, *150*
Tannenbaum, P. H., 136, *149*
Tapp, P. D., 75, 83, *91*
Taranto, M. A., 282, 283, *291*
Tarshish, C., 198, *203*, 340, *349*
Tate, D. F., 75, 78, *89*
Tatemichi, T. K., 374, *379*
Taub, E., 113, *119*
Taussig, I. M., 347, *350*
Taylor, B. J., 29, *37*
Taylor, D. H. J., 315, *321*
Taylor, G. A., 139, *151*
Taylor, M., 339, *349*
Taylor, R. J., 226, *229*
Taylor, R. T., 221, *229*
Taylor, S. E., 191, 197, *205*, 304, *310*
Tchiteya, B. M., 182, *188*
Teachman, B. A., 328, *337*
Teichberg, D., 340, *349*
Teipel, S. J., 78, *87*
Tellegen, A., 33, *39*, 194, *201*
Teng, E. L., 347, *350*, *352*
Teng, H. M., 270, *273*
Ten Have, T. R., 316, *320*
Tennstedt, S., 156, 157, *167*, *171*, 183, 184, 185, *188*, *190*
Tennstedt, S. L., 49, *55*, 156, 159, *171*
Tenover, J., 100, *107*
Tentori, K., 135, *151*
Teresi, J., 314, *323*, 327, *337*
Teri, L., 49, *52*, 347, *352*, 356, *365*
Terracciano, A., 283, *290*
Tesch-Römer, C., 258, *262*, 270, *277*
Tessitore, A., 127, *131*
Thacker, N., 66, 67, 68, *72*
Thal, L. J., 197, *204*, 344, *352*
Thaler, R. H., 137, 145, *150*, *151*
Thayer, J. F., 198, *201*
Thilers, P., 127, 129, *130*
Thomas, G. V., 333, *337*
Thomas, R. G., 347, *351*
Thompson, D., 192, *202*
Thompson, J., 196, *202*
Thompson, L. W., 319, 328, *321*, *336*, *362*
Thompson, P. M., 80, *88*
Thompson, S. C., 178, *190*
Thompson-Brenner, H., 103, *106*
Thorn, R. M., 155, *170*
Thorndike, R. L., 30, *39*
Thorne, S., 47, *50*
Thornton, J. S., 82, *89*
Thornton, L. M., 194, 195, *203*
Thornton, M. C., 180, *187*
Thornton, W. J. L., 135, *151*
Thorpe, R. J., Jr., 208, 210, 211, 213, *215*, *216*, *217*, *218*
Thorson, J. A., 237, *246*, 284, *291*
Thurner, M., 195, *203*
Tighe, L., 225, *232*
Timko, C., 180, 183, *189*
Tiraboschi, P., 344, *352*
Tisak, J., 32, *38*
Tisserand, D. J., 66, *72*, 75, *91*
Titma, M., 48, *54*
Tobi, E. W., 99, *105*
Tobin, S. S., 270, *274*
Todd, E. G., 101, *104*
Tofts, P. S., 82, *90*
Tollefsbol, T. O., 17, *21*, 99, *106*
Tomaka, J., 192, *204*
Tomasello, M., 45, *54*
Tomasik, M. J., 258, *262*
Toner, K., 302, *308*
Tornstam, L., 281, *291*
Toro, R., 67, *72*
Toth, J., 60, 61, 62, 64, 65, 68, *70*
Toth, J. P., 65, *72*
Touboul, P. J., 78, *91*
Toulmin, S., 4, 12, 14, *23*
Touradji, P., 346, 347, *350*
Touron, D. R., 181, *190*
Townsend, A. L., 227, *231*
Townsend, J., 74, *86*
Toyoda, H., 342, *351*
Traipe, E., 82, *85*
Tranel, D., 16, *19*, 138, *146*
Tranh, M., 78, *86*
Tranter, L. J., 162, *170*
Treas, J., 49, *55*
Treece, C., 332, *335*
Triebel, K., 373, *379*
Tripp, K., 370, *377*
Troll, L. E., 220, *232*

Trollor, J. N., 314, 316, *323*
Trostel, P. A., 139, *151*
Trovato, D., 233, *246*
Trunk, D. L., 241, *246*
Tsai, J., 139, *147*
Tsai, J. L., 296, 297, 299, 303, *310*
Tsai, S. J., 100, *107*
Tsai, W. Y., 347, *351*
Tschanz, J. T., 101, *105*, 314, *323*
Tse, C. K., 326, *334*
Tsopelas, N. D., 83, *85*
Tsuang, D., 48, *53*
Tsuang, M. T., 95, *106*
Tu, X. M., 197, *205*
Tuch, D. S., 80, *90*
Tuholksi, S. W., 158, *167*
Tulebaev, S. R., 343, *349*
Tulsky, D., 339, *349*
Tulving, E., 67, *71*, 122, *131*
Tuma, N. B., 48, *54*
Turic, D., 100, *107*
Turner, A., 196, *202*
Turner, J. B., 192, 199, *205*
Turner, J. C., 241, *246*
Turner, J. T., 233, *246*
Turner, R. A., 197, *205*
Turner, R. J., 192, 199, *205*, 209, *218*
Turvey, C., 313, 316, *323*
Tusler, M., 143, 145, *148*
Tversky, A., 133, 137, 139, *148*, *151*
Tweed, R. G., 318, 319, *320*
Twisk, J. W. R., 200, *205*
Tychynski, D., 183, *188*
Tyner, C., 81, 82, *88*
Tyrell, D. A., 209, *215*
Tysoski, S., 237, *245*
Tzourio, C., 78, 79, *86*, *91*

U

Uchino, A., 78, *89*
Uchino, B. N., 196, *205*, 225, *232*, 295, 297, 303, *310*
Uhlenberg, P., 50, *52*, *54*, 219, *230*
Umberson, D., 225, 226, 227, *232*
Uniform Health Decisions Act, 370, *379*
Uno, D., 196, *205*, 303, *310*
Unverzagt, F., 157, *171*, 347, *352*
Updegraff, J. A., 191, *205*
Upton, N., 129, *129*
Ursin, H., 268, *275*
U.S. Bureau of the Census, 209, 210, *218*
U.S. Department of Health and Human Services, 210, *218*
Usui, I., 50, *55*
Uswatte, G., 113, *119*
Uvnas-Moberg, K., 197, *201*, *205*
Uylings, H. B. M., 84, *86*

V

Vahia, I., 282, *289*
Vahtera, J., 304, *308*
Vaillant, G. E., 5, *23*, 175, *190*, 285, *288*, *291*, 318, *323*, 331, *337*
Valentijn, S. A. M., 156, *170*
Valiquette, L., 67, 68, *72*
Valk, R., 297, *309*
Valsasina, P., 82, *85*
Van Alphen, S. P. J., 333, *337*
van Asselen, M., 64, *72*
van Baaren, R. B., 138, *147*
Van Balkom, A. J., 328, *334*
van Beijsterveldt, C. E., 96, 97, *105*
van Boxtel, M. P. J., 75, 84, *86*, *91*, 156, *170*, 265, *273*
Van Broeckhoven, C., 129, *130*
van Buchem, M. A., 82, *91*
Van Cauter, E., 197, *205*
van den Berg, K. E., 75, *86*
Vandenbulcke, M., 84, *89*
VandenHeuvel, A., 268, *277*
Vandeputte, D., 234, *245*
van der Grond, J., 78, *91*
van der Hiele, K., 78, *91*
van der Kolk, B. A., 194, *205*
van der Kouwe, A. J. W., 80, *90*
Van der Linden, M., 69, *69*
van der Mheen, H. D., 209, *218*
Vanderstichele, H., 111, *117*
Vander Weg, M., 157, *171*
van der Welle, A., 78, *91*
van Dyck, J., 184, *189*
van Gool, W. A., 342, *350*
van Groen, T., 17, *21*, 99, *106*
van Harten, B., 78, 79, *89*
Van Hasselt, V. B., 329, 332, *335*, *336*
Van Hooren, S. A. H., 156, *170*
Van Houten, O., 160, *167*
van Ijzendoorn, M. H., 228, *229*
van Lenthe, F. J., 271, *276*
Van Limbeek, J., 327, 328, *334*
Vanmechelen, E., 111, *117*
van Mechelen, W., 200, *205*
Vannorsdall, T. D., 78, 79, *91*
Van Petten, C., 75, 79, *91*
van Praag, H., 164, *167*, *170*, 264, *276*
Van Reenen, J., 268, *273*
Van Solinge, H., 270, *276*
Van Strien, J. W., 302, *308*
van Tilbury, T., 327, *334*
van Tilburg, T. G., 305, *307*
van Tilburg, W., 327, *334*
Van Willigen, M., 179, *188*
Vasil, L., 233, *246*
Vassos, E., 100, *106*
Vasterling, J. J., 198, *205*
Västfjäll, D., 134, 143, *149*
Vasunilashorn, S., 196, *202*
Vaupel, J. W., 95, 99, *104*, *107*, 153, *166*
Vaynman, S., 164, *170*
Vecchi, T., 156, *166*
Vein, A. A., 78, *91*
Venkatraman, V., 111, *117*
Veratti, B., 182, *186*
Verbrugge, L. M., 211, *218*
Verbruggen, A., 84, *89*
Verdelho, A., 342, *350*
Verghese, J., 9, *22*, 75, *91*, 113, *118*, 153, 163, *170*
Verhaeghen, P., 64, *72*, 155, 156, *170*
Verreault, R., 265, *274*
Vicario, F., 319, *321*
Victoroff, J., 78, *88*
Viechtbauer, W., 11, *22*, 265, *275*
Vijg, J., 99, *105*
Vijod, M. A., 196, *203*
Viken, R. J., 98, *107*
Vilkman, H., 111, *118*
Villamarín, F., 183, *189*
Villemagne, V. I., 83, *89*
Villringer, A., 101, 102, *106*, 122, *131*, 138, *149*
Vincent, J. L., 112, *117*
Vinocour, S. M., 47, *55*
Vinokur, A. D., 192, *201*
Vinovskis, M. A., 49, 50, *55*
Vitaliano, P. P., 354, 355, *364*, *365*
Vitiliano, P. P., 198, *201*
Vititoe, E., 313, *321*
Voelcker-Rehage, C., 116, *119*
Voelpel, S., 269, 270, *276*
Vogels, R. L., 78, 79, *89*
Vogler, G. P., 93, 94, *106*, *107*
Volavka, J., 101, *104*
Volicer, L., 368, *377*
von Frijtag, J. C., 164, *165*
von Hippel, W., 61, 66, *71*
von Känel, R., 196, *201*, 361, *364*
von Oertzen, T., 32, *37*, 101, 102, *106*, 122, 125, 127, 129, *130*, *131*, 154, *166*
von Sanden, C., 314, *320*
Voss, M. W., 74, 75, 80, 84, *88*, 115, *117*, 141, *148*, 160, 163, *165*, *167*
Vuurman, E. F. P. M., 84, *86*

W

Wadhwa, R., 116, *118*, 158, 164, *167*
Wadley, V. G., 354, 355, 358, *362*, 374, *377*, *379*
Wadlinger, H. A., 301, 302, *308*
Wager, T., 161, *168*
Wager, T. D., 60, 62, 63, 64, *71*, 114, *118*
Wagner, L., 195, *205*

Author Index

Wagner, L. S., 250, 253, *261*
Wagster, M. V., 345, *349*
Wahl, H.-W., 49, *54*
Wahlin, Å., 6, 11, 14, 17, *21*, *23*, 101, *104*, 121, *129*, *131*
Wais, P., 295, 297, 302, *309*
Waite, L. J., 50, *52*, *222*, *230*
Waldman, D. A., 48, *50*
Waldstein, S. R., 14, *23*, 48, *55*, 77, 78, 79, *91*
Walhovd, K. B., 75, 77, *87*, *91*
Walker, E. F., 183, *187*
Walker, J., 374, *379*
Walkup, J. T., 314, *320*
Wallace, K. A., 299, *309*
Wallace, L. E., 226, *232*
Wallace, R., 345, *350*
Wallace, R. B., 345, *349*
Walsh, D. A., 143, *147*
Walsh, K. T., 249, *262*
Walsh-Riddle, M., 161, *166*
Walters, E. E., 328, *335*
Walthert, J. M., 374, *379*
Walton, K. E., 11, *22*, 265, 266, *275*, *276*
Wan, N., 122, *130*
Wang, H., 223, *231*
Wang, L., 345, *352*
Wang, M., 270, *276*
Wang, S., 83, *90*
Ward, R. A., 220, 226, 227, *232*
Warden, D. R., 101, *105*
Wardlaw, J. M., 82, *85*
Ware, J. H., 160, *170*
Warr, P., 267, *276*
Warr, P. B., 138, *147*
Warren, A., 359, *363*
Wartenburger, I., 138, *149*
Wasik, B., 161, *167*
Wass, H., 233, *246*
Waters, S. J., 139, *147*
Watson, D., 194, *205*, 316, *322*, *323*
Watson, J. A., 266, *274*
Watson, P., 9, *22*
Watson, P. C., 371, *379*
Watts, A., 43, *55*
Watzka, M., 100, *104*
Weale, M. R., 16, *21*
Weale, R. A., 16, *21*
Weatherall, A., 251, *261*
Weaver, L. K., 78, *88*
Weaver, S. L., 177, 179, 183, 184, 185, *188*
Webb, A., 67, *71*, 84, *87*
Webb, A. G., 116, *117*
Webb, H., 253, *260*
Weber, E., 371, *377*, *378*
Weber, E. U., 135, 138, 140, 143, *149*, *151*
Weber, N. S., 313, *323*
Weber, T. A., 164, *168*
Weber-Fahr, W., 125, 126, *129*
Webster, J. D., 284, 287, *291*
Wechsler, D., 339, 343, 344, *352*
Wedervang-Jensen, T., 328, *335*
Wegner, D. M., 198, *205*
Wehling, E., 75, *91*
Wei, J. Y., 180, 181, *188*, 258, 259, *261*
Weich, S., 198, *205*
Weigand, S. D., 83, *88*, 111, *118*
Weil, M., 155, 158, 160, 161, *167*
Weinberger, D. R., 100, 102, *105*, *106*
Weinberger, M. I., 303, *309*, 315, *323*
Weiner, B., 296, *307*
Weiner, M. F., 359, *362*, 373, *377*
Weinstein, H. C., 78, *89*
Weinstein, M., 213, *218*
Weintraub, S., 343, 344, *350*
Weir, D., 345, *350*
Weir, D. R., 345, *351*
Weisner, C., 318, *322*
Weiss, B. D., 346, *352*
Weiss, E. M., 259, *262*, 269, *274*
Weiss, M., 267, *273*
Welch, D. W., 155, *170*
Welch, E. S., 135, *149*
Welch, N., 371, *378*
Weller, J. A., 138, 140, 145, *146*, *151*
Wells, G. D., 183, *190*
Welsh, R. C., 111, *118*, 121, 122, *131*
Wen, W., 78, *86*
Wentura, D., 255, *262*
Wertenbroch, K., 137, *147*
Wesnes, K., 77, *87*
West, N. A., 101, *105*
West, R., 67, 68, *72*, 340, *352*
West, R. F., 135, *150*
West, R. L., 59, 66, *72*, 137, 141, *151*, 155, 156, 159, 164, *165*, *167*, *170*, 181, 182, 183, *186*, *190*
Westberg, L., 101, 102, *105*
Westendorp, R. G., 78, 82, *91*
Westlye, L. T., 75, 77, *87*, *91*
Wetherell, J. L., 297, 305, *307*, *310*, 326, 328, *337*
Wetherell, M. S., 241, *246*
Wethington, E., 192, 200, *205*
Wetter, S. R., 342, *349*
Weuve, J., 160, *170*
Whalley, L. J., 17, *20*,.80, 81, 82, *86*, 96, 99, 100, *105*
Wheaton, B., 192, *205*
Wheeler, S. C., 256, 257, *262*
Whitbourne, S. B., 183, *189*
Whitbourne, S. K., 14, *23*, 183, 184, 185, 193, *205*, 234, *246*, 315, 317, *323*
White, B. Y., 160, *167*
White, D. R., 5, *22*
White, L. E., 80, 81, 82, *86*, *88*, *89*
White, M. F., 374, *379*
Whitfield, K. E., 95, *107*, 208, 209, 211, 213, 214, *215*, *218*
Whitfield, S., 295, 297, 302, *309*
Whiting, W. L., 80, 81, 82, *88*
Whitlatch, C. J., 220, *229*
Whitley, B. E., Jr., 250, 253, 258, *261*
Whitson, J. A., 184, *190*
Whittle, J. D., 138, *149*
Whyte, E. M., 78, 79, *89*
Whyte, H. M., 209, *215*
Wickelgren, E. A., 142, *149*
Wickens, C. D., 158, *166*
Wickrama, K. A. S., 226, *232*, 266, *276*, *277*
Widaman, K. F., 29, 30, 32, *36*, *39*
Widiger, T. A., 333, 326, *337*
Widoe, R. K., 316, *321*
Wieland, G. D., 375, *378*
Wiemann, J., 241, *244*
Wiemels, J. L., 95, *104*
Wierenga, C. E., 343, *349*
Wieser, M. J., 297, *310*
Wight, R. G., 268, *277*
Wildsmith, E. M., 212, *218*
Wilhelm, O., 158, *167*
Wilke, A., 135, *149*
Wilkening, F., 371, *377*
Wilkins, D., 344, *348*
Wilkinson, A., 154, *171*
Willett, J. B., 32, 34, *39*
Williams, A., 233, 237, 238, 239, 240, 242, *244*, *245*, *246*, *247*
Williams, D., 16, *23*, 208, 209, 210, *216*, *217*
Williams, D. R., 208, 209, 210, 211, *215*, *216*, *218*
Williams, G. C., 101, *107*
Williams, G. V., 101, *107*
Williams, I. C., 357, 358, *362*
Williams, J. B., 328, *337*
Williams, J. B. W., 333, *335*
Williams, K. N., 235, 236, 238, *244*, *247*
Williams, L. E., 125, *130*
Williams, L. M., 80, 81, *87*, 101, *104*
Williams, S. C. R., 80, 81, *89*
Williams, T. W., 142, *149*
Williamson, A., 60, 66, *71*, 74, 76, 77, 84, *88*, *90*, 123, 124, *131*, 141, *150*
Williamson, G. M., 354, 359, *362*, *364*
Williamson, S. H., 49, *53*
Willis, R., 345, *350*
Willis, R. J., 304, *308*
Willis, S. L., 42, 43, 45, 46, 48, 49, *54*, *55*, 94, *107*, 154, 155, 156, 157, 159, 163, *167*, *168*, *169*, *170*, *171*, 180, *190*, 367, *379*
Willis, S. W., 4, 6, 7, 8, 9, 10, 12, *19*

Willson, A. E., 220, 225, 226, *232*
Wilner, N. J., 199, *202*
Wilson, H. R., 301, 302, *308*
Wilson, J. A., 46, *55*
Wilson, K., 235, *247*
Wilson, N., 317, *322*
Wilson, R. L., 66, 68, *72*
Wilson, R. S., 30, *39*, 68, *72*, 110, 113, *118*, 154, 159, *167*, *171*, 195, 198, 199, *205*, *206*, 265, *274*, 304, *310*, 345, 347, *348*, *349*, *352*
Wilson, T. D., 136, *151*
Wimmer, G. E., 137, *148*
Winblad, B., 111, *117*, 124, *130*, 164, *168*
Windsor, T. D., 180, *190*, 304, *308*
Wingerson, D., 197, *204*
Wink, P., 284, 285, 286, 287, *291*
Winkleby, M. A., 209, *218*
Winocur, G., 112, *118*, 137, *149*, 159, *166*, *168*, *171*, 257, *262*, 297, *308*, 344, *349*
Wippich, W., 182, *187*
Wiprzycka, U. J., 141, *148*
Wisniewski, S., 344, *350*
Wisocki, P. A., 328, 329, *337*
Wiste, H. J., 83, *88*
Withall, A., 315, *320*
Witthöft, M., 62, *72*
Wittmann, W., 62, *72*
Witzki, A. H., 114, *118*, 161, *168*
Witzkik, A. H., 60, 62, 63, 64, *71*
Wodtke, K., 164, *167*
Wohlheiter, K., 313, *321*
Wohlwill, J. F., 31, *39*, 43, *55*
Wojtowicz, M. A., 60, 66, 67, *70*, *72*, 112, *118*
Wolf, O. T., 182, *187*
Wolf, P. A., 48, *51*, 78, *86*, *91*, 99, *105*
Wolff, F. C., 222, *229*
Wolff, J. L., 219, 223, *232*
Wolff, S. D., 82, *91*
Wolfson, D., 342, *351*
Wolinsky, F., 157, *171*
Wolinsky, F. D., 179, *190*
Wolk, D. A., 77, *86*
Wolkowitz, O. M., 100, *107*, 197, *202*
Wong, J. D., 192, 195, 196, 200, *200*, *206*
Wong, J. G., 371, *379*
Wong, N. D., 196, *202*
Wong, P. T. P., 286, *291*
Wood, D., 265, *275*
Wood, E., 370, 375, *378*, *379*
Wood, P., 33, 34, *39*
Wood, P. K., 284, *289*
Wood, R. A., 158, 159, *168*
Wood, S., 138, 140, 143, 144, 145, *147*, *150*, *151*, 302, *310*, 370, *379*
Woodard, J. L., 65, *72*
Woodburn, S. M., 142, *147*
Woodcock, R. W., 29, 30, 31, 32, *37*, *38*
Wooden, M. W., 268, *277*
Woodhead, E. L., 329, *335*
Woodruff-Borden, J., 316, 317, *321*, *322*
Woods, C. M., 329, *334*
Woods, D. J., 346, *351*
Woodward, M., 343, *352*
Woolf, C. J., 194, *206*
Wortman, C. B., 318, 319, *320*
Wozniak, J. R., 82, *91*
Wrensch, M. R., 95, *104*
Wright, A. F., 17, *20*, 99, *105*
Wright, C. I., 16, *23*
Wright, E., 157, *171*
Wright, K. B., 241, *246*
Wright, M. J., 96, 97, *105*, *106*
Wrosch, C., 177, 178, 181, 183, *187*, *190*, 300, 303, *306*, *308*
Wszalek, T., 67, *71*, 114, *117*
Wu, C., 79, *89*, 209, *217*
Wu, K. D., 332, *335*
Wu, Y., 214, *217*
Wurm, L. H., 145, *151*, 304, *310*
Wurm, S., 258, *262*, 270, *277*

X

Xu, J., 251, 252, *260*
Xuan, L., 80, *87*

Y

Yacubian, J., 101, *107*
Yaffe, K., 75, *86*, 157, 158, 159, 160, *169*, *171*, 197, *204*, 345, *350*
Yamada, H., 80, *85*
Yamada, T. H., 138, 145, *146*
Yamaguchi, S., 179, *190*
Yamamato, K., 7, *19*
Yang, F. M., 220, *231*
Yang, H. K., 318, *322*
Yang, L., 154, 159, *171*
Yang, S.-Y., 281, *291*
Yang, Y., 209, 210, *216*
Yang-Ping, C., 95, *105*
Yao, H., 78, *89*
Yao, M., 100, *106*
Yap, K. B., 125, *131*
Yassuda, M. S., 181, *190*
Yates, M. E., 184, *190*
Yates, W., 331, *336*
Yeager, C., 332, *335*
Yeo, G., 347, *351*, *352*
Yesavage, J. A., 155, *166*, 327, *337*
Ying, Z., 164, *170*
Ylikoski, R., 342, *350*
Yochim, B., 329, *336*
Yonelinas, A. P., 79, *89*, 125, 126, *131*
Yong, L., 333, *337*
Yoon, C., 62, 63, 65, *71*, 134, 142, *150*, *151*, 251, 257, *259*, *262*
York, T. P., 96, 97, *106*
Yoshita, M., 78, *91*
Young, L. J., 197, *202*
Young, R. C., 328, *334*
Young, S. E., 61, 62, 68, 69, *70*
Ystad, M. A., 75, *85*, *91*
Ytsma, J., 236, *247*
Yu, Y. W., 100, *107*
Yun, R. J., 251, *262*
Yuzuriha, T., 78, *89*
Yzerbyt, V., 250, 253, *261*
Yzerbyt, V. Y., 253, *262*

Z

Zabrucky, K. M., 192, *202*
Zack, M. M., 298, *308*
Zacks, R. T., 9, 11, *20*, *21*, *23*, 60, 62, 65, *70*, 137, 141, 143, *147*, *148*, *151*
Zahr, N. M., 81, *91*
Zajonc, R. B., 139, *149*
Zaleta, A. K., 80, *90*
Zamarian, L., 138, *151*
Zamrini, E., 373, *378*, *378*
Zamrini, E. Y., 373, *379*
Zanarini, M. C., 333, *337*
Zandi, P. P., 101, *105*
Zanjani, F. A. K., 46, *54*, 143, *150*
Zanto, T. P., 68, *72*
Zarit, J. M., 223, *232*
Zarit, S. H., 220, 221, 222, 223, 225, 227, *229*, *230*, *232*, 355, 357, 359, 360, 361, *362*, *363*, *365*
Zautra, A. J., 185, *189*, 192, *204*, *206*, 299, *309*
Zebb, B. J., 329, *337*
Zebrowitz, L. A., 253, *262*
Zebuhr, Y., 78, *87*
Zeiss, A. M., 313, *323*
Zeiss, L. M., 358, *362*
Zelinski, E. M., 43, *55*, 122, *131*, 159, 163, *171*
Zemba, Y., 179, *190*
Zettel, L. A., 301, *310*
Zevon, M. A., 33, *39*
Zhan, Y., 270, *276*
Zhang, G., 33, *36*
Zhang, J., 198, *201*, 354, *365*
Zhang, S., 360, *364*
Zhang, Y. B., 239, 240, 241, *245*, *247*, 251, *262*
Zhang, Z., 345, *352*
Zhao, C., 164, *170*
Zhao, S., 314, *322*

Zhao, X., 164, *167*
Zheng, S., 95, *104*
Zhu, S., 164, *168*
Ziegler, M. G., 360, 361, *363*
Zietsch, B. P., 97, *106*
Ziff, M. A., 181, *188*
Zimmer, Z., 208, 210, *218*
Zimmerman, M., 333, *336*
Zimmerman, M. E., 75, *91*, 340, *348*
Zonderman, A. B., 84, *89*, 141, *150*, 175, 180, *188*, 256, 257, 258, 259, *261*, 298, *307*, 327, *336*
Zotti, A. M., 319, *321*
Zrelak, P. A., 79, *89*
Zubek, J. M., 283, *290*
Zubenko, G. S., 17, *23*
Zubenko, W. N., 17, *23*
Zuckerman, A., 193, 194, *201*
Zuderman, A. B., 211, *216*
Zuo, Y. L., 94, *107*
Zvonkovic, A. M., 225, *231*
Zwang-Weissman, Y., 234, *245*
Zweig, R. A., 330, *337*
Zwick, T., 268, *277*

Subject Index

A

ACTIVE, *see* Advanced Cognitive Training for Independent and Vital Elderly
AD, *see* Alzheimer's disease
Adult–parent relationship, *see also* Intergenerational communication
  caregiving relationships, 223
  emotional qualities
    conflict perspective, 224–225
    intergenerational ambivalence theory, 225
    sex and race differences, 226
    solidarity and developmental stake, 224
  overview, 219–220
  prospects for study, 227–228
  support
    exchanges between adults and children, 221
    generational flow, 221–223
  variability, 220–221
  well-being and qualities of tie, 226–227
Advanced Cognitive Training for Independent and Vital Elderly (ACTIVE), 156–157
Affect, *see* Decision making
Age stereotypes
  cultural differences, 251
  negative versus positive, 250–251
  overview, 249–250
  process of stereotyping
    activation, 253–254
    implicit processes, 254–256
  self-stereotyping
    health impact, 257–258
    overview, 256
    stereotype threat, 256–257
  stereotype content model, 251–252
Age stereotypes in interactions model (ASIM), 238
Aging change, psychological aging research theme
  Baltes' view, 8–9
  Birren's view, 7
  general commentaries, 10–11
  overview, 6
  process-specific theories, 11–12
  Salthouse's view, 10
Alcoholism, *see* Substance abuse
Allostatic load, life expectancy and health disparity across socioeconomic groups, 212–213
Alzheimer's disease (AD), *see* Amyloid-β, brain deposition; Dementia
Amyloid-β, brain deposition
  overview, 83
  structure–function studies, 83–84
  cognitive aging studies, 83
  positron emission tomography studies, 111
Anxiety disorders
  assessment, 328–329
  epidemiology, 316
  symptoms in older adults, 316–317
Anxiety, *see* Stress
Apolipoprotein E, behavioral genetics, 100–101, 124
ASIM, *see* Age stereotypes in interactions model
Attention, evaluation in dementia, 342–343
Attrition, *see* Incomplete data

B

Balance of trajectory, psychological aging research theme
  Baltes' view, 8–9
  general commentaries, 10–11
  overview, 6
  process-specific theories, 11–12
BASE, *see* Berlin Aging Study
BDI-II, *see* Beck Depression Inventory-II
BDNF, *see* Brain-derived neurotrophic factor
Beck Depression Inventory-II (BDI-II), 327–328
Behavior from Intergroup Affect and Stereotypes (BIAS), map, 254
Behavioral genetics
  evolution, 94
  gene–environment interactions, 94, 124
  integration of twin and molecular genetics studies
    broad versus narrow phenotypes, 103–104
    construct-measurement fallacy, 102–103
    phenotype definition, 102
  molecular genetics, 98–102
  twin studies, 94–97
Bereavement
  caregivers, 361
  depression risk and protective factors, 317–318
Berlin Aging Study (BASE), 271
BIAS, *see* Behavior from Intergroup Affect and Stereotypes
Brain
  amyloid-β deposition, 83–84, 111
  multimodal imaging, 124–125
  structure changes in aging, *see* Brain morphometry; Magnetic resonance imaging
Brain-derived neurotrophic factor (BDNF), cognitive function, 101
Brain morphometry
  manual morphometry studies of aging, 74
  voxel-based morphometry, 74–75

C

Candidate gene, behavioral genetics, 98
Capacity, *see also* Decision making
  assessment
    guardianship law, 369–370
    health care consent law, 370
    law relationship to decision making science, 370–371
    legal standards, 369
    overview, 375–376
  definition, 368
  driving capacity, 374
  everyday skill-based capacities, 372
  evolution as prominent concern, 368–369
  finance management capacity, 372–373
  independent living capacity, 373–374
  medical treatment consent
    cognitive ability studies, 371
    medical condition studies, 371
  planning for future incapacity, 374–375
  prospects for study, 376
  research consent, 372
  resolution, 368
  sexual relation consent, 372
Cardiovascular disease, cognition impact, 48
Caregiving
  abuse, 359
  adult–parent relationships, 223
  cultural issues
    coping styles, 357–358
    cultural values, 358
    mental health outcomes, 357
    physical health outcomes, 357
    social support, 358
    treatment response differences, 358–359
  grief after loss, 361
  interventions for stress reduction
    clinical significance, 356
    implementation, 356–357
  prospects for study, 361–362
  stages, 359–361
  stress and coping models
    mental health outcomes, 354
    outcome influences
      appraisal of caregiving as stressful, 355
      caregiving stressors, 355
      coping styles, 355
      potential diathesis, 355
      social support, 355–356
    physical health outcomes, 354–355
Catechol-*O*-methyltransferase (COMT), cognitive function, 101–102
CATI, *see* Coolidge Axis II Inventory
Center for Epidemiologic Studies Depression Scale (CES-D), 327
CES-D, *see* Center for Epidemiologic Studies Depression Scale
Chronological age, psychological aging research theme
  Baltes' view, 9
  BioAge, 16–17
  Birren's view, 7–8
  general commentaries, 10–11
  overview, 6
  process-specific theories, 11–12
Chronosystem, three environment system, 43–44
CNV, *see* Copy number variant
Co-constructive framework, cultural learning, 45
Cognition
  behavioral genetics, 100–101
  hormonal factors, 100–102
Cognition, *see also* Executive function
  brain structure changes in aging, *see* Brain morphometry; Magnetic resonance imaging
  chronic disease and health behavior impact, 48–49
  conceptual frameworks
    co-constructive framework, 45
    generational differences, 46
    neurobiological and sociocultural influences, 45
    secular cohort trends, 45–46
    three environment system, 43–45
  decision making, *see* Capacity; Decision making
  educational influences
    GI Bill, 46–47
    historical change in educational curriculum and pedagogy, 47–48
    National Defense Education Act, 47
  interventions
    controls in study, 163
    engagement, 159–160
    lifestyle interventions, 161–162
    mechanisms of long-term effects, 164
    overview, 153–154
    physical activity, 116, 160–161
    research questions, 162–165
    retest effect, 154–155
    timing, 164–165
    training studies
      component-specific training, 156–157
      core capacity training, 157–159
      memory training, 155–156
  memory, *see specific types*
  occupational history influences, 48
  stress and performance effects, 182–183, 198–199
  work and development, 264–265
Cognitive reserve, 59, 347
Communication predicament of aging model (CPAM), 235, 238–239
Competency, *see* Capacity
Complexity, psychological aging research theme
  Baltes' view, 8–9
  Birren's view, 7
  general commentaries, 10–11
  overview, 5
  process-specific theories, 11–12
  Salthouse's view, 10
COMT, *see* Catechol-O-methyltransferase
Consent, *see* Capacity
Control beliefs
  age differences and changes, 177–179
  historical and conceptual overview, 175–177
  interventions, 184–185
  prospects for study, 185–186
  relation to aging-related domains
    high control adaptivity, 180–181
    mechanisms and processes, 181–184
  sociodemographic variations, 179–180
  stress buffering, 183
Coolidge Axis II Inventory (CATI), 332
Coping, styles in caregiving, 355, 357–358
Copy number variant (CNV), behavioral genetics, 98–99
Core capacity, training, 157–159
Cornell Scale for Depression in Dementia (CS), 328
Corticobasal degeneration, *see* Dementia
CPAM, *see* Communication predicament of aging model
CS, *see* Cornell Scale for Depression in Dementia
Cultural differences, *see* Race/ethnicity

D

Decision making, *see also* Capacity
affect influences
affective learning, 138
endowment effects, 137
incidental affect, 139
overview, 136–137
positivity effect, 139–141
risky-choice framing effects, 137–138, 140
time preferences, 138–139
construction of preferences in older adults, 134
deliberation decline in aging
decision tasks, 142–143
numeracy, 143–144
overview, 141–142
perceptions of covariation, 142
Querty Theory, 143
less preference construction in familiar decisions, 135
limitations of studies, 144–145
modes of thinking, 135–136
prospects for study in aging, 145
selectivity and motivated use of deliberative processes, 144
Dehydroepiandrosterone (DHEA), cognitive function, 100
Deliberation, *see* Decision making
Delis Kaplan Executive Function Scale (D-KEFS), 343
Dementia, *see also* Alzheimer's disease; Neuropsychological assessment
age-associated cognitive and age changes, 340–341
differential diagnosis
attention and processing speed, 342–343
executive function, 343
language, 343–344
memory, 342
metacognition, 344–345
visuospatial ability, 344
genetic susceptibility, 100
health behavior risks in Alzheimer's disease, 49
pathology and clinical features, 341
prospects for study, 347–348
special considerations in assessment
acculturation, 346
cognitive reserve, 347
education, 346–347
race/ethnicity, 346
test translation, 347
Depression
assessment, 326–328
bereavement comparison, 318–319
epidemiology, 313–314
risk factors
early life experiences, 315
physical illness, 315
psychosocial risk factors, 315–316
suicide, 316
DET, *see* Differential Emotions Theory
Developmental epidemiological perspectives, psychological theories of aging, 14–15
DFA, *see* Dynamic factor analysis
DHEA, *see* Dehydroepiandrosterone
Diabetes, cognition impact, 48
Differential Emotions Theory (DET), 296
Differential, psychological aging research theme
Baltes' view, 8–9
Birren's view, 7
general commentaries, 10–11
overview, 6
process-specific theories, 11–12
Diffusion tensor imaging (DTI)
cognitive aging studies
episodic memory, 81
executive function, 80
motor performance, 81
processing speed, 81
working memory, 80–81
functional magnetic resonance imaging integration studies, 81–82
principles, 79–80
DIT, *see* Dynamic Integration Theory
D-KEFS, *see* Delis Kaplan Executive Function Scale
Dopamine, neurotransmission studies of cognitive function, 127–128
Driving, capacity, 374
DTI, *see* Diffusion tensor imaging
Durable power of attorney, capacity in appointment, 375
Dynamic factor analysis (DFA), intra-individual variability, 33–34
Dynamic Integration Theory (DIT), emotional regulation, 303

E

Education
cognition influences
GI Bill, 46–47
historical change in educational curriculum and pedagogy, 47–48
National Defense Education Act, 47
dementia assessment considerations, 346–347
relationship with income, 209–210
socioeconomic status measure, 208–209
EF, *see* Executive function
Emotional regulation
age-related strength mechanisms
cognitive and behavioral strategies related to emotional well-being, 301
overview, 300–301
social contexts, 301–302
aging effects
declines in emotional experience, 297–298
emotional complexity, 299
emotional well-being, 298–299
emotion structure and function consistency across adulthood, 296–297
strength and vulnerability integration, 299–300
appraisals of current and past emotional experiences, 302
emotional arousal, 303–304
memory of past vents, 303
overview, 295–296
prospects for study, 305–306
threats to emotional well-being
current situations, 305
early experiences, 304–305
Engagement
cognitive interventions, 159–160
experience-based changes in neural function, 115–116
videogames, 160
Epigenetics
behavioral genetics, 99
theoretical implications in psychology of aging, 17
Episodic memory
diffusion tensor imaging studies, 81
regional brain volume studies in cognitive aging, 75
white matter hyperintensity studies, 79
ERP, *see* Event-related potential
Ethnicity, *see* Race/ethnicity
Event-related potential (ERP), executive function studies, 67–68
Executive function (EF)
conceptualization
construct evolution, 60
dominance of task-based approaches, 61–62

Executive function (EF) (*Continued*)
neuropsychology and cognitive psychology confluence, 61
diffusion tensor imaging studies, 80
diversity in aging, 62–63
evaluation in dementia, 343
mediation and monitoring of cognitive processes, 65–66
neural correlates of training, 114–115
prefrontal cortex
activation patterns, 67
diffuse brain integrity, 66–67
event-related potentials, 67–68
neurodegeneration, 59
volumetric work, 66
Process Dissociation Procedure, 64–65
prospects for study, 68–69
regional brain volume studies in cognitive aging, 75
switching tasks, 64
unity, 62–63
white matter hyperintensity studies, 78
Exosystem, three environment system, 43–44
Experience Corps, cognitive intervention, 161
Expert behavior, experience-based changes in neural function, 113–114

F

Finance management, capacity, 372–373
Finnish Twin Study of Aging (FITSA), 95
FITSA, *see* Finnish Twin Study of Aging
Fluid intelligence
regional brain volume studies in cognitive aging, 76
white matter hyperintensity studies, 79
fMRI, *see* Functional magnetic resonance imaging
Frontotemporal dementia, *see* Dementia
Functional magnetic resonance imaging (fMRI)
BOLD signal and cognitive function in aging, 122–123, 125–126
diffusion tensor imaging integration studies, 81–82
multimodal brain imaging, 124–125
neurotransmission studies of cognitive function, 127–128
working memory studies in aging, 122

G

GDS, *see* Geriatric Depression Scale
Genetic heterogeneity, behavioral genetics, 99
Genome-wide association studies (GWAS), behavioral genetics, 98
Geriatric Depression Scale (GDS), 327
Gerontological Personality Disorders Scale (GPDS), 333
GI Bill, cognition impact, 46–47
Global–local, psychological aging research theme
Baltes' view, 8–9
Birren's view, 7
general commentaries, 10–11
overview, 5
process-specific theories, 11–12
Salthouse's view, 10
GPDS, *see* Gerontological Personality Disorders Scale
Grief, *see* Bereavement
GWAS, *see* Genome-wide association studies

H

Hamilton Rating Scale for Depression (HRSD), 328
Healthcare proxy, capacity in appointment, 375
HPA axis, *see* Hypothalamic-pituitary-adrenal axis
HRSD, *see* Hamilton Rating Scale for Depression
Hypertension
cognition impact, 48
vascular risk in brain aging, 77, 85
Hypothalamic-pituitary-adrenal (HPA) axis, stress response and aging effects, 196–197

I

IAT, *see* Implicit association test
Immigration, aging demographics, 49
Implicit association test (IAT), age stereotyping, 254–255
Incomplete data
attrition causes, 27
classification, 27
methodological approaches for handling, 27–28
planning as design feature, 28–29
Independent living, capacity, 373–374
Informed consent, *see* Capacity
Institutionalization, caregiver impact, 360–361
Intelligence, *see* Cognition; Fluid intelligence
Intergenerational ambivalence theory, adult–parent relationships, 225
Intergenerational communication
communicative constructions of aging, 241–242
overaccomodation
forms and functions, 234–235
management and prevention, 237–238
social and cultural evaluations, 236–237
theoretical models, 238–240
overview, 233–234
problematic elder-to-younger communications, 240–241
prospects for study, 242–243
Intra-individual variability (IV)
statistical models, 33–34
study design, 26–27
Invariance, measurement over time, 29–30
IV, *see* Intra-individual variability

L

Language, evaluation in dementia, 343–344
Latent growth curve (LGC), change modeling, 32
LGC, *see* Latent growth curve
Life transition, stress, 195–196
Life-span model, late-life psychopathology, 311–313
Long-term memory, neural correlates of training, 114
Longitudinal study, advantages and limitations, 26
Longitudinal Study of Aging Danish Twins (LSADT), 95
Loss, *see* Bereavement
LSADT, *see* Longitudinal Study of Aging Danish Twins

M

Magnetic resonance imaging (MRI), *see also* Diffusion tensor imaging; Functional magnetic resonance imaging; Magnetization

transfer imaging; White matter hyperintensity
cortical thinning in cognitive aging, 76–77
regional brain volume studies in cognitive aging
episodic memory, 75
executive function, 75
fluid intelligence, 76
procedural memory, 76
working memory, 76
voxel-based morphometry of brain changes in aging, 74–75
Magnetization transfer imaging (MTI)
cognitive aging studies, 82–83
principles, 82
MCMI-III, *see* Millon Clinical Multiaxial Inventory-III
Medial temporal lobe (MTL), structure–function interactions, 126–127
Memory training, 155–156
Mesosystem, three environment system, 43–45
Millon Clinical Multiaxial Inventory-III (MCMI-III), 332
Missing completely at random, *see* Incomplete data
Missing at random, *see* Incomplete data
MLM, *see* Multilevel model
Mood disorders
affective symptoms in older adults, 314–315
bipolar disorder, 314
depression
epidemiology, 313–314
risk factors
early life experiences, 315
physical illness, 315
psychosocial risk factors, 315–316
suicide, 316
Motor performance, diffusion tensor imaging studies, 81
MRI, *see* Magnetic resonance imaging
MTI, *see* Magnetization transfer imaging
MTL, *see* Medial temporal lobe
Multilevel model (MLM), change modeling, 32

N

National Defense Education Act, cognition impact, 47
Neuropsychological assessment
differential diagnosis of dementia
attention and processing speed, 342–343
executive function, 343
language, 343–344
memory, 342
metacognition, 344–345
visuospatial ability, 344
difficulty in older adults, 340
overview, 339
research applications in cognitive aging, 345
Not missing completely at random, *see* Incomplete data
Numeracy, deliberation decline in aging, 143–144

O

OATS, *see* Older Australian Twins Study
Occupation, *see* Work
Older Australian Twins Study (OATS), 95
Overaccomodation
forms and functions, 234–235
management and prevention, 237–238
social and cultural evaluations, 236–237
theoretical models, 238–240
Oxidative stress, genetics, 100

P

Painful self-disclosure (PSD), elder-to-younger communications, 240–241
Parents, *see* Adult–parent relationship; Caregiving; Intergenerational communication
Parkinson's disease dementia, *see* Dementia
PDP, *see* Process Dissociation Procedure
PDQ-4+, *see* Personality Diagnostic Questionnaire 4+
Personality Diagnostic Questionnaire, 4+ (PDQ-4+), 332
Personality disorders
aging impact on experience and presentation, 331
assessment
Gerontological Personality Disorders Scale, 333
self-report inventories, 332–333
semi-structured interviews, 333
diagnostic criteria, 330
epidemiology, 329–330
personality stability versus change across life span, 330–331
PET, *see* Positron emission tomography
PFC, *see* Prefrontal cortex
Physical activity, cognitive intervention, 116, 160–161
Population of theories, psychological aging, 12–14
Positivity effect, decision making
overview, 139–140
pre-choice information processing, 140–141
risky-choice framing effects, 140
Positron emission tomography (PET)
amyloid-β deposition studies, 111
multimodal brain imaging, 124–125
neurotransmission studies of cognitive function, 127
Poverty
societal interventions, 49–50
socioeconomic status and health, *see* Socioeconomic status
Prefrontal cortex (PFC)
executive function
activation patterns, 67
diffuse brain integrity, 66–67
event-related potentials, 67–68
neurodegeneration, 59
volumetric work, 66
structural changes in aging, 75–76, 122
structure–function interactions, 126
Procedural memory, regional brain volume studies in cognitive aging, 76
Process Dissociation Procedure (PDP), executive function, 64–65
Progressive supranuclear palsy, *see* Dementia
PSD, *see* Painful self-disclosure
Psychological theories of aging, *see* Theories of aging, psychological

Q

Querty Theory, deliberation decline in aging, 143

R

Race/ethnicity
adult–parent relationships
caregiving, 223
emotional qualities, 226
age stereotypes, 251

Race/ethnicity (*Continued*)
caregiving
coping styles, 357–358
cultural values, 358
mental health outcomes, 357
physical health outcomes, 357
social support, 358
treatment response differences, 358–359
chronic disease burden, 211–212
dementia assessment considerations, 346
disability burden, 211–212
genetics in health disparities research, 213–214
life expectancy and health disparity mechanisms
allostatic load, 212–213
weathering hypothesis, 212
overaccomodation, 236–237
socioeconomic status, 210–211
stress response, 195
wisdom definitions, *see* Wisdom
Retest effect
cognitive interventions, 154–155
study design, 30–31
Retirement
health impact, 270–271
transition overview, 269–270
volunteer work, 271–272

S

SAM axis, *see* Sympathetic-adrenal-medullary axis
SATSA, *see* Swedish Adoption/Twin Study of Aging
SAVI, *see* Strength and Vulnerability Integration
Scaffolding theory of aging and cognition (STAC), 59, 68, 112–113
Schedule for Nonadaptive and Adaptive Personality (SNAP-2), 332
Schizophrenia
epidemiology, 317
risk and protective factors, 317
Seattle Longitudinal Study (SLS), 46
Self-stereotyping, *see* Age stereotypes
Senior Odyssey, cognitive intervention, 162
SES, *see* Socioeconomic status
Sex differences
adult-parent relationships, 226
stress response, 197–198
Single nucleotide polymorphism (SNP), behavioral genetics, 98
SNAP-2, *see* Schedule for Nonadaptive and Adaptive Personality
SNP, *see* Single nucleotide polymorphism
Socioeconomic status (SES)
chronic disease burden, 211
definition, 208
genetics in health disparities research, 213–214
life expectancy and health disparity mechanisms
allostatic load, 212–213
weathering hypothesis, 212
measures
education, 208–209
income, 209
relationship between income and education, 209–210
wealth, 210
race effects, 210–211
stress response, 195
STAC, *see* Scaffolding theory of aging and cognition
Stereotypes, *see* Age stereotypes
Strength and Vulnerability Integration (SAVI), emotional regulation, 194, 296, 299–300, 306
Stress
caregiving, *see* Caregiving
changes across middle and later adulthood, 193–194
cognition performance effects, 182–183, 198–199
control belief buffering, 183
coping, *see* Coping
exposure and reactivity pathways, 192–193
genetics of response, 100
individual differences in processes, 194–196
physiology and aging effects
hypothalamic-pituitary-adrenal axis, 196–197
sympathetic-adrenal-medullary axis, 196
prospects for study, 199–200
sex differences in response, 197–198
speedometer of life analogy, 191
Strength and Vulnerability Integration, 194
stressor types, 192
Study design, psychological aging
incomplete data
attrition causes, 27
classification, 27
methodological approaches for handling, 27–28
planning as design feature, 28–29
intra-individual variability
overview, 26–27
statistical models, 33–34
invariance measurement over time, 29–30
longitudinal study advantages and limitations, 26
prospects
model parameter matching to theoretical aging mechanisms, 34–35
time-related sequence identification in aging processes, 35
retest effects, 30–31
statistical modeling for change assessment, 32–34
time definitions, 31–32
Substance abuse, later adulthood, 317–318
Suicide, features in later life, 316
Survival, statistical modeling, 34
Swedish Adoption/Twin Study of Aging (SATSA), 95–97
Switching tasks, executive function, 64
Sympathetic-adrenal-medullary (SAM) axis, stress response and aging effects, 196

T

Testosterone, cognitive function, 100
Theories of aging, psychological
developmental epidemiological perspectives, 14–15
historical influences, 42–43
overview of themes and subthemes, 4–6
perspectives
Baltes, Paul E, 8–9
Birren, James E, 6–8
general commentaries, 10–11
process-specific theories, 11–12
Salthouse, Timothy A., 9–10
population of theories, 12–14
prospects
cause and effect patterns, 17–18
chronological-biological age indexes, 16–17
genetic-epigenetic-environment-process studies, 17
neurosciences impact, 16
Three environment system, historical influences on aging and behavior, 43–45
Time, definitions in study design, 31–32
TMS, *see* Transcranial magnetic stimulation

Transcranial magnetic stimulation (TMS), memory studies, 111
Twin studies, behavioral genetics of aging, 95–97

V

Variable autoregressive moving average (VARMA), intra-individual variability modeling, 34
VARMA, *see* Variable autoregressive moving average
Vascular dementia, *see* Dementia
VBM, *see* Voxel-based morphometry
VETSA, *see* Vietnam Era Twin Study of Aging
Videogames, cognitive interventions, 160
Vietnam Era Twin Study of Aging (VETSA), 95–97
Voxel-based morphometry (VBM), brain changes in aging, 74–75

W

WCST, *see* Wisconsin Card Sorting Task
Wealth, *see* Socioeconomic status
Weathering hypothesis, life expectancy and health disparity across socioeconomic groups, 212
White matter hyperintensity (WMH)
  burden in aging, 77–78, 125–126
  cognitive aging studies
    episodic memory, 79
    executive function, 78
    fluid intelligence, 79
    processing speed, 79
    working memory, 78–79
Will, capacity in execution, 375
Wisconsin Card Sorting Task (WCST)
  behavioral genetics, 101, 103
  executive function, 63, 66
Wisconsin Personality Disorders Inventory (WISPI-IV), 332
Wisdom
  age associations
    empirical associations, 283–285
    hypothetical associations, 282–283
  definitions
    culturally inclusive explicit definitions, 282
    difficulty, 279–280
    Eastern definitions
      explicit theories, 282
      implicit theories, 281
    Western definitions
      explicit theories, 280–281
      implicit theories, 280
  prospects for study, 287
  well-being associations, 285–286
WISPI-IV, *see* Wisconsin Personality Disorders Inventory
WMH, *see* White matter hyperintensity
Work, *see also* Socioeconomic status
  adult development
    cognition, 264–265
    personality
      adjustment, 266
      development, 265–266
      growth and adjustment, 266–267
  aging and outcomes, 267–268
  aging process in work context, 263–264
  attitudes toward older workers, 268–269
  historical changes in complexity and occupational status, 48
  prospects for study, 272
  retirement transition
    health impact, 270–271
    overview, 269–270
    volunteer work, 271–272
  training of older workers, 268
Working memory
  diffusion tensor imaging studies, 80–81
  regional brain volume studies in cognitive aging, 76
  white matter hyperintensity studies, 78–79